FOUNDATIONS OF
ANATOMY AND
PHYSIOLOGY

FREDERIC H. MARTINI

GEORGE KARLESKINT
ST. LOUIS COMMUNITY COLLEGE AT MERAMEC

with

William C. Ober, M.D.
Art Coordinator and Illustrator

Claire W. Garrison, R.N.
Illustrator

Kathleen Welch, M.D.
Clinical Consultant

PRENTICE HALL, Upper Saddle River, NJ 07458

Library of Congress Cataloging-in-Publication Data

Martini, Frederic.
   Foundations of Anatomy & Physiology / Frederic H. Martini, George Karleskint.
        p. cm.
   Includes index.
   ISBN 0-13-592965-2
   1. Human physiology. 2. Human anatomy. 3. Allied health personnel.
   I. Karleskint, George. II. Title. III. Title: Foundations of anatomy and physiology.
   QP34.5.M354 1998
   612—DC21   98-11747
                                                       CIP

Executive Editor: *David Kendric Brake*
Production Editor: *James Buckley*
Editorial Project Manager: *Byron D. Smith*
Special Projects Manager: *Barbara A. Murray*
Director of Creative Services: *Paula Maylahn*
Manufacturing Buyer: *Trudy Pisciotti*
Cover Design: *Bruce Kenselaar*
Interior Design: *Judy Matz-Coniglio*
Assistant Manager of Formatting and Art: *Amy Peltier*
Formatters: *Eric Hulsizer, Ray Caramanna*

©1998 by PRENTICE HALL, Inc.
Simon & Schuster/ A Viacom Company
Upper Saddle River, NJ 07458

Printed in the United States of America
10 9 8 7 6 5 4 3 2 1

ISBN 0-13-592965-2
Prentice-Hall International (UK) Limited, London
Prentice-Hall of Australia Pty. Limited, Sydney
Prentice-Hall Canada, Inc., Toronto
Prentice-Hall Hispanoamericana, S.A., Mexico
Prentice-Hall of India Private Limited, New Delhi
Prentice-Hall of Japan, Inc., Tokyo
Simon & Schuster Asia Pte. Ltd. Singapore
Editora Prentice-Hall do Brasil, Ltda., Rio de Janiero

CONTENTS

PREFACE

The study of anatomy and physiology is both fascinating and challenging. To be successful in your future studies, you need to have a firm grasp of the vocabulary of science and a solid foundation in the basic principles of biology, chemistry, and physics. Many students who attempt a first course in anatomy and physiology do not do well because they are not properly prepared. This text provides you with survival training; that is, it gives you the background necessary to succeed in an anatomy and physiology course. It is designed to be your personal tutor.

Before you begin preparing for your anatomy and physiology course, we would like to introduce the special features of this book that will help you achieve your goals for success. Please take a few minutes to read this important section.

How the Text is Organized

Chapters 1–7 introduce the basic vocabulary you need to study anatomy and physiology. The chapters include the relevant principles of biology, chemistry, and physical science. Chapters 8 and 9 survey the body's 11 organ systems, with an emphasis on vocabulary and basic concepts. The chapters provide you with some familiarity of the organ systems before you encounter them in greater detail in an anatomy and physiology course.

One of the major obstacles for a beginning student in anatomy and physiology is the enormous number of new terms encountered. We have tried to introduce the basic vocabulary in conjunction with aids for learning the terms and their definitions. Important terms are identified with bold type. Terms that generally are not familiar to the introductory student have phonetic pronunciations to help you pronounce the word. The Latin or Greek derivations are also indicated whenever the derivation of a word helps you to remember it more readily.

A unique feature of this book is the incorporation of a variety of exercises for learning and mastering text material after each major section of a chapter. These sections are entitled "Let's Review What You've Just Learned." This combined textbook–workbook approach helps you learn the material a little at a time, mastering one block of information before proceeding to the next. It is our hope that these exercises will not only help you learn and master information that is fundamental to success in the study of anatomy and physiology but that they will also suggest ways to organize and study information when you take an anatomy and physiology course. The major components of these active learning sections are outlined below:

▶ Definitions.

This section is a vocabulary exercise in which you must fill in the proper term for the given definition. This exercise will help you to become more familiar with new terms and their meanings.

▶ Word Roots, Prefixes, Suffixes, and Combining Forms.

This section reviews various word parts (prefixes, suffixes, and word roots) and their meanings. Many terms in anatomy and physiology are based on Latin or Greek, and there are certain word parts that you will encounter again and again. By becoming familiar with these word parts, you can figure out the meaning of many terms, even if you have not seen them before. This skill will be a big help when you continue your study of anatomy and physiology.

▶ Labeling.

In chapters that deal with the learning of anatomy, cell structure, tissues, and chemical formulas, there are sections that ask you to label pictures or to identify structures. These exercises help you visualize important structures and features; they also give you a better understanding of spatial relationships.

▶ Concept Maps.

Concept maps (which are explained inside the front cover of the text) can help you organize information about structures, concepts, or processes. Mapping exercises not only help you learn the relationships but they help you develop an important study skill.

▶ Completion.

Completion sections allow you to answer questions regarding the material you have just learned and to apply it to situations similar to those introduced in the section. There are also tables and charts to complete; these give you another means of organizing information.

We believe that you learn more quickly if you are given immediate reinforcement after completing a task. As a result, we have included the answers to all of the exercises. Be sure to check yourself as soon as you are done, before continuing through the chapter.

Once you complete the exercises from one section, you are ready to move to the next. When you have completed the sections in a chapter, you are ready to take the Self-Check Test that appears at the chapter's end. These short tests are designed to check your mastery of information in the chapter and to give you experience in answering some types of questions encountered in exams from a typical anatomy and physiology course. Most of the test items involve basic recall of facts and terms, but a few at the end of each test ask you to apply the information that you have learned. Answers are provided so that you can check your responses, and there is a grading scale at the end of the test. This format lets you gauge your success before moving on to the next chapter. Most people learn from their mistakes, and in this "friendly" format where you are not penalized for incorrect answers, you can revisit a section until you learn the material to your satisfaction.

It is our hope, that by using this text, you become well-prepared for the challenges of an anatomy and physiology course. Working through this text carefully, you give yourself an edge in future coursework. The study of anatomy and physiology is something to be enjoyed, but first you must build a strong foundation. Good Luck!

Frederic H. Martini
George Karleskint

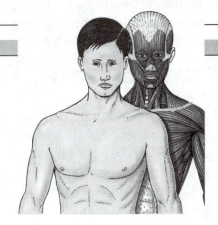

CHAPTER 1

An Introduction to the Study of the Human Body

Why study anatomy and physiology? One reason is that these are fascinating topics. Just about everyone is interested in their own body, how it looks, how it's put together, and what makes it work. We are fascinated by the complexity of our organs and systems and intrigued by the way disease processes can disrupt their functions. We spend a significant amount of our time (and money) trying to ensure that our bodies will look good and function at maximum efficiency. This is the personal side of anatomy and physiology.

In addition to the natural curiosity about the human body, there are other good reasons to study these two fields. For instance, anatomy and physiology form the basis of all of the medical sciences and health-related sports and fitness fields. We also use anatomy and physiology in our everyday lives. To decide whether to use aspirin or ibuprofen for your headache or what exercise is best to develop your leg muscles, you must apply basic concepts of anatomy and physiology. Understanding stories in the media regarding cloning or the effects of diet on disease also requires some knowledge of anatomy and physiology.

As you can see, anatomy and physiology are part of everyone's daily life. A knowledge of these two important fields will allow you not only to understand important issues but also to make better informed decisions about things that affect you and your health.

With this text, you are about to embark on a fascinating journey of discovery. Just as you would use a road map to plan a trip, you can use this book as a guide through the basics that you need to know in order to be successful in your study of anatomy and physiology. In this first chapter we will deal with some basic concepts and terminology that will start you on your way. By the end of this chapter you should have a familiarity with the language of anatomy and physiology, basic anatomical concepts, and the science behind the physiological processes that make human life possible.

WHAT ARE ANATOMY AND PHYSIOLOGY?

The word *anatomy* has its origins in the language of ancient Greece, as do many other anatomical terms and phrases. A literal translation would be "a cutting open." **Anatomy** is *the study of internal and external structure* and the physical relationships between body parts. For instance, someone studying anatomy might examine how a particular muscle attaches to the skeleton or how two bones are connected to each other. **Physiology**, another word adopted from the Greek (*physiologia*, the study of nature), is *the study of how living organisms perform the vital functions of life* such as metabolism, growth, movement, and reproduction. Physiology considers the function of anatomical structures. A physiologist attempts to determine the physical and chemical processes responsible for the body functions that maintain life. Someone studying physiology might consider how a muscle contracts or what chemical processes are involved in the digestion of food.

Anatomy and physiology are closely related in both theory and practice. Anatomical information provides clues about probable functions, and physiological mechanisms can be explained only in terms of the underlying anatomy. This observation leads to a very important concept: *All specific functions are performed by specific structures.*

Anatomists and physiologists approach the relationship between structure and function from different perspectives. To understand the difference, consider a simple analogy. Suppose that an anatomist and a physiologist were asked to examine and report on a pickup truck (Figure 1–1). The anatomist might begin by measuring and photographing the various parts of the truck and, if possible, taking it apart and putting it back together again. The anatomist would then be able to explain its key structural relationships: for example, how the movement of the pistons in the engine cylinders caused the drive shaft to rotate and how that motion was then conveyed to the wheels. The physiologist would note the relationships between the components, but the primary focus would be on functional characteristics, such as the ideal ratio of gasoline to air for the most efficient combustion, the amount of power that the engine could generate, the amount of force transmitted to the wheels in different gears, and so on.

The link between structure and function is always present but not always understood. The superficial anatomy of the heart, for example, was clearly described in the fifteenth century, but almost 200 years passed before the pumping action of the heart was demonstrated.

Figure 1–1

(a) If asked to report on a pickup truck, anatomists would start by measuring the various parts and taking photographs showing how the parts are connected. They would then proceed to carefully take the truck apart and then try to reassemble it. **(b)** Physiologists would approach the task from a different perspective. They would investigate how the gears turn the wheels and how varying the gear ratios affects the truck's movement. They would vary the fuel-air ratio to see what effect it would have on engine efficiency and would monitor exhaust composition when different fuels are used.

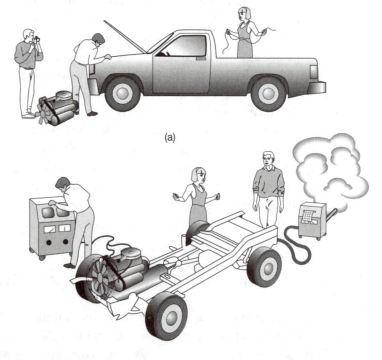

(a)

(b)

THE LANGUAGE OF ANATOMY AND PHYSIOLOGY

Like other sciences, anatomy and physiology use a special language that must be learned from the start. A familiarity with Latin and Greek roots (word parts with specific meanings) and patterns makes these new terms more understandable. As new terms are introduced, notes on pronunciation and relevant word roots will be provided. Additional information on foreign word roots, prefixes, suffixes, and combining forms will be included in the "Let's Review What You've Just Learned" sections in the text.

Latin and Greek words and phrases form the basis for an impressive number of anatomical terms. Many of these were introduced into anatomical literature by Greek and Roman anatomists. Greek physicians between 500 B.C. and A.D. 50 introduced terms such as *prostate* (*prostates*, standing before), *pleura* (*pleura*, rib), and *diaphragm* (*diaphragma*, sheet). Romans between A.D. 50 and 200 translated Greek works and added their own stamp on the vocabulary with regional terms (*fundus:* base, *corpus:* body, *orifice:* opening), names (uterus, coccyx, sacrum), and classifications of joints, muscles, and vessels that remain in use today. During the "Dark Ages" that followed, few anatomical studies were performed in Christian Europe, but Greek and Roman records were translated and preserved by scholars in the Arab world, and the vocabulary diversified further.

The translation of Arabic works that followed the Crusades (the eleventh to thirteenth centuries A.D.) triggered an intense interest in anatomy and an explosive growth in the anatomical literature. During this period, almost all publications were written in classical Latin, so anatomists from many different countries could communicate despite differences in their native languages. Because Latin was only written, and not used in day-to-day communication, the language did not change significantly over time through the introduction of slang terms or other sources of variation.

After the Dark Ages ended, European anatomists were busily naming anatomical structures, and the names assigned were often those of professors. For instance, the Fallopian tube was named for the Italian anatomist Gabrielle Fallopio (1523–1562). Clinical conditions were named after either the most famous victim (Lou Gehrig's disease, a progressive muscle paralysis) or the physician who first described it (Parkinson's disease, Alzheimer's disease). Commemorative names such as these are called **eponyms** (EP-ō-nimz; Greek *eponymos*, from a name), and after 300 or 400 years the eponym situation was out of control. National as well as professional egos were involved, and a common understanding of Latin could not help you recognize the "disease of Philip" or the "ligament of Haller." In addition, when structures are named after people, it is difficult to remember them because there is no connection between the appearance and the name, as there often is when Latin or Greek roots are used.

A series of international meetings have attempted to correct this situation by replacing eponyms with more precise terms. This movement has been reasonably successful, and major anatomical structures such as bones, cartilages, muscles, nerves, ligaments, and tendons no longer bear the names of famous anatomists. The clinical literature still retains many eponyms, but many of the older eponyms are no longer in use. Although reports of new conditions often use the names of physicians or patients, descriptive terms are usually assigned after additional research has been done.

Unfortunately, many eponyms remain as labels for clinical tests, minor anatomical features, and cellular details. A common indication of this type of naming is the capitalization of the term. Thus, the sheath covering nerve fibers is composed of Schwann cells, named for the nineteenth-century German anatomist Theodore Schwann. For those interested in eponyms and historical details, Table 1–1 provides information concerning the origins of the most common anatomical eponyms.

Although the Latin anatomical texts were translated into English and other modern languages centuries ago, many of the Latin names assigned specific structures are still used today. You could visit an anatomical library in Germany, France, or Japan, pick out a text, open to an illustration, and understand the labels without knowing a single word of German, French, or Japanese.

A familiarity with Latin roots and patterns makes anatomical terms more understandable, and the notes included on word derivation in this text are intended to assist you in that regard. In English, when you want to indicate more than one of something, you usually add an *s* to the name: cow/cows, door/doors, and so on. Latin words change their endings. A singular noun that ends in *-us* will have a plural that ends in *-i*; similarly *-um* becomes *-a*, and *-a* becomes *-ae*. You may have already encountered examples such as nucleolus/nucleoli, flagellum/flagella, and fascia/fasciae in your introductory biology courses.

Anatomy and physiology are international disciplines and research reports are published in a variety of languages. During the nineteenth and twentieth centuries, terms with German, French, Spanish and English roots were internationally accepted. This process continues, and the vocabulary continues to expand.

ANATOMY

Anatomy can be divided into **macroscopic** (Greek *macros*, large + *skopein*, to examine) **anatomy** and **microscopic** (Greek *micros*, small + *skopein*, to examine) **anatomy,** on the basis of the size of the object being observed and the degree of structural detail under consideration. As we proceed through the text, we will be considering details at all levels, from macroscopic to microscopic.

Gross Anatomy

Gross anatomy, or **macroscopic anatomy**, considers features of the body that are large enough to be visible to the unaided eye. There are many ways to approach gross anatomy:

- **Surface anatomy** is the study of the body's general form and superficial markings.

- **Regional anatomy** focuses on all the superficial and internal features in a specific area of the body, such as the head, neck, or trunk. Advanced courses in anatomy often stress a regional approach because it emphasizes the spatial relationships between structures already familiar to the students.

- **Systemic anatomy** is concerned with the structure of organ systems such as the skeletal or digestive system. **Organ systems** are *groups of organs that function together* in a coordinated manner. Just as the members of a sports team work together to play a game of baseball or football, the organs that make up an organ system work together to perform a particular task. An example of an organ system is the cardiovascular system, which consists of the heart, blood, and blood vessels and functions in distributing oxygen and nutrients throughout the body. There are 11 organ systems in the human body, and they will be introduced later in the chapter.

Table 1–1 Eponyms in Common Use

Eponym	Equivalent Terms	Individual Referenced
The Cellular Level of Organization		
Golgi apparatus		Camillo Golgi (1844–1926), Italian histologist; shared Nobel Prize in 1906
Krebs cycle	Citric acid, or tricarboxylic, cycle	Hans Adolph Krebs (1900–1981), British biochemist; shared Nobel Prize in 1953
The Skeletal System		
Colles' fracture		Abraham Colles (1773–1843), Irish surgeon
Haversian canals	Central canals	Clopton Havers (1650–1702), English anatomist and microscopist
Haversian systems	Osteons	
Pott's fracture		Percival Pott (1713–1788), English surgeon
Volkmann's canals	Perforating canals	Alfred Wilhelm Volkmann (1800–1877), German surgeon
Wormian bones	Sutural bones	Olas Worm (1588–1654), Danish anatomist
The Muscular System		
Achilles' tendon	Calcaneal tendon	Achilleus, hero of Greek mythology
Cori cycle		Carl Ferdinand Cori (1896–) and Gerty Theresa Cori (1896–1957), American biochemists; shared Nobel Prize in 1947
The Nervous System		
Broca's center	Speech center	Pierre Paul Broca (1824–1880), French surgeon
Foramen of Luschka	Lateral foramina	Hubert von Luschka (1820–1875), German anatomist
Foramen of Magendie	Median foramen	François Magendie (1783–1855), French physiologist
Foramen of Munro	Interventricular foramen	John Cummings Munro (1858–1910), American surgeon
Nissl bodies		Franz Nissl (1860–1919), German neurologist
Purkinje cells		Johannes E. Purkinje (1781–1869), Czechoslovakian physiologist
Nodes of Ranvier	Nodes	Louis Antoine Ranvier (1835–1922), French physiologist
Island of Reil	Insula	Johann Christian Reil (1759–1813), German anatomist
Fissure of Rolando	Central sulcus	Luigi Rolando (1773–1831), Italian anatomist
Schwann cells		Theodor Schwann (1810–1882), German anatomist
Aqueduct of Sylvius	Mesencephalic aqueduct	Jacobus Sylvius (Jacques Dubois, 1478–1555), French anatomist
Sylvian fissure	Lateral sulcus	Franciscus Sylvius (Franz de le Boë, 1614–1672), Dutch anatomist
Pons varolii	Pons	Costanzo Varolio (1543–1575), Italian anatomist
Sensory Function		
Organ of Corti		Alfonso Corti (1822–1888), Italian anatomist
Eustacian tube	Auditory tube	Bartolomeo Eustachio (1520–1574), Italian anatomist
Golgi tendon organs	Tendon organs	*See under* The Cellular Level
Hertz (Hz)		Heinrich Hertz (1857–1894), German physicist
Meibomian glands		Heinrich Meibom (1638–1700), German anatomist
Meissner's corpuscles		Georg Meissner (1829–1905), German physiologist
Merkel's discs		Friedrich Siegismund Merkel (1845–1919), German anatomist
Pacinian corpuscles	Lamellated corpuscles	Fillippo Pacini (1812–1883), Italian anatomist
Ruffini's corpuscles		Angelo Ruffini (1864–1929), Italian anatomist
Canal of Schlemm		Friedrich S. Schlemm (1795–1858), German anatomist
Glands of Zeis		Edward Zeis (1807–1868), German anatomist
The Endocrine System		
Islets of Langerhans	Pancreatic islets	Paul Langerhans (1847–1888), German pathologist
Intersitial cells of Leydig	Interstitial cells	Franz von Leydig (1821–1908), German anatomist

Table 1–1 Eponyms in Common Use

Eponym	Equivalent Terms	Individual Referenced
The Cardiovascular System		
Bundle of His		Wilhelm His (1863–1934), German physician
Purkinje cells		*See under* The Nervous System
Starling's law		Ernest Henry Starling (1866–1927), English physiologist
Circle of Willis		Thomas Willis (1621–1675), English physician
The Lymphatic System		
Hassall's corpuscles		Arthur Hill Hassall (1817–1894), English physician
Kupffer cells		Karl Wilhelm Kupffer (1829–1902), German anatomist
Langerhans cells		*See under* The Endocrine System
Peyer's patches	Aggregate lymphoid nodules	Johann Conrad Peyer (1653–1712), Swiss anatomist
The Respiratory System		
Adam's apple	Thyroid cartilage (laryngeal prominence)	Biblical reference
Bohr effect		Niels Bohr (1885–1962), Danish physicist; won 1922 Nobel Prize
Boyle's law		Robert Boyle (1621–1691), English physicist
Charles' law		Jacques Alexandre César Charles (1746–1823), French physicist
Dalton's law		John Dalton (1766–1844), English physicist
Henry's law		William Henry (1775–1837), English chemist
The Digestive System		
Plexus of Auerbach	Myenteric plexus	Leopold Auerbach (1827–1897), German anatomist
Bruner's glands	Duodenal glands	Johann Conrad Brunner (1653–1727), Swiss anatomist
Kupffer cells	Stellate reticuloendothelial cells	*See under* The Lymphatic System
Crypts of Lieberkühn	Intestinal crypts	Johann Nathaniel Lieberkühn (1711–1756), German anatomist
Plexus of Meissner	Submucosal plexus	*See under* Sensory Function
Sphincter of Oddi	Hepatopancreatic sphincter	Ruggero Oddi (1864–1913), Italian physician
Peyer's patches		*See under* The Lymphatic System
Duct of Santorini	Accessory pancreatic duct	Giovanni Domenico Santorini (1681–1737), Italian anatomist
Stensen's duct	Parotid duct	Niels Stensen (1638–1686), Danish physician-priest
Ampulla of Vater	Duodenal ampulla	Abraham Vater (1684–1751), German anatomist
Wharton's duct	Submandibular duct	Thomas Wharton (1614–1673), English physician
Foramen of Winslow	Epiploic foramen	Jacob Benignus Winslow (1669–1760), French anatomist
Duct of Wirsung	Pancreatic duct	Johann Georg Wirsung (1600–1643), German physician
The Urinary System		
Bowman's capsule	Glomerular capsule	Sir William Bowman (1816–1892), English physician
Loop of Henle		Friedrich Gustav Jakob Henle (1809–1885), German histologist
The Reproductive System		
Bartholin's glands	Greater vetibular glands	Casper Bartholin Jr. (1655–1738), Danish anatomist
Cowper's glands	Bulboourethral glands	William Cowper (1666–1709), English surgeon
Fallopian tube	Uterine tube (oviduct)	Gabriele Falloppio (1523–1562), Italian anatomist
Graafian follicle	Tertiary follicle	Reijnier de Graaf (1641–1673), Dutch physician
Interstitial cells of Leydig	Interstitial cells	*See under* The Endocrine System
Glands of Littre	Lesser vestibular glands	Alexis Littre (1658–1726), French surgeon
Sertoli cells	Sustentacular cells	Enrico Sertoli (1842–1910), Italian histologist

Microscopic Anatomy

Microscopic anatomy deals with structures that cannot be seen without magnification. The boundaries of microscopic anatomy are established by the limits of the equipment used. A **light microscope** uses visible light to illuminate an object and can show you basic details about cell structure. Getting a clear view of objects that are smaller than a human cell requires an electron microscope. An electron microscope uses electron beams instead of light to make an object visible. (See Figures 4–2 and 4–3 on p. 134–135 for pictures and further descriptions of these microscopes.) An electron microscope enables you to see individual structures only a few nanometers across (1 nanometer [nm] = 0.000000001 meter (10^{-9} meter), or 0.000001 millimeter (10^{-6} millimeter); see Figure 1–2).

Microscopic anatomy can be subdivided into specialties that consider features within a characteristic range of sizes. **Cytology** (sī-TOL-uh-jē; Greek *kytos*, a hollow vessel + *logia*, the study of) is *the study of the structure and function of living cells*, the simplest units of life. Living cells are composed of chemical substances in various combinations, and our lives depend on the chemical processes occurring in the trillions of cells that form our body. **Histology** (his-TOL-uh-jē; Greek *histos*, web, loom) is *the study of tissues; tissues* are groups of specialized cells and cell products that work together to perform a particular function. The trillions of cells in the human body can be assigned to four tissue types that are the focus of Chapter 4. Tissues combine to form **organs**, such as the heart, kidney, liver, and brain. Many organs are easily examined without a microscope, and at the organ level we cross the boundary into gross anatomy.

Developmental Anatomy

Developmental anatomy examines the changes in form that occur during the period between conception and physical maturity. Because it considers anatomical structures over such a broad range of sizes (from a single cell to an adult human), techniques used in developmental anatomy are similar to those used in both microscopic and gross anatomy. Developmental anatomy is important in medicine because many structural abnormalities can result from errors in development. The most extensive structural changes occur during the first two months of development. The study of these early developmental processes is called **embryology** (em-brē-OL-uh-jē; Greek *embryon*, to swell, grow inside).

Clinical Anatomy

There are a number of anatomical specialties that are most important in a clinical setting. Examples include **medical anatomy** (anatomical changes that occur during illness), **radiographic anatomy** (anatomical structures as seen using specialized imaging techniques, such as X-rays or CT scans, which are discussed later in this chapter, and **surgical anatomy** (anatomical landmarks important in surgery).

PHYSIOLOGY

Human physiology is the study of the functions of the human body or, in other words, how the body parts work. Body functions are complex and much more difficult to examine than most anatomical structures. As a result, there are even more specialties in physiology than in anatomy.

Figure 1–2
A comparison of the ranges of the human eye and light and electron microscopes.

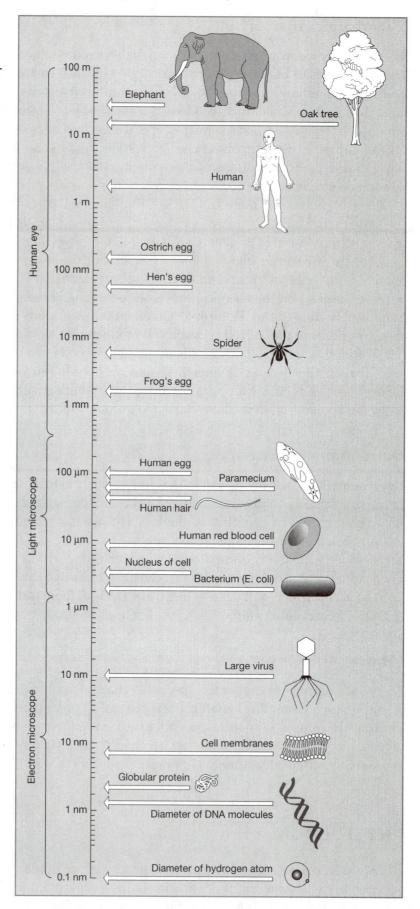

- **Cell physiology**, the study of the functions of living cells, is the cornerstone of human physiology. Cell physiology deals with events at the chemical and molecular levels: both chemical processes within cells and chemical interactions between cells. The term **metabolism** (me-TAB-uh-lizm; Greek *metabole*, change) is used in reference to all of the chemical reactions that occur within a living cell. Chapters 2 to 6 will focus on the chemical structure, internal organization, and control mechanisms of living cells and tissues.

- **Special physiology** is the study of the physiology of specific organs. Cardiac physiology, for example, is the study of heart function.

- **Systemic physiology** considers all aspects of the function of specific organ systems. Cardiovascular physiology, respiratory physiology, and reproductive physiology are examples of systemic physiology.

- **Pathophysiology** (path-ō-fiz-ē-OL-uh-jē; Greek *pathos*, disease) is the study of the effects of diseases on organ or system functions. Modern medicine depends on an accurate understanding of both normal physiology and pathophysiology; the health practitioner must know not only what is wrong but also how to correct it.

There are also specialties in physiology that deal with specific functions of the human body as a whole. These specialties focus on physiological interactions between multiple organ systems. Exercise physiology, for example, studies the physiological adjustments to exercise.

Let's Review What You've Just Learned

▶ Definitions

In the space provided, write the term for each of the following definitions.

_____ **1.** The study of cells and cell parts.

_____ **2.** The study of development that focuses on the first two months after fertilization.

_____ **3.** The study of the structure of the body.

_____ **4.** The study of tissues.

_____ **5.** The study of the functions of living organisms and their parts.

_____ **6.** A collection of specialized cells and cell products that performs a specific function.

_____ **7.** The sum of all the chemical processes that occur within an organism.

_____ **8.** Combinations of tissues that perform complex functions.

► Word Roots, Prefixes, Suffixes, and Combining Forms

In the space provided, list the boldfaced terms introduced in this section that contain the indicated word part.

Word Part	Meaning		Examples
-logy	study of	**9.**	_____
-tomy	to cut	**10.**	_____
histo-	tissue	**11.**	_____
physio-	nature	**12.**	_____
patho-	disease	**13.**	_____
ana-	up	**14.**	_____
cyto-	cell	**15.**	_____
embryo-	to grow inside	**16.**	_____

► Concept Mapping

Using the following terms, fill in the blank spaces next to the circled numbers to complete the concept map. Follow the numbers to comply with the organization of the map.

Surgical anatomy
Embryology
Tissues
Structure of organ systems

Regional anatomy
Cytology
Macroscopic anatomy

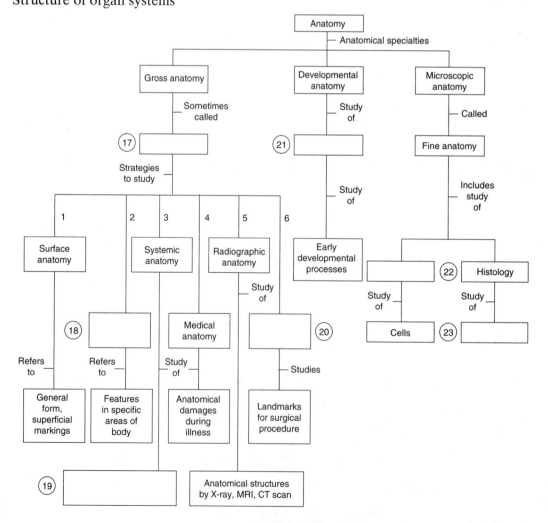

Using the following terms, fill in the blank spaces next to the circled numbers to complete the concept map. Follow the numbers to comply with the organization of the map.

Pathophysiology

Functions of living cells

Exercise physiology

Functions of anatomical structures

Histophysiology

Specific organ systems

Body function response to athletics

Body function response to changes in atmospheric pressure

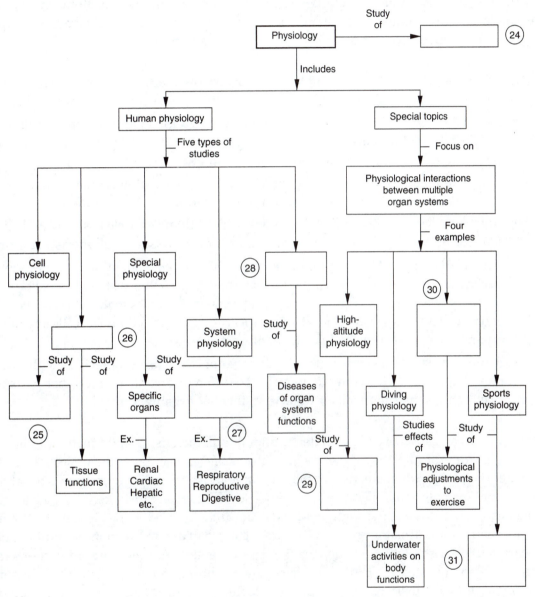

LEVELS OF ORGANIZATION

Many familiar objects exhibit different levels of organization. A carpet, for instance, is woven from fibers, which in turn are formed from threads that are composed of certain chemicals. In this case, we could talk about the chemical level of carpet organization, referring to the kinds of chemicals in the threads, or the thread level, the fiber level, or the carpet level.

The human body also exhibits levels of organization, from the tiny atoms that make up molecules to the entire organism. Figure 1–3 presents an example of the relationships among the various levels of organization in the human body.

- All the organ systems of the body work together to maintain life and health. This is the highest level of organization, that of the **organism**, in this case a human being.

- Groups of organs function together to perform specific vital functions within the body. This is the **organ system level of organization**. The heart, blood, and blood vessels form the cardiovascular system, an example of an organ system.

- Layers of muscle tissue form the bulk of the heart, a hollow, three-dimensional organ. We are now at the **organ level of organization**.

- Heart muscle cells are components of one form of tissue, muscle tissue. Muscle tissue, one of the four tissue types, is an example of the **tissue level of organization**.

- Cells are the smallest living units of the body. Human cells contain structures known as **organelles** (or-gan-ELZ; Latin *organella*, small organ). Just as the human body is made up of organs, each responsible for a specific job, the human cell is composed of organelles, internal structures that perform a specific function. The cells and their organelles represent the **cellular level of organization**.

- **Atoms**, the smallest stable units of matter, combine to form **molecules** with complex shapes. Molecules interact to form the different organelles and other parts of a cell. This is the **chemical**, or **molecular**, **level of organization**.

The organization of each level determines the characteristics and functions of higher levels. For example, the arrangement of atoms and molecules at the molecular level creates the protein filaments that, at the cellular level, give cardiac muscle cells the ability to contract powerfully. Because at the tissue level these cells are linked together, forming heart muscle tissue, the contractions are coordinated, producing a heartbeat. When that beat occurs, the anatomy of the heart, an organ, enables it to function as a pump. The heart is filled with blood and connected to blood vessels, and the pumping action circulates blood through the cardiovascular system. Through interactions with the respiratory, digestive, urinary, and other systems, the cardiovascular system performs a variety of functions essential to the survival of the organism.

Something that affects a particular system will ultimately affect all of the system's components. The heart, for example, cannot pump blood effectively after a massive blood loss if there is not enough blood to fill the circulatory system. If the heart cannot pump and blood cannot flow, oxygen and nutrients cannot be distributed. In a very short time, the tissue begins to break down as heart muscle cells die from oxygen and nutrient starvation. Of course, these changes will not be restricted to the cardiovascular system; all the cells, tissues, and organs in the body will be affected.

Figure 1–3   Levels of Organization.

Interacting atoms form molecules that combine in the protein fibers of heart muscle cells. These cells interlock, creating heart muscle tissue that constitutes most of the walls of a three-dimensional organ, the heart. The heart is one component of the cardiovascular system, which also includes the blood and blood vessels. The combined organ systems form an organism, a living human being.

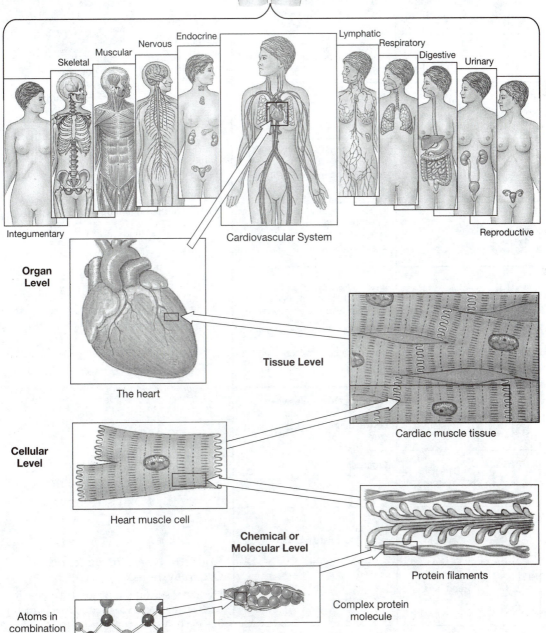

Organism Level

Organ System Level

Integumentary
Skeletal
Muscular
Nervous
Endocrine
Cardiovascular System
Lymphatic
Respiratory
Digestive
Urinary
Reproductive

Organ Level

The heart

Tissue Level

Cardiac muscle tissue

Cellular Level

Heart muscle cell

Chemical or Molecular Level

Protein filaments

Complex protein molecule

Atoms in combination

AN INTRODUCTION TO ORGAN SYSTEMS

Figure 1–4 introduces the 11 organ systems in the human body. This figure indicates the major functions of each system and the system's relative contribution to the total body weight. Figure 1–5 provides an overview of the individual systems and their major components.

Organ System		Major Functions
	Integumentary system	Protection from environmental hazards; temperature control
	Skeletal system	Support; protection of soft tissues; mineral storage; blood formation
	Muscular system	Locomotion; support; heat production
	Nervous system	Directing immediate responses to stimuli, generally by coordinating the activities of other organ systems
	Endocrine system	Directing long-term changes in the activities of other organ systems
	Cardiovascular system	Internal transport of cells and dissolved materials, including nutrients, wastes, and gases
	Lymphatic system	Defense against infection and disease
	Respiratory system	Delivery of air to sites where gas exchange can occur between the air and circulating blood
	Digestive system	Processing of food and absorption of nutrients, minerals, vitamins, and water
	Urinary system	Elimination of excess water, salts, and waste products
	Reproductive system	Production of sex cells and hormones

(a)

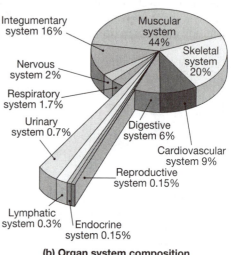

(b) Organ system composition of the human body by weight

Figure 1–4   An Introduction to Organ Systems.

Here you see **(a)** the major functions of each system and **(b)** the relative percentage each system contributes to total body weight.

**Figure 1–5
The Organ
Systems of
the Human
Body.**

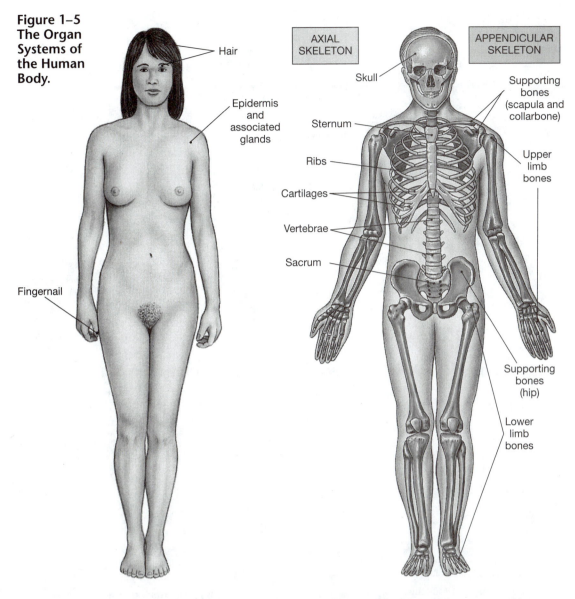

Hair

Epidermis
and
associated
glands

Fingernail

AXIAL
SKELETON

APPENDICULAR
SKELETON

Skull

Supporting
bones
(scapula and
collarbone)

Sternum

Upper
limb
bones

Ribs

Cartilages

Vertebrae

Sacrum

Supporting
bones
(hip)

Lower
limb
bones

(a)   The Integumentary System (skin)

Organ	Primary Functions
CUTANEOUS MEMBRANE	
Epidermis	Covers surface; protects underlying tissues
Dermis	Nourishes epidermis; provides strength; contains glands
HAIR FOLLICLES	Produce hair
Hairs	Provide sensation; provide some protection for head
Sebaceous glands	Secrete lipid coating that lubricates hair shaft
SWEAT GLANDS	Produce perspiration for evaporative cooling
NAILS	Protect and stiffen distal tips of digits
SENSORY RECEPTORS	Provide sensations of touch, pressure, temperature, pain
SUBCUTANEOUS LAYER	Stores lipids; attaches skin to deeper structures

(b)   The Skeletal System

Organ	Primary Functions
BONES (206), CARTILAGES, AND LIGAMENTS	Support, protect soft tissues; store minerals
Axial skeleton (skull, vertebrae, sacrum, ribs, sternum)	Protects brain, spinal cord, sense organs, and soft tissues of thoracic cavity; supports the body weight over the lower limbs
Appendicular skeleton (limbs and supporting bones)	Provides internal support and positioning of the limbs; supports and moves axial skeleton
BONE MARROW	Primary site of blood cell production

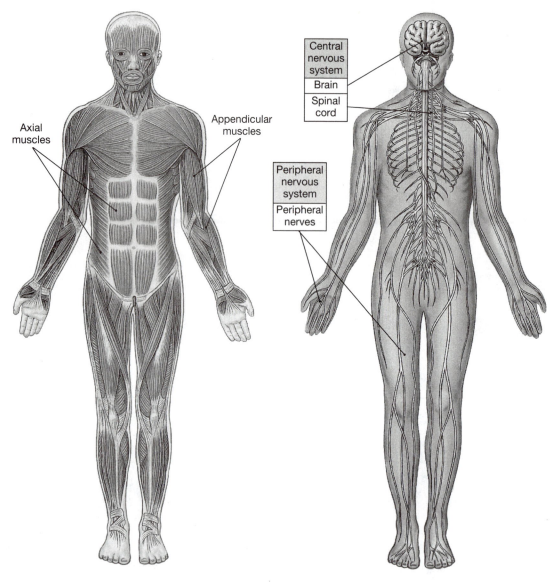

(c)   **The Muscular System**

Organ	Primary Functions
SKELETAL MUSCLES (700)	Provide skeletal movement; control entrances and exits of digestive tract; produce heat; support skeletal position; protect soft tissues
Axial muscles	Support and position axial skeleton
Appendicular muscles	Support, move, and brace limbs
TENDONS, APONEUROSES	Harness forces of contraction to perform specific tasks

(d)   **The Nervous System**

Organ	Primary Functions
CENTRAL NERVOUS SYSTEM (CNS)	Control center for nervous system: processes information; provides short-term control over activities of other systems
Brain	Performs complex integrative functions; controls voluntary activities
Spinal cord	Relays information to and from the brain; performs less-complex integrative functions; directs many simple involuntary activities
PERIPHERAL NERVOUS SYSTEM (PNS)	Links CNS with other systems and with sense organs

Figure 1–5   **(continued)**

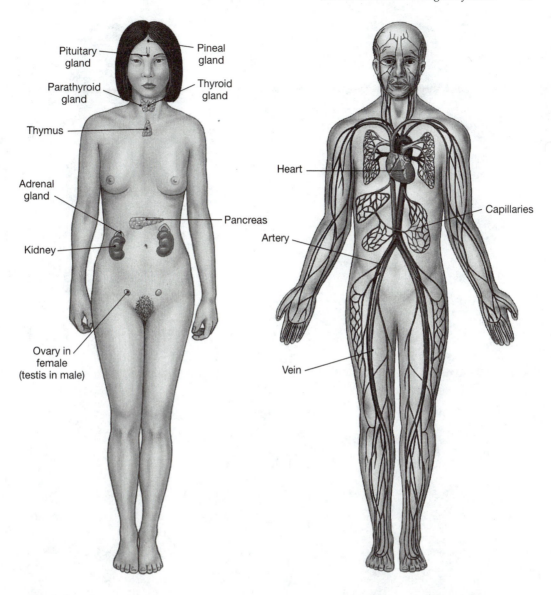

(e) The Endocrine System

Organ	Primary Functions
PINEAL GLAND	May control timing of reproduction and set day/night rhythms
PITUITARY GLAND	Controls other endocrine glands; regulates growth and fluid balance
THYROID GLAND	Controls tissue metabolic rate; regulates calcium levels
PARATHYROID GLAND	Regulates calcium levels (with thyroid)
THYMUS	Controls maturation of lymphocytes
ADRENAL GLANDS	Adjust water balance, tissue metabolism, and cardiovascular and respiratory activity
KIDNEYS	Control red blood cell production and elevate blood pressure
PANCREAS	Regulates blood glucose levels
GONADS	
Testes	Support male sexual characteristics and reproductive functions *(see Figure 1–5k)*
Ovaries	Support female sexual characteristics and reproductive functions *(see Figure 1–5k)*

(f) The Cardiovascular System

Organ	Primary Functions
HEART	Propels blood; maintains blood pressure
BLOOD VESSELS	Distribute blood around the body
Arteries	Carry blood from heart to capillaries
Capillaries	Site of diffusion between blood and interstitial fluids
Veins	Return blood from capillaries to the heart
BLOOD	Transports oxygen, carbon dioxide, and blood cells; delivers nutrients and hormones; removes waste products; assists in temperature regulation and defense against disease

Figure 1–5   (continued)

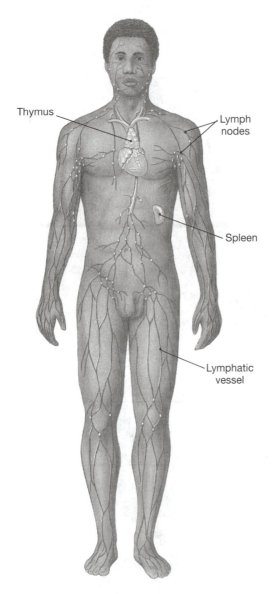

Thymus

Lymph nodes

Spleen

Lymphatic vessel

Nasal cavity

Sinus

Pharynx

Larynx

Trachea

Bronchi

Lung

Diaphragm

(g) The Lymphatic System

(h) The Respiratory System

Organ	Primary Functions
LYMPHATIC VESSELS	Carry lymph (water and proteins) and lymphocytes from peripheral tissues to the veins of the cardio-vascular system
LYMPH NODES	Monitor the composition of lymph; engulf pathogens; stimulate immune response
SPLEEN	Monitors circulating blood; engulfs pathogens; stimulates immune response
THYMUS	Controls development and mainte-nance of one class of lymphocytes (T cells); immature lymphocytes and other blood cells are produced in the bone marrow

Organ	Primary Functions
NASAL CAVITIES, PARANASAL SINUSES	Filter, warm, humidify air; detect smells
PHARYNX	Chamber shared with digestive tract; conducts air to larynx
LARYNX	Protects opening to trachea and contains vocal cords
TRACHEA	Filters air, traps particles in mucus; cartilages keep airway open
BRONCHI	Same functions as trachea
LUNGS	Include airways and alveoli; volume changes due to move-ments of ribs and diaphragm are responsible for air movement
ALVEOLI	Sites of gas exchange between air and blood

Figure 1–5   **(continued)**

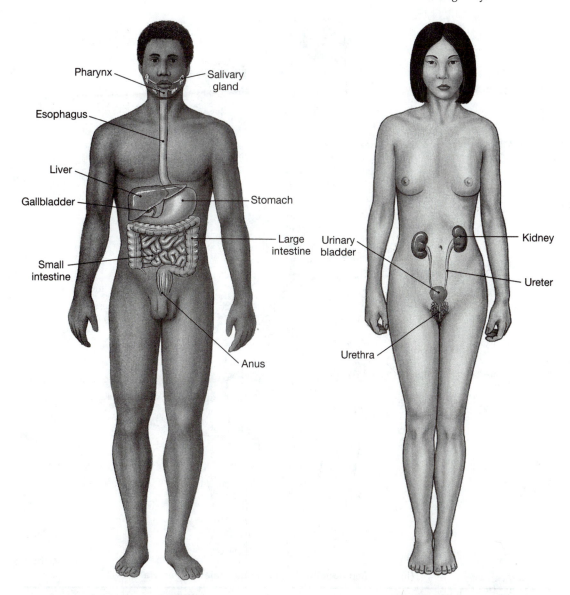

(i) The Digestive System

Organ	Primary Functions
SALIVARY GLANDS	Provide buffers and lubrication; produce enzymes that begin digestion
PHARYNX	Passageway connected to esophagus and trachea
ESOPHAGUS	Delivers food to stomach
STOMACH	Secretes acids and enzymes
SMALL INTESTINE	Secretes digestive enzymes, buffers, and hormones; absorbs nutrients
LIVER	Secretes bile; regulates blood composition of nutrients
GALLBLADDER	Stores bile for release into small intestine
PANCREAS	Secretes digestive enzymes and buffers; contains endocrine cells (*see Figure 1–5e*)
LARGE INTESTINE	Removes water from fecal material; stores wastes

(j) The Urinary System

Organ	Primary Functions
KIDNEYS	Form and concentrate urine; regulate blood pH and ion concentrations; endocrine functions noted in *Figure 1–5e*
URETERS	Conduct urine from kidneys to urinary bladder
URINARY BLADDER	Stores urine for eventual elimination
URETHRA	Conducts urine to exterior

Figure 1–5 (continued)

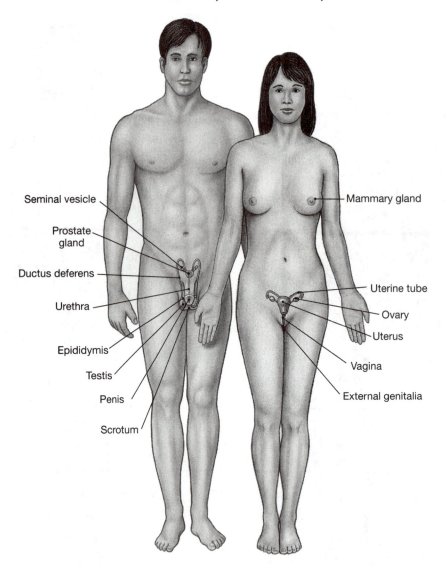

Seminal vesicle

Prostate gland

Ductus deferens

Urethra

Epididymis

Testis

Penis

Scrotum

Mammary gland

Uterine tube

Ovary

Uterus

Vagina

External genitalia

(k) The Reproductive System of the Male and Female

Organ	Primary Functions	Organ	Primary Functions
TESTES	Produce sperm and hormones (*see Figure 1–5e*)	**OVARIES**	Produce oocytes and hormones (*see Figure 1–5e*)
ACCESSORY ORGANS		**UTERINE TUBES**	Deliver ova or embryo to uterus; normal site of fertilization
Epididymis	Site of sperm maturation	**UTERUS**	Site of embryonic development and
Ductus deferens (sperm duct)	Conducts sperm between epididymis and prostate		diffusion between maternal and embryonic bloodstreams
Seminal vesicles	Secrete fluid that makes up much of the volume of semen	**VAGINA**	Site of sperm deposition; birth canal at delivery; provides passage of fluids during menstruation
Prostate gland	Secretes fluid and enzymes		
Urethra	Conducts semen to exterior	**EXTERNAL GENITALIA**	
EXTERNAL GENITALIA		**Clitoris**	Erectile organ; produces pleasurable sensations during sexual act
Penis	Erectile organ used to deposit sperm in the vagina of a female; produces pleasurable sensations during sexual act	**Labia**	Contain glands that lubricate entrance to vagina
Scrotum	Surrounds the testes and controls their temperature	**MAMMARY GLANDS**	Produce milk that nourishes newborn infant

Figure 1–5 (continued)

Let's Review What You've Just Learned

▶ **Definitions**

In the space provided, write the term for each of the following definitions.

_____ **32.** An intracellular structure that performs a specific function or group of functions.

_____ **33.** The smallest stable unit of matter.

_____ **34.** A compound containing two or more atoms that are held together by chemical bonds.

35. *Arrange the following levels of organization into the proper order from least complex to most complex.*

a. epithelial cell   **d.** proteins
b. skin   **e.** epithelial tissue
c. atoms

The following is a list of major functions for selected organ systems. Identify the organ system that is being described.

_____ **36.** Elimination of excess water, salts, and waste products.

_____ **37.** Directing long-term changes in the activities of other organ systems.

_____ **38.** Defense against infection and disease.

_____ **39.** Locomotion, support, heat production

_____ **40.** Processing of food and absorption of nutrients.

Complete the following statements concerning organs, organ systems, and their functions.

41. The stomach, which is part of the _____ system, secretes acids and enzymes.

42. The _____ of the integumentary system produce hair.

43. The arteries of the cardiovascular system function in _____.

44. The _____ of the skeletal system is the primary site of blood cell production.

45. The urethra of the _____ system conducts urine to the exterior of the body.

46. The _____ of the reproductive system is the site of embryonic development.

47. The _____ gland of the endocrine system controls tissue metabolic rate.

48. The larynx of the respiratory system functions in _____ and contains _____.

49. The _____ of the nervous system performs complex integrative functions and controls voluntary activity.

50. The spleen of the _____ system monitors circulating blood, engulfs pathogens, and stimulates immune responses.

MAINTAINING A STABLE ENVIRONMENT

Organ systems are interconnected and depend on each other. The cells, tissues, organs, and systems of the body exist together in a shared environment like the inhabitants of a large city. City dwellers breathe the city air and drink the water provided by the local water company; cells in the human body absorb oxygen and nutrients from fluids that surround them. If a city is blanketed in smog, or the water is contaminated, the inhabitants will become ill. Similarly, if body fluid composition becomes abnormal, cells will be injured or destroyed. Maintaining a stable environment is absolutely vital; a failure to maintain a relatively constant environment for the body's cells will result in illness and, in many cases, death within a relatively short period. Suppose, for example, there are changes in the temperature or salt content of the blood. The effect on the heart could range from a minor adjustment (heart muscle tissue contracts more often, and the heart rate goes up) to a total disaster (the heart stops beating altogether, and the individual dies).

Regulating the Internal Balance

A central principle of physiology is that the normal function of physiological systems is to maintain fairly constant internal conditions. A variety of physiological mechanisms act to prevent potentially disruptive changes from occurring in the environment inside the body. **Homeostasis** (hō-mē-ō-STĀ-sis; Greek *homoios*, like, similar + *stasis*, fixation, standing) refers to the existence of a stable internal environment. To survive, every living organism must maintain homeostasis. The term **homeostatic regulation** refers to the adjustments in physiological systems that are responsible for preserving homeostasis. The physiological processes that control homeostasis operate to keep vital characteristics within the relatively narrow limits required for normal body function. Examples include the mechanisms responsible for controlling levels of oxygen, carbon dioxide, glucose, pH, blood pressure, and other factors.

Physiological values usually vary within a normal range. For this reason most laboratory reports indicate the values determined and the normal ranges for each. In many cases, the ranges can change over time (from infancy to old age) or from moment to moment, depending on the activity under way. For instance, people often use 72 beats per minute (bpm) as an ideal heart rate, but that value is actually the average for young adults at rest. The real, measured values can be quite different. This variation becomes very apparent when you consider the normal ranges. The typical heart rate of resting young adults (60–80 bpm) differs from that of infants (70–170 bpm), and the adult heart rate during deep sleep (45–60 bpm) is very different from that found during heavy exercise (160–180 bpm).

An understanding of how homeostasis is regulated will help you make accurate predictions about the body's responses to normal and abnormal conditions. Two general mechanisms are involved in homeostatic regulation: autoregulation and extrinsic regulation.

- **Autoregulation** (*auto*, self) occurs when the activities of a cell, tissue, organ, or system change automatically when there is some change in its environment. When the cells within a tissue need more oxygen, they release chemicals that cause an increase in blood flow to the area, providing more oxygen to the region.

- **Extrinsic** (outside) **regulation** results from the activities of the nervous or endocrine system, organ systems that can control or adjust the activities of many different systems simultaneously. When you are exercising, the nervous system issues commands that increase the heart rate so that blood will circulate faster. The nervous system also reduces blood flow to organs, such as the digestive tract, that are relatively inactive. The oxygen in the circulating blood is thus saved for the active muscles.

In general, the nervous system directs rapid, short-term, and very specific responses. When you accidentally set your hand on a hot stove, the rising temperature produces a painful, localized disturbance of homeostasis. The nervous system responds by ordering the contraction of specific muscles that will pull the hand away from the stove. The effects last only as long as the neural activity continues, usually a matter of seconds.

By contrast, the endocrine system releases chemical messengers, called **hormones**, that affect tissues and organs throughout the body. The responses may not be immediately apparent, but when the effects appear they often persist for days or weeks. Examples of endocrine function include the long-term regulation of blood volume and composition and the adjustments of organ system function during starvation or stress.

Regardless of which system is involved, homeostatic regulation always functions to stabilize a particular aspect of the internal environment. An abnormality in a controlled condition (such as blood pressure) acts as a stimulus that activates the regulatory mechanism, which in turn acts to change the controlled condition back to the normal state. The mechanism itself consists of a **receptor** sensitive to that particular stimulus and an **effector** whose activity has an effect on the same stimulus. A **control center**, or **integration center**, is placed between the receptor and the effector. You are probably already familiar with several examples of homeostatic regulation, although not in those terms. As an example, consider the operation of the thermostat in a house or apartment (Figure 1–6).

The thermostat is a control center that monitors room temperature. The dial on the thermostat establishes the **set point**, or optimal level for the controlled condition—in this case, the temperature you find most comfortable. In our example, the set point is 22°C (about 72°F). The function of the thermostat is to keep room temperature within acceptable limits, usually within a degree or so of the set point. This thermostat receives information from a receptor (a thermometer exposed to the air in the room), and it controls an effector (an air conditioner).

When the temperature at the thermometer (a receptor) increases outside the normal range, the thermostat (a control center) turns on the air conditioner (an effector). The air conditioner then cools the room. When the temperature at the thermometer approaches the set point, the thermostat turns off the air conditioner.

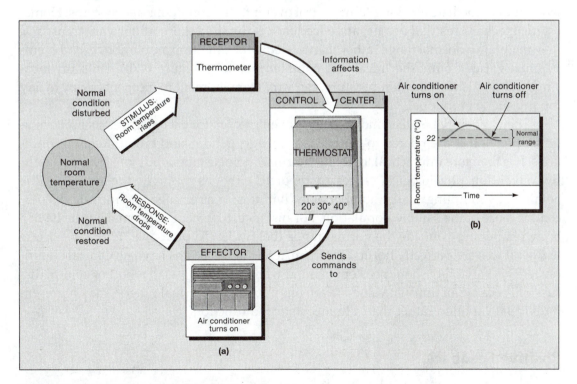

Figure 1–6   The Control of Room Temperature.
(a) A thermostat stabilizes room temperature by turning on an air conditioner (or heater) as needed to keep room temperature near the desired set point. Whether the room temperature rises or falls, the thermostat (a control center) triggers an effector response that restores normal temperature. When room temperature rises, the thermostat turns on the air conditioner, and the room temperature returns to normal levels. **(b)** With this regulatory system, room temperature oscillates around the set point.

Negative Feedback

The essential feature of the example we have been discussing can be summarized very simply: A variation outside of normal limits triggers an automatic response that restores homeostasis. This method of homeostatic regulation is called **negative feedback** because an effector activated by the control center acts to eliminate the stimulus or reduce its magnitude.

Most homeostatic mechanisms in the body involve negative feedback. For example, consider the control of body temperature, a process called **thermoregulation** (Figure 1–7a) Thermoregulation involves altering the relationship between heat loss, which occurs primarily at the body surface, and heat production, which occurs in all active tissues.

The control center for thermoregulation is located in the brain. It receives information from two temperature receptors, one in the skin and the other in the control center of the brain. At the set point, the general body temperature will be approximately 37°C (98.6°F). If body temperature rises above 37.2°C, activity in the control center targets two different effectors: (1) smooth muscles in the walls of blood vessels supplying the skin and (2) sweat glands. The muscles in the walls of the blood vessels relax, allowing the blood vessels to dilate. This dilation increases blood flow through vessels near the body surface. The sweat glands increase their rate of secretion, moving more water to the skin surface. The skin then acts as a radiator, losing heat to the environment, and the evaporation of sweat speeds the process. When body temperature returns to normal, the control center becomes inactive, and superficial blood flow and sweat gland activity return to previous levels.

Negative feedback is the primary mechanism for regulating homeostasis and provides both immediate and long-term control over internal conditions and systems. Homeostatic mechanisms that use negative feedback normally ignore minor variations, and they maintain a normal range rather than a fixed value. In the example above, body temperature varies around the "ideal" set-point temperature (Figure 1–7b). Thus any measured value, such as body temperature, can vary from moment to moment or day to day for any single individual.

The variability between individuals is even greater, for each person has homeostatic set points that are related to genetic factors, age, gender, and environmental conditions. It is therefore impractical to define "normal" homeostatic conditions very precisely. By convention, physiological values are reported either as averages, the average value obtained by sampling a large number of individuals, or as a range that includes 95 percent or more of the sample population. For instance, 5 percent of normal adults have a body temperature outside the normal range (below 36.7°C or above 37.2°C). But these temperatures are perfectly normal for them, and the variations have no clinical significance. This variability should be kept in mind when reviewing a lab report or clinical discussion, because an unusual value—even one outside the normal range—may represent individual variation rather than a homeostatic malfunction.

Positive Feedback

In **positive feedback**, the initial stimulus produces a response that exaggerates the stimulus. Suppose that the thermostat in our previous example were wired so that when the temperature rose it would turn on a heater rather than the air conditioner. In that case, the initial stimulus (rising room temperature) would cause a response (heater turns on)

Maintaining a Stable Environment

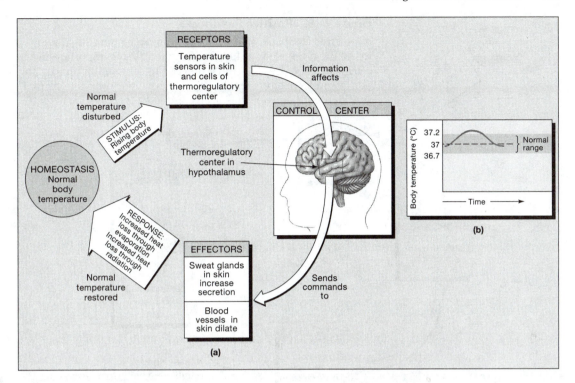

Figure 1–7   Negative Feedback in Body Temperature Control.
(a) Events comparable to those shown in Figure 1–6 occur in the regulation of body temperature. A control center in the brain functions as a thermostat with a set point of 37°C. If body temperature climbs above 37.2°C, heat loss is increased through enhanced blood flow to the skin and increased sweating. **(b)** The thermoregulatory center keeps body temperature oscillating within an acceptable range, usually between 36.7° and 37.2°C.

that would exaggerate the stimulus. The room temperature would continue to rise until some external factor switched off the thermostat, unplugged the heater, or interrupted the process in some other way.

Control mechanisms relying on positive feedback are not nearly as common as those involving negative feedback. However, positive feedback is important in controlling physiological processes that, once initiated, must be completed quickly. Consider the process of labor that results in the delivery of a newborn infant. Once labor begins, it is important that it be completed as soon as possible to avoid unduly stressing both mother and infant. A major stimulus initiating labor and delivery is stretching of the uterus by the growing fetus. The trigger for the initiation of labor contractions is a rise in the uterine level of **oxytocin** (ok-si-TŌ-sin; Greek *okytokios*, quick childbirth), a hormone that stimulates the contractions of uterine muscles. One source of oxytocin, and the regulatory mechanism that controls its secretion, has been diagrammed in Figure 1–8. Stretch receptors in the uterine wall are monitored by a control center in the brain. When sufficient uterine stretching occurs, the control center releases oxytocin. As uterine contractions occur, the fetus is pushed toward the vagina. The movement causes extreme stretching of the lower portion of the uterus, triggering the release of additional oxytocin. The uterine contractions then become more forceful, leading to greater movement and stretching. Each time the control center responds, the action of the effectors causes an increase in receptor stimulation. This kind of cycle, a positive feedback loop, can be broken only by some external force or process—in this instance, the delivery of the newborn infant, which eliminates the uterine stretching. Blood clotting is another important example of a positive feedback mechanism.

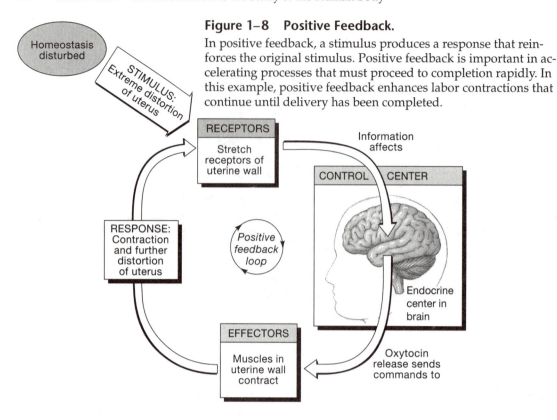

Figure 1–8 Positive Feedback.

In positive feedback, a stimulus produces a response that reinforces the original stimulus. Positive feedback is important in accelerating processes that must proceed to completion rapidly. In this example, positive feedback enhances labor contractions that continue until delivery has been completed.

HOMEOSTASIS AND DISEASE

Physiological mechanisms do a remarkably good job of maintaining a constant internal environment, regardless of our ongoing activities. The ability to maintain homeostasis depends on two interacting factors: (1) the status of the physiological systems involved and (2) the nature of the stress imposed. Homeostasis is a balancing act, and each person is like a tightrope walker. Homeostatic systems must adapt to sudden or gradual changes in the environment, such as the arrival of disease-causing organisms or accidental injuries, just as a tightrope walker must make allowances for gusts of wind, frayed segments of the rope, and thrown popcorn.

The ability to maintain homeostatic balance varies with the age, general health, and genetic makeup of the individual. If homeostatic mechanisms cannot cope with a particular stress, physiological values will begin to drift outside of the normal range. This deviation can ultimately affect all other systems with potentially fatal results; after all, a person unable to maintain balance will eventually fall off the tightrope.

Consider a specific example. A young adult exercising heavily may have a heart rate of 180 bpm for several minutes. But such a heart rate can be disastrous for an older person already suffering from cardiovascular and respiratory problems. If the heart rate cannot be reduced because of problems with the pacemaking or conducting system of the heart, there will be damage to the heart muscle tissue, leading to decreased pumping efficiency and a decline in blood pressure.

This process represents a serious threat to homeostasis. Other systems soon become involved, and the situation worsens. Filtration at the kidneys occurs at the normal range of arterial blood pressures. When the blood pressure becomes abnormally low, blood flow through the kidneys declines and they may stop working. Toxins then begin accumulating in the bloodstream. The reduced blood flow in other tissues soon leads to a low tissue oxygen level. Cells throughout the body then begin to suffer from oxygen starvation. The person is now in serious trouble, and unless steps are taken to correct the situation, survival is threatened.

Disease is *the failure to maintain homeostatic conditions*. The disease process may initially affect cells in a single tissue, organ, or system, but it will ultimately lead to changes in the function or structure of cells throughout the body. A disease can often be overcome through appropriate automatic adjustments in physiological systems. In a case of the flu, the disease develops because the immune system cannot defeat the influenza virus before it has infected cells of the respiratory passageways. For most people, the physiological adjustments made in response to the presence of the disease will lead to the elimination of the virus and the restoration of homeostasis. Some diseases cannot be easily overcome. In the case of the person with acute cardiovascular problems, some outside intervention must be provided to restore homeostasis and prevent fatal complications.

Diseases may result from:

- **Pathogens (organisms that cause disease) or parasites that invade the body:** Examples include the flu, mumps, measles, pinworm, and tapeworms.

- **Inherited genetic conditions that disrupt normal physiological mechanisms:** These conditions make normal homeostatic control difficult or impossible. Examples include sickle-cell anemia, hemophilia, and muscular dystrophy.

- **The loss of normal regulatory control mechanisms:** Cancer involves the rapid, unregulated multiplication of abnormal cells. Many cancers have been linked to abnormalities in genes responsible for controlling the rates of cell division. A variety of other diseases occur when regulatory mechanisms of the immune system fail and normal tissues are attacked.

- **Degenerative changes in vital physiological systems:** Many systems become less adaptable and less efficient as part of the aging process. As an individual ages, there are significant reductions in bone mass, respiratory capacity, cardiac efficiency, and kidney filtration. If these individuals are exposed to stresses that their weakened systems cannot tolerate, disease results.

- **Trauma, toxins, or other environmental hazards:** Accidents may damage internal organs, impairing their function. Toxins consumed in the diet or absorbed through the skin may disrupt normal cellular activities.

- **Nutritional factors:** Diseases may result from diets inadequate in important nutrients, including proteins, essential fats, vitamins, minerals, or water. *Kwashiorkor* (kwah-shē-OR-kor; Swahili, displaced child), a protein deficiency disease, and *scurvy*, a disease caused by vitamin C deficiency, are two examples. Excessive consumption of high-calorie foods, fats, or fat-soluble vitamins can also cause disease.

Pathology is *the study of disease*. Different diseases can often result in the same alteration of function and produce the same symptoms. For example, a patient with pale skin and complaining of a lack of energy and breathlessness may have (1) respiratory problems that prevent normal oxygen transfer to the blood or (2) cardiovascular problems that interfere with normal oxygen transport *(anemia)* or circulation *(heart failure)*. Clinicians must ask questions and collect appropriate information to make a proper diagnosis. This process often involves eliminating possible causes until a specific diagnosis is reached.

This brings us to a key concept: *All diagnostic procedures assume an understanding of normal anatomy and physiology.* An understanding of normal homeostatic mechanisms can usually enable you to draw conclusions about what might be responsible for observed symptoms.

Let's Review What You've Just Learned

▶ **Definitions**

In the space provided, write the term for each of the following definitions.

_____ **51.** Mechanism that increases a deviation from normal limits after an initial stimulus.

_____ **52.** A chemical secreted by one cell that travels through the circulatory system to affect the activities of cells in another part of the body.

_____ **53.** The failure of physiological mechanisms to maintain homeostasis.

_____ **54.** Homeostatic maintenance of body temperature.

_____ **55.** The maintenance of a relatively constant internal environment.

_____ **56.** A hormone that stimulates muscle contractions of the uterus.

_____ **57.** Alterations in activity that maintain homeostasis in direct response to changes in the local environment.

_____ **58.** Corrective mechanism that opposes or cancels a variation from normal limits.

▶ **Feedback**

For each of the following examples, indicate whether the process is an example of negative feedback or positive feedback.

59. A rise in the level of calcium ions in the blood stimulates the release of a hormone that causes bone cells to deposit more of the calcium in bone.

60. An increase in blood pressure triggers an neural response that results in lowering the blood pressure.

61. When platelets in the blood stick to an injured area, they release chemicals that causes more platelets to stick in the area.

AN INTRODUCTION TO ANATOMICAL STUDIES

Early anatomists faced serious problems in communicating with each other. Stating that a bump is "on the back" does not give very precise information about the location. To solve the problem, anatomists created maps of the human body. The landmarks for these maps are prominent anatomical structures. Distances are measured in centimeters or inches, and special terms are used to indicate direction. As indicated earlier in this chapter, anatomy uses a special language that must be learned from the start. Although at first the names might be hard to associate with an area of the body, such as carpal for wrist, it is necessary to learn these terms now, so that they will become familiar and easy to relate to when you encounter them again in other coursework.

Superficial Anatomy

A familiarity with anatomical landmarks and directional terms will make your study of anatomy more understandable because none of the organ systems except the skin (integument) can be seen from the body surface. You will find it helpful to try creating your own mental maps from the information and anatomical illustrations that accompany this discussion. Your maps will help you apply the information effectively in future coursework and actual practice.

Anatomical Landmarks

Important anatomical landmarks are presented in Figure 1–9. The anatomical terms are given in boldface, the common names in plain type, and the anatomical adjectives in parentheses. You should become familiar with all three terms. The term **brachium** (BRĀ-kē-um; Latin *brachium*, arm) for example, refers to the arm. The brachial artery is located in the arm, as is the brachial nerve. An understanding of the terms and their origins will help you remember the location of a particular structure as well as its name.

Standard anatomical illustrations show the human form in the **anatomical position**. In this position, the hands are at the sides with the palms facing forward. Figure 1–9 shows an individual in the anatomical position as seen from the front and the back. Unless otherwise noted, all the descriptions given in this text refer to the body in the anatomical position. A person lying down is said to be **supine** (sū-PĪN; Latin *supinus*, lying back) when lying face up and **prone** (Latin *pronus*, leaning forward) when lying face down.

Anatomical Regions

Major regions of the body are listed in Table 1–2 and shown in Figure 1–9. When dealing with the abdomen, anatomists and clinicians often need to use regional terms, in addition to specific landmarks, to describe a general area of interest or injury. Two approaches have been developed for mapping the surface of the abdominal area, specifically referred to as the abdominopelvic region.

Workers in clinical fields divide the abdominopelvic region into four segments using a pair of imaginary lines that intersect at the **umbilicus** (um-BIL-i-kus; Latin *umbilicus*, navel). These four regions are called **abdominopelvic quadrants**. This simple method, shown in Figure 1–10a provides useful references for the description of aches, pains, and injuries. The location can assist a doctor in deciding the possible cause; for example, tenderness in the **right lower quadrant (RLQ)** is a symptom of appendicitis, whereas tenderness in the **right upper quadrant (RUQ)** may indicate gallbladder or liver problems.

Anatomists prefer to use more-precise regional terms to describe the location and orientation of internal organs. They divide the abdominopelvic area into nine regions (Figure 1–10b). Figure 1–10c shows the relationship among quadrants, regions, and internal organs.

Anatomical Directions

Table 1–3 and Figure 1–11 show the principal directional terms and examples of their use. There are many different terms, and some can be used interchangeably. The term **anterior**, for example, refers to the front of the body. When humans are viewed in the anatomical position, the term *anterior* is equivalent to **ventral**, which actually refers to the belly. Before continuing, take the time to review Table 1–3 in detail, and practice using these terms at every opportunity. If you are familiar with the basic vocabulary, you will find all the description in anatomy and physiology courses easier to follow. You will find it useful to remember that the terms *left* and *right* always refer to the left and right sides of the subject, not of the observer.

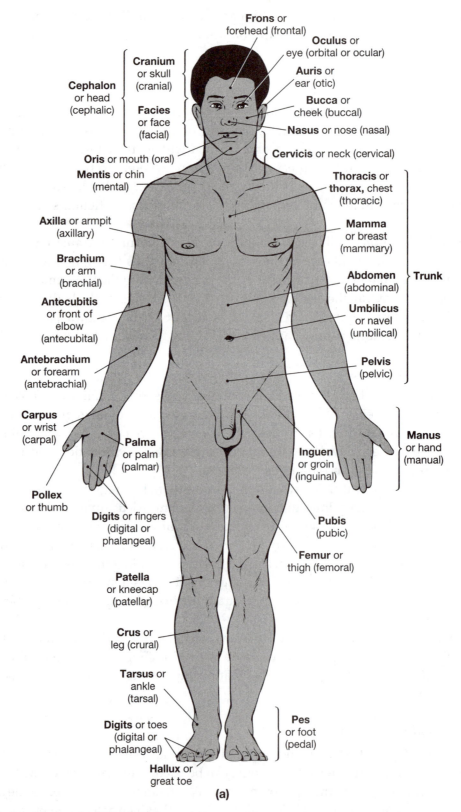

(a)

Figure 1–9 Anatomical Landmarks.
The anatomical terms are shown in boldface type, the common names in plain type, and the anatomical adjectives in parentheses.

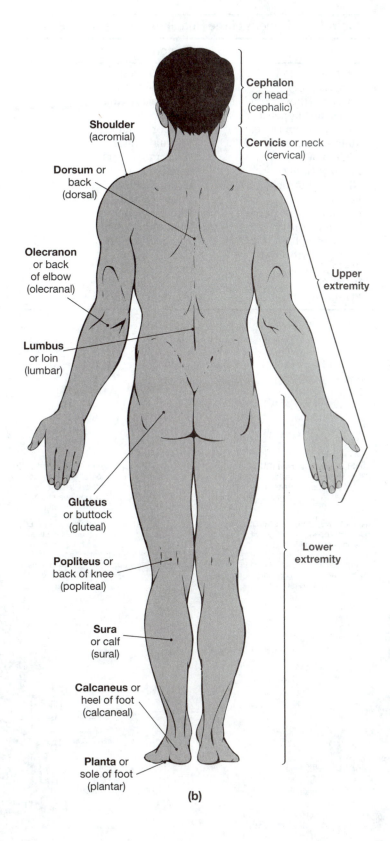

Cephalon
or head
(cephalic)

Shoulder
(acromial)

Cervicis or neck
(cervical)

Dorsum or
back
(dorsal)

Olecranon
or back
of elbow
(olecranal)

**Upper
extremity**

Lumbus
or loin
(lumbar)

Gluteus
or buttock
(gluteal)

Popliteus or
back of knee
(popliteal)

**Lower
extremity**

Sura
or calf
(sural)

Calcaneus or
heel of foot
(calcaneal)

Planta or
sole of foot
(plantar)

(b)

Figure 1–9 (continued)

Table 1–2   Regions of the Human Body (*see Figure 1–9*)

Structure	Region
Cephalon (head)	Cephalic region
Cervicis (neck)	Cervical region
Thoracis (thorax or chest)	Thoracic region
Brachium (upper arm)	Brachial region
Antebrachium (forearm)	Antebrachial region
Manus (hand)	Manual region
Abdomen	Abdominal region
Lumbus (loin)	Lumbar region
Gluteus (buttock)	Gluteal region
Pelvis	Pelvic region
Pubis (anterior pelvis)	Pubic region
Inguen (groin)	Inguinal region
Femur (thigh)	Femoral region
Crus (anterior leg)	Crural region
Sura (calf)	Sural region
Pes (foot)	Pedal region
Planta (sole)	Plantar region

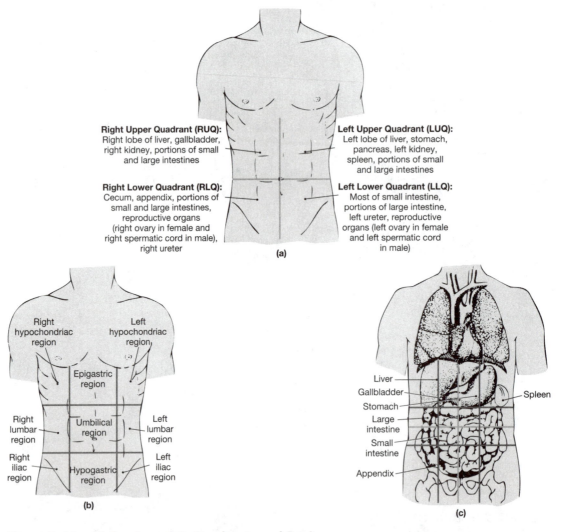

Right Upper Quadrant (RUQ):
Right lobe of liver, gallbladder, right kidney, portions of small and large intestines

Left Upper Quadrant (LUQ):
Left lobe of liver, stomach, pancreas, left kidney, spleen, portions of small and large intestines

Right Lower Quadrant (RLQ):
Cecum, appendix, portions of small and large intestines, reproductive organs (right ovary in female and right spermatic cord in male), right ureter

Left Lower Quadrant (LLQ):
Most of small intestine, portions of large intestine, left ureter, reproductive organs (left ovary in female and left spermatic cord in male)

(a)

Right hypochondriac region

Left hypochondriac region

Epigastric region

Right lumbar region

Umbilical region

Left lumbar region

Right iliac region

Hypogastric region

Left iliac region

(b)

Liver
Gallbladder
Stomach
Large intestine
Small intestine
Appendix
Spleen

(c)

Figure 1–10   Abdominopelvic Quadrants and Regions.

(a) Abdominopelvic quadrants divide the area into four sections. These terms, or their abbreviations, are most often used in clinical discussions. **(b)** More-precise regional descriptions are provided by reference to the appropriate abdominopelvic region. **(c)** Quadrants or regions are useful because there is a known relationship between superficial anatomical landmarks and underlying organs.

Table 1–3 Directional Terms (*see Figure 1–11*)

Term	Region or Reference	Example
Anterior	The front; before	The navel is on the *anterior* surface of the trunk.
Ventral	The belly side (equivalent to anterior when referring to human body)	In humans, the navel is on the *ventral* surface.
Posterior	The back; behind	The shoulder blade is located *posterior* to the rib cage.
Dorsal	The back (equivalent to posterior when referring to human body)	The *dorsal* body cavity encloses the brain and spinal cord.
Cranial or cephalic	The head	The *cranial*, or *cephalic*, border of the pelvis is on the side toward the head rather than toward the foot.
Superior	Above; at a higher level (in human body, toward the head)	In humans, the cranial border of the pelvis is superior to the thigh.
Caudal	The tail (coccyx in humans)	The hips are *caudal* to the waist.
Inferior	Below; at a lower level	The knees are *inferior* to the hips.
Medial	Toward the body's longitudinal axis	The *medial* surfaces of the thighs may be in contact; moving medially from the arm across the chest brings you to the sternum.
Lateral	Away from the body's longitudinal axis	The thigh articulates with the *lateral* surface of the pelvis; moving laterally from the nose brings you to the eyes.
Proximal	Toward an attached base	The thigh is *proximal* to the foot; moving proximally from the wrist brings you to the elbow.
Distal	Away from an attached base	The fingers are *distal* to the wrist; moving distally the elbow brings you to the wrist.
Superficial	At, near, or relatively close to the body surface	The skin is *superficial* to underlying structures.
Deep	Farther from the body surface	The bone of the thigh is *deep* to the surrounding muscles.

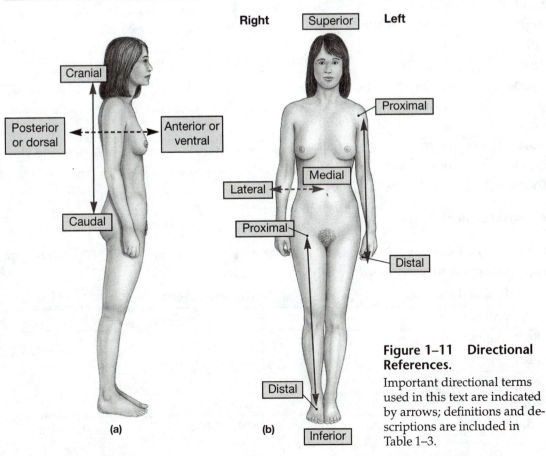

Figure 1–11 Directional References.

Important directional terms used in this text are indicated by arrows; definitions and descriptions are included in Table 1–3.

Let's Review What You've Just Learned

▶ **Definitions**

In the space provided, write the term for each of the following definitions.

_____   **62.** Movement away from the point of attachment or origin; for a limb away from the point of attachment to the trunk.

_____   **63.** Lying face up, with palms facing anteriorly.

_____   **64.** An anatomical reference position, the body viewed from the anterior surface with the palms facing forward.

_____   **65.** Toward the back; dorsal.

_____   **66.** Pertaining to the side.

▶ **Word Roots, Prefixes, Suffixes, and Combining Forms**

In the space provided, list the boldfaced terms introduced in this section that contain the indicated word part.

Word Part	Meaning	Examples
al-	pertaining to	**67.** _____
ante-	before	**68.** _____
brachi-	arm	**69.** _____
cephal-	head	**70.** _____
cervic-	neck	**71.** _____
crani-	skull	**72.** _____
cubit-	elbow	**73.** _____
digit-	a finger or toe	**74.** _____
epi-	on	**75.** _____
gastr-	stomach	**76.** _____
hypo-	under	**77.** _____
nas-	nose	**78.** _____
oculo-	eye	**79.** _____
post-	after	**80.** _____
quadr-	one quarter	**81.** _____
thorac-	chest	**82.** _____

▶ **Anatomical Parts**

Complete the following table by inserting either the common name or the proper name for each anatomical structure listed.

	Proper Term	Common Term
83.	pollex	
84.	manus	
85.		foot
86.	mentis	
87.		armpit
88.		sole of foot

	Proper Term	Common Term
89.		buttock
91.	calcaneus	
92.	oris	
93.		forearm
94.	popliteus	
95.	mamma	
96.		wrist
97.		back of elbow
98.	hallux	
99.	brachium	

▶ **Labeling Exercises**

Label the body regions indicated on the following diagram.

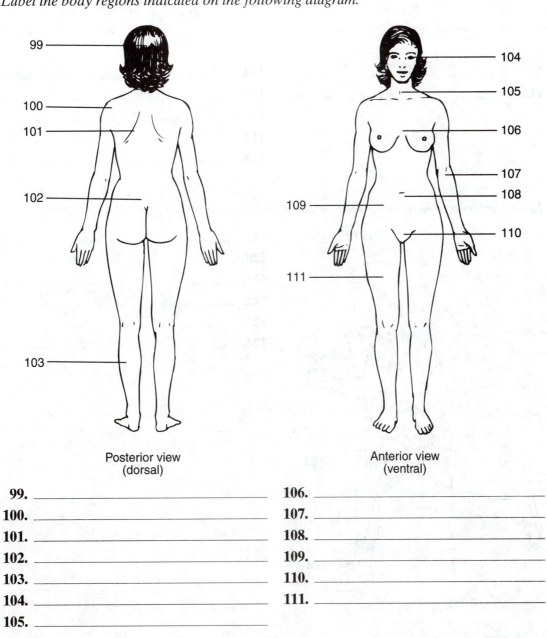

Posterior view
(dorsal)

Anterior view
(ventral)

  99. _____
 100. _____
 101. _____
 102. _____
 103. _____
 104. _____
 105. _____

 106. _____
 107. _____
 108. _____
 109. _____
 110. _____
 111. _____

Label the areas of the human body shown on the following diagram.

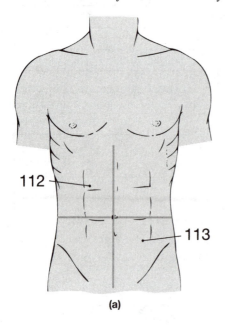

(a)

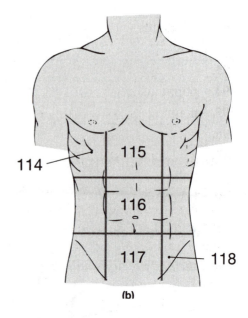

(b)

112. _____
113. _____

114. _____
115. _____
116. _____
117. _____
118. _____

Label the terms used to indicate orientation and direction on the following diagram.

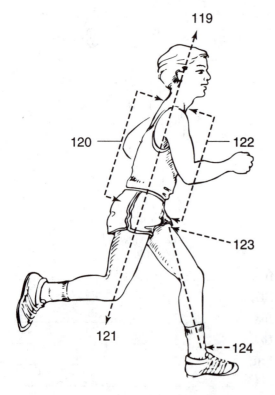

119. _____
120. _____
121. _____
122. _____
123. _____
124. _____

THE BODY IN SECTIONS

Sometimes the best way to show the relationships among the parts of a three-dimensional object, such as the human body, is to show the object in sectional view (i.e. to show the object as several pieces). An ability to understand and interpret sectional views of the human body has become increasingly important since the development of electronic imaging techniques, such as X-rays and CT scans, that allow us to see inside the living body without resorting to surgery.

Planes and Sections

Any slice through a three-dimensional object can be described with reference to the three sectional planes, indicated in Table 1–4, and Figure 1–12. The **transverse plane** lies at right angles to the long axis of the body and divides it into superior and inferior sections. A cut in this plane is called a **transverse section**, or **cross section**. The **frontal**, or **coronal**, **plane** and the **sagittal plane** are parallel to the long axis of the body. The frontal plane extends from side to side, dividing the body into anterior and posterior sections. The sagittal plane is one that divides the body into right and left sides. There is only one sagittal plane that divides the body into exactly equal left and right sections and that is called the **midsagittal plane**. Any other sagittal plane is referred to as a **parasagittal plane**.

Sometimes it is helpful to compare the information provided by sections made along different planes. You can experiment with this procedure by mentally sectioning this book as in Figure 1–13a. (Performing this experiment is not recommended unless you

Table 1–4 Terms That Indicate Planes of Section (see Figure 1–12)

Orientation of Plane	Plane	Directional Reference	Description
Perpendicular to long axis	Transverse or horizontal	Transversely or horizontally	A *transverse*, or *horizontal*, *section* separates superior and inferior portions of the body.
Parallel to long axis	Sagittal	Sagittally	A *sagittal section* separates right and left portions. You examine a sagittal section, but you section sagittally.
	Midsagittal		In a *midsagittal section* the plane passes through the midline, dividing the body in half and separating right and left sides.
	Parasagittal		A *parasagittal section* misses the midline, separating right and left portions of unequal size.
	Frontal or coronal	Frontally or coronally	A *frontal*, or *coronal*, *section* separates anterior and posterior portions of the body; coronal usually refers to sections passing through the skull.

Figure 1–12   Planes of Section.

The three primary planes of section are indicated here. Table 1–4 defines and describes them.

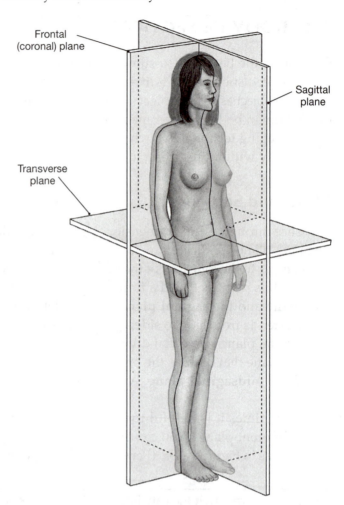

Frontal (coronal) plane

Sagittal plane

Transverse plane

are willing to buy another copy of the book.) Each sectional plane provides a different perspective on the structure of the book; when combined with observations of the external structure, they create a reasonably complete picture.

Obtaining a more accurate and detailed picture would entail choosing one sectional plane and making a series of sections at small intervals. This process, called **serial reconstruction**, permits the analysis of relatively complex structures. Figure 1–13b shows

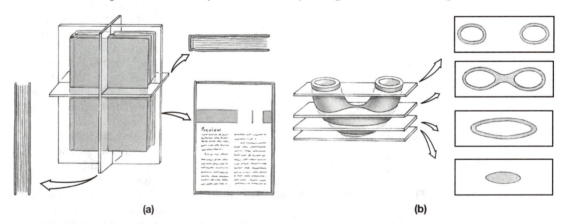

(a)   (b)

Figure 1–13   Sectional Planes and Visualization.

(a) Taking three different sections through a book provide detailed information about its three-dimensional structure. **(b)** More-complete pictures can be assembled by taking a series of sections at small intervals. This process is called serial reconstruction.

the serial reconstruction of a simple bent tube. The same procedure could be used to visualize the path of a small blood vessel or to follow a loop of the intestine. Serial reconstruction is an important method for studying tissue structure and for analyzing the images produced by sophisticated clinical procedures.

Body Cavities

The human body is not a solid object, as a rock, in which all of the parts are fused together. Many vital organs, collectively called **viscera** (VIS-e-ra; Latin *viscus*, internal organ), are suspended in internal chambers called **body cavities**. These cavities have two essential functions: (1) They protect delicate organs, such as the brain and spinal cord, from accidental shocks and cushion them from the bumps that occur during walking, jumping, and running; and (2) they permit significant changes in the size and shape of visceral (VIS-uh-rul) organs. Because they are situated within body cavities, the lungs, heart, stomach, intestines, urinary bladder, and many other organs can expand and contract without distorting surrounding tissues and disrupting the activities of nearby organs.

A **dorsal body cavity** surrounds the brain and spinal cord, and a much larger **ventral body cavity**, or **coelom** (SĒ-lom; Greek *koila*, cavity), surrounds organs of the respiratory, cardiovascular, digestive, urinary, and reproductive systems. Relationships between the dorsal and ventral cavities and their various subdivisions are indicated in Figure 1–14 and are shown in Figure 1–15.

- **Dorsal body cavity:** The dorsal body cavity is a fluid-filled space whose limits are established by the **cranium**, the bones of the skull that surround the brain, and the vertebrae, the bones that surround the spinal cord. The dorsal body cavity is subdivided into the **cranial cavity**, which encloses the brain, and the **spinal cavity**, which surrounds the spinal cord.

- **Ventral body cavity:** As development proceeds, internal organs grow and change their relative positions. These changes lead to the subdivision of the ventral body cavity. The **diaphragm** (DĪ-uh-fram; Greek *diaphragma*, a sheet), a flat muscular sheet,

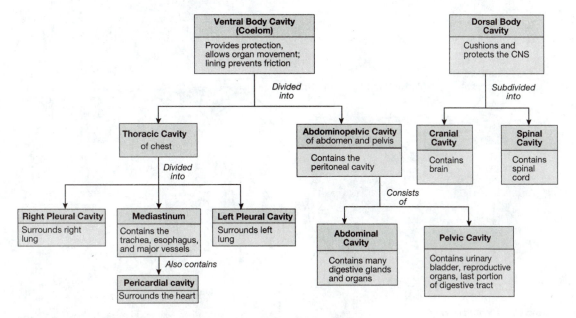

Figure 1–14   Relationships of the Various Body Cavities.

POSTERIOR   ANTERIOR

Figure 1–15   Body Cavities.

(a) The dorsal body cavity is bounded by the bones of the skull and vertebral column. The muscular diaphragm divides the ventral body cavity into a superior thoracic (chest) cavity and an inferior abdominopelvic cavity. The pericardial cavity is located inside the chest cavity. **(b)** The heart is suspended within the pericardial cavity like a fist pushed into a balloon. The attachment site, corresponding to the wrist of the hand in the model, lies at the connection between the heart and major blood vessels. **(c)** Anterior and sectional views of the ventral body cavity, showing the central location of the pericardial cavity within the chest cavity. The sectional plane shows how the mediastinum divides the thoracic cavity into two pleural cavities.

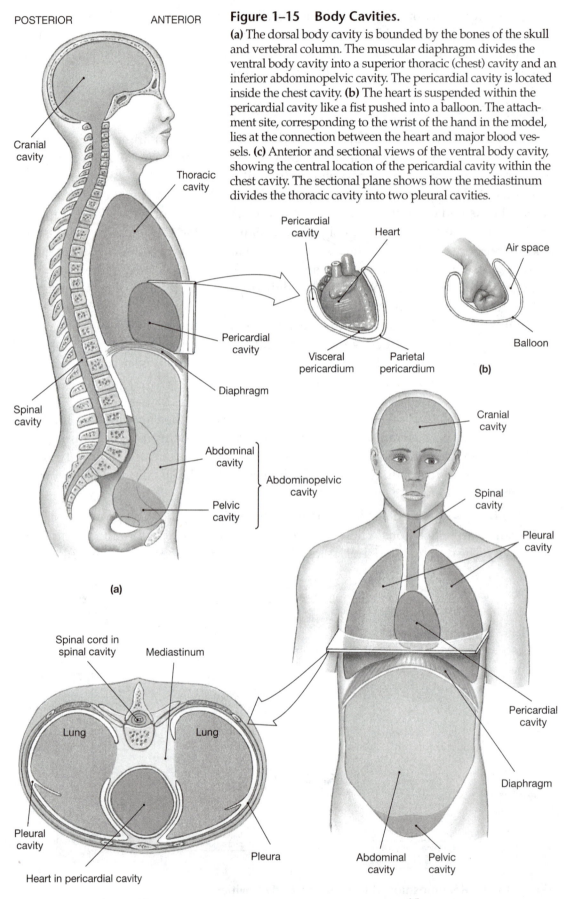

Cranial cavity

Thoracic cavity

Pericardial cavity

Diaphragm

Spinal cavity

Abdominal cavity

Abdominopelvic cavity

Pelvic cavity

(a)

Pericardial cavity   Heart

Air space

Visceral pericardium   Parietal pericardium   **(b)**   Balloon

Cranial cavity

Spinal cavity

Pleural cavity

Pericardial cavity

Diaphragm

Abdominal cavity   Pelvic cavity

(d)

Spinal cord in spinal cavity   Mediastinum

Lung   Lung

Pleural cavity

Heart in pericardial cavity

Pleura

(c)

divides the ventral body cavity into a superior **thoracic cavity**, enclosed by the chest wall, and an inferior **abdominopelvic cavity**, enclosed by the abdomen and pelvis. Many of the organs within these cavities change size and shape as they perform their functions. The stomach swells at each meal, and the heart contracts and expands with each beat. Organs such as these project into moist internal spaces that permit expansion and limited movement but prevent friction. There are three of these spaces (chambers) in the thoracic cavity and one in the abdominopelvic cavity.

The Thoracic Cavity

The walls of the thoracic cavity surround the lungs and heart and organs associated with the respiratory, cardiovascular, and lymphatic systems. The inferior portions of the esophagus and the thymus gland are also located here. The thoracic cavity contains three internal chambers; a single **pericardial cavity** (per-i-KAR-dē-al; Greek *perikardios*, around the heart) and a pair of **pleural cavities** (PLOO-ral; Greek *pleura*, rib). Each of these cavities is lined by a shiny, delicate membrane with a slippery surface. The lining of the pericardial cavity is called the **pericardium** (per-i-KAR-dē-um), and each lung is lined by its own **pleura** (PLOO-ra; plural *pleurae* or *pleuras*).

The heart is located in the pericardial cavity. The relationship between the heart and the cavity resembles that of a fist pushing into a balloon (Figure 1–15b). The wrist corresponds to the base (superior portion) of the heart, and the balloon corresponds to the pericardium. During each beat, the heart changes in size and shape. The pericardial cavity permits these changes, and the slippery lining of the cavity (the pericardium) prevents friction between the heart and neighboring structures.

The pericardial cavity lies within the **mediastinum** (mē-dē-as-TĪ-num, or mē-dē-AS-ti-num; Latin *mediastinum*, middle of the chest). The mediastinum is the portion of the thoracic cavity that lies between the left and right pleural cavities (Figure 1–15c). The connective tissue of the mediastinum surrounds the pericardial cavity and heart, the large arteries and veins attached to the heart, the thymus gland, trachea, and esophagus.

The thoracic cavity contains two pleural cavities. Each pleural cavity contains a lung, and the relationship between a lung and its pleural cavity is the same as that between the heart and the pericardial cavity.

The Abdominopelvic Cavity

The abdominopelvic cavity can be divided into a superior abdominal cavity and an inferior pelvic cavity (Figure 1-15d):

- **The abdominal cavity:** The **abdominal cavity** extends from the inferior surface of the diaphragm to an imaginary plane extending from the inferior surface of the lowest spinal vertebra to the anterior and superior margin of the pelvic girdle. The abdominal cavity contains the liver, stomach, spleen, kidneys, pancreas, small intestine, and most of the large intestine. The positions of these organs can be seen in Figure 1–10c. Many of these organs are partially or completely covered by a membrane known as the **peritoneum** (per-i-tō-NĒ-um; Greek *peritonaion*, to stretch around), much as the heart or lungs are covered by the pericardial or pleural membranes.

- **The pelvic cavity:** The portion of the ventral body cavity inferior to the abdominal cavity is the pelvic cavity. The pelvic cavity is enclosed by the bones of the pelvis and contains the last segments of the large intestine, the urinary bladder, and various reproductive organs. The pelvic cavity of a female contains the *ovaries, uterine tubes,* and *uterus;* in a male, it contains the *prostate gland* and the *seminal vesicles.*

VISUALIZING ANATOMICAL STRUCTURES

In this chapter you learned the locations of some of the major components of each organ system. You were also introduced to the anatomical vocabulary you will need to follow the more detailed anatomical descriptions you will encounter in other coursework. Figures 1–16 and 1–17 summarize some modern methods that are used to visualize anatomical structures in living individuals. Some of the figures in later chapters contain images produced by the procedures outlined in these figures.

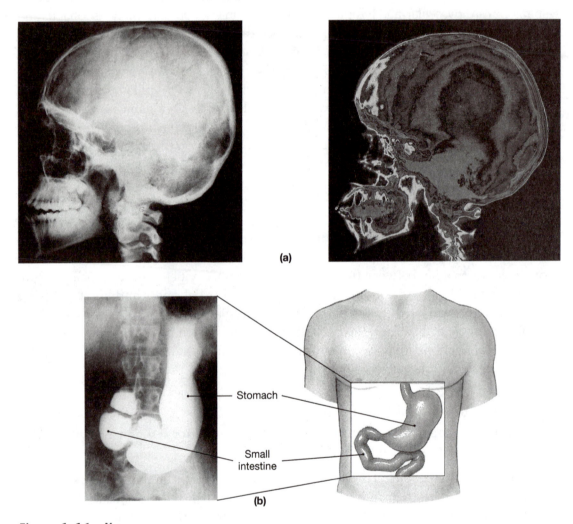

(a)

Stomach

Small intestine

(b)

Figure 1–16   X-rays.

(a) X-rays of the skull, taken from the left side. **X-rays** are a form of high-energy radiation that can penetrate living tissues. In the most familiar procedure, a beam of X-rays travels through the body and strikes a photographic plate. All the projected X-rays do not arrive at the film; some are absorbed or deflected as they pass through the body. The resistance to X-ray penetration is called **radiodensity**. In the human body, the order of increasing radiodensity is as follows: air, fat, liver, blood, muscle, bone. The result is an image with radiodense tissues, such as bone, appearing in white, and less-dense tissues in shades of gray to black. (The image on the right has been comupter-enhanced.) These are two-dimensional images of a three-dimensional object. In such an image it is difficult to decide whether a particular feature is on the left side (toward the viewer) or on the right side (away from the viewer). **(b)** A barium-contrast X-ray of the upper digestive tract. Barium is very dense, and the contours of the gastric and intestinal lining can be seen outlined against the white of the barium solution.

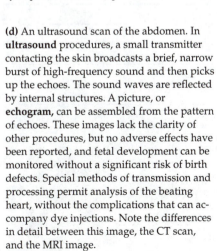

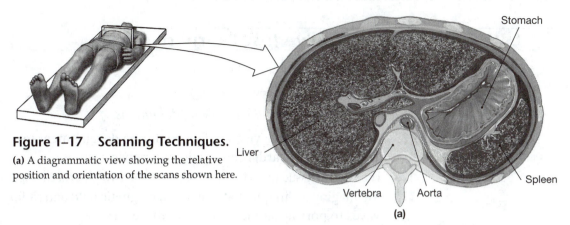

Figure 1–17   Scanning Techniques.

(a) A diagrammatic view showing the relative position and orientation of the scans shown here.

Stomach

Liver

Vertebra   Aorta

Spleen

(a)

(b) A CT scan of the abdomen. **CT** (computerized tomography), formerly called **CAT** (computerized axial tomography), uses computers to reconstruct sectional views. A single X-ray source rotates around the body, and the X-ray beam strikes a sensor monitored by the computer. The source completes one revolution around the body every few seconds; it then moves a short distance and repeats the process. The result is usually displayed as a sectional view in black and white, but it can be colorized for visual effect. CT scans show three-dimensional relationships and soft-tissue structure more clearly than do standard X-rays.

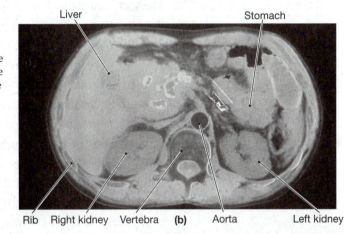

Liver

Stomach

Rib   Right kidney   Vertebra   **(b)**   Aorta   Left kidney

(c) An MRI scan of the same region. **Magnetic resonance imaging (MRI)** surrounds part or all of the body with a magnetic field about 3000 times as strong as that of Earth. This field affects protons within atomic nuclei throughout the body. The protons line up along the magnetic lines of force like compass needles in Earth's magnetic field. When struck by a radio wave of the proper frequency, a proton will absorb energy. When the wave pulse ends, that energy is released, and the source of the radiation is detected. Each element differs in terms of the radio frequency required to affect its protons.

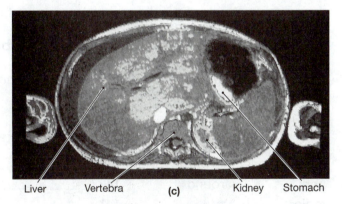

Liver   Vertebra   **(c)**   Kidney   Stomach

(d) An ultrasound scan of the abdomen. In **ultrasound** procedures, a small transmitter contacting the skin broadcasts a brief, narrow burst of high-frequency sound and then picks up the echoes. The sound waves are reflected by internal structures. A picture, or **echogram,** can be assembled from the pattern of echoes. These images lack the clarity of other procedures, but no adverse effects have been reported, and fetal development can be monitored without a significant risk of birth defects. Special methods of transmission and processing permit analysis of the beating heart, without the complications that can accompany dye injections. Note the differences in detail between this image, the CT scan, and the MRI image.

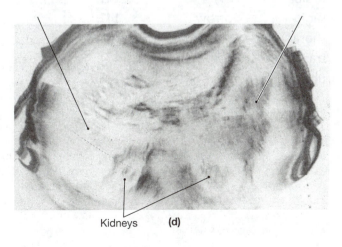

Kidneys   **(d)**

Let's Review What You've Just Learned

► **Definitions**

In the space provided, write the term for each of the following definitions.

_____ **125.** The ventral body cavity subdivided during development into the pleural, pericardial, and abdominopelvic cavities.

_____ **126.** The central tissue mass that lies between the two pleural cavities.

_____ **127.** An imaging technique that employs a magnetic field and radio waves to portray subtle structural differences.

_____ **128.** The sectional plane that divides the body into right and left portions.

_____ **129.** A collective term for organs in the ventral body cavity.

_____ **130.** A collective term for the skull bones that surround the brain.

_____ **131.** A sectional plane that divides the body into anterior and posterior portions.

_____ **132.** An image created by ultrasound.

_____ **133.** The inferior subdivision of the abdominopelvic cavity.

_____ **134.** Subdivisions of the thoracic cavity that contain the lungs.

_____ **135.** An imaging technique that uses brief bursts of high-frequency sound reflected by internal structures.

_____ **136.** Any muscular partition; often used to refer to the muscle that separates the thoracic from the abdominopelvic cavity.

_____ **137.** An imaging technique that reconstructs the three-dimensional structure of the body.

► **Word Roots, Prefixes, Suffixes, and Combining Forms**

In the space provided, list the boldfaced terms introduced in this section that contain the indicated word part.

Word Part	Meaning		Examples
cranio-	skull	**138.**	_____
para-	beyond	**139.**	_____
peri-	around	**140.**	_____
radio-	ray	**141.**	_____
sagit-	arrow	**142.**	_____
thorac-	chest	**143.**	_____
trans-	through, across	**144.**	_____
ultra-	beyond	**145.**	_____

► Labeling Exercises

Label the planes of the body indicated in the following diagram.

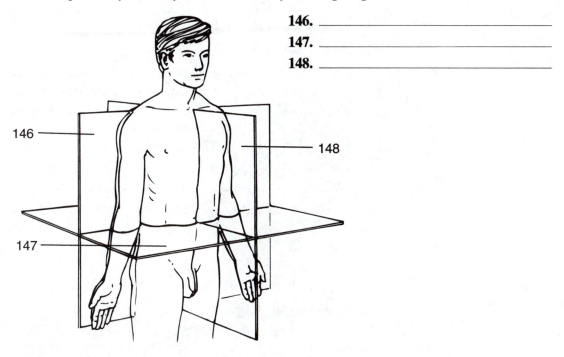

146. _____

147. _____

148. _____

Label the body cavities shown in the following diagram.

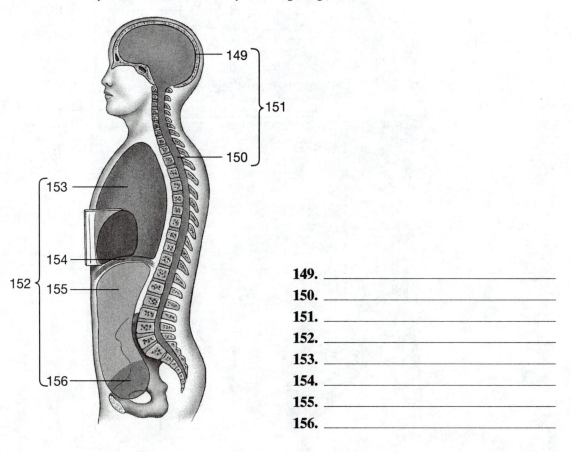

149. _____

150. _____

151. _____

152. _____

153. _____

154. _____

155. _____

156. _____

Label the body cavities shown in the following diagram.

157. _____

158. _____

159. _____

160. _____

161. _____

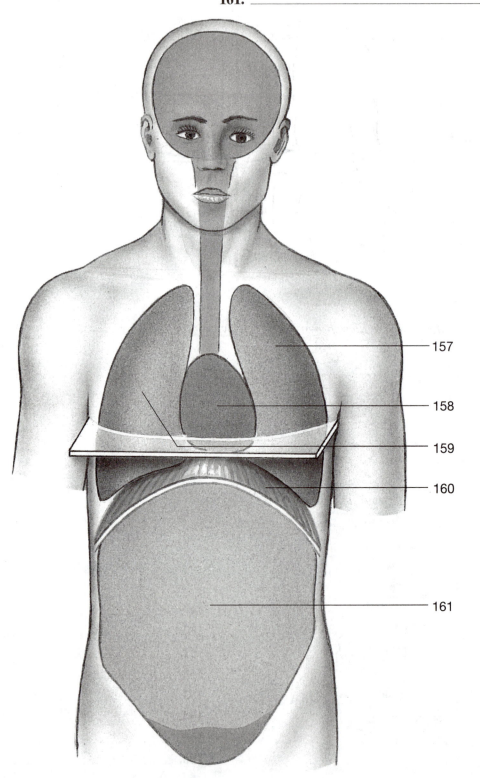

► Concept Mapping

Using the following terms, fill in the blank spaces next to the circled numbers to complete the concept map. Follow the numbers that comply with the organization of the concept map.

Pelvic cavity   Spinal cord
Cranial cavity   Heart
Abdominopelvic cavity   Two pleural cavities

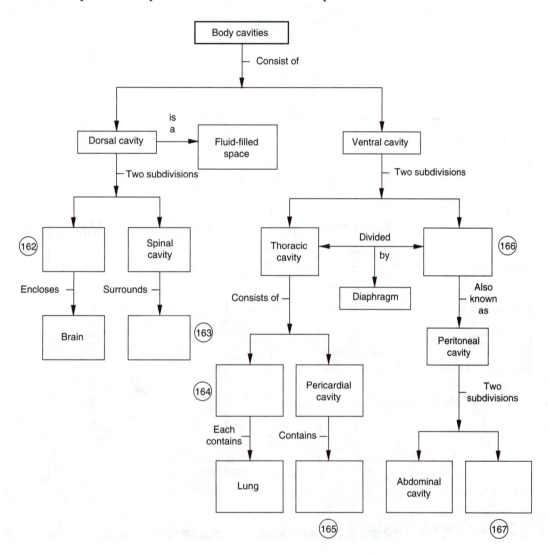

Using the following terms, fill in the blank spaces next to the circled numbers to complete the concept map. Follow the numbers to comply with the organization of the map.

Angiogram   High-energy radiation
CT scans   Echogram
Radio waves   Radiologist

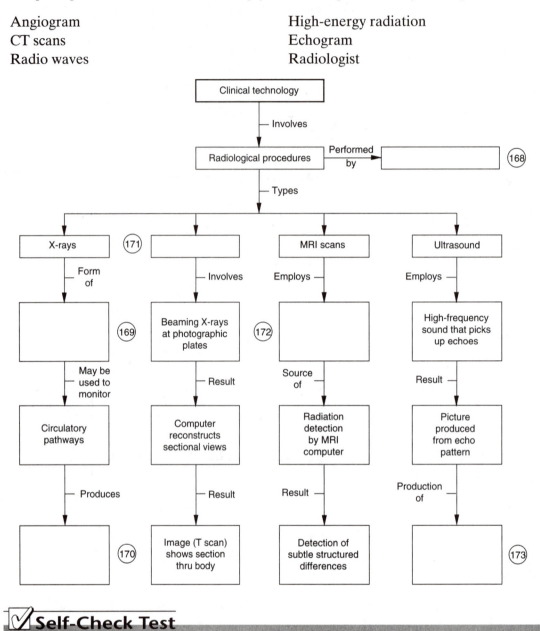

☑ Self-Check Test

The following test will allow you to determine how well you have mastered the vocabulary and basic concepts of this chapter. It will also help you prepare for the type of questions you are likely to encounter on a test in an anatomy and physiology course. The self-check test will help you assess your understanding of the chapter material, and will help you develop good test-taking skills. The following questions test your ability to use vocabulary and to recall facts.

1. The study of the structure of individual cells is called
  a. cytology
  b. histology
  c. embryology
  d. physiology
  e. anatomy

2. The study of early developmental processes is termed

   a. histology

   b. embryology

   c. cytology

   d. pathology

   e. organology

3. The branch of physiology that deals with the changes in function that result from disease is called

   a. histophysiology

   b. special physiology

   c. system physiology

   d. pathophysiology

   e. physiological chemistry

4. The following is a list of several levels of organization that make up the human body

   1. tissue

   2. cell

   3. organ

   4. molecule

   5. organism

   6. organ system

   The correct order from the simplest to the most complex level is

   a. 2,4,1,3,6,5

   b. 4,2,1,3,6,5

   c. 4,2,1,6,3,5

   d. 4,2,3,1,6,5

   e. 2,1,4,3,5,6

5. Support, protection of soft tissue, mineral storage, and blood formation are functions of which system?

   a. integumentary

   b. muscular

   c. skeletal

   d. nervous

   e. circulatory

6. Skin, hair, and nails are associated with the

   a. skeletal system

   b. muscular system

   c. integumentary system

   d. endocrine system

   e. nervous system

7. When body temperature rises, a center in the brain initiates physiological changes to decrease the body temperature. This is an example of

   a. negative feedback

   b. positive feedback

   c. nonhomeostatic regulation

   d. diagnostic regulation

   e. disease

8. A woman who is facing forward with hands at her sides and palms facing forward is said to be in the
   a. supine position
   b. prone position
   c. anatomical position
   d. frontal position
   e. sagittal position
9. Which of the following terms refers to the front of the body?
   a. anterior
   b. posterior
   c. superior
   d. inferior
   e. dorsal
10. Which of the following structures is lateral to the nose?
    a. eye
    b. forehead
    c. scalp
    d. chin
    e. chest
11. The wrist is considered _____ to the elbow.
    a. proximal
    b. distal
    c. lateral
    d. medial
    e. superior
12. Which of the following regions corresponds to the lower back?
    a. pelvic
    b. cephalic
    c. gluteal
    d. lumbar
    e. thoracic
13. A cut through the body that passes parallel to the long axis of the body and divides the body into equal left and right halves is known as a
    a. frontal section
    b. coronal section
    c. transverse section
    d. midsagittal section
    e. parasagittal section
14. The cranial cavity and spinal cavity are found in the
    a. dorsal body cavity
    b. pericardial cavity
    c. peritoneal cavity
    d. ventral body cavity
    e. abdominopelvic cavity
15. The thoracic cavity contains the
    a. coelom
    b. pericardial cavity
    c. pelvic cavity
    d. cranium
    e. all of the above

16. The muscle known as the diaphragm separates the _____ from the _____.
  a. pleural cavity; mediastinum
  b. thoracic cavity; pelvic cavity
  c. pericardial cavity; pleural cavity
  d. abdominal cavity; pelvic cavity
  e. thoracic cavity; abdominopelvic cavity
17. Mary, who is 6 months pregnant, goes to her physician for a test to check the development of her fetus. The physician uses a device that employs sound waves to produce an image of the fetus. The technique is known as
  a. X-ray
  b. CT
  c. MRI
  d. ultrasound
  e. radiography

The following questions are more challenging and require you to synthesize the information that you have learned in this chapter.

 18. Which sectional plane could divide the body so that the face remains intact?
  a. sagittal plane
  b. coronal plane
  c. equatorial plane
  d. midsagittal plane
  e. none of the above
 19. A chemical imbalance in a heart muscle cell can cause the heart to cease pumping blood; cessation of the heart's pumping action will, in turn, cause other tissues and organs to cease functioning. This observation supports the view that
  a. all organisms are composed of cells
  b. all levels of organization within an organism are interdependent
  c. chemical molecules make up cells
  d. all cells are independent of each other
  e. birth defects can be life-threatening
 20. Each of the following is an example of negative feedback except one. Identify the exception.
  a. Increased blood pressure in the aorta triggers mechanisms to lower blood pressure.
  b. A rise in estrogens during the menstrual cycle increases the number of progesterone receptors in the uterus.
  c. A rise in blood calcium levels triggers the release of a hormone that lowers blood calcium levels.
  d. Increased blood sugar stimulates the release of a hormone from the pancreas that stimulates the liver to store blood sugar.
  e. A decrease in body temperature triggers a neural response that initiates physiological changes to increase body temperature.

☑ Self-Assessment

If your score was

between 18 and 20, you are ready to proceed to the next chapter.

between 15 and 17, you have a good general idea of the chapter content, but you should review sections of the chapter that deal with items that you missed before proceeding to the next chapter.

less than 14, you have not mastered the chapter content well enough to proceed. Reread the chapter and rework the exercises. Then retake the self check test. Repeat this process until you achieve a score that will allow you to continue.

Answers

1. cytology
2. embryology
3. anatomy
4. histology
5. physiology
6. tissue
7. metabolism
8. organs
9. physiology, embryology, cytology, etc.
10. anatomy
11. histology
12. physiology
13. pathophysiology
14. anatomy
15. cytology
16. embryology
17. macroscopic anatomy
18. regional anatomy
19. structure of organ systems
20. surgical anatomy
21. embryology
22. cytology
23. tissues
24. functions of anatomical structures
25. functions of living cells
26. histophysiology
27. specific organ systems
28. pathophysiology
29. body function response to changes in atmospheric pressure
30. exercise physiology
31. body function response to athletics
32. organelle
33. atom
34. molecule
35. c, d, a, e, b
36. urinary system
37. endocrine system
38. lymphatic system
39. muscular system
40. digestive system
41. digestive system
42. hair follicles
43. carrying blood from heart to capillaries
44. bone marrow
45. urinary system
46. uterus
47. thyroid gland
48. protect opening to the trachea; vocal cords
49. brain
50. lymphatic system
51. positive feedback
52. hormone
53. disease
54. thermoregulation
55. homeostasis
56. oxytocin
57. autoregulation
58. negative feedback
59. negative feedback
60. negative feedback
61. positive feedback
62. distal
63. supine
64. anatomical position
65. posterior
66. lateral
67. ventral, distal, lateral, etc.
68. anterior
69. brachium
70. cephalic
71. cervicis
72. cranium
73. antecubitus
74. digits
75. epigastric
76. hypogastric
77. hypogastric
78. nasus
79. ocular
80. posterior
81. quadrant
82. thoracis
83. thumb
84. hand
85. pes

86. chin
87. axilla
88. plantus
89. gluteus
90. heel
91. mouth
92. antebrachium
93. back of knee
94. breast
95. carpus
96. olecranon
97. great toe
98. arm
99. head
100. shoulder
101. dorsum
102. loin
103. calf
104. eye
105. cervicis
106. thoracis
107. antecubitus
108. umbilicus
109. pelvis
110. pubis
111. thigh
112. right upper quadrant
113. left lower quadrant
114. right hypochondriac region
115. epigastric region
116. umbilical region
117. hypogastric region
118. left iliac region
119. superior (cephalad)
120. posterior (dorsal)
121. inferior (caudal)
122. anterior (ventral)
123. proximal
124. distal
125. coelom
126. mediastinum
127. MRI
128. sagittal plane
129. viscera
130. cranium
131. frontal or coronal plane

132. echogram
133. pelvic cavity
134. pleural cavities
135. ultrasound
136. diaphragm
137. CT, or CAT, scan
138. cranium
139. parasaggital
140. pericardium
141. radiologist, radiological
142. sagittal
143. thoracic
144. transverse
145. ultrasound
146. frontal or coronal plane
147. transverse plane
148. midsaggital plane
149. cranial cavity
150. spinal cavity
151. dorsal cavity
152. ventral cavity
153. thoracic cavity
154. diaphragm
155. abdominal cavity
156. pelvic cavity
157. left thoracic cavity
158. pericardial cavity
159. right thoracic cavity
160. diaphragm
161. abdominal cavity
162. cranial cavity
163. spinal cord
164. two pleural cavities
165. heart
166. abdominopelvic cavity
167. pelvic cavity
168. radiologist
169. high-energy radiation
170. angiogram
171. CT scans
172. radio waves
173. echogram

Answers to Self-Check Test

1. a 2. b 3. d 4. b 5. c 6. c 7. a 8. c 9. a 10. a 11. b 12. d
13. d 14. a 15. b 16. e 17. d 18. b 19. b 20. b

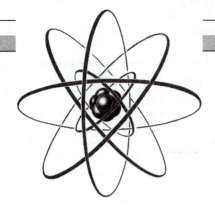

CHAPTER 2

An Introduction to Chemistry

Air, elephants, oranges, oceans, rocks, and people are all composed of various combinations of basic units of matter called **atoms.** The unique characteristics of each object, living or nonliving, result from the types of atoms that make them up and the ways those atoms combine and interact. **Chemistry** is the branch of science that *deals with atoms and their interactions.* To be successful in your study of anatomy and physiology you will need to know some basic chemistry. In this chapter we will examine the chemical principles and concepts that are needed to understand the anatomy and physiology of the cells, tissues, organs, and organ systems of the human body.

UNITS OF MEASUREMENT

Before we begin a study of chemistry, you need to become familiar with the different units that are used when making scientific measurements. Units are an important part of any measurement. For example, to say that an organ has a length of three or a mass of five has no meaning unless some unit such as centimeter (a unit of length) or kilogram (a unit of mass) is added. The system of measurement used in all of the sciences, including anatomy and physiology, is a metric-based system. Since 1960 the *International System of Units,* or *SI units* (from the French le Système International d'Unités), a modified version of the older metric system, has been in use in science. Table 2–1 lists some of the common base units of the SI system. During the course of your studies in anatomy and physiology, you will encounter many if not all of these units.

Table 2–1 Common SI Base Units

Physical Quantity	Name of Unit	Symbol
Mass	Gram	g
Length	Meter	m
Volume	Liter	L or l
Time	Second	s
Temperature	Kelvin	K
Amount of substance	Mole	mol

Table 2–2 Common SI Prefixes		
Factor	Prefix	Symbol
10^{-12}	Pico-	p
10^{-9}	Nano-	n
10^{-6}	Micro-	μ
10^{-3}	Milli-	m
10^{-2}	Centi-	c
10^{-1}	Deci-	d
10^{3}	Kilo-	k

Frequently the SI base units are not of a convenient size for a particular measurement. In these cases the base unit is modified by some factor of 10, and prefixes are used to indicate the order of magnitude. For instance 1/100 of a unit is indicated by the prefix **centi-** (Latin *centum*, 100) as in *centimeter* (1/100 of a meter), and the prefix **kilo-** (Greek *chilioi*, 1000) indicates 1000 times the base unit, as in *kilogram*. Table 2–2 lists some common SI prefixes, and Table 2–3 gives some examples of how the prefixes are used to indicate size relative to the SI base units.

In anatomy and physiology, we regularly measure mass, length, volume, and temperature. The units that we generally use to express these are **gram** (g), **meter** (m), **liter** (L or l), and **degree Celsius** (°C), respectively. The liter, the base unit of volume in the SI system, is defined as exactly 1000 cubic centimeters (cm^3 or cc). Since there are 1000 **milliliters** (ml) in 1 liter, the size of a milliliter and a cubic centimeter are the same; they are identical. The cubic centimeter, or cc, is frequently used in medical practice instead of the milliliter. The SI unit for temperature is a **Kelvin.** One unit on the Kelvin scale is equal to one degree on the Celsius scale. The difference between the two scales is the zero point. On the Celsius scale, zero is the freezing point of water, whereas on the Kelvin scale, the zero point is absolute zero (–273.15°C, a theoretical point at which molecular

Table 2–3 Modifying the Size of SI Units with Prefixes			
Prefix	Multiplication Factor	Examples	Symbol
Pico-	1/1,000,000,000,000 (10^{-12})	1 picometer = 0.000 000 000 001 meter (10^{-12}m)	pm
		1 picogram = 0.000 000 000 001 gram (10^{-12}g)	pg
Nano-	1/1,000,000,000 (10^{-9})	1 nanometer = 0.000 000 001 meter (10^{-9} m)	nm
		1 nanogram = 0.000 000 001 gram (10^{-9} g)	ng
Micro-	1/1,000,000 (10^{-6})	1 micrometer = 0.000 001 meter (10^{-6} m)	μm
		1 microgram = 0.000 001 gram (10^{-6} g)	μg
Milli-	1/1,000 (10^{-3})	1 millimeter = 0.001 meter (10^{-3} m)	mm
		1 millisecond = 0.001 second (10^{-3} s)	ms
		1 milligram = 0.001 gram (10^{-3} g)	mg
Centi-	1/100 (10^{-2})	1 centimeter = 0.01 meter (10^{-2} m)	cm
Deci-	1/10 (10^{-1})	1 decimeter = 0.1 meter (10^{-1} m)	dm
Kilo-	1000 (10^{3})	1 kilometer = 1000 meter (10^{3} m)	km
		1 kilogram = 1000 gram (10^{3} g)	kg

motion would cease, there would be no heat, and gases would have a volume of zero). The Kelvin temperature scale is the only temperature scale where zero really means zero. The benefit of using the Kelvin temperature unit is that all temperatures will be positive numbers, a definite advantage in many calculations involving temperature. Although both the Kelvin and the Celsius degree units are used in physiology, you will encounter the Celsius degree in introductory A&P courses and in allied health professions.

Let's Review What You've Just Learned

In the space provided, give the proper SI unit for each of the following measurements.

_____ **1.** mass
_____ **2.** volume
_____ **3.** length
_____ **4.** amount of substance
_____ **5.** temperature

In the space provided, write the name for the unit that is being defined.

_____ **6.** 1/1000 of a liter
_____ **7.** 10^{-3} gram
_____ **8.** 1/100 meter
_____ **9.** 1000 grams
_____ **10.** 1/10 of a liter

In the space provided, identify each of the following units.

_____ **11.** millisecond
_____ **12.** microgram
_____ **13.** millimeter
_____ **14.** nanometer
_____ **15.** kiloliter

MATTER AND ELEMENTS

All things whether living or nonliving are composed of matter. **Matter** is defined as *anything that has mass and occupies space.* **Mass** is a measure of *the amount of matter* in an object. Frequently we use the term *weight* to mean mass, although the two are not really the same. The **weight** of an object is the *gravitational force* that acts on the object's mass. For instance, an astronaut in space has no weight but still has mass.

The basic building blocks of matter are **chemical elements,** substances that cannot be broken down into simpler substances by ordinary chemical processes. Only 92 elements occur in nature (although 17 more have been made by means of nuclear reactions in the laboratory). Each element is represented by a chemical symbol, an abbreviation recognized by scientists everywhere. Most of the symbols are easily connected with the

English names of the elements, such as H for hydrogen and O for oxygen. A few symbols, such as Na for sodium are abbreviations of their Latin names (Latin *natrium*, float on water). Figure 2–1 indicates the 13 most abundant elements in the human body and their relative contributions to the total body weight. This list is incomplete, for the human body contains another 13 elements that are found in such small amounts that their percentage values are meaningless.

Figure 2–1   Principal Elements in the Human Body.

(a) The percentages given are estimates of the contribution made by each elements to the total number of atoms in the body. Note that just four elements (C, H, O, and N) contribute over 99 percent to the total. Among the so-called trace elements present in quantities too small to show are silicon (Si), fluorine (F), copper (Cu), manganese (Mn), zinc (Zn), selenium (Se); cobalt (Co), molybdenum (Mo), cadmium (Cd), chromium (Cr), tin (Sn), aluminum (Al), and boron (B). The functions of some of these in the body are still poorly understood. (b) Representative functions of each major element in the body; the percentages indicate the contribution of each element to total body weight.

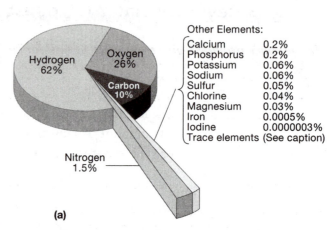

Other Elements:
Calcium	0.2%
Phosphorus	0.2%
Potassium	0.06%
Sodium	0.06%
Sulfur	0.05%
Chlorine	0.04%
Magnesium	0.03%
Iron	0.0005%
Iodine	0.0000003%
Trace elements (See caption)	

Hydrogen 62%
Oxygen 26%
Carbon 10%
Nitrogen 1.5%

(a)

Element (% of body weight)	Significance
Hydrogen (9.7)	A component of water and most other compounds in the body.
Oxygen (65)	A component of water and other compounds; oxygen gas essential for respiration.
Carbon (18.6)	Found in all organic molecules.
Nitrogen (3.2)	Found in proteins, nucleic acids, and other organic compounds.
Calcium (1.8)	Found in bones and teeth; important for membrane function, nerve impulses, muscle contraction, and blood clotting.
Phosphorus (1)	Found in bones and teeth, nucleic acids, and high-energy compounds.
Potassium (0.4)	Important for proper membrane function, nerve impulses, and muscle contraction.
Sodium (0.2)	Important for membrane function, nerve impulses, and muscle contraction.
Chlorine (0.2)	Important for membrane function and water absorption.
Magnesium (0.06)	A cofactor for several enzymes.
Sulfur (0.04)	Found in many proteins.
Iron (0.007)	Essential for oxygen transport and energy capture.
Iodine (0.0002)	A component of hormones of the thyroid gland.

(b)

ATOMS

Atoms (AT-umz; Greek *atomos*, indivisible) are the smallest portions of an element that exhibit the chemical characteristics of that element; no chemical change can alter their identities. Atoms are composed of tiny units of matter called **subatomic particles.** Although there are dozens of different subatomic particles, only three are important for understanding chemical properties. These three fundamental particles are *protons, neutrons,* and *electrons.*

Protons are relatively large particles that carry a positive (+) electrical charge. They are located in the center of the atom, a region called the **nucleus** (Figure 2–2a). The number of protons in an atom is known as its **atomic number.** Since all of the atoms of any given element have the same number of protons in their nucleus, they all have the same atomic number. The number of protons in the nucleus of an atom then identifies that atom as a specific element. For instance, atoms with one proton are hydrogen atoms (Figure 2–2b), and hydrogen atoms have an atomic number of one. Atoms with two protons are helium atoms, and helium has an atomic number of two. Oxygen has an atomic number of eight, which means each oxygen atom has eight protons in its nucleus.

Like planets orbiting the sun, electrons travel around the nucleus at various levels. **Electrons** are lighter than protons (only 1/1836th as massive) and they carry a negative (–) electrical charge. In an electrically neutral atom, there are equal numbers of protons and electrons. For example, in a neutral atom of sodium (atomic number 11) there are 11 protons and 11 electrons. Electrons are responsible for the chemical properties of an element.

Neutrons are similar to protons in size and mass, but neutrons are neutral—that is, uncharged. Neutrons add mass to atoms and are responsible for the different isotopes that exist. **Isotopes** of an element are atoms that contain different numbers of neutrons.

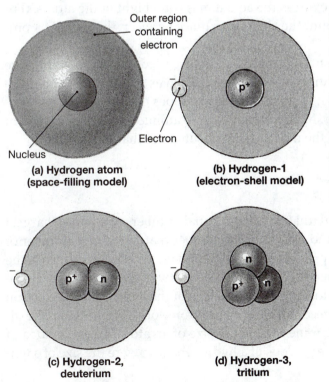

Outer region containing electron

Electron

Nucleus

(a) Hydrogen atom
(space-filling model)

(b) Hydrogen-1
(electron-shell model)

(c) Hydrogen-2,
deuterium

(d) Hydrogen-3,
tritium

Figure 2–2   Hydrogen Atoms.
(a) In a three-dimensional model, the zone surrounding the nucleus indicates the probable location of the electron orbiting the nucleus. **(b)** A two-dimensional model depicting the electron in a fixed location makes it easier to visualize the components of the atom and diagram the structure of the nucleus. A typical hydrogen nucleus contains a single proton and no neutrons. **(c)** A deuterium (^2H) nucleus contains a proton and a neutron. **(d)** A tritium (^3H) nucleus contains a pair of neutrons in addition to the proton.

When neutrons are present in an atom they are found in the nucleus together with the protons. Most hydrogen nuclei lack neutrons, but a small number of hydrogen nuclei and the nuclei of all other atoms contain neutrons. The number of neutrons present does not affect the properties of an atom, other than its mass. The number of neutrons in the nucleus can vary among the atoms of a single element. For example, although most hydrogen nuclei consist of a single proton, 0.015 percent also contain one neutron, and a very small percentage contain two. Because the presence or absence of neutrons has very little effect on the chemical properties of an atom, isotopes are usually indistinguishable except on the basis of mass. The **mass number**—the total number of protons and neutrons in the nucleus—is used to designate a particular isotope. Thus, the three isotopes of hydrogen are hydrogen-1, or ^{1}H; hydrogen-2, or ^{2}H (also known as deuterium); and hydrogen-3, or ^{3}H (also known as tritium) (Figure 2–2c, d).

Radioisotopes are isotopes with unstable nuclei that emit subatomic particles in measurable amounts. **Alpha particles** are generally released by the nuclei of large radioactive atoms, such as uranium. Each alpha particle consists of a helium nucleus: two protons and two neutrons. **Beta particles** are electrons, most often released by radioisotopes of lighter atoms. **Gamma rays** are very-high-energy electromagnetic waves comparable to the X-rays used in clinical diagnosis. The **half-life** of any radioactive isotope is the time required for a 50 percent reduction in the amount of radiation it emits. The half-lives of radioisotopes range from fractions of a second to thousands of years.

Atomic Weights

A typical atom of oxygen, which has an atomic number of 8, contains eight protons and eight neutrons. The mass number of this isotope is therefore 16. The mass numbers of other isotopes of oxygen will be different, depending on the number of neutrons present. Such mass numbers, however, simply tell us the number of subatomic particles in the nuclei of different atoms. They do not express the actual mass or weight of the atoms. (For example, they do not take into account the slight difference between the mass of a proton and that of a neutron.)

Because an individual atom is so small, special units are used to indicate its relative mass. This unit is the **atomic mass unit**, or **amu** (also known as a **dalton**.) When referring to the atomic mass of an element, which includes isotopes of differing mass numbers, the term **atomic weight** is used. In most instances, the atomic weight of an element is very close to the mass number of the most common isotope of that element.

Structure of the Atom

All atoms that are electrically neutral (that is, contain equal numbers of + and – charges) contain equal numbers of protons and electrons. Remember that the atomic number of an element indicates the number of protons in an atom of that element. Hydrogen is the simplest atom, with an atomic number of 1. A neutral atom of hydrogen contains one proton and one electron. The proton is located in the nucleus of the atom, and the electron whirls around the nucleus at high speed, forming an electron cloud (Figure 2–3). The dimensions of the electron cloud determine the overall size of an atom. To get an idea of the scale involved, consider that if the nucleus of a hydrogen atom were the size of a ten-

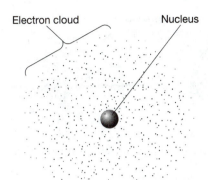

(a) Hydrogen atom

Figure 2–3   Structure of an Atom.
(a) A representation of a hydrogen atom. Electrons travel rapidly around the nucleus of an atom, forming electron clouds. **(b)** If the nucleus of a hydrogen atom were the size of a tennis ball, then the electron cloud surrounding the nucleus would have a radius of 6 miles.

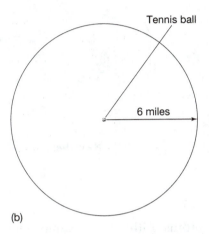

(b)

nis ball the electron cloud would have a radius of 6 miles! In reality, atoms are so small that atomic measurements are most conveniently reported in terms of **nanometers** (nm) (NA-nō-mē-terz, 0.000000001, or 10^{-9} meter). The very largest atoms approach 0.5 nm in diameter (0.0000005 cm, or 0.00000002 in.).

Electrons orbit the nucleus because of the electrical attraction between their negative charge and the positive charge on the protons. This attraction is an example of an *electrical force*. Ordinarily, atoms are electrically neutral because every positively charged proton is balanced by a negatively charged electron. Note that each increase in the atomic number (number of protons) is accompanied by a comparable increase in the number of electrons orbiting the nucleus.

For convenience, atomic structure is often illustrated in the simplified form shown in Figure 2–4. In this representation, the electrons are shown in circular paths around the nucleus, much like planets orbiting the sun. These paths form concentric rings that are referred to as **orbitals** or **electron shells.** It requires a certain amount of energy to hold an electron in position in a given orbit. Each orbital can be identified by the specific amount of energy associated with it, and the orbitals are frequently referred to as **energy levels.**

The number and arrangement of electrons in an atom's outermost energy level determine the chemical properties of that element. Each energy level can accommodate a specific number of electrons. For example, the innermost level can hold only two electrons. As indicated in Figure 2–4a, a hydrogen atom has one electron in this energy level, but a helium atom has two. Because it has a full outer energy level, a helium atom is

Figure 2–4 Atoms and Energy Levels.
(a) A typical hydrogen atom has one proton and one electron. The electron orbiting the nucleus occupies the first energy level, diagrammed as an electron shell. (b) An atom of helium has two protons, two neutrons, and two electrons. The two electrons orbit in the same energy level.
(c) The first energy level can hold only two electrons. In a lithium atom, with three protons, four neutrons, and three electrons, the third electron occupies a second energy level. (d) The second level can hold up to eight electrons. A neon atom has 10 protons, 10 neutrons, and 10 electrons; thus both the first and second energy levels are filled.

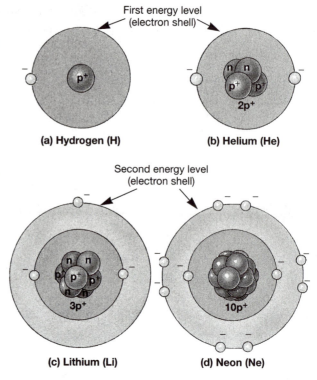

very stable, and it will not ordinarily react with other atoms. Lithium has three electrons, so in a lithium atom the first level is filled and the third electron occupies a second energy level. The second level can hold up to eight electrons, and this level is filled in a neon atom with an atomic number of 10. Neon atoms, like helium atoms, are thus very stable. Each successive energy level accommodates a specific number of electrons, but with the exception of the first level, the outermost levels can only accommodate a maximum of eight electrons. When the energy level is filled with those eight electrons, the resulting atom is chemically inert.

Let's Review What You've Just Learned

▶ **Definitions**

In the space provided, write the term for each of the following definitions.

_____ **16.** Atoms of an element whose nuclei contain different numbers of neutrons.

_____ **17.** Substances that cannot be broken down into simpler substances by ordinary chemical processes.

_____ **18.** Anything that has mass and occupies space.

_____ **19.** The time required for a 50% reduction in the amount of radiation emitted by a radioactive isotope.

_____   **20.** The number of protons and neutrons in the nucleus of an atom.

_____   **21.** A measure of the amount of matter in an object.

_____   **22.** The smallest portions of an element that exhibit the chemical characteristics of that element.

_____   **23.** The part of an atom that contains its protons and neutrons.

_____   **24.** The relative weight of an atom.

_____   **25.** The gravitational force that acts on an object's mass.

_____   **26.** The number of protons in the nucleus of an atom.

_____   **27.** The unit used to measure atomic weight.

_____   **28.** A particular energy that an electron can have in an atom.

_____   **29.** Tiny units of matter that make up atoms.

Complete the following chart of element names and symbols.

	Element	Symbol
30.	Oxygen	
31.	Nitrogen	
32.		K
33.		Ca
34.	Sodium	
35.		C
36.		H
37.	Sulfur	
38.		P
39.	Chlorine	
40.	Magnesium	
41.		I
42.		Fe

Complete the following table.

	Subatomic Particle	Mass	Charge
43.	Proton		
44.	Neutron		
45.	Electron		

For each of the following elements, indicate the number of protons, the number of electrons, the number of neutrons, and mass number.

46. ^{14}C

Number of protons _____   Number of electrons _____

Number of neutrons _____   Mass number _____

47. ^{4}He

Number of protons _____   Number of electrons _____

Number of neutrons _____   Mass number _____

48. ^{24}Na

Number of protons _____   Number of electrons _____

Number of neutrons _____   Mass number _____

CHEMICAL BONDS AND CHEMICAL COMPOUNDS

Helium, neon, and argon are called *inert gases* because their atoms, having full outer energy levels, neither react with one another nor combine with atoms of other elements. Atoms with unfilled outer energy levels are relatively unstable. Such atoms can achieve stability by gaining, losing, or sharing electrons to achieve a full outer energy level. The processes of gaining, losing, or sharing electrons create **chemical bonds** that hold the atoms together. When such chemical bonding occurs between atoms of different elements, the result is a chemical compound. A **compound** is a new chemical *substance consisting of two or more elements*. The physical and chemical properties of a compound can be quite different from those of its component elements. For example, a mixture of hydrogen and oxygen is highly flammable, but chemically combining hydrogen and oxygen atoms produces water, a compound used to put out fires.

Ionic Bonds

Ionic bonds are created by *the electrical attraction between atoms* that have gained or lost electrons and thus carry an electrical charge. If we assign a value of +1 to the charge on a proton, the charge on an electron will be –1. As long as the number of protons is equal to the number of electrons, an atom will be electrically neutral (net charge = 0). If an atom loses an electron, it will exhibit a charge of +1 because there will be one proton without a corresponding electron. Losing a second electron would leave the atom with a charge of +2, losing a third would leave the atom with a charge of +3, and so on. Adding an extra electron to an atom will give it a charge of –1; adding a second electron will produce a charge of –2, and so on. Atoms or particles that have + or – charges are called **ions.** Ions with a positive charge are **cations** (KAT-ī-onz; Greek *katienai,* to go down); those with a negative charge are **anions** (AN-ī-onz; Greek *anienai,* to go up).

In an **ionic** (ī-ON-ik; Greek *ienai,* to go) **bond,** anions and cations are held together by the attraction between positive and negative charges. In forming an ionic bond:

- One atom loses one or more electrons, becoming a cation with a positive charge.
- Another atom gains those electrons, becoming an anion with a negative charge.
- The opposite charges draw the two ions together, just as oppositely charged ends of two magnets attract each other.

The formation of a representative ionic bond is illustrated in Figure 2–5. The sodium atom diagrammed in Figure 2–5 (Step 1) has an atomic number of 11, so this atom normally contains 11 protons and 11 electrons. Electrons fill the first and second energy levels, and a single electron occupies level 3. Losing that outermost electron would give the sodium atom a full outer energy level (energy level 2) and produce a sodium ion with a +1 charge. But the electron cannot simply be thrown away; it must be donated to

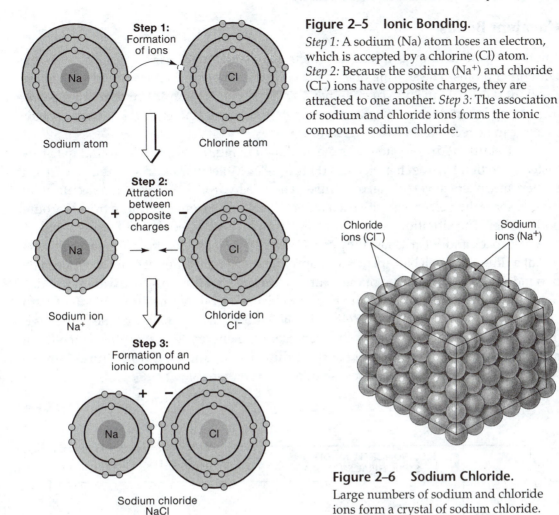

Step 1:
Formation
of ions

Sodium atom

Chlorine atom

Step 2:
Attraction
between
opposite
charges

Sodium ion
Na$^+$

Chloride ion
Cl$^-$

Step 3:
Formation of an
ionic compound

Sodium chloride
NaCl

Figure 2–5   Ionic Bonding.
Step 1: A sodium (Na) atom loses an electron, which is accepted by a chlorine (Cl) atom. *Step 2:* Because the sodium (Na$^+$) and chloride (Cl$^-$) ions have opposite charges, they are attracted to one another. *Step 3:* The association of sodium and chloride ions forms the ionic compound sodium chloride.

Chloride
ions (Cl$^-$)

Sodium
ions (Na$^+$)

Figure 2–6   Sodium Chloride.
Large numbers of sodium and chloride ions form a crystal of sodium chloride.

another atom. A chlorine atom has seven electrons in its outer energy level. An additional electron would fill this energy level, and a sodium atom can provide it. In the process (Step 2) the chlorine atom becomes a *chloride ion* with a –1 charge.

Both atoms have now become stable ions with filled outer energy levels. The two ions do not move apart after the electron transfer, because the positively charged sodium ion is attracted to the negatively charged chloride ion (Step 3). The combination of oppositely charged ions forms the ionic compound sodium chloride, otherwise known as table salt. Large numbers of sodium and chloride ions interact to form highly structured crystals held together only by the electrical attraction of oppositely charged ions (Figure 2–6).

The number of electrons an atom will lose or gain when it forms ions depends on the number of electrons that are present in the outermost energy level. In general, if there are fewer than four electrons in the outermost level, the atom will lose them and form a positive ion (cation). On the other hand, if there are five, six, or seven electrons in the outermost level, the atom will generally gain enough electrons to fill the available spaces, forming a negative ion (anion). As we have already noted, atoms with full outer energy levels exhibit no tendency to either lose or gain electrons.

Covalent Bonds

Another way that atoms can complete their outer electron shells is by sharing electrons with other atoms. The sharing of electrons creates a type of chemical bond known as a **covalent** (kō-VĀ-lent; Latin *co-* together + *valentia,* power) **bond.** The result of this type of bonding is a **molecule**—two or more *atoms held together by covalent bonds* that behave as and can be recognized as a single unit.

Individual hydrogen atoms, as diagrammed in Figure 2–4, are not found in nature. Instead, we find hydrogen molecules (Figure 2–7). Molecular hydrogen is a gas present in the atmosphere in very small quantities. The two hydrogen atoms in a molecule of hydrogen share their electrons with each other. The electron from each atom travels around both nuclei. The situation is similar to one in which two people are tossing a pair of baseballs back and forth as fast they can. On the average, each person has just one baseball at a time, and each ball spends an approximately equal amount of time between the two individuals. The sharing of one pair of electrons creates a **single covalent bond.**

Notice that three different methods can be used to show the structure of a hydrogen molecule (Figure 2–7): (1) the electron-shell model, which diagrams the positions of the electrons in concentric shells that represent the energy levels; (2) the space-filling model, which shows the molecule in three dimensions; and (3) the structural formula, which uses a solid line to indicate a shared electron pair.

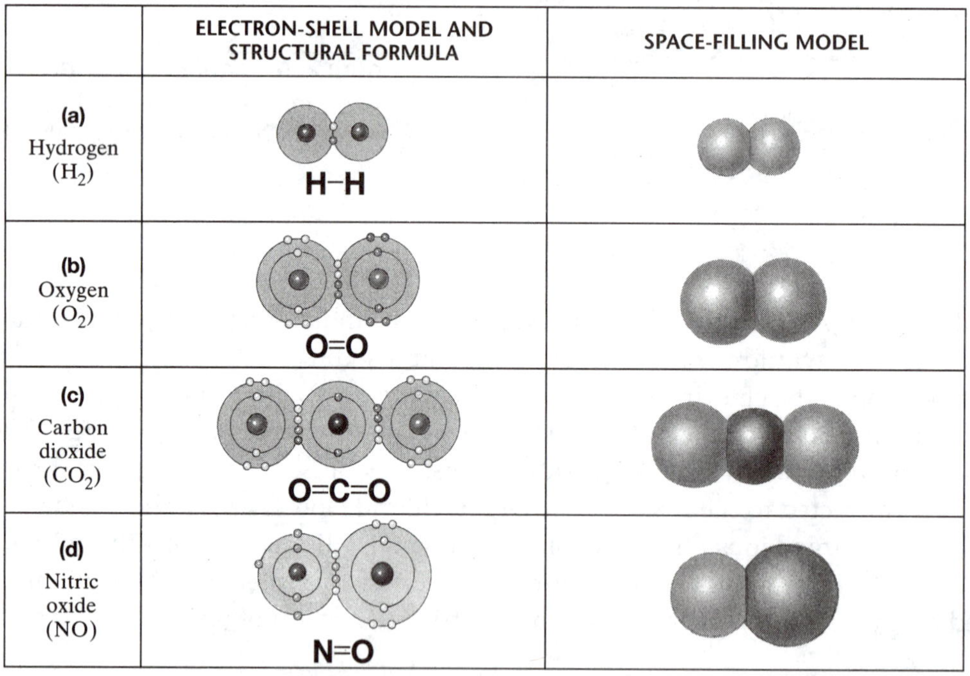

Figure 2–7 Covalent Bonds.
(a) In a molecule of hydrogen, two hydrogen atoms share their electrons such that each has a filled outer electron shell. This sharing creates a single covalent bond. (b) A molecule of oxygen consists of two oxygen atoms that share two pairs of electrons. The result is a double covelent bond. (c) In a molecule of carbon dioxide, a central carbon atom forms double covalent bonds with a pair of oxygen atoms. (d) A molecule of nitric oxide is held together by a double covelent bond, but the outer electron shell of the nitrogen atom requires an additional electron to be complete. Thus, nitric oxide is a *free radical,* which will readily react with another atom or molecule.

Oxygen, with an atomic number of 8, has two electrons in its first energy level and six in the second. The oxygen atoms diagrammed in Figure 2–7 attain a stable electron configuration by sharing two pairs of electrons, forming a **double covalent bond.** Molecular oxygen is an atmospheric gas that is very important to living organisms; our cells would die without a relatively constant supply of oxygen.

The chemical reactions in our bodies that consume oxygen also produce a waste product, *carbon dioxide.* The oxygen atoms in a carbon dioxide molecule form double covalent bonds with the carbon atom, as indicated in Figure 2–7.

Covalent bonds are very strong because the electrons hold the atoms together. In typical covalent bonds, the atoms remain electrically neutral because each shared electron spends equal time between the two nuclei (recall the baseball analogy). Covalent bonds, especially between carbon atoms, create the stable framework of the large molecules that make up most of the structural components of the human body.

Covalent bonds usually form molecules that complete the outer electron shells of the atoms involved. An atom or molecule that contains unpaired electrons in its outer shell is called a **free radical.** Free radicals are highly reactive and persist only for a very short time before additional reactions occur. Free radicals sometimes form as intermediaries in chemical reactions. Living cells usually have mechanisms to tie up or eliminate free radicals to prevent the damage or destruction of vital compounds, such as proteins. However, *nitric oxide* (Figure 2–7) is a free radical that has important functions in the body. It is involved in chemical communication in the nervous system, the control of blood vessel diameter, blood clotting, and the defense against bacteria and other pathogens.

Polar Covalent Bonds

Many covalent bonds involve relatively equal sharing of electrons. Some, however, do not, because elements differ in how strongly they hold shared electrons. An unequal sharing of electrons creates a **polar covalent bond.** For example, in a molecule of water (Figure 2–8), an oxygen atom forms covalent bonds with two hydrogen atoms. The oxygen atom has a much stronger attraction for the shared electrons than the hydrogen atoms do, so the electrons spend most of their time orbiting around the oxygen nucleus. Because it has two extra electrons part of the time, the oxygen atom develops a slight

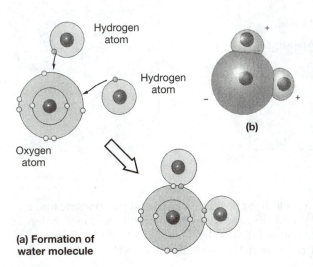

(a) Formation of water molecule

(b)

Figure 2–8   Polar Covalent Bonds and the Structure of Water.

(a) In forming a water molecule, an oxygen atom completes its outer energy level by sharing electrons with a pair of hydrogen atoms. The sharing is unequal because the oxygen atom holds the electrons more tightly than do the hydrogen atoms. **(b)** Because the oxygen atom has two extra electrons much of the time, it develops a slight negative charge, and the hydrogen atoms become weakly positive. The bonds in a water molecule are polar covalent bonds.

negative charge. At the same time, the hydrogen atoms develop slight positive charges, since their electrons are away part of the time. This unequal sharing makes polar covalent bonds somewhat weaker than other covalent bonds.

Hydrogen Bonds

Covalent and ionic bonds tie atoms together in a relatively stable framework. Comparatively weak attractive forces act between atoms in different parts of a large molecule as well as between adjacent molecules. *Hydrogen bonds* are the most important of these attractive forces. A **hydrogen bond** is the attraction between a hydrogen atom and an atom such as oxygen or nitrogen that is either part of another molecule or located at a distant site on the same molecule. Both the hydrogen and the other atom must be involved in a polar covalent bond. Because the atoms are involved in polar covalent bonds, the hydrogen will have a slight positive charge and the oxygen or nitrogen will have a slight negative charge. The opposite charges cause the atoms to be attracted to each other. The hydrogen bond that is created is a very weak attractive force that reflects the attraction between opposite charges.

Hydrogen bonds do not create molecules, but they can change molecular shapes or pull molecules together. For example, hydrogen bonding occurs between water molecules (Figure 2–9). At the water surface the attraction between molecules slows the rate of evaporation and creates the phenomenon known as **surface tension** (Figure 2–9). Surface tension acts as a barrier that keeps small objects from entering the water: it is surface tension that enables insects to "walk" across the surface of a pond or puddle. Surface tension in a layer of tears keeps small objects such as dust particles from touching the surface of the eye. At the cellular level, hydrogen bonds affect the shapes and properties of complex molecules, such as proteins; they may also determine the three-dimensional relationships between molecules.

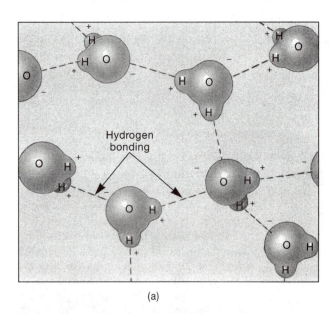

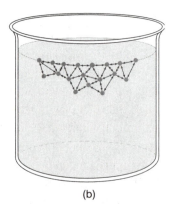

(a)   (b)

Figure 2–9   Hydrogen Bonds.
(a) The hydrogen atoms of a water molecule have a slight positive charge, and the oxygen atom has a slight negative charge (*see Figure 2–8*). Attraction between a hydrogen atom of one water molecule and the oxygen atom of another is a hydrogen bond (indicated by dashed lines). **(b)** Hydrogen bonding between water molecules at a free surface restricts evaporation and creates surface tension.

✏️ Let's Review What You've Just Learned

▶ Definitions

In the space provided, write the term for each of the following definitions.

_____ **49.** An atom or molecule that contains one or more unpaired electrons in its outer shell.

_____ **50.** An electrically charged atom or group of atoms.

_____ **51.** A substance consisting of two or more elements.

_____ **52.** The weak attraction between a positively charged hydrogen atom and a negatively charged atom on the same or another molecule.

_____ **53.** A positively charged ion.

_____ **54.** A negatively charged ion.

_____ **55.** Two or more atoms held together by covalent bonds that behave as and can be recognized as a single unit.

_____ **56.** The force of attraction that holds ions together in an ionic compound.

_____ **57.** A chemical bond formed by the sharing of electrons between two atoms.

▶ Completion

Complete each of the following items.

58. A _____ covalent bond occurs when there is unequal sharing of the electrons in the bond.

59. The _____ between water molecules account for water's relatively slow rate of evaporation and the phenomenon known as surface tension.

CHEMICAL NOTATION

Before we can consider the specific compounds found in the human body, we must be able to describe chemical compounds and reactions effectively. Using sentences to describe chemical structures and events often leads to confusion, and a simple form of "chemical shorthand" makes communication much more efficient.

The chemical shorthand we will use is known as **chemical notation.** Chemical notation enables us to describe complex events in a brief and precise fashion. An atom is represented in chemical notation by the chemical symbol for the element. For instance, H (the chemical symbol for hydrogen) represents one atom of hydrogen. If we want to indicate more than one atom, we can place a number in front of the symbol. Thus 2 H represents two hydrogen atoms. When more than one atom of an element occurs in a compound, a subscript is used to indicate the number of atoms. The formula for water (H_2O), for example, tells us that the compound contains two atoms of hydrogen and one atom of oxygen.

The substances participating in a chemical reaction are called **reactants,** and the substances generated by a reaction are called **products.** An arrow is used to indicate the direction of the reaction, with the reactants at the "tail" of the arrow and the products at the "head." In order to be able to calculate amounts using a chemical equation, we must balance the equation. Atoms (and mass) must be conserved during a chemical reaction; in other words, chemical reactions cannot create or destroy atoms. The existing atoms are simply rearranged into different combinations. Therefore, the numbers of atoms must always be the same on both sides of the equation. Balancing a chemical equation requires the addition of coefficients to the compounds on each side until the number of each kind of atom is equal on both sides. For example, nitrogen and hydrogen gas can combine to form a compound called *ammonia*. We can write a chemical equation for the process as follows:

$$N_2 + H_2 \longrightarrow NH_3$$

Nitrogen and hydrogen are reactants and are written on the tail side of the arrow. Ammonia (NH_3) is the product and is written on the head side of the arrow. The equation is an accurate description of the chemical process, but it is not balanced. Although each side of the equation indicates that four atoms are present, the reactant side shows two nitrogen atoms whereas the product side shows only one. Likewise there are two hydrogen atoms on the reactant side and three on the product side. To balance the equation, we need to add coefficients that will give us the same number of nitrogen and hydrogen atoms on both sides. Since there are two nitrogen atoms on the left, we put a coefficient of 2 in front of the ammonia on the right. Now the nitrogens are equal on both sides. However, now there are six hydrogens on the right side. We can balance the hydrogens by placing the coefficient 3 in front of the hydrogen molecule on the left. The balanced equation appears as follows:

$$N_2 + 3\,H_2 \longrightarrow 2\,NH_3$$

The rules of chemical notation are summarized in Table 2–4.

You cannot actually handle individual atoms or molecules, nor could you easily count the billions of atoms and molecules that take part in ordinary chemical processes in the lab or in the body. As an example, suppose you wanted to create water from hydrogen and oxygen, using the balanced equation

$$2\,H_2 + O_2 = 2\,H_2O$$

The first step in performing such an experiment would be to calculate the molecular weights involved. The **molecular weight** is equal to the sum of the atomic weights of the components of the molecule. The atomic weight of hydrogen is close to 1, so one hydrogen molecule (H_2) has a molecular weight of 2. Oxygen has an atomic weight of around 16, so the molecular weight of an oxygen molecule (O_2) is roughly 32. In practical terms, if you wanted to perform the experiment you would take 4 g of hydrogen, combine it with 32 g of oxygen, and produce 36 g of water. You could also work with ounces, pounds, or tons, as long as the proportions remained the same.

CHEMICAL REACTIONS

Living cells remain alive and functional by controlling internal chemical reactions. In a chemical reaction, chemical bonds between atoms are broken as atoms in the reacting substances, or reactants, are rearranged in different combinations to form new substances, the products. In effect, each cell is a chemical factory. For example, growth, maintenance and repair, secretion, and contraction all involve complex chemical reactions. The term

Table 2–4	Rules of Chemical Notation

1. The symbol of an element indicates one atom of that element:

   H = one atom of hydrogen; O = one atom of oxygen

2. A number preceding the symbol of an element indicates more than one atom:

   2 H = two individual atoms of hydrogen
   2 O = two individual atoms of oxygen

3. A subscript following the symbol of an element indicates a molecule with that number of atoms of that element:

   H_2 = a hydrogen molecule, composed of two hydrogen atoms

   O_2 = an oxygen molecule, composed of two oxygen atoms

   H_2O = a water molecule, composed of two hydrogen atoms and one oxygen atom

4. In a description of a chemical reaction, the interacting participants are called reactants, and the reaction generates one or more products. An arrow indicates the direction of the reaction, from reactants (usually on the left) to products (usually on the right). In the following reaction, two atoms of hydrogen combine with one atom of oxygen to produce a single molecule of water:

   $$2\,H + O \rightarrow H_2O$$

5. A superscript plus or minus sign following the symbol of an element indicates an ion. A single plus sign indicates a cation with a charge of +1 (the original atom has lost one electron). A single minus sign indicates an anion with a charge of –1 (gain of one electron). If more than one electron has been lost or gained, the charge on the ion is indicated by a number preceding the plus or minus:

   Na^+ = one sodium ion (the sodium atom has lost 1 electron)

   Cl^- = one chloride ion (the chlorine atom has gained 1 electron)

   Ca^{2+} = one calcium ion (the calcium atom has lost 2 electrons)

6. Chemical reactions neither create nor destroy atoms—they merely rearrange atoms into new combinations. Therefore, the numbers of atoms of each element must always be the same on both sides of the equation for a chemical reaction. When this is the case, the equation is balanced:

   Unbalanced: $H_2 + O_2 \rightarrow H_2O$
   Balanced: $2\,H_2 + O_2 \rightarrow 2\,H_2O$

metabolism (meh-TAB-o-lizm; Greek *metabole,* change) refers to all the chemical reactions that occur in the body. Living cells use chemical reactions to provide the energy needed to maintain homeostasis and perform essential functions.

Types of Reactions

Three types of chemical reactions are important to the study of physiology: decomposition reactions, synthesis reactions, and exchange reactions.

Decomposition Reactions

A **decomposition reaction** breaks larger compounds into smaller components. You could diagram a typical decomposition reaction as:

$$AB \longrightarrow A + B$$

Decomposition reactions involve the breaking of chemical bonds and can occur outside cells as well as inside. For example, a typical meal contains molecules of fats, sugars, and proteins that are too large and too complex to be absorbed and used by our bodies. Decomposition reactions in the digestive tract break these down into smaller molecules before absorption begins.

Synthesis Reactions

Synthesis (SIN-the-sis; Greek *syn-*, together + *thesis*, setting or placing) is the opposite of decomposition. A synthesis reaction assembles larger compounds from smaller components. Relatively simple synthetic reactions could be diagrammed as:

$$A + B \longrightarrow AB$$

Synthesis reactions may involve individual atoms or the combination of molecules to form even larger products. The formation of water from hydrogen and oxygen molecules is an example of synthesis. Synthesis always involves the formation of new chemical bonds, whether the reactants are atoms or molecules.

Exchange Reactions

In an **exchange reaction** parts of the reacting substances are shuffled around, as in:

$$AB + CD \longrightarrow AD + CB$$

You will notice that there are two reactants and two products. Although the reactants and products contain the same components (A, B, C, and D), those components are present in different combinations. In an exchange reaction, the reactant compounds AB and CD break apart (a decomposition) before they interact with one another to form AD and CB (a synthesis).

Reversible Reactions

Chemical reactions are at least theoretically reversible, so that if $A + B \longrightarrow AB$, then $AB \longrightarrow A + B$. Many important biological reactions are freely reversible. Such reactions can be represented as an equation:

$$A + B \xrightleftharpoons{} AB$$

This equation reminds you that there are really two reactions occurring simultaneously, one a synthesis ($A + B \longrightarrow AB$) and the other a decomposition ($AB \longrightarrow A + B$). At **equilibrium** (ē-kwi-LIB-rē-um; Latin *aequilibrium*, uniform) the rate of synthesis is equal to the rate of decomposition. The two rates are in balance. As fast as a molecule of AB forms, another degrades into $A + B$.

   Not all chemical reactions are easily reversed. The requirements for the two reactions may differ, so that at any given time and place the reaction will proceed mainly in one direction. For example, the synthesis reaction may occur when the A and B molecules are heated, and the decomposition reaction when AB molecules are placed in water. In this case the reaction would be written as:

$$A + B \xrightleftharpoons[H_2O]{heat} AB$$

   Decomposition reactions involving water are important in the breakdown of complex molecules in the body; several examples of this process, called **hydrolysis** (hī-DROL-i-sis; Greek *hydor*, water + *lyein*, loosen), will be encountered in the next chapter. In hydrolysis, one of the bonds in a complex molecule is broken, and the components of a water molecule (H and OH) are added to the resulting fragments:

$$A\text{-}B\text{-}C\text{-}D\text{-}E + H_2O \longrightarrow A\text{-}B\text{-}C\text{-}H + HO\text{-}D\text{-}E$$

Let's Review What You've Just Learned

► **Definitions**

In the space provided, write the term for each of the following definitions.

_____ **60.** All of the chemical reactions that occur in a living cell or organism.

_____ **61.** The substances generated by a chemical reaction.

_____ **62.** The point in a chemical reaction at which the rate of synthesis is equal to the rate of decomposition.

_____ **63.** The substances participating in a chemical reaction.

_____ **64.** A decomposition reaction involving water.

► **Chemical Notation**

In the space provided, indicate whether the reaction is a decomposition reaction (mark D), a synthesis reaction (mark S) or an exchange reaction (mark E).

_____ **65.** $C + O_2 \longrightarrow CO_2$

_____ **66.** $C_6H_{12}O_6 \longrightarrow 6C + 6H_2O$

_____ **67.** $HCl + NaOH \longrightarrow NaCl + H_2O$

In the space provided, write the formula for each indicated molecule.

68. nitrogen (contains 2 atoms of nitrogen): Formula = _____

69. sucrose (contains 12 atoms of carbon, 22 atoms of hydrogen, and 11 atoms of oxygen in that order): Formula = _____

70. hydrochloric acid (contains 1 atom of hydrogen and 1 atom of chlorine in that order): Formula = _____

SOME BASICS ABOUT ENERGY

Work occurs when a force moves matter some distance. **Energy** is the *capacity to perform work;* movement or physical change will not occur unless energy is provided. There are two major forms of energy: kinetic energy and potential energy (Figure 2–10).

- **Kinetic energy** is the *energy of motion.* When a car hits a tree, it is kinetic energy that does the damage.
- **Potential energy** is *stored energy.* It may result from the position of an object (a book on a high shelf) or its physical or chemical structure (a stretched spring or a charged battery).

Kinetic energy must be used to lift a book, stretch a spring, or charge a battery. The potential energy is converted back into kinetic energy when the book falls, the spring recoils, or the battery discharges, and the kinetic energy can be used to perform work. A conversion between potential energy and kinetic energy is never 100 percent efficient. Each time an energy exchange occurs, some of the energy is released in the form of heat.

Living cells perform work in many forms. For example, a resting skeletal muscle contains potential energy in the form of the positions of protein filaments and the attachments between molecules inside the cell. When a muscle contracts, it performs work;

Figure 2–10 Potential and Kinetic Energy.
(a) Energy (kinetic energy) is required to set the arm on the mousetrap. **(b)** Once the catch is set, the energy (potential energy) is stored in the spring-operated arm. **(c)** If the mousetrap is tripped, the potential energy is transformed into kinetic energy.

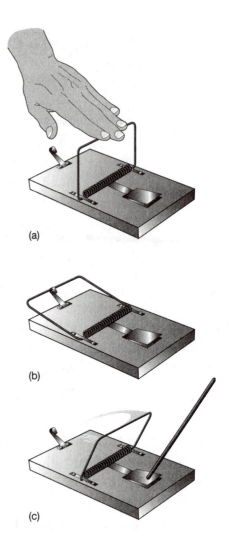

(a)

(b)

(c)

potential energy is converted to kinetic energy, and heat is released. The amount of heat is proportional to the amount of work done. As a result, when we exercise, our body temperature rises.

Types of Energy

There are several categories of energy, including light, thermal, mechanical, electrical, and chemical to name a few. The different kinds of energy are all related, and one kind can readily be converted into another. For instance, electrical energy can be converted to thermal energy and chemical energy can be converted into light energy. Four forms of energy are particularly important in the function of the human body. They are electromagnetic energy, electrical energy, chemical energy, and thermal energy.

Electromagnetic Energy

Electromagnetic energy is *a form of energy that travels through space as a wave* (Figure 2–11). The distance between successive peaks or troughs of a wave is called the **wavelength.** The number of wave cycles (peak to peak) that occur per second is the **frequency** of the wave. Wavelength and frequency are inversely proportional to each other. In other words,

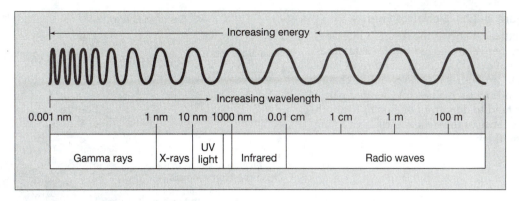

Figure 2–11   The Electromagnetic Spectrum.
Electromagnetic energy travels through space as a wave. High-energy waves have high frequencies and short wavelengths; low-energy waves have low frequencies and short wavelengths; low-energy waves have low frequencies and long wavelengths. X-rays, ultraviolet (UV) light, radio waves, and visible light are just some examples of electromagnetic energy.

as the wavelength increases the frequency decreases and vice versa. Wavelengths are usually measured in nanometers, and frequencies are measured in **hertz (Hz)** (1 hertz = 1 cycle per second).

Energy waves of different wavelengths form a continuum called the **electromagnetic spectrum.** At one end of the spectrum are energy waves such as gamma radiation, X-rays, and ultraviolet radiation. These waves have short wavelengths and high frequencies. On the opposite end of the spectrum are waves with long wavelengths and low frequencies, such as radio waves for radio and television broadcasts and the waves used in MRI (magnetic resonance imaging) procedures.

The portion of the spectrum that we can perceive with our eyes is called **visible light** and consists of energy with wavelengths between 400 nm (violet light) and 700 nm (red light). Energy in this range can stimulate chemicals in special cells, called **photoreceptors,** found in the retina of our eyes. Stimulation of these cells results in vision. Electromagnetic energy in the range adjacent to violet light with shorter wavelengths (and higher frequencies) than violet light is called **ultraviolet radiation (UV light).** This radiation is responsible for phenomena such as suntanning and sunburns. On the other end of the visible spectrum is energy with longer wavelengths and lower frequencies than red light. This is **infrared radiation (IR),** and it is associated with heat loss or gain.

Electrical Energy

Electrical energy is *the result of the interactions between charged particles* and involves the movement of ions or electrons (Figure 2–12). Bodies that carry a like charge (both positive or both negative) will repel each other. On the other hand, bodies that carry unlike charges (one positive and one negative) will attract each other. The force of attraction or repulsion depends on the amount of charge (positive or negative) and the distance between the charged bodies. The more charge a body carries, the greater will be its attraction for unlike charges and its repulsion of like charges. Also, the greater the distance between two charged bodies the less the force exerted between them. Charged particles tend to move or flow from one point to another because of the electrical forces acting upon them. When charged particles move, an **electrical current** is created.

Figure 2–12 Electrical Energy.

Electrical energy is the result of interactions between charged particles. **(a)** Bodies that carry like charges will repel each other. **(b)** Bodies that carry unlike charges will attract each other. **(c)** Charged particles tend to flow from one point to another because of the electrical charges acting upon them.

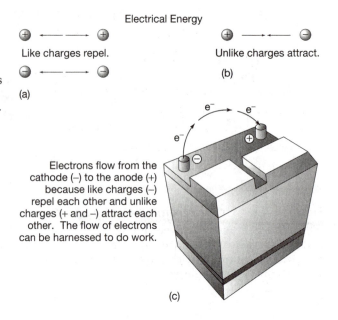

Electrons flow from the cathode (–) to the anode (+) because like charges (–) repel each other and unlike charges (+ and –) attract each other. The flow of electrons can be harnessed to do work.

Information is carried along the processes of neurons by electrical impulses that result from the movement of ions into and out of the cell. Electrical energy is important not only in the functioning of neurons but also in the contraction of muscle tissue.

Charged particles that are separated by a barrier still tend to attract or repel each other on the basis of their charge. This force of attraction or repulsion is a form of potential energy. The **volt (V)** is the unit used to measure this type of potential energy. For most physiological work, the volt is too large a unit, so a smaller unit, the **millivolt (mV =** 1/1000 of a volt), is used.

Chemical Energy

Chemical energy is *energy that is stored (potential energy) in a chemical bond* (Figure 2–13). **Catabolism** (kah-TAB-o-lizm; Greek *katabole*, a throwing down) is the decomposition of molecules within cells. Since a chemical bond contains potential energy, when such a bond is broken, it releases kinetic energy that can perform work. By harnessing the energy released in this way, living cells perform vital functions such as growth, movement, and reproduction. **Anabolism** (a-NAB-o-lizm; Greek *anabole*, a throwing upward) is the synthesis of new compounds within the body. Because energy is required to form a

Figure 2–13 Chemical Energy.

Chemical energy is potential energy that is stored in the bonds that hold atoms together. In catabolic reactions, chemical bonds are broken and energy is released (exergonic reaction). In anabolic reactions, energy is required to form new chemical bonds (endergonic reaction).

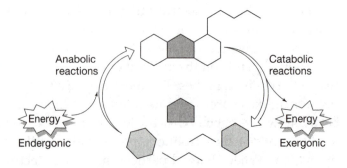

chemical bond, anabolism is usually an "uphill" process. Living cells must "balance their energy budgets," with catabolism providing the energy to support anabolism as well as other vital functions.

If breaking the old bonds releases more energy than it takes to create the new ones, the reaction will release energy, usually in the form of heat. Reactions that release energy are said to be **exergonic** (ek-ser-GON-ik; Greek *exo-*, outside + *ergon*, work). If the energy required for synthesis exceeds the amount released by the associated decomposition reaction, additional energy must be provided. Reactions that absorb energy are termed **endergonic** (end-er-GON-ik; Greek *endo-*, inside + *ergon*, work).

Thermal Energy

Thermal energy results from the *random motions of atoms and molecules* (Figure 2–14). As these random movements increase so does thermal energy. When the random movements of atoms and molecules decrease, thermal energy decreases. **Heat** is thermal energy passing from one substance to another. **Temperature** is an indication of heat transfer (heat is always transferred from a warmer body to a cooler one). At higher temperatures, atomic and molecular movements are more rapid and the thermal content is greater. On the other hand, as temperature decreases, atomic and molecular movements are slower and the thermal content is less. When a warm object is placed next to a cold one, thermal energy is transferred: The warm object loses heat and the cold object gains heat. All other kinds of energy can be converted into thermal energy. For instance, in exergonic reactions, the energy that is released when chemical bonds are broken is frequently in the form of heat. The heat released by exergonic reactions in the human body is responsible for maintaining our body temperature.

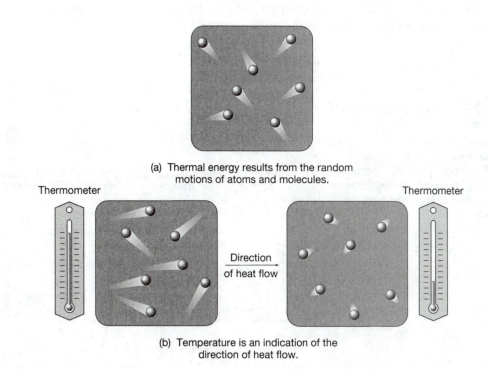

(a) Thermal energy results from the random
motions of atoms and molecules.

(b) Temperature is an indication of the
direction of heat flow.

Figure 2–14   Thermal Energy.
(a) Thermal energy results from the random motions of atoms and molecules. **(b)** Temperature is an indication of the direction of heat flow.

Measuring Thermal Energy and Heat

All forms of energy ultimately are transformed into thermal energy, which is transferred as heat. The measurement of heat involves temperature. Heat is thermal energy being transferred from one object to another. The relative temperatures of the two objects define the direction and rate of heat flow. Heat flows from a body of higher temperature to one of lower temperature.

The unit of heat energy is the **calorie (cal).** Originally, this unit was defined as the amount of heat energy necessary to raise the temperature of water 1°C from 14.5°C to 15.5°C. However, the **kilocalorie (kcal)** is a more appropriate unit for dealing with the energy changes that occur in chemical reactions. A kilocalorie is equal to 1000 calories. In nutrition, the term **Calorie** (notice the spelling with a capital **C**) is the same unit as the kilocalorie.

ENZYMES AND CHEMICAL REACTIONS

Most chemical reactions do not occur spontaneously, or they occur so slowly that they would be of little value to living cells. Before a reaction can proceed, enough energy must be provided to activate the reactants. **Activation energy** is the *amount of energy required to start a reaction* (Figure 2–15). Although many reactions can be activated by changes in temperature or acidity, such changes are deadly to cells. For example, to break down a complex sugar you must boil it in an acid solution.

Enzymes are *special proteins that promote chemical processes* by lowering the activation energy requirements and so allow most physiological reactions to occur at body temperature. Enzymes belong to a class of substances called **catalysts** (KAT-a-lists; Greek *katalysis,* dissolution), *compounds that accelerate chemical reactions* without themselves being permanently changed. Each enzyme is made by a living cell to promote a specific reaction. These reversible reactions can be written as:

$$A + B \xrightarrow{\text{enzyme 1}} AB$$

Figure 2–15 Enzyme-Catalyzed Reaction.

The activation energy is the energy required for a chemical reaction to occur. Enzymes speed up chemical reactions in the body by lowering the activation energy required for the reaction.

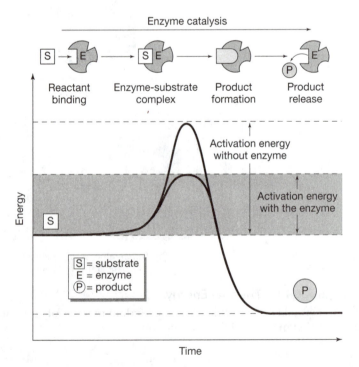

Although the presence of an appropriate enzyme can accelerate a reaction, an enzyme affects only the rate of a reaction, not the direction of the reaction or the products that will be formed. An enzyme cannot bring about a reaction that would otherwise be impossible.

The complex reactions that support life proceed in a series of interlocking steps, each step controlled by a different enzyme. Such a reaction sequence is called a **pathway.** A synthetic pathway could be written as:

$$A \xrightarrow[\text{Step 1}]{\text{enzyme 1}} B \xrightarrow[\text{Step 2}]{\text{enzyme 2}} C \xrightarrow[\text{Step 3}]{\text{enzyme 3}} \text{etc.}$$

Sometimes the steps in the synthetic pathway differ from those of the decomposition pathway, and separate enzymes are involved.

Let's Review What You've Just Learned

► **Definitions**

In the space provided, write the term for each of the following definitions.

_____ **71.** The breakdown of complex molecules into simpler components.

_____ **72.** The capacity to do work.

_____ **73.** The distance between the crests of two successive waves.

_____ **74.** Proteins that act as biological catalysts.

_____ **75.** The term for reactions that release energy.

_____ **76.** That which occurs when a force moves matter some distance.

_____ **77.** Energy that results from the interactions between charged particles.

_____ **78.** The synthesis of new compounds within the body.

_____ **79.** The energy of motion.

_____ **80.** Energy that results from the random motions of atoms and molecules.

_____ **81.** The term for reactions that absorb energy.

_____ **82.** Stored energy.

_____ **83.** The amount of energy required to start a chemical reaction.

_____ **84.** Energy that travels through space as waves.

_____ **85.** An indicator of the direction and rate of heat flow.

_____ **86.** The number of wave cycles that occur per second.

_____ **87.** A compound that can accelerate the rate of chemical reactions without itself being permanently changed.

_____ **88.** Electromagnetic energy with wavelengths slightly shorter than violet light.

_____ **89.** The energy that is stored in a chemical bond.

_____ **90.** The unit used to measure wave frequency.

_____ **91.** The basic unit of heat.

_____ **92.** The unit used to measure electrical potential energy.

_____ **93.** A reaction sequence in which each step is catalyzed by a specific enzyme.

_____ **94.** The continuum formed by energy waves of different wavelengths.

_____ **95.** Energy with wavelengths slightly longer than red light.

► **Completion**

In the space provided, complete each of the following statements.

96. When a glass is placed on a shelf, it has _____ energy by virtue of its position.

97. When a sperm cell moves, energy stored in chemical compounds is being converted to _____ energy.

98. There is a(n) _____ relationship between the wavelength and frequency of electromagnetic energy.

99. Bodies that carry like charges will _____ each other, whereas bodies that carry unlike charges will _____ each other.

INORGANIC COMPOUNDS

Although the human body is complex, it contains a relatively small number of elements, as indicated in Figure 2–1. But knowing the identity and quantity of each element will not help you understand a human being any more than studying the alphabet will help you understand this text. A better approach would be to develop an understanding of nutrients and metabolites (me-TAB-o-līts; Greek *metabole,* change). **Nutrients** are the essential elements and molecules obtained from the diet. **Metabolites** include all the molecules synthesized or broken down by chemical reactions inside our bodies. Nutrients and metabolites can be broadly categorized as inorganic or organic (Figure 2–16). **Inorganic compounds** are *compounds whose structure is not primarily determined by the linking together of carbon atoms.* **Organic compounds** are *compounds whose structure is determined primarily by the linking together of carbon atoms.* We will focus on inorganic compounds in this chapter and organic compounds in the next chapter.

The most important inorganic compounds in the body are (1) carbon dioxide, a byproduct of cell metabolism; (2) oxygen, an atmospheric gas required in important metabolic reactions; (3) water, which accounts for most of the body weight; and (4) inorganic acids, bases, and salts, compounds held together partially or completely by ionic bonds.

Water and Its Properties

Water, H_2O, is the single most important component of the body, accounting for almost two-thirds of the body's total weight. A change in body water content can have fatal consequences because virtually all physiological systems will be affected. Although familiar to everyone, water really has some very unusual properties. The properties of water are a direct result of the hydrogen bonding that occurs between neighboring water molecules.

1. *Water is a medium for most chemical reactions and a participant in many reactions.* Most chemical reactions in the body take place in water. Water molecules participate in some of these reactions, especially catabolic reactions that break large molecules into smaller ones. Specific examples will be encountered later in this chapter and in the following chapter.

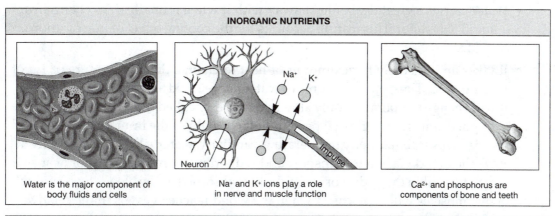

INORGANIC NUTRIENTS

Water is the major component of body fluids and cells

Na⁺ and K⁺ ions play a role in nerve and muscle function

Ca²⁺ and phosphorus are components of bone and teeth

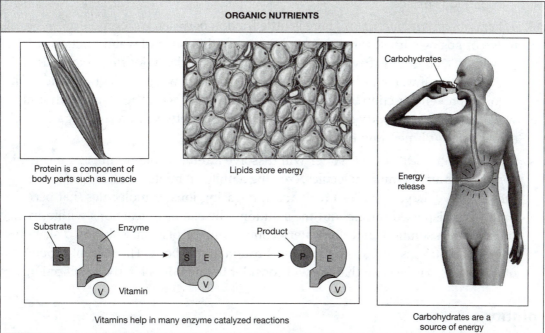

ORGANIC NUTRIENTS

Protein is a component of body parts such as muscle

Lipids store energy

Carbohydrates

Energy release

Vitamins help in many enzyme catalyzed reactions

Carbohydrates are a source of energy

Figure 2–16   Nutrients.
Nutrients can be divided into two broad groups. **(a)** Inorganic nutrients include water and the various minerals. **(b)** Organic nutrients include proteins, lipids, vitamins, and carbohydrates.

2. *Water has a very high heat capacity, and its freezing and boiling points are far apart.* **Heat capacity** is the ability to absorb and retain thermal energy, transferred as heat. For example, a large body of water, such as a lake or an ocean, can absorb and store large quantities of heat. That is why coastal regions and areas near large lakes are usually cooler in the summer and warmer in the winter than are areas that are not close to a large body of water. During the summer, the water absorbs and stores heat, keeping the air cooler. On the other hand, during the winter, the gradual release of the heat that was stored during the summer warms the nearby air, keeping air temperatures slightly higher. The reason that water has a high heat capacity is that water molecules in the liquid state are attracted to one another through hydrogen bonding. Important consequences of this attraction include:

- The temperature must be quite high before individual molecules have enough energy to break free and become water vapor. Consequently, water stays in the liquid state over a broad range of environmental temperatures.

- Water carries a great deal of heat away with it when it finally does change from a liquid to a vapor. This feature accounts for the cooling effect of perspiration on the skin.

- It takes an unusually large amount of heat to change the temperature of 1 g of water by 1°C. Thus, once a volume of water has reached a particular temperature, it will change temperature only slowly, a property called *thermal inertia*. Because water accounts for roughly 66 percent of the weight of the human body, thermal inertia helps stabilize body temperature. Similarly, water's high heat capacity allows the blood plasma to transport and redistribute large amounts of heat as it circulates within the body. For example, heat absorbed as the blood flows through active muscles will be released when the blood reaches vessels in the relatively cool body surface.

3. *Water is an effective lubricant.* There is little friction between water molecules. Thus, if two opposing surfaces are separated by even a thin layer of water, friction will be very low. (That is why driving on wet roads can be tricky; your tires may start sliding on a layer of water, rather than maintaining contact with the road.) Liquid within joints prevents friction between opposing body surfaces, and a small amount of water in the ventral body cavities prevents friction between internal organs, such as the heart or lungs, and body wall.

4. *Water is an excellent solvent.* Water will dissolve a remarkable number of inorganic compounds and organic molecules, creating a uniform mixture called a **solution.** As they dissolve, large particles break apart, releasing ions or molecules that become uniformly dispersed throughout the solution. The chemical reactions within living cells occur in solution, and the watery component, or plasma, of blood distributes dissolved nutrients and waste products throughout the body. The solvent properties of water are so important that we will consider them in detail in the next section.

Solutions

Every solution consists of a medium, or **solvent,** in which atoms, ions, or molecules of another substance, or **solute,** are dispersed. In an **aqueous solution** water is the solvent. Water is particularly effective as a solvent because of its chemical structure. Since the hydrogen atoms are attached to the oxygen atom by polar covalent bonds, the hydrogen atoms have a slight positive charge and the oxygen atom has a slight negative charge (Figure 2–8). The bonds in a water molecule are oriented so as to place the hydrogen atoms relatively close together. As a result, the water molecule has a positive end and a negative end. We refer to the charged ends of a molecule such as water as poles. A water molecule is therefore called a *polar molecule.*

Many inorganic compounds held together by ionic bonds will undergo **ionization** (ī-on-i-ZĀ-shun), or **dissociation** (di-sō-sē-Ā-shun) in water. In this process, shown in Figure 2–17, ionic bonds are broken as the individual ions interact with the positive or negative ends of polar water molecules. The result is a mixture of cations and anions surrounded by water molecules held by the attraction between opposite charges. The water molecules form a **hydration sphere,** a zone of water molecules, that completely surrounds each ion. The hydration sphere helps to ensure that the ions will stay in solution and not re-form crystals.

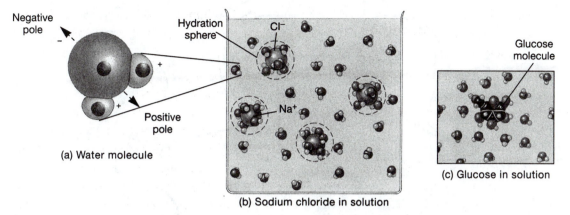

Figure 2–17   Water Molecules and Solutions.
(a) In a water molecule, oxygen forms polar covalent bonds with two hydrogen atoms. Because the hydrogen atoms are positioned toward one end of the molecule, the molecule has an uneven distribution of charges that creates positive and negative poles. **(b)** Ionic compounds dissociate in water as the polar water molecules disrupt the ionic bonds. Each ion in solution is surrounded by water molecules, creating hydration spheres. **(c)** Hydration spheres also form around an organic molecule containing polar covalent bonds. If the molecule is small, it will be carried into solution, as shown here with glucose.

A solution containing anions and cations will conduct an electrical current: cations (+) move toward the negative terminal, and anions (−) move toward the positive terminal (Figure 2–18). Electrical forces across cell membranes affect the functioning of all cells, and small electrical currents carried by ions are essential to muscle contraction and nerve function.

Soluble inorganic compounds whose ions will conduct an electrical current in solution are called **electrolytes** (ē-LEK-trō-līts). Sodium ions (Na^+), potassium ions (K^+), calcium ions (Ca^{2+}), and chloride ions (Cl^-) are released by the dissociation of electrolytes in blood and other body fluids. Table 2–5 contains a more complete listing of important electrolytes found in the human body and the ions released by their dissociation. Alterations in the body fluid concentrations of these ions will disturb almost every vital function. For example, declining potassium levels will lead to a general muscular paralysis, and rising concentrations will cause weak and irregular heartbeats. The concentrations of ions in body fluids are carefully regulated, primarily by coordinating activities at the kidneys (excretion of ions), the digestive tract (absorption of ions), and the skeletal system (storage or release of ions).

Organic molecules often contain polar covalent bonds, which also attract water molecules. The hydration spheres that form then carry these molecules into solution. Molecules that readily associate with water molecules are called **hydrophilic** (hī-drō-FI-lik; Greek *hydro-*, water + *philos*, loving). Molecules that do not readily associate with water are called **hydrophobic** (hī-drō-FŌ-bik; Greek *hydro-*, water + *phobos*, fear). Hydrophobic molecules have few if any polar covalent bonds. When placed in contact with water molecules, hydration spheres do not form and the molecules do not dissolve. Body fat deposits consist of large insoluble droplets of hydrophobic molecules trapped in the watery interior of cells. Gasoline, heating oil, and diesel fuel are examples of hydrophobic molecules not found in the body.

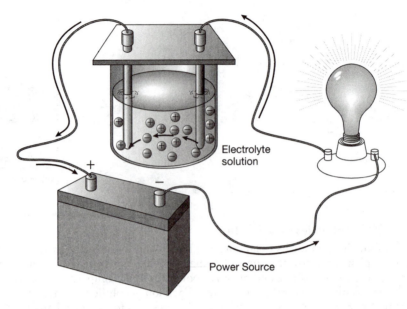

Figure 2–18   Electrolytes.
Because solutions containing electrolytes contain positive and negative ions, they are capable of conducting an electrical current.

Colloids and Suspensions

Body fluids may contain large and complex organic molecules, such as proteins and protein complexes, that are held in solution by their association with water molecules, as in Figure 2–19. A solution containing dispersed proteins or other large molecules is called a **colloid.** Liquid and solid gelatin are familiar examples of a rather viscous (thick) colloid. The particles or molecules in a colloid will remain in solution indefinitely. A **suspension** contains even larger particles that will, if undisturbed, settle out of solution because of the force of gravity. Stirring beach sand into a bucket of water creates a temporary suspension that ends as the sand settles to the bottom. Whole blood is an example of a suspension because the cells circulating in the bloodstream are suspended in the plasma. If clotting is prevented, the cells in a blood sample will settle to the bottom of the container.

Salts

A **salt** is an ionic compound consisting of a cation that is not a hydrogen ion (H^+) and an anion that is not a hydroxide ion (OH^-). Because they are held together by ionic bonds, many salts ionize completely in water, releasing cations and anions. For example, sodium chloride, or table salt, immediately ionizes into Na^+ and Cl^- when placed in water.

Table 2–5	Important Electrolytes That Dissociate in Body Fluids			
NaCl (sodium chloride)	$\rightarrow$	Na^+	+	Cl^-
KCl (potassium chloride)	$\rightarrow$	K^+	+	Cl^-
CaCl$_2$ (calcium chloride)	$\rightarrow$	Ca^{2+}	+	$2Cl^-$
NaHCO$_3$ (sodium bicarbonate)	$\rightarrow$	Na^+	+	HCO_3^-
MgCl$_2$ (magnesium chloride)	$\rightarrow$	Mg^{2+}	+	$2Cl^-$
Na2HPO4 (disodium phosphate)	$\rightarrow$	$2Na^+$	+	HPO_4^{2-}
Na$_2$SO$_4$ (sodium sulfate)	$\rightarrow$	$2Na^+$	+	SO_4^{2-}

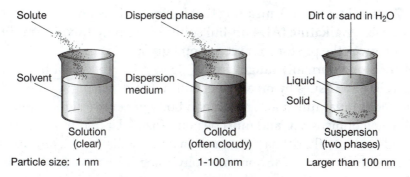

Figure 2–19   Solutions, Suspensions, Colloids.
(a) A solution is a uniform mixture containing a solute dissolved in a solvent. (b) If the particles in solution are large, such as proteins, the mixture is called a colloid. (c) Very large particles form a suspension. If left undisturbed, these particles will eventually settle out of solution.

Sodium and chloride are the most abundant ions in body fluids. However, many other ions are present in lesser amounts released by the ionization of various other compounds.

Hydrogen Ions in Body Fluids

The concentration of hydrogen ions (H^+) in body fluids is precisely regulated. Hydrogen ions are extremely reactive in solution; in excessive numbers they can break chemical bonds, change the shapes of complex molecules, and disrupt cell and tissue functions.

A few hydrogen ions are normally present, even in a sample of pure water, because some of the water molecules dissociate, releasing cations and anions. The dissociation of water is a reversible reaction that can be represented as:

$$H_2O \rightleftharpoons H^+ + OH^-$$

The dissociation of a water molecule yields a hydrogen ion (H^+) and a **hydroxide** (hī-DROK-sīd) **ion, OH$^-$**. Very few water molecules ionize in pure water, and the number of hydrogen and hydroxide ions is very small. A liter of pure water contains around 0.0000001 (10^{-7}) moles of hydrogen ions and an equal number of hydroxide ions. (A mole is a quantity of items. Just as there are 12 items in a dozen, there are 6.02×10^{23} items in one mole [mol]). In other words, the concentration of hydrogen ions in that solution is 0.0000001 moles per liter. This can be written:

$$[H^+] = 1 \times 10^{-7} \text{ mol/l}$$

The brackets around H^+ indicate "the concentration of," another example of chemical notation.

The hydrogen ion concentration is so important to physiological processes that a special shorthand is used to express it. The **pH** of a solution is defined as the negative logarithm of the hydrogen ion concentration expressed in moles per liter. Thus, instead of using the above expression, we would state that the pH of pure water is –(–7), or 7. (The logarithm is the exponent of 10, –7 in this case, and it is multiplied by a –1 as per the definition of pH.) This shorthand saves space, but you must always remember that the pH number is an exponent. Thus a pH of 6, for example ($[H^+] = 1 \times 10^{-6}$, or 0.000001), means that the concentration of hydrogen ions is 10 times as great as it is at a pH of 7 ($[H^+] = 1 \times 10^{-7}$, or 0.0000001).

Although pure water has a pH of 7, solutions display a wide range of pH values (0 to 14), depending on the nature of the solutes involved. A solution with a pH of 7 is neutral because it contains equal numbers of hydrogen and hydroxide ions. A solution with a pH below 7 is **acidic** (a-SI-dik), meaning that hydrogen ions predominate. A pH above 7 indicates a basic, or **alkaline** (AL-kuh-lin) solution, with hydroxide ions in the majority. Figure 2–20 gives the pH for some common liquids.

The pH of blood normally ranges from 7.35 to 7.45. Abnormal fluctuations in pH can damage cells and tissues by breaking chemical bonds, changing the shapes of proteins, or altering cellular function. The human body generates significant quantities of acids that threaten homeostasis and must be neutralized. Under unusual circumstances, the loss of acids in body fluids may promote an equally disruptive increase in pH.

The term **acidosis** refers to an abnormal physiological state caused by low blood pH (below 7.35); a pH below 7 can produce coma. **Alkalosis** results from an abnormally high pH (above 7.45); a blood pH above 7.8 usually causes uncontrollable, sustained skeletal muscle contractions.

Inorganic Acids and Bases

The body contains both inorganic and organic acids and bases. We will discuss acids and bases here because the inorganic acids and bases generated in the body are often responsible for producing acidosis or alkalosis.

An **acid** is any solute that dissociates to release hydrogen ions. Because a hydrogen atom that loses its electron consists solely of a proton, hydrogen ions are often referred to simply as protons, and acids as "proton donors." A strong acid ionizes completely, and the reaction is essentially one-way. Hydrochloric acid (HCl) is an excellent example, for in water it ionizes as:

$$HCl \longrightarrow H^+ + Cl^-$$

The stomach produces this powerful acid to assist in breakdown of food. Hardware stores sell HCl, as "muriatic acid," for cleaning sidewalks and swimming pools.

A **base** is a solute that removes hydrogen ions from a solution. Many common bases are compounds that dissociate in solution to liberate a hydroxide ion. Hydroxide ions have a strong affinity for hydrogen ions and quickly react with them, tying them up in water molecules. For example, sodium hydroxide, NaOH, is a strong base, because in solution it

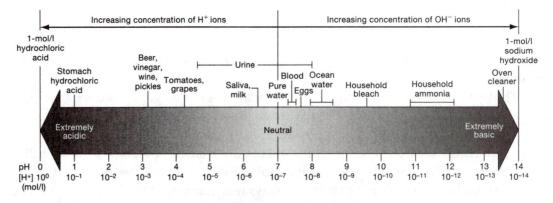

Figure 2–20   pH and Hydrogen Ion Concentration.
Note that the scale is logarithmic; an increase or decrease of one unit corresponds to a 10-fold change in H^+ concentration.

ionizes completely. The reaction that releases sodium and hydroxide ions can be written as:

$$NaOH \longrightarrow Na^+ + OH^-$$

Strong bases have a variety of industrial and household uses; drain openers and lye are two familiar examples.

Weak acids and weak bases fail to ionize completely, and a significant number of molecules remain intact. For the same number of molecules in solution, weak acids and weak bases therefore have less of an impact on pH than do strong acids and strong bases. Carbonic acid (H_2CO_3) which forms when carbon dioxide dissolves in water, is an example of a weak acid found in body fluids.

Buffers and pH Control

Buffers are compounds that stabilize the pH of a solution by removing or replacing hydrogen ions. Buffers and buffer systems in body fluids maintain pH within normal limits: Figure 2–20 includes the pH of several body fluids. Buffer systems typically involve a weak acid and its related salt, which functions as a weak base. For example, the carbonic acid–bicarbonate buffer system consists of carbonic acid and its disassociation products, a hydrogen ion and a bicarbonate ion. The reaction consists of: $H_2CO_3 \longrightarrow H^+ + HCO_3^-$. When there are excess hydrogen ions in body fluids such as blood, they can combine with bicarbonate ions to form carbonic acid, which then dissociates into carbon dioxide and water as shown below.

$$H^+ + HCO_3^- \longrightarrow H_2CO_3 \longrightarrow CO_2 + H_2O$$

The bicarbonate ion acts as a base and removes the hydrogen ion from solution. This action prevents hydrogen ions from accumulating and lowering the pH. On the other hand, if there is excess base the carbonic acid removes the excess hydroxide ions as shown below.

$$H_2CO_3 \longrightarrow H^+ + HCO_3^- + OH^- \longrightarrow H_2O + HCO_3^-$$

In this case the bicarbonate buffer prevents an increase in the pH.

Antacids such as Alka-Seltzer® and Rolaids® use sodium bicarbonate to neutralize excess hydrochloric acid in the stomach. The effects of neutralization are most evident when you add a strong acid to a strong base. For example, adding hydrochloric acid to sodium hydroxide results in the neutralization of both the strong acid and the strong base.

$$HCl + NaOH \longrightarrow H_2O + NaCl$$

This reaction produces water and a salt, in this case sodium chloride.

Let's Review What You've Just Learned

▶ Definitions

In the space provided, write the term for each of the following definitions.

_____ **100.** A solute that dissociates in water to release hydrogen ions.

_____ **101.** A homogeneous mixture.

_____ **102.** The negative logarithm of the hydrogen ion concentration in a solution.

_____ **103.** The term for molecules that do not readily associate with water.

_____ 104. Essential elements and molecules obtained from the diet.

_____ 105. A solution containing dispersed proteins or other large molecules.

_____ 106. A compound that stabilizes the pH of a solution by removing or replacing hydrogen ions.

_____ 107. All of the molecules synthesized or broken down by chemical reactions in the body.

_____ 108. A solute that removes hydrogen ions from solution.

_____ 109. The process by which ionic bonds are broken and individual ions interact with water molecules.

_____ 110. Compounds whose structure is not primarily determined by the linking together of carbon atoms.

_____ 111. A term for solutions containing a majority of hydroxide ions.

_____ 112. A substance dispersed in a solvent.

_____ 113. Compounds whose structure is determined primarily by the linking together of carbon atoms.

_____ 114. An ion with a single positive or negative charge.

_____ 115. An ionic compound that consists of a cation that is not a hydrogen ion and an anion that is not a hydroxide ion.

_____ 116. A zone of water molecules that surrounds ions in solution.

_____ 117. A substance's ability to absorb and retain heat.

_____ 118. A liquid mixture containing large particles that will settle on standing.

_____ 119. The term for a molecule that will readily associate with water.

_____ 120. An abnormal physiological state caused by low blood pH.

_____ 121. A medium in which atoms, ions, or molecules of another substance are dispersed to form a solution.

_____ 122. A substance that forms ions in solution producing a solution that will conduct electricity.

_____ 123. An abnormal physiological state that results from an abnormally high blood pH.

_____ 124. A solution in which water is the solvent.

► Completion

Answer or complete each of the following items.

125. Why is water such an important compound in human bodies?

    a. _____

    b. _____

    c. _____

    d. _____

126. Which of the following substances would be the stronger acid: solution A (pH = 6.0) or solution B (pH = 4.5)? _____

☑ Self-Check Test

The following test will allow you to determine how well you have mastered the vocabulary and basic concepts of this chapter. It will also help you prepare for the type of questions you are likely to encounter on a test in an anatomy and physiology course. The self-check test will help you assess your understanding of the chapter material, and will help you develop good test-taking skills.

The following questions test your ability to use vocabulary and to recall facts.

1. A nanometer is
   a. 10^{-6} meter
   b. 10^{-8} meter
   c. 10^{-9} meter
   d. 10^{-10} meter
   e. 10^{-12} meter
2. The smallest chemical units of matter are
   a. atoms
   b. molecules
   c. protons
   d. neutrons
   e. electrons
3. Isotopes of an element differ in the number of
   a. protons in the nucleus
   b. electrons in the nucleus
   c. neutrons in the nucleus
   d. electron clouds
   e. energy levels they contain
4. The atomic number of an element represents the number of
   a. protons in an atom of the element
   b. electrons in an ion
   c. neutrons in an atom of the element
   d. protons and neutrons in an atom of the element
   e. neutrons and electrons in an atom of the element
5. The chemical behavior of an atom is determined by
   a. the number of protons
   b. the number of neutrons
   c. the number and arrangement of electrons
   d. the size of the atom
   e. the mass of the atom
6. Ions with a positive charge are called
   a. cations
   b. anions
   c. radical ions
   d. polyatomic ions

7. Ionic bonds are formed when
   a. atoms share electrons
   b. electrons are completely transferred from one atom to another
   c. a pair of electrons is shared unequally by two atoms
   d. hydrogen forms bonds with negatively charged atoms in the same or a different molecule
   e. two or more atoms lose electrons at the same time

8. If a pair of electrons is unequally shared between two atoms, a _____ occurs.
   a. single covalent bond
   b. double covalent bond
   c. triple covalent bond
   d. polar covalent bond
   e. hydrogen bond

9. Which of the following statements about the reaction $H_2 + Cl_2 \longrightarrow 2\,HCl$ is not correct?
   a. H_2 and Cl_2 are the reactants
   b. HCl is the product
   c. one molecule of hydrogen contains two atoms
   d. two molecules of HCl are formed in the reaction
   e. one mole of chlorine molecules contains one mole of chlorine atoms

10. The reaction in Question 9 is an example of a(n)
    a. exchange reaction
    b. synthesis reaction
    c. decomposition reaction
    d. equilibrium reaction
    e. enzyme-catalyzed reaction

11. Chemical reactions that require an input of energy, such as heat, are said to be
    a. endergonic
    b. exergonic
    c. energy neutral
    d. in equilibrium
    e. enzyme-catalyzed

12. Energy that is stored is called
    a. kinetic energy
    b. potential energy

13. Light is a example of
    a. chemical energy
    b. electrical energy
    c. electromagnetic energy
    d. mechanical energy
    e. nuclear energy

14. The random motion of atoms and molecules results in
    a. electrical energy
    b. thermal energy
    c. chemical energy
    d. electromagnetic energy
    e. mechanical energy

15. Each of the following is an example of an inorganic compound except one. Identify the exception.

    a. water

    b. acids

    c. bases

    d. salts

    e. enzymes

16. Which of the following statements about water is not correct?

    a. Water is composed of polar molecules.

    b. Water accounts for about two-thirds of the mass of the human body.

    c. Water has a relatively low heat capacity.

    d. Water will dissolve many compounds.

    e. Water molecules can attach to each other by hydrogen bonds.

17. If a solution has a pH that is greater than 7, it is

    a. neutral

    b. acidic

    c. alkaline

    d. a buffer

    e. a salt solution

The following questions are more challenging and require you to synthesize the information that you have learned in this chapter.

18. Elements that have seven electrons in their outermost shell

    a. will usually form cations

    b. will usually form anions

    c. will not form any compounds

    d. will generally form hydrogen bonds

    e. will most likely transfer electrons to other atoms

19. Magnesium atoms have two electrons in the outermost shell and chlorine atoms have seven. The compound magnesium chloride would contain

    a. 1 magnesium and 1 chlorine

    b. 1 magnesium and 2 chlorine

    c. 2 magnesium and 1 chlorine

    d. 2 magnesium and 7 chlorine

    e. impossible to tell without more information

20. When a small amount of hydrochloric acid is added to a solution of Na_2HPO_4, the pH of the solution does not change. The pH does not change when a small amount of NaOH is added either. On the basis of these observations, the compound Na_2HPO_4 is

    a. able to accept extra hydrogen ions from HCl

    b. able to donate hydrogen ions to the OH^- from NaOH

    c. acting as a buffer

    d. a salt formed from reacting a strong base with a weak acid

    e. all of the above

☑ Self-Assessment

If your score was

between 18 and 20, you are ready to proceed to the next chapter.

between 15 and 17, you have a good general idea of the chapter content, but you should review sections of the chapter that deal with items that you missed before proceeding to the next chapter.

less than 14, you have not mastered the chapter content well enough to proceed. Reread the chapter and rework the exercises. Then retake the self-check test. Repeat this process until you achieve a score that will allow you to continue.

Answers

1. gram
2. liter
3. meter
4. mole
5. Kelvin
6. milliliter
7. milligram
8. centimeter
9. kilogram
10. deciliter
11. 10^{-3} second
12. 10^{-6} gram
13. 10^{-3} meter
14. 10^{-9} meter
15. 1000 liters
16. isotopes
17. chemical elements
18. matter
19. half-life
20. atomic mass
21. mass
22. atoms
23. nucleus
24. atomic weight
25. weight
26. atomic number
27. atomic mass unit (amu), or dalton
28. energy level
29. subatomic particles
30. O
31. N
32. potassium
33. calcium
34. Na
35. carbon
36. hydrogen
37. S
38. phosphorus
39. Cl
40. Mg
41. iodine
42. iron
43. 1; +
44. 1; 0

45. 1/1836; -
46. protons = 6 electrons = 6 neutrons = 8 mass number = 14
47. protons = 2 electrons = 2 neutrons = 8 mass number = 14
48. protons = 11 electrons = 11 neutrons = 13 mass number = 24
49. free radical
50. ion
51. compound
52. hydrogen bond
53. cation
54. anion
55. molecule
56. ionic bond
57. covalent bond
58. polar
59. hydrogen bonds
60. metabolism
61. products
62. equilibrium
63. reactants
64. hydrolysis
65. S (synthesis)
66. D (decomposition)
67. E (exchange)
68. N_2
69. $C_{12}H_{22}O_{11}$
70. HCl
71. catabolism
72. energy
73. wavelength
74. enzymes
75. exergonic
76. work
77. electrical energy
78. anabolism
79. kinetic energy
80. heat energy
81. endergonic
82. potential energy
83. activation energy
84. electromagnetic energy
85. temperature

86. frequency
87. catalyst
88. ultraviolet radiation
89. chemical energy
90. hertz
91. calorie
92. volt
93. pathway
94. electromagnetic spectrum
95. infrared radiation
96. potential energy
97. kinetic
98. inverse
99. repel; attract
100. acid
101. solution
102. pH
103. hydrophobic
104. nutrients
105. colloid
106. buffer
107. metabolites
108. base
109. ionization
110. inorganic compounds

111. alkaline
112. solute
113. organic compounds
114. monovalent ion
115. salt
116. hydration sphere
117. heat capacity
118. suspension
119. hydrophilic
120. acidosis
121. solvent
122. electrolyte
123. alkalosis
124. aqueous solution
125. a. Water is a medium for most chemical reactions.
     b. Water has a very high heat capacity.
     c. Water is an effective lubricant.
     d. Water is an excellent solvent.
126. solution B

Answers to Self-Check Test

1. c 2. a 3. c 4. a 5. c 6. a 7. b 8. d 9. e 10. b 11. a
12. b 13. c 14. b 15. e 16. c 17. c 18. b 19. b 20. e

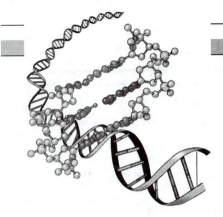

CHAPTER 3

An Introduction to Organic Compounds

The molecules that make up our cells, tissues, and body parts and control their functions are organic compounds. **Organic compounds** are compounds whose structure is determined primarily by the linking together of carbon atoms. Organic molecules often contain long chains of carbon atoms linked by covalent bonds. These carbon atoms typically form additional covalent bonds with hydrogen or oxygen atoms and less often with nitrogen, phosphorus, sulfur, iron, or other elements.

Many organic molecules are soluble in water. Simple sugars such as glucose dissolve readily in water, and they are rapidly distributed throughout the body by the blood and other body fluids. Although the discussion in the preceding chapter focused on inorganic acids and bases, there are also important organic acids and bases. For example, lactic acid is an organic acid generated by active muscle tissues that must be neutralized by the buffers in body fluids.

There are four major classes of organic compounds found in the human body: carbohydrates, lipids, proteins, and nucleic acids (Figure 3–1). In addition, the human body contains small quantities of many other organic molecules whose structures and functions will be considered in later chapters.

CARBOHYDRATES

A **carbohydrate** (kar-bō-HĪ-drāt; *carbo-*, carbon + *hydra-*, water) molecule contains atoms of carbon, hydrogen, and oxygen in a ratio near 1:2:1. Familiar carbohydrates include the sugars and starches that make up roughly half of the typical American diet. Our tissues can break down many carbohydrates, and, although they may have other functions, carbohydrates are most important as sources of energy. We will focus on three groups of carbohydrates: monosaccharides, disaccharides, and polysaccharides.

Monosaccharides

A **simple sugar**, or **monosaccharide** (mon-ō-SAK-uh-rīd; Greek *monos*, alone + *sakchar*, sugar), is a carbohydrate containing from three to seven carbon atoms. A simple sugar may be called a **triose** (three-carbon), **tetrose** (four-carbon), **pentose** (five-carbon), **hexose** (six-carbon), or **heptose** (seven-carbon). The hexose **glucose** (GLOO-kōs), $C_6H_{12}O_6$,

(a) Carbohydrates such as sugars and starches are sources of energy for cells

(b) Lipids such as triglycerides function in energy storage

(c) Proteins are important components of many body tissues, like muscle

(d) Nucleic acids function in the storage of information and controlling the synthesis of proteins

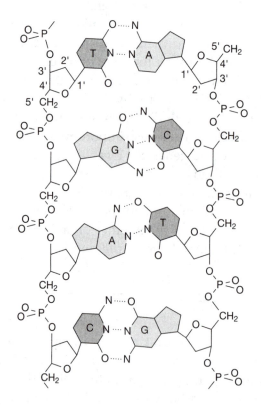

Figure 3–1   Four Major Classes of Biological Molecules.

(a) Carbohydrate. (b) Lipid. (c) Protein. (d) Nucleic acid. C, A, T and G = Cytosine, Adenine, Thymine and Guanine, three nitrogenous bases.

is the most important metabolic "fuel" in the body. The arrangement of the atoms, which determines the specific shape of each molecule, is shown by the **structural formula**. Figure 3–2 diagrams the structure of a glucose molecule in several ways. The straight-chain

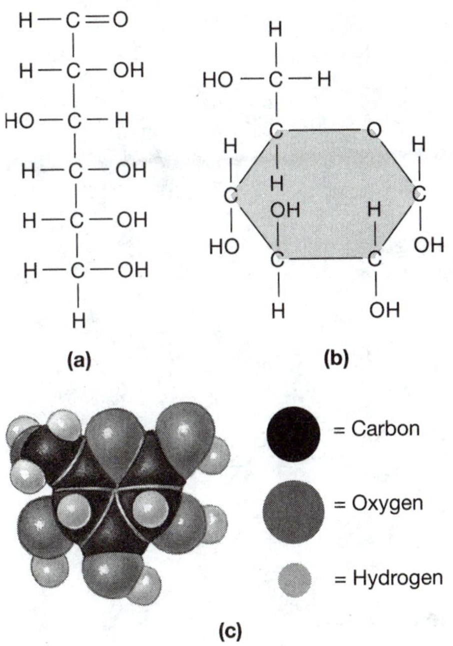

Figure 3-2   Different Ways to Represent a Glucose Molecule.
(a) The straight-chain structural formula. (b) The ring form that is most common in nature. (c) A space-filling model that shows the actual three-dimensional organization of the atoms in the ring.

form (Figure 3–2a) shows the component atoms clearly, but in the body the ring form (Figure 3–2b) is more common. The actual arrangement of atoms in three dimensions is shown most realistically in a space-filling model (Figure 3–2c).

It is important to note that each organic molecule has a specific three-dimensional shape and that molecular shape is an important characteristic. **Isomers** are molecules that have the same chemical formula but different structural formulas. That is, the molecules have different shapes. Although the molecules contain the same atoms, those atoms are bonded together in different arrangements. The body generally treats different isomers as distinct molecules, and they have different chemical properties and are metabolized differently. For example, the simple sugars glucose and fructose are isomers. **Fructose** is found in many fruits and in secretions of the male reproductive tract. Although its chemical formula is the same as that of glucose, the atoms are arranged differently and the two molecules have different shapes. As a result, separate enzymes and reaction sequences control the breakdown and synthesis of glucose and fructose.

Disaccharides and Polysaccharides

Carbohydrates other than simple sugars are complex molecules composed of monosaccharide building blocks. Two simple sugars join together for a **disaccharide** (dī-SAK-uh-rīd; Greek *dis*, twice). Disaccharides such as **sucrose** (table sugar) have a sweet taste, and they are also quite water- soluble. Figure 3–3a diagrams the reaction responsible for the formation of sucrose. This reaction is an example of **dehydration synthesis**, the linking together of chemical units by the removal of water to create a more complex molecule. The reverse of this process, shown in Figure 3–3b, is an example of hydrolysis, a process introduced in Chapter 2.

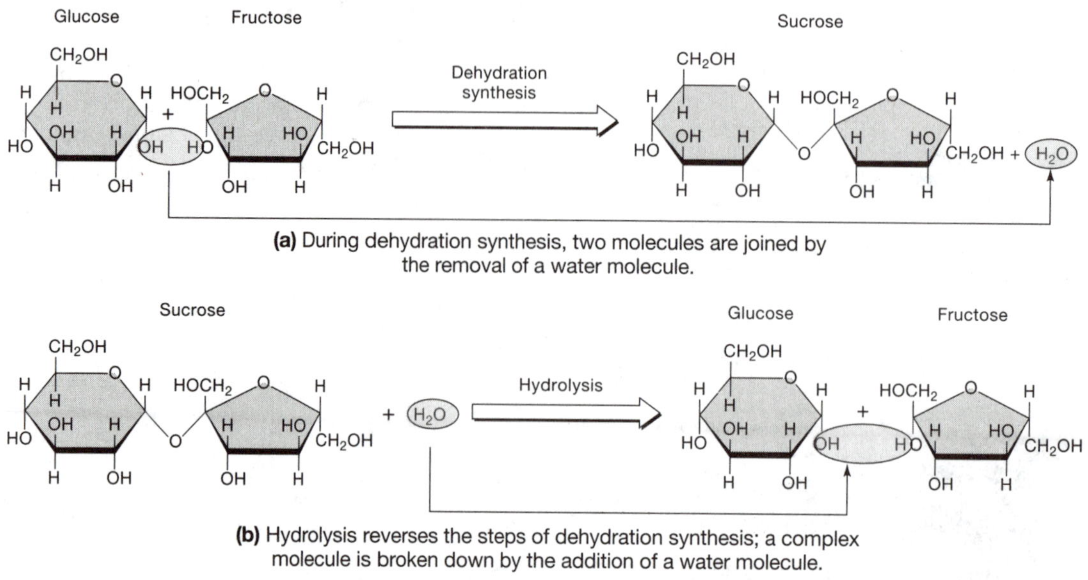

Glucose   Fructose   Sucrose

(a) During dehydration synthesis, two molecules are joined by
the removal of a water molecule.

Sucrose   Glucose   Fructose

(b) Hydrolysis reverses the steps of dehydration synthesis; a complex
molecule is broken down by the addition of a water molecule.

Figure 3–3   The Formation and Breakdown of Complex Sugars.
(a) During dehydration synthesis, two molecules are joined by the removal of a water molecule.
(b) Hydrolysis reverses the steps of dehydration synthesis; a complex molecule is broken down by
the addition of a water molecule.

Many foods contain disaccharides, but they must be disassembled by hydrolysis before their monosaccharide subunits can be broken down to provide useful energy. Most popular "junk foods," such as candies and sodas, abound in simple sugars (often fructose) and disaccharides such as sucrose. Some people cannot tolerate sugar for medical reasons; others avoid it in an effort to control their weight. (Excess sugars are converted to fat for long-term storage.) Many of these people are using artificial sweeteners in their foods and beverages. These compounds have a very sweet taste, but either they cannot be broken down in the body or they are used in insignificant amounts. Nutrasweet and saccharin are the two most popular artificial sweeteners in current use.

The process of dehydration synthesis can continue adding monosaccharides to each other or combining disaccharides to create very complex molecules. These large molecules are called **polysaccharides** (pol-ē-SAK-uh-rīdz; Greek *polys*, many). Polysaccharide chains may be straight or highly branched (Figure 3–4). **Starches** are glucose-based polysaccharides. Most starches are manufactured by plants. The digestive tract can break these molecules into simple sugars, and starches such as those found in potatoes and grains represent a major dietary energy source. **Cellulose**, a structural component of many plants, is a polysaccharide that our bodies cannot digest at all. Cellulose makes up most of the bulk or fiber in the human diet.

Glycogen (GLĪ-kō-jen), or animal starch, is a branched polysaccharide composed of interconnected glucose molecules. Like most other large polysaccharides, glycogen will not dissolve in water or other body fluids. Liver and muscle tissues manufacture and store large quantities of glycogen. When these tissues have a high demand for energy, glycogen molecules are broken down into glucose; when demands are low, the tissues absorb glucose and rebuild glycogen reserves.

Despite their metabolic importance, carbohydrates account for less than 3 percent of our total body weight. Table 3–1 summarizes information concerning the carbohydrates.

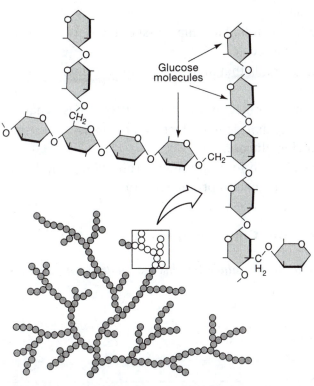

Figure 3–4   Structure of a Polysaccharide.
Liver and muscle cells store glucose as the polysaccharide glycogen, a long, branching chain of glucose molecules. This figure introduces a different method of representing a carbon ring structure; at each corner of the solid hexagon is a carbon atom. The position of an oxygen atom in each glucose ring is shown.

Table 3–1   Carbohydrates in the Body

Structure	Example(s)	Primary Function	Remarks
Monosaccharides (simple sugars)	Glucose, fructose	Energy source	Manufactured in the body and obtained from food; found in body fluids
Disaccharides	Sucrose, lactose, maltose	Energy source	Sucrose is table sugar, lactose is present in milk; all must be broken down to monosaccharides before absorption
Polysaccharides	Glycogen	Storage of glucose molecules	Glycogen is found in animal cells; other starches and cellulose occur in plant cells.

Let's Review What You've Just Learned

► Definitions

In the space provided, write the term for each of the following definitions.

_____ **1.** Molecules that have the same chemical formula but different structural formulas.

_____ **2.** A carbohydrate that is formed by joining together many monosaccharides.

_____ **3.** An organic compound that contains the elements carbon, hydrogen, and oxygen in a ratio that approximates 1:2:1.

_____ **4.** A disaccharide formed by combining glucose and fructose; also known as table sugar.

_____ **5.** A large, undigestible polysaccharide that is a structural component of plants.

_____ **6.** A simple sugar.

_____ **7.** A polysaccharide found in animal tissues that serves as an energy-storage molecule.

_____ **8.** A chemical formula that indicates the arrangement of atoms in a molecule.

_____ **9.** A carbohydrate formed by the union of two monosaccharides.

_____ **10.** A large polysaccharide manufactured by plants for the purpose of storing glucose.

_____ **11.** A monosaccharide found in many fruits, "junk food," and secretions of the male reproductive tract.

▶ **Word Roots, Prefixes, Suffixes, and Combining Forms**

In the space provided, list the boldfaced terms introduced in this section that contain the indicated word part.

Word Part	Meaning	Examples
tri-	three	**12.** _____
poly-	many	**13.** _____
glyco-	sugar	**14.** _____
hex-	six	**15.** _____
iso-	equal	**16.** _____
hept-	seven	**17.** _____
sacch-	sugar	**18.** _____
pent-	five	**19.** _____
tetr-	four	**20.** _____

▶ **Identification of Organic Molecules and Reactions**

In the space provided, identify the type of molecule that is shown or the type of reaction that is illustrated.

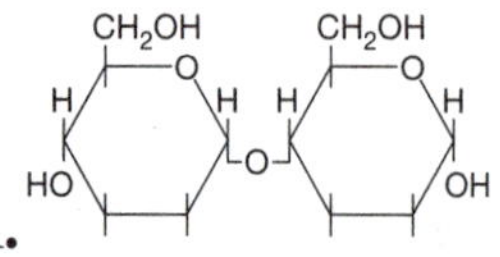

21.

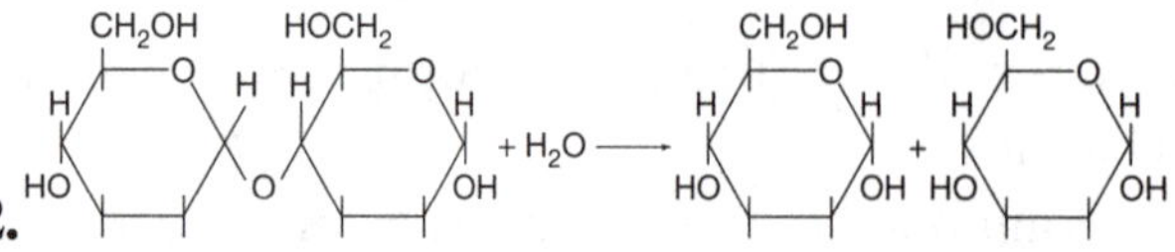

_____

22.

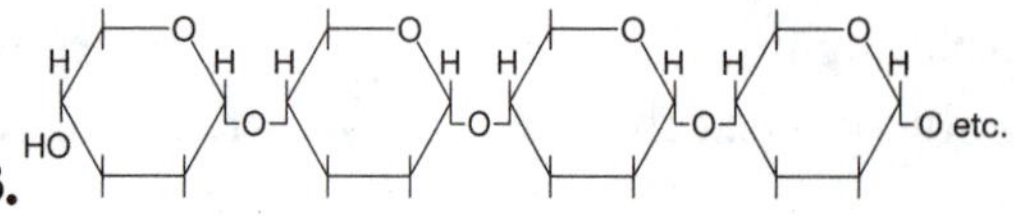

_____

23.

_____

24.

▶ Concept Mapping

Using the following terms, fill in the blank spaces next to the circled numbers to complete the concept map. Follow the numbers to comply with the organization of the map.

Monosaccharides	Sucrose	Complex carbohydrates
Glucose	Glycogen	Bulk, fiber
Disaccharides		

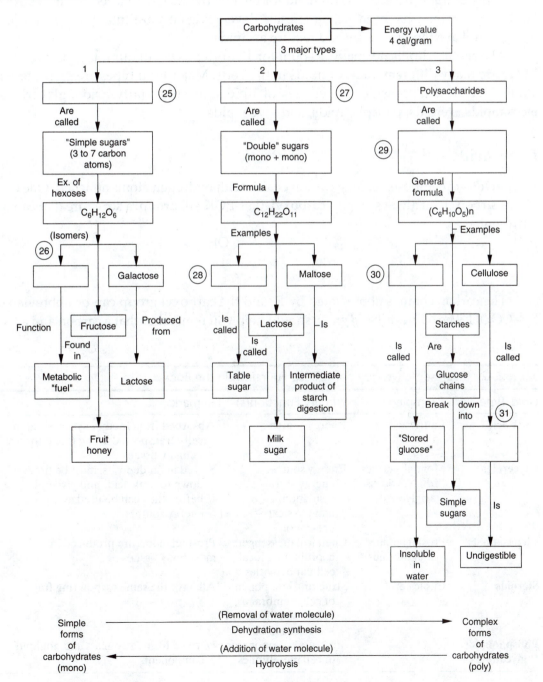

LIPIDS

Lipids (Greek *lipos*, fat) also contain the elements carbon, hydrogen, and oxygen, but the ratios do not approximate 1:2:1. In general, a lipid molecule contains much less oxygen than a carbohydrate having the same number of carbon atoms. In addition to carbon, hydrogen, and oxygen, lipids may contain small quantities of other elements, such as phosphorus, nitrogen, or sulfur. Familiar lipids include fats, oils, and waxes. Most lipids are insoluble in water, but special transport mechanisms exist to carry them in the circulating blood.

Lipids form essential structural components of all cells. In addition, lipid deposits are important as energy reserves, for on the average lipids provide roughly twice as much energy as carbohydrates, gram for gram, when broken down in the body. When the supply of lipids exceeds the demand for energy, the excess is stored in fat deposits. For this reason there has been great interest in developing fat substitutes that provide less energy but have the same taste and texture as lipids.

All together, lipids normally account for 12 to 15 percent of our total body weight. There are many different kinds of lipids in the body. Major lipid types are presented in Table 3–2. We will consider six classes of lipid molecules: fatty acids, glycerides, eicosanoids, steroids, phospholipids, and glycolipids.

Fatty Acids

Fatty acids are composed of long carbon chains with hydrogen atoms attached. One end of the carbon chain always bears a **carboxyl** (kar-BOK-sil) **group**, a structure that can be represented as

$$\underset{\text{R...}}{\qquad}\!\!-\!\!\underset{\text{C=O}}{\overset{\overset{\text{OH}}{|}}{}}$$

The carbon chain is abbreviated by *R*, and the carboxyl group can be abbreviated by –COOH. The name *carboxyl group* should help you remember that a carbon and a **hy-**

Table 3–2   Representative Lipids and Their Functions in the Body

Lipid Type	Example(s)	Primary Function(s)	Remarks
Fatty acids	Lauric acid	Energy source	Absorbed from food or synthesized in cells; transported in the blood for use in many tissues
Glycerides	Monoglycerides, diglycerides, triglycerides	Energy source; energy storage; insulation; and physical protection	Stored in fat deposits; must be broken down to fatty acids and glycerol before they can be used as an energy source
Eiconsanoids	Prostaglandins, leukotrienes	Chemical messengers coordinating local cellular activities	Prostaglandins are produced in most body tissues
Steroids	Cholesterol	Structural component of cell membranes, hormones, digestive secretions in bile	All have the same carbon ring frame
Phospholipids, glycolipids		Structural components of cell membranes	Derived from fatty acids and nonlipid components

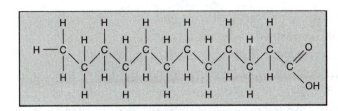

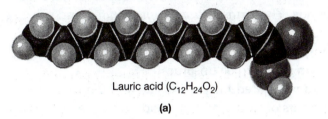

Lauric acid (C$_{12}$H$_{24}$O$_2$)

(a)

Figure 3–5 Fatty Acids.
(a) Lauric acid demonstrates two structural characteristics common to all fatty acids; a long backbone of carbon atoms and a carboxyllic acid group (–COOH) at one end. **(b)** A fatty acid may be saturated or unsaturated. Unsaturated fatty acids have double covalent bonds, and their presence causes a sharp bend in the molecule. **(c)** An omega-3 fatty acid has an unsaturated bond three carbons before the end of the carbon chain.

Saturated

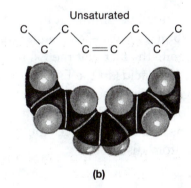

Unsaturated

(b)

Omega-3
double bond

Omega
carbon

#1
carbon

(c)

droxyl (**–OH**) group are the important structural features. Figure 3–5a shows a representative fatty acid, *lauric acid*.

In a fatty acid, the polar covalent bond between the oxygen and hydrogen atoms of the carboxyl group breaks down in solution, releasing a hydrogen ion. This reaction can be summarized as:

$$R \ldots - \overset{\displaystyle \overset{OH}{|}}{C}{=}O \longrightarrow R \ldots - \overset{\displaystyle \overset{O^-}{|}}{C}{=}O + H^+$$

When a fatty acid is placed in solution, only its carboxyl end associates with water molecules, for this is the only hydrophilic portion of the molecule. The rest of the carbon chain is hydrophobic, so fatty acids have a very limited solubility in water.

In a **saturated fatty acid** each carbon atom in the hydrocarbon chain has four single covalent bonds (Figure 3–5b). If one of the carbon-to-carbon bonds is a double covalent bond, the fatty acid is said to be **unsaturated** (or **monounsaturated**). A **polyunsaturated fatty acid** contains multiple double bonds. The terms *saturated*, *unsaturated*, and *polyunsaturated* refer to the number of hydrogen atoms in the fatty acid. Replacing a double bond between carbon atoms with a single bond allows the molecule to accept two more hydrogens; hence a double-bonded chain is said to be unsaturated.

Saturated, unsaturated, and polyunsaturated fatty acids can all be broken down for energy. A diet containing large amounts of saturated fatty acids, however, increases the risk of heart disease and other circulatory problems. Butter, fatty meat, and ice cream are popular dietary sources of saturated fatty acids. Vegetable oils, such as olive oil and corn oil, contain a mixture of unsaturated and polyunsaturated fatty acids. Current research indicates that the monounsaturated fats may be more effective than polyunsaturated fats in lowering the risk of heart disease. In fact, the manufacture of margarine and vegetable shortening from polyunsaturated fats produces compounds called **trans fatty acids** that may actually increase the risk of heart disease. Increasing the proportion of oleic acid, an 18-carbon monounsaturated fatty acid, in cooking oils and other products could therefore yield health benefits.

The carbons in a fatty acid molecule are numbered beginning at the carboxyl end; the last carbon in the chain is called the **omega carbon** (Figure 3–5c). Eskimos have lower rates of heart disease than other populations, despite the fact that the Eskimo diet contains high quantities of fats and cholesterol. The fatty acids in the Eskimo diet have an unsaturated bond three carbons before the omega carbon, a position known as "omega minus 3," or omega-3. **Omega-3 fatty acids** are found in fish flesh and fish oils. For unknown reasons the presence of omega-3 fatty acids in the diet reduces the risks of heart disease, rheumatoid arthritis, and other inflammatory diseases.

Glycerides

Individual fatty acids cannot be strung together in a chain by dehydration, as simple sugars can. But they can be attached to another compound, **glycerol** (GLI-se-rōl), through a similar reaction. As illustrated in Figure 3–6, dehydration synthesis can produce a **monoglyceride** (mo-nō-GLI-se-rīd) consisting of glycerol plus one fatty acid. Subsequent reactions can yield a **diglyceride** (glycerol + two fatty acids), and then a **triglyceride** (glycerol + three fatty acids). Hydrolysis breaks the glycerides into fatty acids and glycerol. A comparison of Figure 3–3 with Figure 3–6 demonstrates the fact that dehydration synthesis and hydrolysis operate in the same way, whether the molecules involved are carbohydrates or lipids.

Triglycerides, otherwise known as **neutral fats**, have several important functions.

1. Fatty deposits in specialized sites represent a significant energy reserve. In times of need the triglycerides are disassembled to yield fatty acids that can be broken down to provide energy.

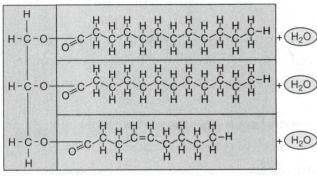

Figure 3–6 Triglyceride Formation.
The formation of a triglyceride involves the attachment of fatty acids to the carbons of a glycerol molecule. This example shows the formation of a triglyceride by the attachment of one unsaturated and two saturated fatty acids to a glycerol molecule.

2. Fat deposits under the skin serve as insulation, preventing heat loss to the environment. Heat loss across a layer of lipids is only about one-third of that through other tissues.

3. A fat deposit around a delicate organ such as a kidney provides a cushion that protects against shocks or blows.

Triglycerides are stored in the body as lipid droplets within cells. The lipids absorb and accumulate lipid-soluble vitamins, drugs, or toxins that appear in body fluids. This activity has both positive and negative effects. For example, the body's lipid reserves retain both valuable lipid-soluble vitamins (A, D, E, and K) and potentially dangerous lipid-soluble pesticides such as DDT.

Eicosanoids

Eicosanoids (ī-KŌ-sa-noydz; Greek *eicos*, twenty) are polyunsaturated fatty acids that contain 20 carbon atoms. They have a five-carbon ring at one end, and their overall shape resembles a hairpin (Figure 3–7). These compounds coordinate or direct local cellular activities and are often called "local hormones." (Hormones are chemical messengers produced at one site to regulate activities under way in a different part of the body.) Eicosanoids are extremely powerful and effective in minute quantities. Almost every tissue in the body contains eicosanoids, and the effects vary depending on the nature of the molecule and the site of release. Examples of important eicosanoids include the following:

Figure 3–7 Eicosanoids.
Prostaglandins, a type of eicosanoid, are unusual short-chain fatty acids. Compare the complete structural formula of a typical prostaglandin with the abbreviated formula.

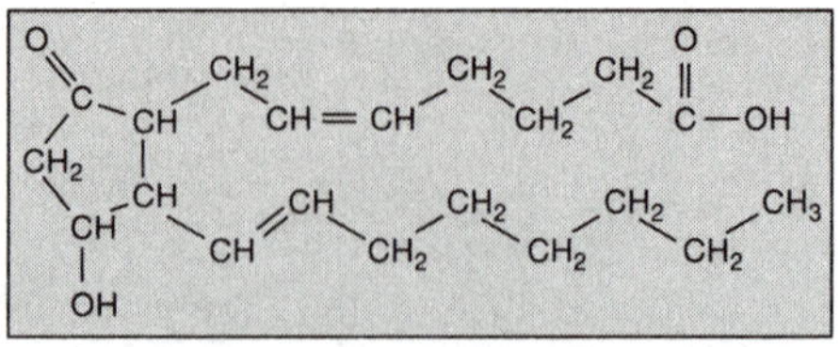

Complete structural formula

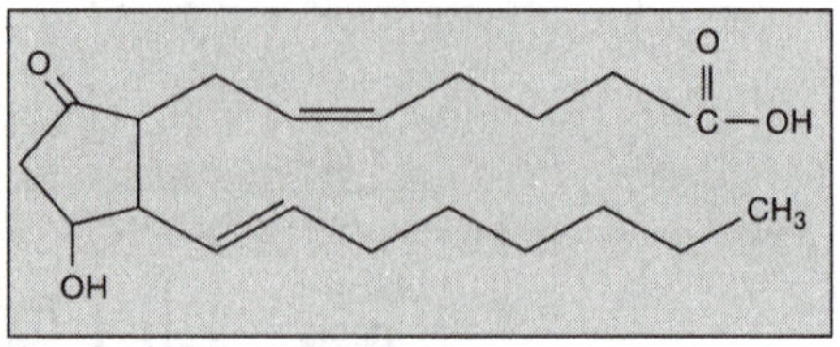

Abbreviated structural formula

- **Prostaglandins** (pros-tuh-GLAN-dinz) are produced in most tissues of the body and are involved primarily in coordinating local cellular activities. For example,
  1. Prostaglandins released by damaged tissues stimulate nerve endings and produce the sensation of pain.
  2. Prostaglandins released in the uterus help trigger the start of labor contractions.
  3. Prostaglandins released in the stomach may help prevent stomach ulcers.
- **Leukotrienes** (loo-kō-TRĪ-ēnz) are released by activated white blood cells called leukocytes (LOO-kō-sīts). Leukotrienes are important in coordinating tissue responses to injury or disease.
- **Thromboxanes** (throm-BOX-ānz) and **prostacyclins** (pros-ta-SĪ-klinz) are released by circulating platelets when blood clotting occurs. (Platelets are normal components of the blood and function in the process of blood clotting.)

Steroids

Steroids are large lipid molecules that share a distinctive carbon framework composed of four interconnected rings. They differ from one another in the chemical groups that are attached to this basic structure. Figure 3–8 shows the structural formulas for **cholesterol** (kō-LES-ter-ol; Greek *chole-*, bile + *stereos*, solid) and some other representative steroids. Cholesterol and related steroids are important for the following reasons:

- The membrane that surrounds each animal cell contains cholesterol. Cells need cholesterol to maintain their cell membranes over time, as well as for cell growth and division.
- Steroid hormones are involved in the regulation of sexual function. Examples include the male sex hormones, such as **testosterone**, and female sex hormones, such as the **estrogens**.
- Steroid hormones are important in the regulation of tissue metabolism and mineral balance. Examples include the hormones of the adrenal gland, called **corticosteroids**, and **calcitriol**, a hormone important in calcium ion regulation.
- Steroids called **bile salts** are required for the normal processing of dietary fats. Bile salts are produced in the liver and secreted in a liquid called bile. These steroids interact with lipids in the intestinal tract and facilitate their digestion and absorption.

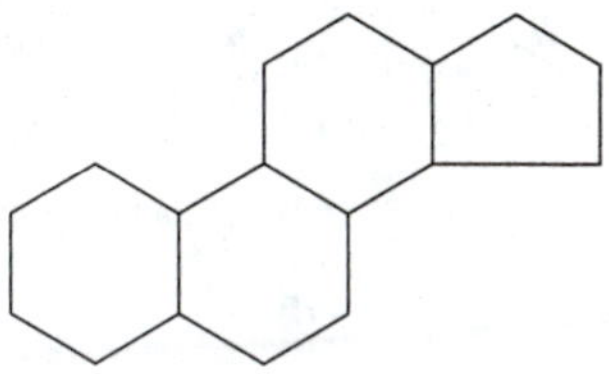

(a) Basic steroid ring structure

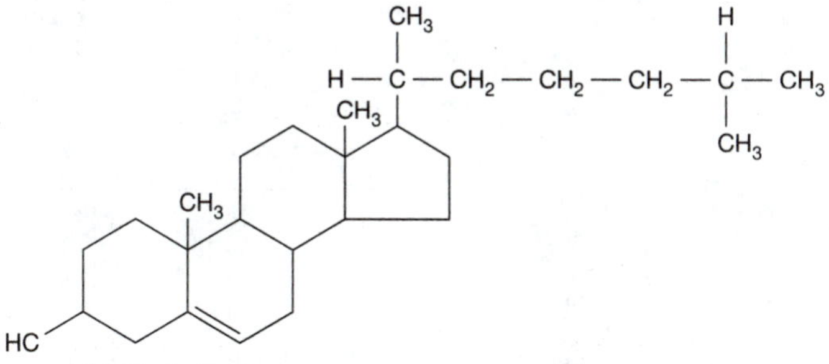

Figure 3–8 Steroids.
(a) All steroids share this complex
four-ring structure. Individual
steroids differ in the side chains attached to the carbon rings.
  (b) Cholesterol. **(c)** Testosterone.
(d) Estradiol.

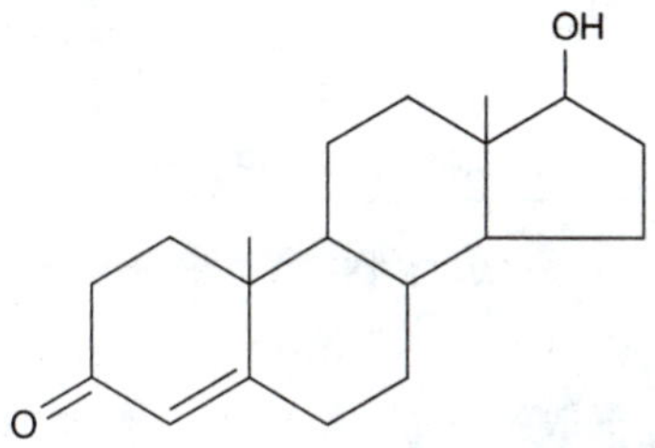

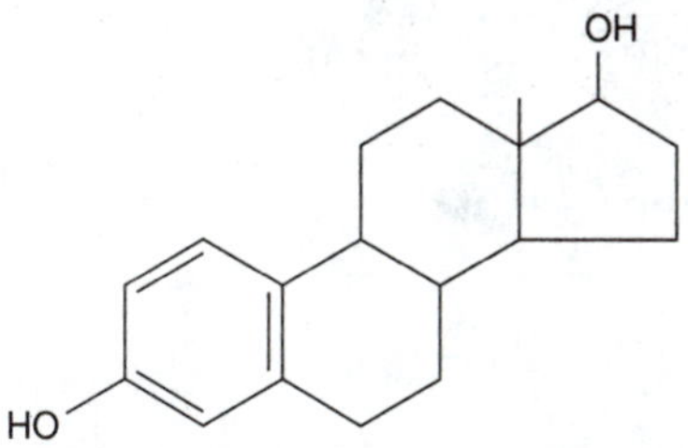

(b) Cholesterol

(c) Testosterone

(d) Estradiol

Cholesterol is obtained from two sources: (1) by absorption from the diet and (2) by synthesis within the body. Meat, cream, and egg yolks are especially rich dietary sources of cholesterol. A diet high in cholesterol can be harmful, because a strong link exists between high blood cholesterol levels and heart disease. Current nutritional advice suggests reducing cholesterol intake to under 300 mg per day; this represents a 40 percent reduction for the average American adult. Unfortunately, because the body can synthesize cholesterol as well, it is sometimes difficult to control blood cholesterol levels by dietary restriction alone.

Phospholipids and Glycolipids

Phospholipids (FOS-fō-lip-idz) and **glycolipids** (GLĪ-cō-lip-idz) are structurally related, and both can be synthesized from fatty acids. In a phospholipid (Figure 3–9a) a *phosphate group* (PO_4^{3-}) serves as a link between a diglyceride and a nonlipid group. In a glycolipid (Figure 3–9b) a carbohydrate is attached to a diglyceride. Note that placing -*lipid* last in these names indicates that the molecule consists primarily of lipid. The long, fatty acid "tails" of these molecules are hydrophobic, but the nonlipid "heads" are hydrophilic.

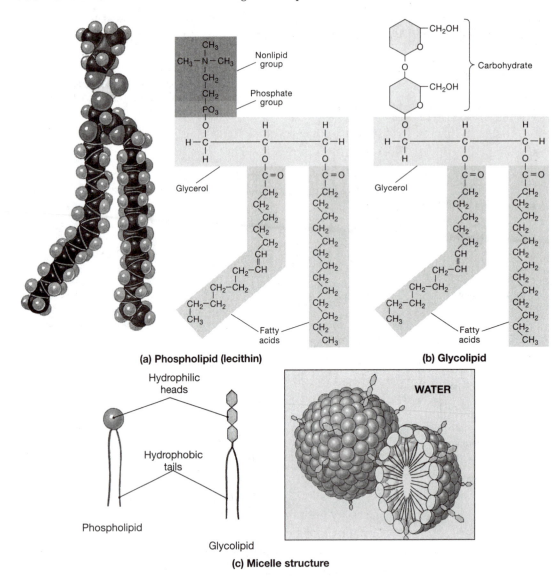

(a) Phospholipid (lecithin)

(b) Glycolipid

(c) Micelle structure

Figure 3–9   Phospholipids and Glycolipids.

(a) In a phospholipid, a phosphate group links a nonlipid molecule to a diglyceride. This phospholipid is a molecule of *lecithin*. **(b)** In a glycolipid, a carbohydrate is attached to a diglyceride. **(c)** When present in large numbers, these molecules will form micelles, with the hydrophilic heads facing the water molecules and the hydrophobic tails on the inside of each droplet.

In water, large numbers of these molecules tend to form droplets, or **micelles** (mī-SELLS; Latin *micella*, little crumb), with the hydrophilic portions on the outside (Figure 3–9c). Most meals contain a mixture of lipids and other organic molecules, and micelles form as the food breaks down in the digestive tract. In addition to phospholipids and glycolipids, micelles may contain other insoluble lipids, such as steroids, glycerides, and long-chain fatty acids.

Cholesterol, phospholipids, and glycolipids are called **structural lipids** because they form and maintain cellular membranes. Membranes composed of hydrophobic lipids are important components of living cells. These include the membrane that surrounds each cell as well as internal membranes that subdivide the interior of the cell. Because they are separated by hydrophobic membranes, each of the intracellular compartments can have a distinctive chemical composition, and the watery interior of the cell is relatively isolated from the watery environment outside the cell.

Let's Review What You've Just Learned

▶ **Definitions**

In the space provided, write the term for each of the following definitions.

_____ **32.** Spherical droplets formed during digestion that contain various lipids.

_____ **33.** Organic compounds containing carbon, hydrogen, and oxygen that are not very soluble in water but are soluble in oils.

_____ **34.** A lipid composed of glycerol and one fatty acid.

_____ **35.** A fatty acid in which all of the carbon-to-carbon bonds are single covalent bonds.

_____ **36.** Another term for triglyceride fats.

_____ **37.** A common steroid hormone in males.

_____ **38.** Molecules composed of hydrocarbon chains that end in a carboxyl group.

_____ **39.** A lipid composed of a diglyceride and a carbohydrate.

_____ **40.** A fatty acid in which one carbon-to-carbon bond is a double covalent bond.

_____ **41.** A three-carbon molecule that combines with fatty acids to form glycerides.

_____ **42.** Large lipid molecules that have a carbon framework composed of four interconnected rings.

_____ **43.** A lipid composed of glycerol and three fatty acids.

_____ **44.** Steroid molecules produced by the liver and secreted in bile that play an important role in fat digestion.

_____ **45.** The terminal carbon atom in a fatty acid.

_____ **46.** Steroid hormones produced by the adrenal glands that regulate mineral balance and tissue metabolism.

_____ **47.** Eicosanoids released by white blood cells to coordinate responses to tissue injury.

_____ **48.** Eicosanoids found in almost every tissue of the body that coordinate local cellular activities.

_____ **49.** A fatty acid that contains more than one carbon-to-carbon double covalent bond.

_____ **50.** A collective term for lipids that are components of membranes.

_____ **51.** Fatty acids that contain a double covalent bond three carbons before the terminal carbon atom.

_____ **52.** A steroid that is both absorbed in the diet and synthesized in the liver and that is implicated in heart disease.

_____ **53.** A lipid composed of a diglyceride and a nonlipid molecule linked to the glycerol by a phosphate group.

_____ **54.** A steroid hormone important in regulating calcium ion levels in the body.

_____ **55.** Compounds formed from polyunsaturated fats during the production of products such as margarine and vegetable shortening.

_____ **56.** A lipid composed of glycerol and two fatty acids.

_____ **57.** Eicosanoids released by platelets during blood clotting.

_____ **58.** A group of female steroid hormones.

► Word Roots, Prefixes, Suffixes, and Combining Forms

In the space provided, list the boldfaced terms introduced in this section that contain the indicated word part.

Word Part	Meaning	Examples
calci-	calcium	**59.** _____
poly-	many	**60.** _____
mono-	single	**61.** _____
phospho-	phosphorus	**62.** _____
di-	two	**63.** _____
glyco-	sugar	**64.** _____
tri-	three	**65.** _____
eicos-	twenty	**66.** _____

► Identification of Organic Molecules and Groups

In the space provided, identify the molecule or chemical group that is illustrated.

67.

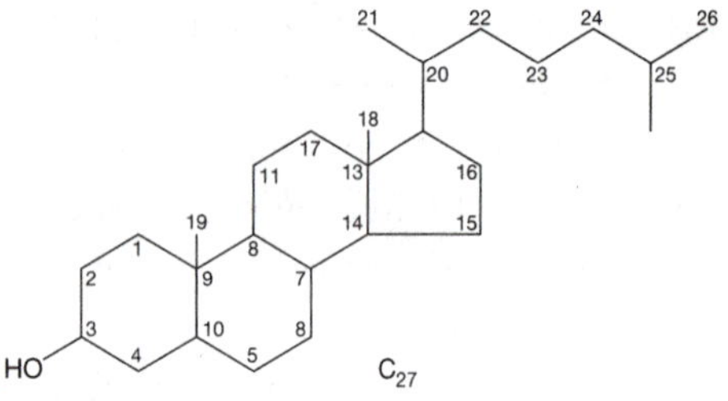

_____

68.

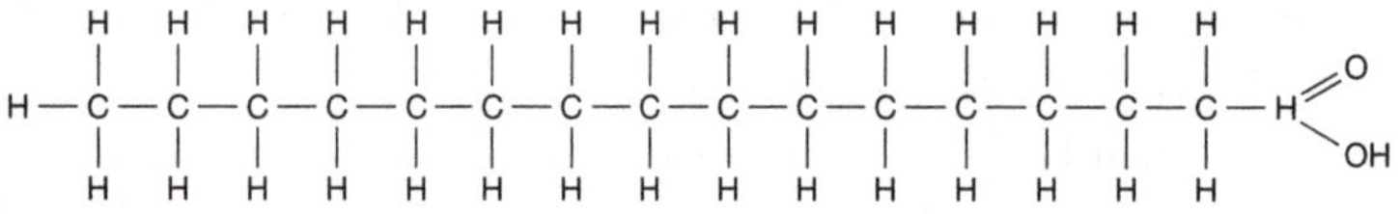

_____

69.

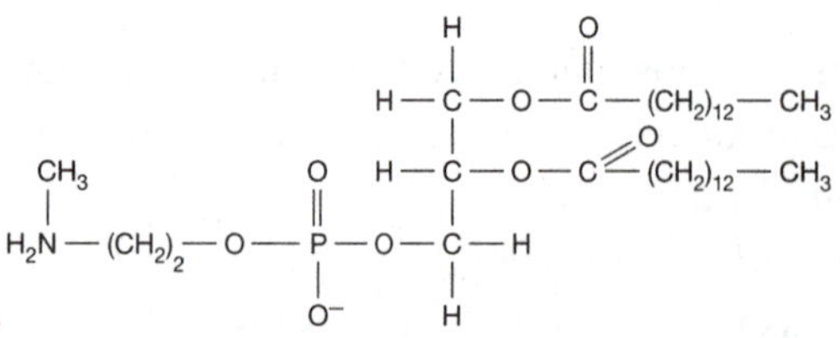

_____

70. $-C\overset{O}{\underset{OH}{\lessgtr}}$

_____

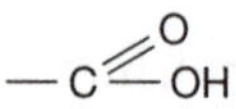

71.

72.

73.

—OH

PROTEINS

Proteins are the most abundant organic components of the human body, and in many ways the most important. There are roughly 100,000 different kinds of proteins, and they account for about 20 percent of the total body weight. All proteins contain carbon, hydrogen, oxygen, and nitrogen; smaller quantities of sulfur may also be present. Table 3–3 identifies the major types of proteins in the body. Proteins perform a variety of essential functions. These include seven major functional categories.

1. **Support: Structural proteins** create a three-dimensional framework for the body, providing strength, organization, and support for cells, tissues, and organs.

2. **Movement: Contractile proteins** are responsible for muscular contraction; related proteins are responsible for the movement of individual cells.

3. **Transport:** Insoluble lipids, respiratory gases, special minerals, such as iron, and several hormones are carried in the blood attached to special **transport proteins**. Other specialized proteins transport materials from one part of a cell to another.

4. **Buffering:** Proteins provide a considerable buffering action, helping to prevent changes in pH.

5. **Metabolic regulation:** Enzymes are proteins that accelerate chemical reactions in living cells. The sensitivity of enzymes to environmental factors is extremely important in controlling the speed and direction of metabolic operations.

6. **Coordination and control:** Protein hormones can influence the metabolic activities of every cell in the body or affect the function of specific organs or organ systems.

7. **Defense:** The tough, waterproof proteins of the skin, hair, and nails protect the body from environmental hazards. The proteins of the immune system known as *antibodies* protect us from disease. Special *clotting proteins* restrict bleeding after an injury to the blood vessels.

Table 3–3 Representative Proteins and Their Functions

Protein Type	Example(s)	Representative Location(s)	Function(s)
Structural proteins	Keratin	Skin surface, hair, nails	Provides strength and waterproofing
	Collagen	Dermis of skin, tendons	Provides tensile strength
Contractile proteins	Actin, myosin	Muscle cells	Perform contraction and movement
Transport proteins	Albumin	Circulating blood	Transports fatty acids and steroid and thyroid hormones
	Transferrin	Circulating blood	Transports iron
	Apolipoproteins	Circulating blood	Transport glycerides
	Hemoglobin	Circulating blood	Transports oxygen in blood (within red blood cells)
Buffers	Intracellular and extracellular proteins	Within cells and body fluids	Stabilize pH
Enzymes	Hydrolases	All cells	Catalyze hydrolysis of organic molecules
	Kinases	All cells	Attach phosphate groups to organic substrates
	Proteases	All cells; digestive secretions of stomach, pancreas	Break down proteins
	Carbohydrates	All cells; digestive secretions of salivary glands, pancreas	Break down carbohydrates
	Lipases	All cells; digestive secretions of pancreas	Break down lipids
Antibodies (immuno- globulins)	Gamma globulins	Circulating blood	Attack foreign proteins and pathogens
Hormones	Insulin, glucagon	Circulating blood	Coordinate and/or control metabolic activities

Structure of Proteins

Proteins consist of chains of small organic molecules called **amino acids**. The human body contains significant quantities of 20 different amino acids. A typical protein contains 1000 amino acids, but the largest protein complexes may have a hundred thousand or more. Each amino acid consists of a central carbon atom to which four groups are attached: (1) a hydrogen atom, (2) an **amino group** ($-NH_2$), (3) a carboxyl group ($-COOH$), and (4) a variable group, known as an **R group**, or side chain (Figure 3–10a). Different R groups distinguish one amino acid from another, giving each its individual chemical properties. The name *amino acid* refers to the presence of the amino group and the carboxyl group. Figure 3–10b shows two representative amino acids, glycine and alanine.

As indicated in Figure 3–10b, dehydration synthesis can link two amino acids. This process creates a covalent bond between the carboxyl group of one amino acid and the amino group of another. This covalent bond is called a **peptide bond**, and the molecule created is a **dipeptide**. The chain can be lengthened by the addition of more amino acids. Attaching a third produces a **tripeptide**, and there are **tetrapeptides**, **pentapeptides**, and so forth. Tripeptides and larger peptide chains are called **polypeptides**. Polypeptides

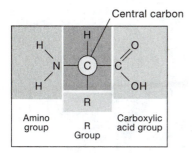

(a) Structure of an amino acid

Figure 3–10   Amino Acids and Peptide Bonds.

(a) Each amino acid consists of a central carbon atom to which four different groups are attached: a hydrogen atom, an amino group ($-NH_2$), a carboxyl group ($-COOH$), and a variable group generally designated R. **(b)** Peptides form as dehydration synthesis creates a peptide bond between the carboxyl group of one amino acid and the amino group of another. In this example, the amino acids glycine and alanine are linked to form a dipeptide.

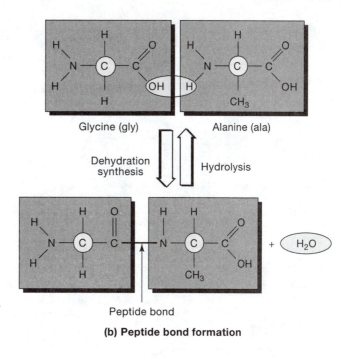

(b) Peptide bond formation

containing more than 100 amino acids are usually called **proteins**. You are probably already familiar with the names of several important proteins, including hemoglobin in red blood cells and keratin in fingernails and hair.

The characteristics of a particular protein are determined in part by the R groups on its component amino acids. But the properties of a protein are more than just the sum of the properties of its parts, for polypeptides and proteins can have very complex shapes that also influence the way they behave. There are four levels of structural complexity:

1. The **primary structure** of a protein is the sequence of amino acids along its length. The primary structure of a short peptide chain has been diagrammed in Figure 3–11a.

2. The **secondary structure** appears as hydrogen bonding occurs between parts of the polypeptide chain. This bonding often creates a simple spiral, known as an **alphahelix**, shown in Figure 3–11b. Less often, hydrogen bonding produces a flat **pleated sheet**. A single polypeptide chain may have both helical and pleated sections.

3. The **tertiary structure** of a protein is the complex coiling and folding that gives the protein its unique shape. Tertiary structure results partly from interactions between the polypeptide chain and the surrounding water molecules and partly from interactions between the R groups of amino acids in different parts of the molecule. Figure 3–11c shows the tertiary structure of myoglobin, a protein found in muscle cells. Myoglobin is an example of a globular protein. **Globular proteins** are compact, usually rounded, and water-soluble.

4. Some proteins contain several polypeptide chains, each with its own secondary or tertiary structure. Interactions between these polypeptides determine the **quaternary structure** of the functional protein. The protein hemoglobin (Figure 3–12a)

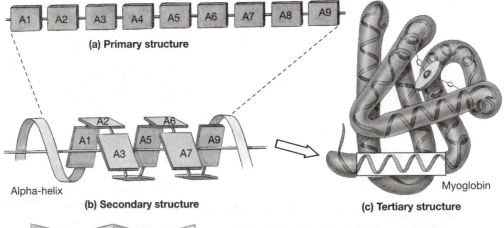

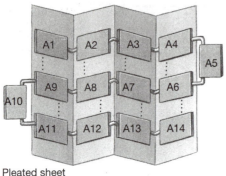

Pleated sheet

Figure 3–11 Protein Structure.
(a) The primary structure of a polypeptide is the sequence of amino acids along its length. **(b)** The secondary structure is primarily the result of hydrogen bonding along the length of the polypeptide chain. Such bonding often produces a simple spiral (an alpha-helix) or a flattened arrangement known as a pleated sheet. **(c)** The tertiary structure is the coiling and folding of a polypeptide. This is the structure of myoglobin, a globular protein involved in the storage of oxygen in muscle tissue. Within the cylindrical segments, the polypeptide chain is arranged in an alpha-helix.

contains four globular subunits, each structurally similar to myoglobin. Hemoglobin is found within red blood cells, where it binds and transports oxygen. In keratin (Figure 3–12b) three helical polypeptides are wound together like the strands of a rope. **Keratin** is the tough, water-resistant protein found in skin, nails, and hair. Keratin is an example of a fibrous protein. **Fibrous proteins** are tough, durable, and generally insoluble. **Collagen** (COL-a-jen; Greek *kolla*, glue), another fibrous protein, forms a strong supporting framework in tissues and organs throughout the body.

Figure 3–12 Quaternary Proteins.
The quaternary structure develops when separate polypeptide subunits interact to form a larger molecule. **(a)** A single hemoglobin molecule contains four globular subunits, each structurally similar to myoglobin. Hemoglobin transports oxygen in the blood; the oxygen binds reversibly to the heme units. **(b)** In keratin and collagen, three fibrous subunits intertwine. Keratin is a tough, water-resistant protein found in skin, hair, and nails. Collagen is the principal extracellular protein in most organs.

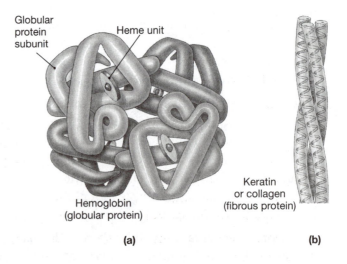

The Relationship between Protein Shape and Function

Proteins are versatile, and they have a variety of functions. The shape of a protein determines its functional properties, and the primary factor that determines protein shape is the sequence of amino acids. The 20 major amino acids can be linked in an astonishing number of combinations, creating proteins with a wide variety of shapes and functions. Changing the identity of a single amino acid out of the hundreds or thousands found in a protein may significantly alter the protein's functional properties. For example, several cancers and *sickle-cell anemia*, a blood disorder, result from single changes in the amino acid sequences of complex proteins.

The tertiary and quaternary shapes of complex proteins depend not only on the amino acid sequence but also on the local environmental characteristics. Small changes in the ionic composition, temperature, or pH of their surroundings can thus affect the function of proteins. Protein shape can also be affected by hydrogen bonding to other molecules in solution. The significance of these factors is most striking when one considers the function of enzymes, for these proteins are essential to the metabolic operations under way in every cell in the body.

Enzyme Function

The reactants in enzymatic reactions are called **substrates**. Before an enzyme can function as a catalyst, the substrate must bind to a special region of the enzyme called the **active site**. The tertiary or quaternary structure of an enzyme molecule determines the shape of the active site, typically a groove or pocket into which the substrate fits. This physical fit is reinforced by weak electrical attractive forces such as hydrogen bonding.

Figure 3–13 diagrams enzyme function in a synthesis reaction. Substrate binding occurs at the active site (Step 1). The enzyme then promotes product formation (Step 2). It appears likely that substrate binding results in a change in the shape of the protein and that this shape change promotes the reaction by placing physical stresses on the substrate molecules. The completed product then detaches from the active site and enters the surrounding environment (Step 3). The enzyme is then ready to repeat the cycle.

Our example was an enzyme that catalyzed a synthesis reaction. However, other enzymes may catalyze decomposition reactions or exchange reactions. The specific binding of an enzyme to its substrate is determined by the ability of a particular substrate to combine with the enzyme's active site, a relatively small portion of the entire protein.

Cofactors and Enzyme Function

Cofactors are ions or molecules that must bind to an enzyme before substrate binding can occur. Examples of such cofactors include ions such as calcium (Ca^{2+}) and magnesium (Mg^{2+}), which bind at the active site. Cofactors may also bind at other sites, as long as they produce the necessary change in the shape of the active site.

Coenzymes are nonprotein organic molecules that participate in enzymatic reactions, sometimes as cofactors, and, like enzymes, they are not used up in the chemical reaction. Many of the *vitamins* that we need in our diet are converted by the body into essential coenzymes. **Vitamins** are organic compounds that in most cases are not synthesized by the body and must come from the diet. They are required in small amounts and are essential for body functions.

Figure 3–13 A Simplified View of Enzyme Structure and Function.

Each enzyme contains a specific active site somewhere on its exposed surface. **Step 1:** A pair of substrate molecules (S_1 and S_2) bind to the active site. **Step 2:** The subtrates interact, forming a product. **Step 3:** That product detaches from the active site. Because the structure of the enzyme has not been affected, the entire process can be repeated.

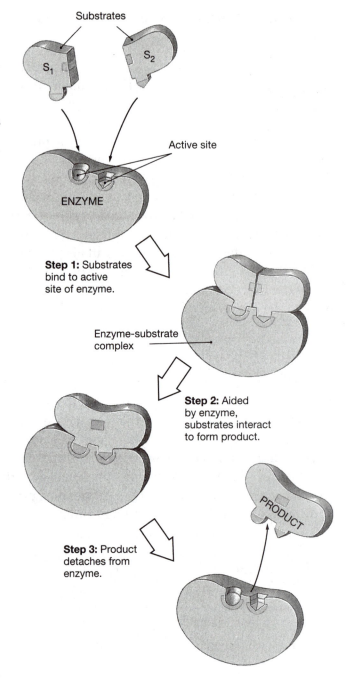

Substrates

S_1 S_2

Active site

ENZYME

Step 1: Substrates bind to active site of enzyme.

Enzyme-substrate complex

Step 2: Aided by enzyme, substrates interact to form product.

Step 3: Product detaches from enzyme.

PRODUCT

The relationship between enzymes and cofactors is one example of how enzyme activity can be controlled. Without a cofactor, the enzyme is intact but nonfunctional; with the cofactor, the enzyme can catalyze a specific reaction. In this case, binding the cofactor makes the active site functional. Other factors can activate or inactivate an enzyme. In fact, virtually any factor that changes the tertiary or quaternary shape of an enzyme may switch it "on" or "off."

Effects of Temperature and pH on Enzyme Function

Each enzyme works best at an optimal combination of temperature and pH. As temperatures rise, proteins change shape, and enzyme function deteriorates. Very high body temperatures (over 42°C, or 107°F) cause death because at these temperatures proteins undergo **denaturation**, a change in tertiary or quaternary shape. Denatured proteins are nonfunctional, and the loss of structural proteins and enzymes causes irreparable damage to organs and organ systems. You see denaturation in progress each time you fry an egg, for the clear egg white contains large amounts of dissolved proteins. As the temperature rises, the protein structure changes (denatures). Eventually the egg proteins become completely and permanently denatured, forming an insoluble white mass.

Enzymes are equally sensitive to pH changes. Pepsin, an enzyme that breaks down proteins in the stomach contents, works best at a pH of 2.0 (strongly acid). The small intestine contains trypsin, another enzyme that attacks proteins. Trypsin works only in an alkaline environment, with an optimum pH of 7.7 (somewhat basic).

Controlling Enzyme Activity

Each cell contains an assortment of enzymes, and any particular enzyme may be active under one set of conditions and inactive under another. Because the change is immediate, enzyme activation or inactivation is an important method for short-term control over reaction rates and pathways. There are four major factors that determine the rate at which a particular enzymatic reaction occurs.

1. **Substrate and product concentration:** Consider a situation in which there are many enzymes but no substrate molecules. No reaction occurs. Figure 3–14 plots the effect of increasing substrate concentrations on the reaction rate. At low concentrations, substrate availability limits the reaction rate. The higher the substrate concentration, the faster the reaction proceeds. This acceleration does not continue. As product concentration rises, the chances increase that a product molecule instead of substrate molecules will contact the active site. When all the active sites are bound to substrate or product molecules, the enzyme system is saturated. Any further increase in substrate concentration will have no effect on the reaction rate. The graph in Figure 3–14 is a typical enzyme saturation curve.

2. **Enzyme concentration:** The concentration of enzymes has a direct effect on the rate of reaction (Figure 3–14). The higher the enzyme concentration, the faster the initial reaction rate. Enzyme concentrations in a cell may change by varying rates of enzyme synthesis or destruction. Turning enzymes ON or OFF can also regulate the concentration of functional enzymes.

3. **Competitive inhibition:** The binding of a specific substrate by its enzyme results from the shape and charge characteristics of the enzyme's active site. That specificity is not perfect. Molecules that resemble the normal substrate can bind to the active site and interfere with substrate binding. This process is called **competitive inhibition** because substrate molecules must compete for a space on the active site. The higher the concentration of competitive inhibitors, the lower the rate of reaction. Figure 3–14 diagrams the effects of competitive inhibition on reaction rates.

4. **Enzyme activation states:** An activated enzyme will catalyze a particular reaction and an inactivated enzyme will not. In an inactive enzyme the active site cannot interact with substrate molecules. During activation, the shape of the active site changes. Activation or inactivation may occur as a result of environmental changes, such as changes in temperature or pH, or the presence or absence of cofactors. Figure 3–15 diagrams the function of a cofactor.

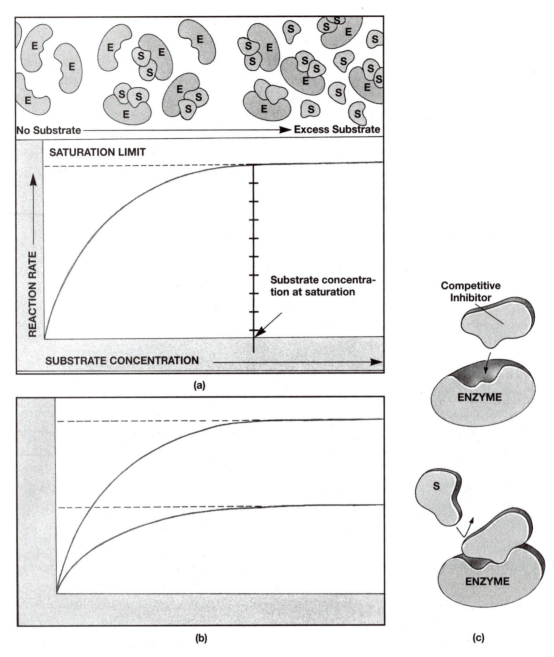

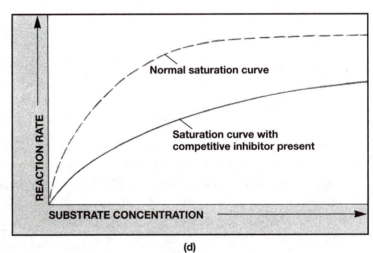

Figure 3–14 Factors That Affect Enzymatic Reaction Rates.

(a) A saturation curve, showing the effects of changing substrate concentrations. Here E = enzyme and S = substrate. (b) The effect of altering the concentration of enzymes on a reaction rate. Curve 2 has a higher enzyme concentration and therefore a faster initial reaction rate than curve 1 has. (c) A competitive inhibitor blocks the enzyme's active site, so the substrate cannot bind. (d) The effects of competitive inhibitors on reaction rates.

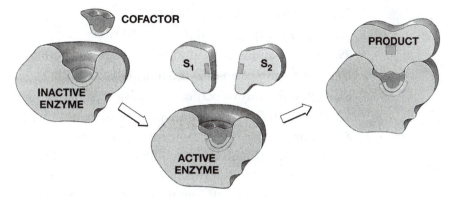

Figure 3–15   Cofactors and Enzyme Activity.
In some cases, a cofactor must bind to the active site before the enzyme can bind substrate molecules and function normally.

Chemicals that affect enzyme activity can have powerful effects on cells throughout the body. For example, several deadly compounds, such as hydrogen cyanide (HCN) and hydrogen sulfide (H_2S), kill cells by inhibiting enzymes involved with energy release from food molecules. Many inhibitors with less drastic effects are in clinical use. For example, the drug warfarin slows blood clotting by inhibiting liver enzymes responsible for the synthesis of proteins necessary for clotting. Several of the beneficial effects of aspirin, such as the reduction of inflammation, are related to the inhibition of an enzyme involved with prostaglandin synthesis. Many important antibiotics, such as penicillin, kill bacteria by inhibiting enzymes that are essential to bacteria but absent from our cells.

Glycoproteins and Proteoglycans

Glycoproteins (GLĪ-kō-prō-tēns) and **proteoglycans** (prō-tē-ō-GLĪ-kans) are combinations of protein and carbohydrate molecules. Glycoprotein molecules are large proteins with small carbohydrate groups attached. Glycoproteins may function as enzymes, antibodies, hormones, or protein components of cell membranes. Glycoproteins in cell membranes play a major role in the identification of normal and abnormal cells and in the initiation and coordination of the immune response. Proteoglycans are large polysaccharide molecules connected to short polypeptide chains. Proteoglycan secretions coat the surfaces of the respiratory and digestive tracts, providing lubrication. Proteoglycans dissolved in tissue fluids give them a syrupy consistency.

 Let's Review What You've Just Learned

▶ **Definitions**

In the space provided, write the term for each of the following definitions.

_____ **74.** Organic compounds that are not synthesized by the body, are required in small amounts, and are essential for body functions.

_____ **75.** The covalent bond formed between the carboxyl group of one amino acid and the amino group of another.

_____ **76.** Small organic molecules that are the basic constituents of proteins.

_____ 77. The reactants in an ezymatic reaction.

_____ 78. A change in the tertiary or quaternary shape of a protein.

_____ 79. A polypeptide containing more than 100 amino acids.

_____ 80. The region of an enzyme that binds the substrate.

_____ 81. A tough, fibrous protein found in skin hair, and nails.

_____ 82. The term for the variable portion of an amino acid.

_____ 83. Nonprotein organic molecules that participate in enzymatic reactions, sometimes as cofactors, and that, like enzymes are not used up in the reaction.

_____ 84. Large proteins with small carbohydrate molecules attached.

_____ 85. A molecule formed by the union of two amino acids.

_____ 86. Large polysaccharide molecules connected to short polypeptide chains.

_____ 87. Compact, usually rounded, water-soluble proteins.

_____ 88. The process in which a molecule similar in structure to an enzyme's substrate competes with the substrate for the enzyme's active site.

_____ 89. A spiral shape produced by hydrogen bonding within a polypeptide chain.

_____ 90. An ion or molecule that must bind to an enzyme before substrate binding can occur.

_____ 91. Peptide chains that are larger than tripeptides.

_____ 92. Tough, durable, ropelike proteins that are generally insoluble.

► Word Roots, Prefixes, Suffixes, and Combining Forms

In the space provided, list the boldfaced terms introduced in this section that contain the indicated word part.

Word Part	Meaning	Examples
glyco-	sugar	93. _____
poly-	many	94. _____
co-	together	95. _____

► Identification of Organic Molecules and Groups

In the space provided, identify the molecule or chemical group that is illustrated.

96. —NH$_2$

_____

$$H_2N-\overset{\overset{\displaystyle H}{|}}{\underset{\underset{\displaystyle R_1}{|}}{C}}-\overset{\overset{\displaystyle O}{\|}}{C}-\overset{\overset{\displaystyle H}{|}}{\underset{\underset{\displaystyle H}{|}}{N}}-\overset{\overset{\displaystyle H}{|}}{\underset{\underset{\displaystyle R_2}{|}}{C}}-\overset{\overset{\displaystyle O}{\|}}{C}-OH$$

97.

_____

98.

H₂N—CH(R)—C(H)(OH)—C(=O)—OH

(structure)

▶ **Completion**

Complete each of the following statements.

  99. The primary structure of a protein is determined by _____.

 100. The _____ structure of a protein is the complex coiling and folding that gives a protein its unique shape.

 101. _____ proteins are responsible for muscular contractions.

 102. Some substances such as lipids and iron are carried in the blood attached to _____.

 103. Two examples of secondary structure in proteins are the _____ and the _____.

 104. _____ create a three-dimensional framework for the body.

 105. Proteins that regulate metabolic processes are _____.

 106. Proteins containing two or more polypeptide chains each with its own secondary and tertiary structure are said to have a _____ structure.

 107. The secondary structure of a protein is the result of _____ between parts of the polypeptide chain.

NUCLEIC ACIDS

Nucleic (noo-KLĀ-ik) **acids** are large organic molecules composed of carbon, hydrogen, oxygen, nitrogen, and phosphorus. Nucleic acids store and process information at the molecular level, inside living cells. There are two classes of nucleic acid molecules, **deoxyribonucleic** (dē-ok-sē-rī-bō-noo-KLĀ-ik) **acid**, or **DNA**, and **ribonucleic** (rī-bō-noo-KLĀ-ik) **acid**, or **RNA**.

The DNA in our cells determines our inherited characteristics, such as eye color, hair color, blood type, and so on. It affects all aspects of body structure and function because DNA molecules encode the information needed to build proteins. By directing the synthesis of structural proteins, DNA controls the shape and physical characteristics of our bodies. By controlling the manufacture of enzymes, DNA regulates not only protein synthesis but all aspects of cellular metabolism, including the creation and destruction of lipids, carbohydrates, and other vital molecules.

Several forms of RNA cooperate to manufacture specific proteins using the information provided by DNA. The functional relationships between DNA and RNA will be detailed in Chapter 5.

The Structure of Nucleic Acids

A nucleic acid consists of a series of **nucleotides** linked by dehydration synthesis. A single nucleotide has three basic components: a sugar, a phosphate group, and a nitrogenous (nitrogen-containing) base (Figure 3–16). The sugar is always a pentose (five-carbon sugar), either **ribose** (in RNA) or **deoxyribose** (in DNA). Each pentose is attached to a

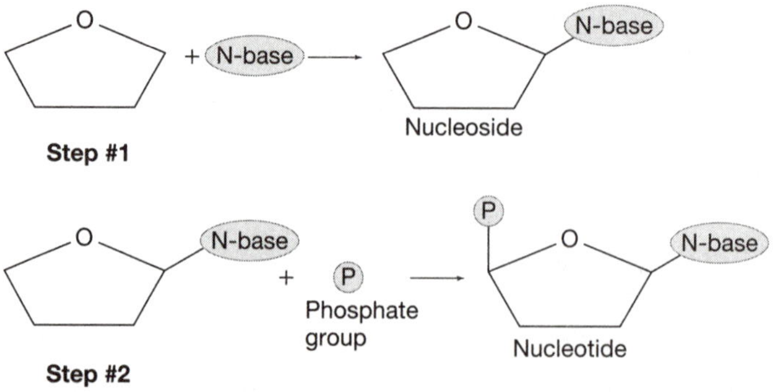

Figure 3–16 Nucleotide Formation.

Step 1: A nitrogenous base (adenine, guanine, cytosine, thymine, or uracil) is attached to the 1′ carbon of a ribose sugar to form a nucleoside. *Step 2:* An inorganic phosphate group is attached to the 5′ carbon of the nucleoside to form a nucleotide.

phosphate group (PO_4^{3-}) and a nitrogenous base. There are five nitrogenous bases found in nucleic acids: adenine (A), guanine (G), cytosine (C), thymine (T), and uracil (U). **Adenine** and **guanine** have two rings in their structural formulas, a six-membered ring fused to a five-membered ring, and are called **purines**; the others have only a single, six-membered ring and are called **pyrimidines**. Both RNA and DNA contain adenine, guanine, and cytosine. Uracil is found only in RNA, and thymine only in DNA.

In the formation of a nucleic acid (Figure 3–16), attachment of a nitrogenous base to a carbohydrate (Step 1) creates a **nucleoside** that is named after the nitrogenous base. For example, attaching a guanine molecule produces a guanine nucleoside. A nucleotide forms when a phosphate group binds to the carbohydrate of the nucleoside (Step 2). Dehydration synthesis then attaches the phosphate group of one nucleotide to the carbohydrate of another. The "backbone" of a nucleic acid molecule is a linear sugar-to-phosphate-to-sugar sequence with the nitrogenous bases projecting to one side (Figure 3–17).

RNA and DNA

There are important structural differences between RNA and DNA. A molecule of RNA consists of a single chain of nucleotides (Figure 3–17a). Its shape depends on the order of the nucleotides and the interactions between them. There are three main types of RNA in our cells: messenger RNA (mRNA), transfer RNA (tRNA), and ribosomal RNA (rRNA). These types have different shapes and functions, but all three are required for the synthesis of proteins, a process that will be detailed in Chapter 5.

A DNA molecule consists of a pair of nucleotide chains (Figure 3–17b). Hydrogen bonding between opposing nitrogenous bases holds the two strands together. Because of their shapes, adenine can bond only with thymine, and cytosine only with guanine. As a result, adenine-thymine and cytosine-guanine are known as **complementary base pairs**. The two strands of DNA twist around one another in a double helix that resembles a spiral staircase. The stair steps correspond to the nitrogenous base pairs. Figure 3–17c presents a three-dimensional view of a DNA molecule. Table 3–4 summarizes the differences between DNA and RNA.

HIGH-ENERGY COMPOUNDS

Catabolism releases energy, and living cells can use that energy in constructive ways. The energy released by catabolic reactions is first harnessed to create high-energy bonds. A **high-energy bond** is a covalent bond that, when broken, releases a useful amount of energy. In our cells a high-energy bond usually connects a phosphate group (PO_4^{3-}), also

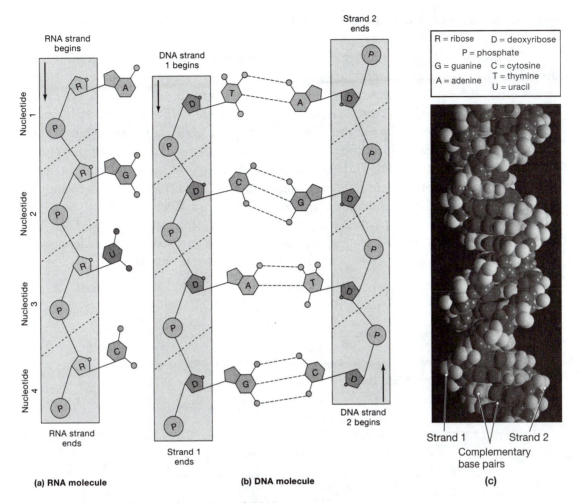

Figure 3–17   Nucleic Acids: RNA and DNA.

Nucleic acids are long chains of nucleotides. Each molecule starts at the sugar-nitrogenous base of the first nucleotide and ends at the phosphate group as the last member of the chain. An RNA molecule **(a)** consists of a single nucleotide chain. Its shape is determined by the sequence of nucleotides and the interactions between them. A DNA molecule **(b)** consists of a pair of nucleotide chains linked by hydrogen bonding between complementary base pairs. **(c)** A three-dimensional model of a DNA molecule shows the double helix formed by the two DNA strands.

Table 3–4   A Comparison of RNA and DNA

Characteristic	RNA	DNA
Sugar	Ribose	Deoxyribose
Nitrogenous bases	Adenine	Adenine
	Guanine	Guanine
	Cytosine	Cytosine
	Uracil	Thymine
Number of nucleotides in typical molecule	Varies from fewer than 100 to about 50,000	Always more than 45 million
Shape of molecule	Varies, depending on hydrogen bonding along the length of the strand; 3 main types (mRNA, rRNA, tRNA)	Paired strands coiled in a double helix
Function	Performs protein synthesis as directed by DNA	Stores genetic information that controls protein synthesis by RNA

symbolized as P_i (for inorganic phosphate) to an organic molecule. The resulting complex is called a **high-energy compound**.

The creation of a high-energy compound requires (1) a phosphate group, (2) appropriate enzymes, and (3) suitable organic substrates. The most important substrate is an adenine nucleoside, adenosine, with two phosphate groups attached. This combination is called **adenosine diphosphate**, or **ADP**. ADP is created by adding a phosphate group (a process known as **phosphorylation**) to the nucleotide **adenosine monophosphate**, or **AMP**, one of the building blocks of nucleic acids. It takes a significant energy input to convert AMP to ADP, and the second phosphate is attached by a high-energy bond. An even greater amount of energy is required to add a third phosphate and create the high-energy compound **adenosine triphosphate**, or **ATP**.

Figure 3–18 details the structure of ATP. Within our cells the conversion of ADP to ATP represents the primary method of energy storage, and the reverse reaction provides a mechanism for controlled energy release. The arrangement can be summarized as:

$$ATP + H_2O \rightarrow ADP + P_i + energy$$

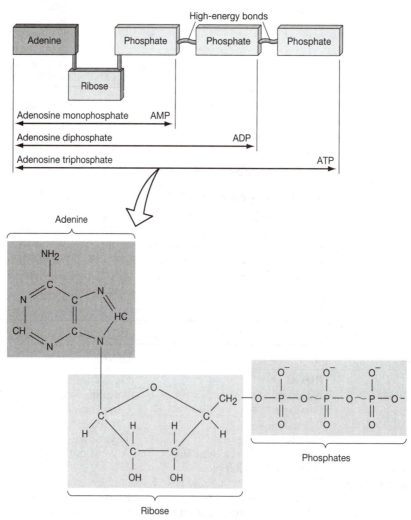

Figure 3–18   The Structure of ATP.
A molecule of ATP consists of an adenine nucleoside to which three phosphate groups have been joined. Cells most often transfer energy by attaching a third phosphate group to ADP with a high-energy bond and then removing that phosphate group at another site, where the associated release of energy performs cellular work.

Table 3–5   Turnover Rates

Cell Type	Component	Average Recycling Time*
Liver	Total protein	5–6 days
	Enzymes	1 hour to several days, depending on the enzyme
	Glycogen	1–2 days
	Cholesterol	5–7 days
Muscle cell	Total protein	30 days
	Glycogen	12–24 hours
Neuron	Phospholipids	200 days
	Cholesterol	100+ days
Fat cell	Triglycerides	15–20 days

*Most values were obtained from studies on mammals other than humans.

When energy sources are available, our cells make ATP from ADP; when energy is required, the reverse reaction occurs.

Although ATP is the most abundant high-energy compound, there are others. These compounds are typically other nucleotides that have undergone phosphorylation. For example, guanosine triphosphate (**GTP**) and uridine triphosphate (**UTP**) are nucleotide-based high-energy compounds that transfer energy in specific enzymatic reactions.

CHEMICALS AND LIVING CELLS

The human body is more than a collection of chemicals. Biochemical building blocks form functional units called **cells**. Each cell behaves like a miniature organism, responding to internal and external stimuli. A lipid membrane separates the cell from its environment, and internal membranes create compartments with specific functions. Proteins form an internal supporting framework and act as enzymes to accelerate and control the chemical reactions that maintain homeostasis. Nucleic acids direct the synthesis of all cellular proteins, including the enzymes that enable the cell to synthesize a wide variety of other substances. Carbohydrates provide energy for vital activities and form part of specialized compounds, such as proteoglycans and glycolipids.

Cells are dynamic structures that adapt to changes in their environment. That adaptation may involve changes in the chemical organization of the cell. These changes are easily made because organic molecules other than DNA are temporary rather than permanent components of the cell. Their continual removal and replacement are part of the process of **metabolic turnover**.

Most of the organic molecules in a cell are replaced at intervals ranging from hours to months. The average time between synthesis and recycling is known as the **turnover rate**. Table 3–5 indicates the turnover rate for representative cells.

Let's Review What You've Just Learned

▶ **Definitions**

In the space provided, write the term for each of the following definitions.

_____ **108.** An organic molecule consisting of a pentose sugar, a nitrogenous base, and a phosphate group.

_____ **109.** A nitrogen-containing compound that contains a six-membered ring.

_____ **110.** A covalent bond that releases useful energy when broken.

_____ **111.** The continual removal and replacement of organic molecules other than DNA in cells.

_____ **112.** A high-energy compound consisting of adenosine and three phosphate groups.

_____ **113.** The molecule that contains genetic information.

_____ **114.** The functional unit of living organisms.

_____ **115.** Pairs of nitrogenous bases, such as adenine-thymine and guanine-cytosine, that are held together by hydrogen bonds.

_____ **116.** A high-energy compound consisting of adenosine and two phosphate groups.

_____ **117.** The average time between synthesis and recycling of an organic molecule in a cell.

_____ **118.** Large organic molecules composed of carbon, hydrogen, nitrogen, oxygen, and phosphorus.

_____ **119.** The pentose found in DNA.

_____ **120.** A nitrogen-containing compound that contains two rings, a six-membered ring fused to a five-membered ring.

_____ **121.** A compound consisting of adenosine and a single phosphate group.

_____ **122.** A nucleic acid that contains the pentose ribose.

_____ **123.** The compound formed when a pentose is bonded to a purine or pyrimidine base.

▶ Identification of Organic Molecules and Groups

In the space provided, identify the molecule or chemical group that is illustrated.

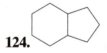

124.

_____

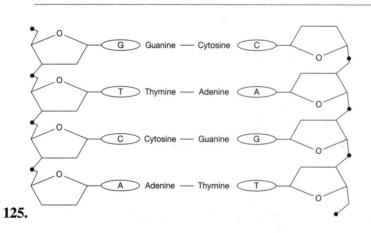

125.

_____

126.

► Concept Mapping

Using the following terms, fill in the blank spaces next to the circled numbers to complete the concept map. Follow the numbers to comply with the organization of the map.

Ribonucleic acid

Nitrogenous (N) bases

Guanine (G)

Deoxyribose

Ribose

Deoxyribonucleic acid

Pyrimidines

Thymine (T)

Purines

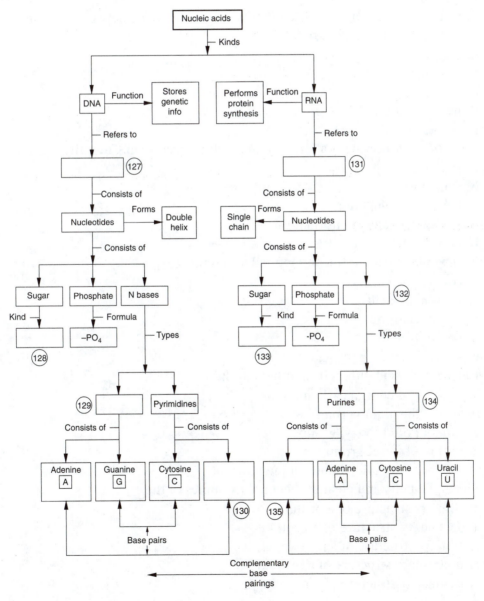

☑ Self-Check Test

The following test will allow you to determine how well you have mastered the vocabulary and basic concepts of this chapter. It will also help you prepare for the type of questions you are likely to encounter on a test in an anatomy and physiology course. The self-check test will help you assess your understanding of the chapter material and will help you develop good test-taking skills.

The following questions test your ability to use vocabulary and to recall facts.

1. Organic compounds containing carbon, hydrogen, and oxygen in a near 1:2:1 ratio are
   a. carbohydrates
   b. lipids
   c. proteins
   d. nucleic acids
   e. enzymes

2. A fatty acid that contains three double covalent bonds between carbon atoms in its carbon chain is said to be
   a. saturated
   b. monounsaturated
   c. polyunsaturated
   d. hydrogenated
   e. carboxylated

3. Each of the following is a function of proteins except one. Identify the exception.
   a. support
   b. transport
   c. metabolic regulation
   d. storage of genetic information
   e. movement

4. You would expect to find a peptide bond linking
   a. two simple sugars
   b. two amino acids
   c. two nucleotides
   d. two fatty acids
   e. a steroid and a fatty acid

5. Each amino acid differs from others in the
   a. number of central carbon atoms
   b. size of the amino group
   c. number of carboxyl groups
   d. nature of the R group
   e. number of peptide bonds in the molecule

6. The alpha-helix and pleated sheet are examples of the
   a. primary structure of a protein
   b. secondary structure of a protein
   c. tertiary structure of a protein
   d. quaternary structure of a protein
   e. pentanary structure of a protein

7. Nucleic acids are composed of units called

    a. amino acids

    b. fatty acids

    c. purines

    d. pyrimidines

    e. nucleotides

8. Molecules that have the same chemical formula but different structural formulas are called

    a. isozymes

    b. isomers

    c. cofactors

    d. coenzymes

    e. apoenzymes

9. The prefix *poly-* means

    a. equal

    b. whole

    c. many

    d. five

    e. sugar

10. According to the rules of complementary base pairing, a nucleotide containing the base cytosine would pair only with a nucleotide containing the base

    a. thymine

    b. adenine

    c. uracil

    d. cytosine

    e. guanine

11. Which of the following structural formulas represents a simple sugar?

a.

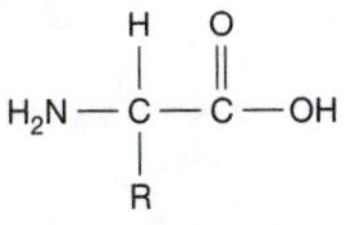

$$H_2N - C - C - OH$$

with H and O above, R below

b. $CH_3 - CH_2 - CH_2 - CH_2 - CH_2 - CH_2 - CH_2 - CH_2 - CH_2 - COOH$

c. (six-membered ring sugar structure with CH_2OH, OH, H groups)

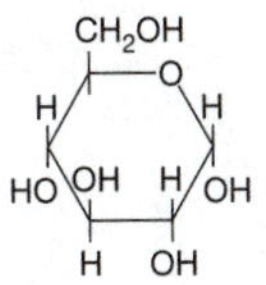

d. (steroid ring structure with OH and HO groups)

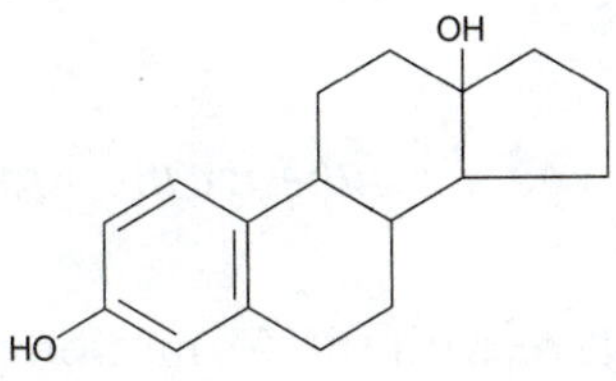

e. (disaccharide structure with CH_2OH, OH, H groups)

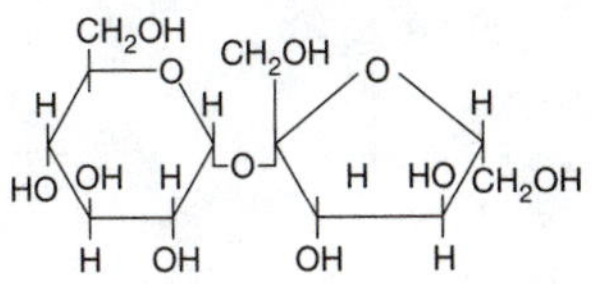

12. A nucleotide consists of
    a. a five-carbon sugar and phosphate group
    b. a five-carbon sugar and a nitrogenous base
    c. a five-carbon sugar and an amino acid
    d. a phosphate group and a nitrogenous base
    e. a five-carbon sugar, a nitrogenous base, and a phosphate group

13. The most important high-energy compound in cells is
    a. glucose
    b. fructose
    c. protein
    d. ATP
    e. DNA

14. All fatty acids contain an arrangement of atoms called a(n) _____ at one end of the chain.
    a. amino group
    b. omega carbon
    c. carboxyl group
    d. hydroxyl group
    e. nitrogenous base

15. Large lipid molecules that have a carbon framework composed of four interconnected rings are
    a. fatty acids
    b. triglycerides
    c. prostaglandins
    d. steroids
    e. phospholipids

16. The reactants in an enzyme catalyzed reaction are called
    a. coenzymes
    b. cofactors
    c. substrates
    d. products
    e. nutrients

17. A common disaccharide is
    a. glucose
    b. fructose
    c. sucrose
    d. cellulose
    e. starch

The following questions are more challenging and require you to synthesize the information that you have learned in this chapter.

18. A shortage of cholesterol in the body would interfere with the formation of
    a. sex hormones
    b. proteins
    c. glycogen
    d. nucleic acids
    e. triglycerides

19. Blocking the active site of an enzyme
    a. is the first step in an enzyme-catalyzed reaction
    b. is the role of a cofactor
    c. will prevent the enzyme from binding substrate
    d. will increase the rate of an enzyme-catalyzed reaction
    e. will have no effect on enzyme function
20. Disease and possibly death can occur when
    a. the body hydrolyzes ATP
    b. proteins become denatured
    c. peptide bonds are formed
    d. proteins assume a quaternary structure
    e. prostaglandins are synthesized

✓ Self-Assessment

If your score was

between 18 and 20, you are ready to proceed to the next chapter.

between 15 and 17, you have a good general idea of the chapter content, but you should review sections of the chapter that deal with items that you missed before proceeding to the next chapter.

less than 14, you have not mastered the chapter content well enough to proceed. Reread the chapter and rework the exercises. Then retake the self-check test. Repeat this process until you achieve a score that will allow you to continue.

Answers

1. isomers
2. polysaccharide
3. carbohydrate
4. sucrose
5. cellulose
6. monosaccharide
7. glycogen
8. structural formula
9. disaccharide
10. starch
11. fructose
12. triose
13. polysaccharide
14. glycogen
15. hexose
16. isomer
17. heptose
18. monosaccharide; disaccharide; polysaccharide
19. pentose
20. tetrose
21. disaccharide
22. hydrolysis
23. polysaccharide
24. monosaccharide
25. monosaccharides
26. glucose
27. disaccharides
28. sucrose
29. complex carbohydrates
30. glycogen
31. bulk, fiber
32. micelles
33. lipids
34. monoglyceride
35. saturated fatty acid
36. neutral fat
37. testosterone
38. fatty acids
39. glycolipid
40. unsaturated or monounsaturated fatty acid
41. glycerol
42. steroids
43. triglyceride
44. bile salts
45. omega carbon
46. corticosteroids
47. leukotrienes
48. prostaglandins
49. polyunsaturated fatty acid
50. structural lipids
51. omega-3 fatty acids
52. cholesterol

53. phospholipid
54. calcitriol
55. trans fatty acids
56. diglyceride
57. thromboxanes; prostacyclins
58. estrogens
59. calcitriol
60. polyunsaturated
61. monoglyceride, monounsaturated
62. phospholipid
63. diglyceride
64. glycolipid
65. triglyceride
66. eicosanoid
67. steroid
68. saturated fatty acid
69. phospholipid
70. carboxyl group
71. polyunsaturated fatty acid
72. eicosanoid
73. hydroxyl group
74. vitamins
75. peptide bond
76. amino acids
77. substrates
78. denaturation
79. protein
80. active site
81. keratin
82. R group
83. coenzymes
84. glycoproteins
85. dipeptide
86. proteoglycans
87. globular proteins
88. competitive inhibition
89. alpha-helix
90. cofactor
91. polypeptides
92. fibrous proteins
93. glycoprotein
94. polypeptide
95. cofactor, coenzyme
96. amino group
97. dipeptide
98. amino acid
99. the sequence of amino acids
100. tertiary
101. Contractile
102. transport proteins
103. alpha-helix; pleated sheet
104. Structural proteins
105. enzymes
106. quaternary
107. hydrogen bonding
108. nucleotide
109. pyrimidine
110. high-energy bond
111. metabolic turnover
112. ATP (adenosine triphosphate)
113. DNA (deoxyribonucleic acid)
114. cell
115. complementary base pairs
116. ADP (adenosine diphosphate)
117. turnover rate
118. nucleic acid
119. deoxyribose
120. purine
121. AMP (adenosine monophosphate)
122. RNA (ribonucleic acid)
123. nucleoside
124. purine
125. DNA
126. ATP
127. deoxyribonucleic acid
128. deoxyribose
129. purines
130. thymine (T)
131. ribonucleic acid
132. nitrogenous bases
133. ribose
134. pyrimidines
135. guanine (G)

Answers to Self-Check Test

1. a 2. c 3. d 4. b 5. d 6. b 7. e 8. b 9. c 10. e 11. c 12. e
13. d 14. c 15. d 16. c 17. c 18. a 19. c 20. b

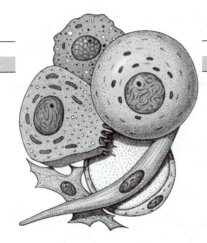

CHAPTER 4

The Cell

Just as atoms are the building blocks of molecules, cells are the building blocks of the human body. Cells were first described by the English scientist Robert Hooke, around 1665. Hooke used an early version of a light microscope to examine dried cork. He observed thousands of tiny empty chambers in the cork, which he named **cells.** Later that decade other scientists, observing the structure of living plants, realized that in life the cells were filled with a gelatinous material. Research over the next 175 years led to the **cell theory,** the concept that cells are the fundamental units of all plant and animal tissues. Since that time, the cell theory has been expanded to incorporate the following basic concepts important to our discussion of the human body.

1. Cells are the building blocks of all plants and animals.
2. Cells are produced by the division of preexisting cells.
3. Cells are the smallest units that perform all vital physiological functions.
4. Each cell maintains homeostasis (internal balance) at the cellular level.
5. Homeostasis at the tissue, organ, system, and organism levels reflects the combined and coordinated actions of many cells.

Cells have a variety of forms and functions. Figure 4–1 gives examples of the range of cell sizes and shapes found in the human body. The relative proportions of the cells in this figure are correct, but all have been magnified roughly 500 times. Together, these and other types of cells create and maintain all anatomical structures and perform all vital physiological functions in the human body.

The human body contains trillions of cells, and all our activities, from running to thinking, result from the combined and coordinated responses of millions or even billions of cells. Yet each cell also functions as an individual entity, responding to a variety of environmental cues. As a result, anyone interested in understanding how the human body functions must first become familiar with basic concepts in cell biology.

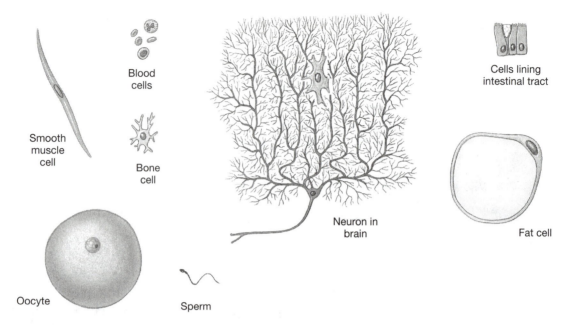

Figure 4–1 The Diversity of Cells in the Human Body.
The cells of the body have many different shapes and a variety of special functions. These examples give an indication of the range of forms. All the cells are shown with the dimensions they would have if magnified approximately 500 times.

STUDYING CELLS

Cytology is *the study of the structure and function of cells.* What we have learned over the past 40 years has given us new insights into cellular physiology and the mechanisms of homeostatic control, and today the study of cell biology incorporates aspects of biology, chemistry, and physics. The two most common methods used to study cell and tissue structure are light microscopy and electron microscopy.

Before the 1950s most information about the structure of cells was provided by **light microscopy.** In light microscopy, a specimen is illuminated by a light source, usu-

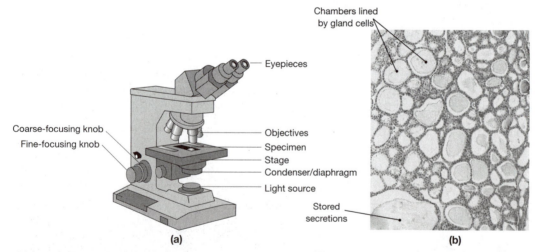

Figure 4–2 Light Microscope.
(a) The light microscope uses light to illuminate the image. The image is then magnified once by the objective lens and then again by the lens in the eyepiece. **(b)** A light micrograph of tissue from the thyroid gland.

ally a light bulb, and then magnified by a series of lenses. Figure 4–2a shows the structure of a generalized light microscope. A photograph taken through a light microscope is called a **light micrograph (LM)** (Figure 4–2b). Light microscopy can magnify cellular structures about 1000 times and show details as fine as 0.25 μm. The symbol μm stands for **micrometer** (also known as a micron); 1 μm = 0.001 mm, or 0.00004 inch. With a light microscope one can identify cell types, such as muscle cells or nerve cells, and see large intracellular (within the cell) structures. Because individual cells are relatively transparent, they are treated with dyes that stain intracellular structures. This staining makes the intracellular structures easier to see.

Although special staining techniques can show the general distribution of protein, lipid, carbohydrate, or nucleic acids in a cell, many fine details of intracellular structure remained a mystery until investigators began using **electron microscopy.** Electron microscopy uses a focused beam of electrons, rather than a beam of light, to examine cell structure. In **transmission electron microscopy,** electrons pass through an ultrathin section of a tissue to strike a photographic plate (Figure 4–3a). The result is a **transmission**

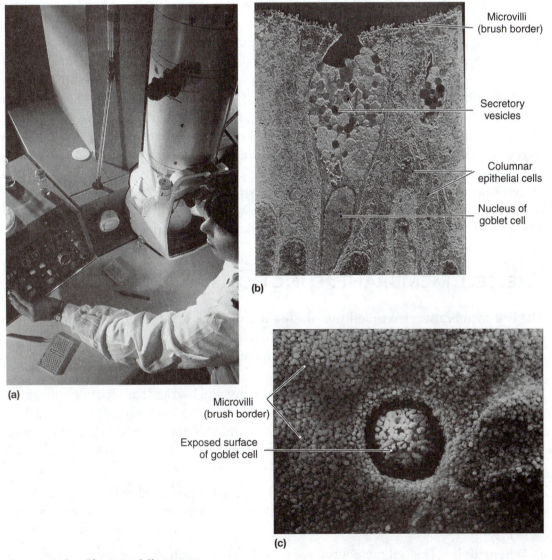

Figure 4–3 Electron Microscope.
(a) An electron microscope. **(b)** A transmission electron micrograph of a goblet cell. **(c)** The cell surface of the same type of goblet cell as seen in a scanning electron micrograph.

electron micrograph (TEM) (Figure 4–3b). Transmission electron microscopy shows the fine structure of cell membranes and intracellular structures. In **scanning electron microscopy** electrons bouncing off exposed surfaces create a **scanning electron micrograph (SEM)** (Figure 4–3c). Although scanning microscopy provides less magnification, it provides a three-dimensional picture of cell structure.

Many other methods can be used to examine cell and tissue structure, and examples will be found in the pages that follow. Each method gives a different perspective, but none tells the entire story. This chapter describes the structure of a typical animal cell and some of the ways in which cells interact with their environment. The next chapter considers cellular metabolism and how cells reproduce.

AN OVERVIEW OF CELLULAR STRUCTURE

The human body contains two classes of cells: somatic cells and sex cells. There are only two types of **sex cells**, or **reproductive cells:** (1) the **sperm** of a male and (2) the **ova** (eggs) of a female. **Somatic cells** (sō-MAT-ik; Greek *soma*, body) include all of the other cells in the human body. This chapter will be looking at somatic cells; sex cells will be considered in Chapter 7, which deals with reproduction.

The "typical" somatic cell is like the "average" person. Any description masks enormous individual variations. For this discussion we will refer to a model cell that shares features with most cells of the body without being identical to any. Figure 4–4 shows such a cell, and Table 4-1 summarizes the structures and functions of its parts.

Our typical cell floats in a watery medium known as the **extracellular fluid.** The extracellular fluid found in most tissues is called **interstitial fluid** (in-ter-STISH-al; Latin *interstitium*, something standing between). A **cell membrane** separates the cell contents, or **cytoplasm** (SĪ-tō-plaz-um), from the interstitial fluid. The cytoplasm, which surrounds the membranous nucleus, can be further subdivided into a liquid, the **cytosol** (SĪ-tō-sol), and intracellular structures collectively known as **organelles** (or-gan-ELZ).

THE CELL MEMBRANE: FUNCTIONS AND STRUCTURE

The cell membrane, also called the **plasma membrane,** or **plasmalemma** (plaz-mah-LEM-uh; Greek *plassein*, to mold + *lemma*, a husk), forms the outer boundary of the cell. The general functions of the cell membrane include:

1. **Physical isolation:** The cell membrane is a physical barrier that separates the inside of a cell from the surrounding extracellular fluid. Conditions inside and outside of a cell are very different, and those differences must be maintained to preserve homeostasis. For example, the cell membrane is a barrier that keeps enzymes and structural proteins inside the cell.

2. **Regulation of exchange with the environment:** The cell membrane controls the entry of ions and nutrients, the elimination of wastes, and the release of secretory products.

3. **Sensitivity:** The cell membrane is the first part of a cell affected by changes in the extracellular fluid. It also contains a variety of receptors that allow a cell to recognize and respond to specific molecules in its environment. For example, the cell

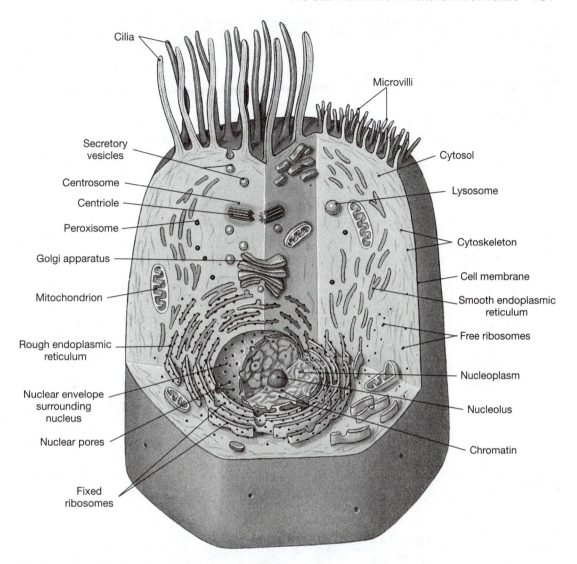

Figure 4–4   The Anatomy of a Representative Cell.
See Table 4-1 for a summary of the functions associated with the various cell structures.

membrane may bind chemical signals from other cells or nutrients in the interstitial fluid. A single alteration in the cell membrane may trigger the activation or de-activation of enzymes that affect many cellular activities.

4. **Structural support:** Specialized connections between cell membranes or between membranes and extracellular materials give tissues a stable structure. For example, the cells at the surface of the skin hold onto one another, and those in the deepest layers are attached to extracellular (outside of the cell) protein fibers in underlying tissues.

The cell membrane is extremely thin and delicate, ranging from 6 to 10 nanometers (nm) in thickness (1 nm = 0.001 μm, 0.000001 mm, or 0.00000004 in.). The cell membrane contains lipids, proteins, and carbohydrates. In terms of relative abundance, phospholipids are the largest contributors to membrane structure, followed by proteins, glycolipids, and cholesterol.

Table 4–1   Organelles of a Representative Cell

Appearance	Structure	Composition	Function
	CELL MEMBRANE	Lipid bilayer, containing phospholipids, steroids and proteins	Isolation; protection; sensitivity; support; controls entrance/exit of materials
	CYTOSOL	Fluid component of cytoplasm	Distributes materials by diffusion
	NONMEMBRANOUS ORGANELLES		
	Cytoskeleton Microtubule Microfilament	Proteins organized in fine filaments or slender tubes	Strength and support; movement of cellular structures and materials
	Microvilli	Membrane extensions containing microfilaments	Increase surface area to facilitate absorption of extracellular materials
	Cilia	Membrane extensions containing microtubule doublets in a 9 + 2 array	Movement of materials over cell surface
	Centrosome Centrioles	Cytoplasm containing two centrioles, at right angles; each centriole cytoskeleton microtubule triplets	Essential for movement of chromosomes during cell division organization of microtublules in cytoskeleton
	Ribosomes	RNA + proteins; fixed ribosomes bound to endoplasmic reticulum, free ribosomes scattered in cytoplasm	Protein synthesis
	MEMBRANOUS ORGANELLES		
	Mitochondria	Double membrane, with inner membrane folds (cristae) enclosing important metabolic enzymes	Produce 95% of the ATP required by the cell
	Endoplasmic reticulum (ER)	Network of membranous channels extending throughout the cytoplasm	Synthesis of secretory products; intracellular storage and transport
	Rough ER	Has ribosomes bound to membranes	Modification and packaging of newly synthesized proteins
	Smooth ER	Lacks attached ribosomes	Lipid and carbohydrate synthesis
	Golgi apparatus	Stacks of flattened membranes (saccules) containing chambers (cisternae)	Storage, alteration, and packaging of secretory products and lysosomal enzymes
	Lysosomes	Vesicles containing powerful digestive enzymes	Intracellular removal of damaged organelles or of pathogens
	Peroxisomes	Vesicles containing degradative enzymes	Neutralization of toxic compounds

Table 4–1	Organelles of a Representative Cell (Continued)		
Appearance	Structure	Composition	Function
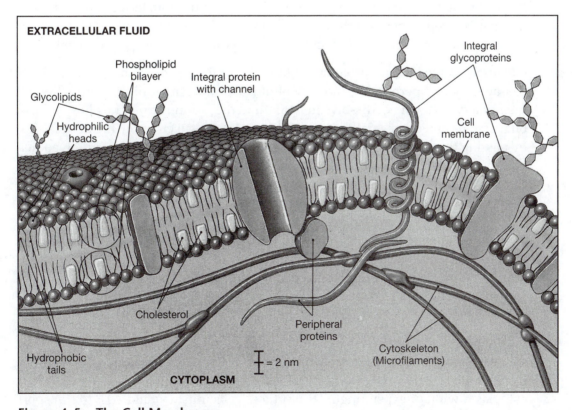Nuclear pore — **NUCLEUS** — **Nucleolus** — Nuclear membrane		Nucleoplasm containing nucleotides, enzymes, nucleoproteins, and chromatin; surrounded by double membrane (nuclear envelope)	Control of metabolism; storage and processing of genetic information; control of protein synthesis
		Dense region in nucleoplasm containing DNA and RNA	Site of rRNA synthesis and assembly of ribosomal subunits

Membrane Lipids

Figure 4–5 is a diagrammatic sketch that highlights important aspects of cell membrane structure. The cell membrane is called a phospholipid bilayer because the phospholipids form two distinct layers. In one layer the phospholipid molecules lie so that the hydrophilic (able to associate with water) heads face outward toward the extracellular fluid, and in the other layer the heads face inward toward the intracellular fluid. The hydrophobic (unable to associate with water) tails turn away from the water and orient toward each other. Associated with the hydrophobic tails are cholesterol and small quantities of other lipids.

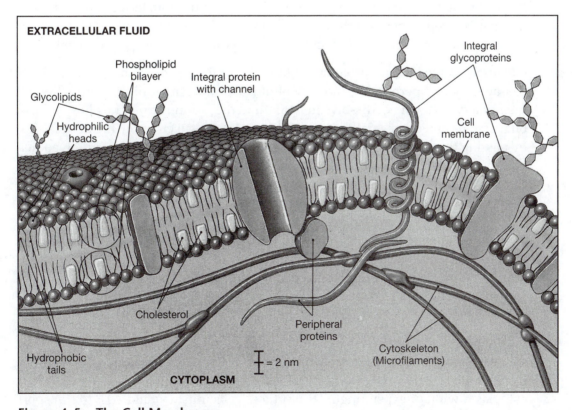

Figure 4–5   The Cell Membrane.

Note the similarities in lipid organization between a micelle, described in Chapter 3 (Figure 3–9, p. 108), and the cell membrane. Ions and water-soluble compounds cannot enter the interior of a micelle because the lipid tails of the phospholipid molecules are highly hydrophobic and will not associate with water molecules. For the same reason, ions and water-soluble compounds cannot cross the lipid portion of a cell membrane. This arrangement makes the membrane very effective in isolating the cytoplasm from the surrounding fluid environment.

Membrane Proteins

Several types of proteins are associated with the membrane. **Integral proteins** are part of the membrane structure. Integral proteins span the entire width of the membrane one or more times and are therefore known as **transmembrane proteins. Peripheral proteins** are bound to the inner or outer surfaces of the membrane and are easily separated from it. Integral proteins greatly outnumber peripheral proteins. A membrane protein (Figure 4–6) can function as a receptor, a channel, a carrier, an enzyme, an anchor, or an identifier.

1. **Receptors:** Receptor proteins in the cell membrane are sensitive to the presence of specific extracellular materials, called **ligands** (LIG-andz; Latin *ligare*, to bind). A receptor protein exposed to an appropriate ligand will bind to it, and that binding may trigger changes in the activity of the cell. For example, binding of the hormone insulin to a specific membrane receptor is the key step that leads to an increase in the rate of glucose uptake by the cell. Cell membranes differ in terms of the type and number of receptor proteins they contain, and this difference accounts for their differing sensitivities to hormones and other compounds in their environment.

2. **Channels:** Some integral proteins contain a central pore, or channel, that forms a passageway that permits the movement of water and small solutes across the cell membrane. Ions will not dissolve in lipids, and they cannot cross the phospholipid bilayer; ions and other small water-soluble materials can cross the membrane only by passing through a channel. Ion movements through channels are involved in a variety of physiological mechanisms, and physiologists speak of sodium channels, calcium channels, potassium channels, and so forth, to refer to channels with specific permeability properties. There are two major kinds of channels: (1) **Leak channels** are essentially pores that are always open and permit water and ion movement at all times, although the rate may vary from moment to moment; (2) **gated channels** are pores that can open or close to regulate ion passage. Channels account for around 0.2 percent of the total membrane surface area.

3. **Carriers:** Carrier proteins bind solutes and transport them across the cell membrane. The transport process involves a change in the shape of the carrier protein; the shape change occurs when solute binding occurs, and it reverses when the solute is released. Carrier proteins may or may not require ATP as an energy source. For example, virtually all cells have carrier proteins that can bring glucose into the cytoplasm without expending ATP, but these cells must expend ATP to transport ions such as sodium, potassium, and calcium across the cell membrane.

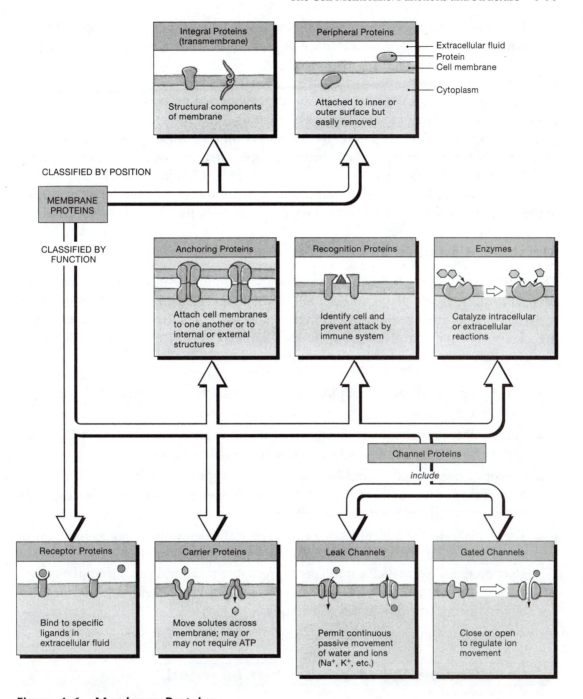

Figure 4–6 Membrane Proteins.

4. **Enzymes:** Enzymes in cell membranes may be integral or peripheral proteins. These enzymes catalyze reactions in the extracellular fluid or within the cytosol, depending on the location of the enzyme and its active site. For example, dipeptides are broken down into amino acids by enzymes on the exposed membranes of cells lining the intestinal tract.

5. **Anchors:** Membrane proteins may attach the cell membrane to other structures and stabilize its position. Inside the cell, membrane proteins are bound to the **cytoskeleton,** a network of supporting filaments within the cytoplasm. Outside the cell, other membrane proteins may attach the cell to extracellular protein fibers or to another cell.

6. **Identifiers:** The cells of the immune system recognize other cells as normal or abnormal on the basis of the presence or absence of characteristic recognition proteins, many of which are glycoproteins.

Membrane structure is not rigid, and the embedded proteins drift from place to place across the surface of the membrane like ice cubes in a punch bowl. In addition, the composition of the cell membrane can change over time, because of the removal and replacement of the membrane surface through processes described later in the chapter.

The inner and outer surfaces of the cell membrane differ in protein and lipid composition. For example, some cytoplasmic enzymes are found only on the inner surface of the membrane, whereas some receptors are exclusively found on its outer surface.

Membrane Carbohydrates

The carbohydrates in the cell membrane are found as components of complex molecules such as proteoglycans, glycoproteins, and glycolipids. The carbohydrate portions of these large molecules extend away from the outer surface of the cell membrane, forming a layer known as the **glycocalyx** (glī-kō-KAL-iks; Greek *glycos*, sugar + *kalyx*, cup). The glycocalyx has a variety of important functions:

1. The glycoproteins and glycolipids form a viscous layer that lubricates and protects the cell membrane.

2. Because the components are sticky, the glycocalyx can help anchor the cell in place, and it also participates in the locomotion of specialized cells.

3. Glycoproteins and glycolipids can function as receptors, binding specific extracellular compounds. Such binding can alter the properties of the cell surface and indirectly affect the behavior of the cell.

4. The characteristics of the glycocalyx are genetically determined. For example, your blood type (A, B, AB, or O) is determined by the presence or absence of membrane glycoproteins. Normal glycoproteins are recognized by the body's immune system as "self" rather than "foreign," and this recognition system keeps the immune system from attacking the tissues of the body.

Let's Review What You've Just Learned

► Definitions

In the space provided, write the term for each of the following definitions.

_____ 1. The fluid found inside a living cell.

_____ 2. Protein channels found in cell membranes that permit water and ion movement at all times.

_____ 3. All of the cells of the body except the reproductive cells.

_____ 4. A unit of measurement equal to 0.001 mm.

_____ 5. A network of supporting filaments within the cytoplasm.

_____ 6. Male reproductive cells.

_____ 7. A layer formed on the outside of a cell membrane by the carbohydrate portion of glycoproteins and glycolipids.

_____ **8.** The smallest living unit of the human body.

_____ **9.** A protein channel in a cell membrane that can open or close to regulate ion passage.

_____ **10.** The branch of biological science that deals with the study of cells.

_____ **11.** The structure that forms the outer boundary of a cell.

_____ **12.** Proteins that are part of the cell membrane structure.

_____ **13.** A general term for the contents of a cell.

_____ **14.** Specific extracellular substances that can bind to receptors on the cell surface.

_____ **15.** Structures that perform specific functions within cells.

_____ **16.** The watery environment around a cell.

_____ **17.** A protein that is attached to the inner or outer surface of the cell membrane.

_____ **18.** Female sex cells.

▶ Word Roots, Prefixes, Suffixes, and Combining Forms

In the space provided, list the boldfaced terms introduced in this section that contain the indicated word part.

Word Part	Meaning	Examples
cyt-	cell	**19.** _____
micro-	small	**20.** _____
glyco-	sugar	**21.** _____
som-	body	**22.** _____
-lemma	husk	**23.** _____
liga-	to bind	**24.** _____

▶ Completion

Complete each of the following statements.

25. A plasma membrane is composed of a bilayer of _____.

26. A _____ can be used to obtain a three-dimensional perspective of a cell.

27. Four important functions of the glycocalyx are

    a. _____

    b. _____

    c. _____

    d. _____

28. Four functions of a cell membrane are

    a. _____

    b. _____

    c. _____

    d. _____

29. Five basic points of the cell theory that are important to a study of human anatomy and physiology are

    a. _____

    b. _____

c. _____

d. _____

e. _____

30. Membrane proteins can function as

  a. _____

  b. _____

  c. _____

  d. _____

  e. _____

  f. _____

▶ **Labeling**

Label the indicated structures on the following diagram of a cell membrane.

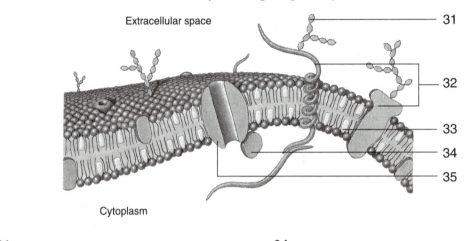

31. _____   **34.** _____

32. _____   **35.** _____

33. _____

THE CYTOPLASM

Cytoplasm is a general term for the material inside the cell membrane and outside of the membrane surrounding the nucleus. There is more protein in cytoplasm than in the interstitial fluid, and the cytoplasmic proteins account for 15–30 percent of the cell's weight. The cytoplasm includes two major subdivisions:

1. **Cytosol, or intracellular fluid:** The cytosol contains dissolved nutrients, ions, soluble and insoluble proteins, and waste products. The cell membrane separates the cytosol from the surrounding extracellular fluid.

2. **Organelles:** Organelles are structures that perform specific functions within the cell.

The Cytosol

Table 4-2 compares the composition of cytosol with the composition of interstitial (tissue) fluid. The three most important differences between cytosol and interstitial fluid are:

1. Cytosol contains a relatively high concentration of potassium ions, whereas interstitial fluid contains a high concentration of sodium ions.

Table 4–2 A Comparison of Cytosol and Tissue Fluid

	Cytosol	Tissue Fluid
Ions (mmol/l)1[†]		
Na$^+$ (sodium)	10	145
K$^+$ (potassium)	160	4
Cl$^-$ (chloride)	3	114
Dissolved proteins (g/dl)[††]	16	1.8
Nutrients (mg/dl)[†††]		
Carbohydrates	0–20	90
Amino acids	200	30
Lipids (g/dl)	2–95	0.6

[†] 0.001 mol of solute per liter of solution = 1 mmol/l.

[††] 1 g protein per 100 ml = 1 g/dl.

[†††] 1 mg (0.001 g) per 100 ml = 1 mg/dl.

2. Cytosol contains a relatively high concentration of suspended proteins. Many of the proteins are enzymes that regulate metabolic operations; others are associated with the various organelles. The cytosol is a colloid with a consistency that varies between that of thin maple syrup and almost-set gelatin.

3. Cytosol usually contains relatively small quantities of carbohydrates and large reserves of amino acids and lipids. Carbohydrates are broken down to provide energy, and the amino acids are used to manufacture proteins. Lipids are primarily used as an energy source when carbohydrates are unavailable.

The cytosol may also contain masses of insoluble materials known as **inclusions**. Among the most common inclusions are stored nutrients: for example, glycogen granules in liver or skeletal muscle cells and lipid droplets in fat cells.

Organelles

Organelles are structures found in the cytoplasm. Each organelle performs specific functions that are essential to normal cell structure, maintenance, and metabolism. Cellular organelles can be divided into two broad categories.

1. **Nonmembranous organelles** are always in direct contact with the cytosol. The cell's nonmembranous organelles include the cytoskeleton, microvilli, centrioles, cilia, flagella, and ribosomes.

2. **Membranous organelles** are surrounded by lipid membranes that isolate them from the cytosol, just as the cell membrane isolates the cytosol from the extracellular fluid. Membranous organelles include the mitochondria, the endoplasmic reticulum, the Golgi apparatus, lysosomes, and peroxisomes. The nucleus, which is also surrounded by a membranous envelope, will be the focus of a separate section.

The Cytoskeleton

The **cytoskeleton** (Figure 4–7) is an internal protein framework that gives the cytoplasm strength and flexibility. It has four major components: microfilaments, intermediate filaments, thick filaments, and microtubules.

Microfilaments are slender protein strands, usually under 6 nm in diameter. The most abundant microfilaments are composed of the protein **actin.** In most cells, microfilaments are scattered throughout the cytoplasm, and they form a dense layer under the cell membrane. Microfilaments attach the cell membrane to the enclosed cytoplasm, and the microfilaments composed of actin play a role in cellular movement.

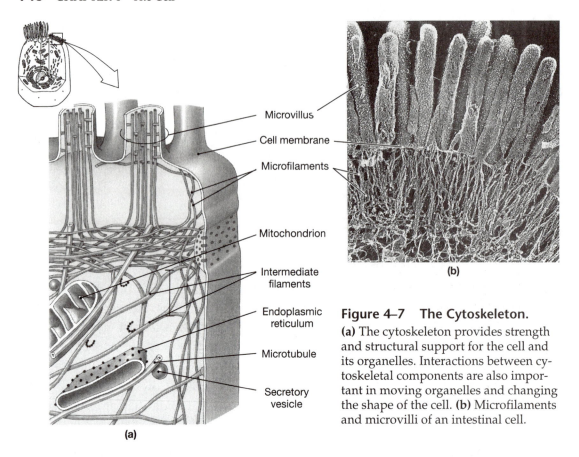

Figure 4–7   The Cytoskeleton.
(a) The cytoskeleton provides strength and structural support for the cell and its organelles. Interactions between cytoskeletal components are also important in moving organelles and changing the shape of the cell. (b) Microfilaments and microvilli of an intestinal cell.

Intermediate filaments are intermediate in size between microfilaments and thick filaments. The composition of intermediate filaments, which range from 7 to 11 nm in diameter, varies from one cell type to another. Intermediate filaments (1) provide strength, (2) stabilize the positions of organelles, and (3) transport materials within the cytoplasm. Nerve cells contain **neurofilaments,** specialized intermediate filaments that provide structural support and assist in the movement of materials within the cytoplasm.

Thick filaments are relatively massive bundles of the protein myosin that may be 15 nm in diameter. Thick filaments are abundant in skeletal and cardiac muscle cells, where they interact with actin filaments to produce powerful contractions.

Microtubules are found in all our cells. They are hollow tubes built from the globular protein **tubulin** (TOO-bū-lin). Microtubules are the largest elements of the cytoskeleton, with diameters around 25 nm. The number and distribution of microtubules within a cell change over time. A microtubule forms through the aggregation of tubulin molecules; it persists for a time and then disassembles into individual tubulin molecules once again.

Microtubules have a variety of functions:

1. Microtubules form the primary components of the cytoskeleton, giving the cell strength and rigidity and anchoring the position of major organelles.

2. Disassembly of microtubules provides a mechanism for changing the shape of the cell, perhaps assisting in cell movement.

3. Microtubules can attach to organelles and other intracellular materials and move them around within the cell.

4. Microtubules move chromosomes during the process of cell division. (Cell division will be considered in more detail in the next chapter.)

5. Microtubules form structural components of other organelles such as centrioles, cilia, and flagella.

The cytoskeleton as a whole incorporates microfilaments, intermediate filaments, and microtubules into a network that extends throughout the cytoplasm. The organizational details are as yet poorly understood, because the network is extremely delicate and thus hard to study in an intact state. Figure 4–7 is based on our current knowledge of cytoskeletal structure. Table 4–3 summarizes the characteristics of the components of the cytoskeleton.

Microvilli

Microvilli are small, finger-shaped projections of the cell membrane (Figure 4–7). Microvilli greatly increase the surface area of the cell exposed to the extracellular environment. They cover the surfaces of cells that are actively absorbing materials from the extracellular fluid, such as the cells lining the digestive tract. A network of microfilaments stiffens each microvillus and anchors it to the underlying cytoskeleton. Interactions between these microfilaments and the cytoskeleton can produce a waving or bending action. Their movements help circulate fluid around the microvilli, bringing dissolved nutrients into contact with receptors on the membrane surface.

Table 4–3 The Cytoskeleton

Cytoskeletal Element	Diameter	Protein Composition	Location	Remarks	Functions	Examples
Microfilaments	Under 6 nm	Actin	In bundles beneath the cell membrane and throughout the cytoplasm	Present in most cells; best organized in skeletal and cardiac muscle cells	Provide strength; alter cell shape; bind the cytoskeleton to the cell membrane; tie cells together	Thin filaments in muscle cells
Intermediate filaments	7–11 nm	Variable	In cytoplasm	Present in most cells; at least 5 types known	Provide strength; move materials through cytoplasm	Neurofilaments in nerve cells; keratin in skin
Thick filaments	15 nm	Myosin	In cytoplasm	Found in skeletal and cardiac muscle cells cells	Interact with thin filaments to produce muscle contraction	Thick filaments in skeletal muscle
Microtubules	25 nm	Tubulin	In cytoplasm radiating away from centrosome	Present in most cells	Provide strength, move organelles	Cilia, centrioles

Centrioles, Cilia, and Flagella

The cytoskeleton contains numerous microtubules that function individually. Microtubules can also combine to form more-complex structures known as centrioles, cilia, and flagella.

All animal cells that are capable of reproducing themselves contain a pair of centrioles. The centrioles direct the movement of DNA strands during cell division (a process discussed in the next chapter). A **centriole** (Figure 4–8a) is a cylindrical structure composed of short microtubules. There are nine groups of microtubules, with three in each group. Each group is connected to the center of the centriole, and in section these connections resemble the spokes of a bicycle wheel. The **centrosome** is the cytoplasm surrounding the centrioles and is the heart of the cytoskeletal system. Microtubules of the cytoskeleton usually begin at the centrosome and radiate through the cytoplasm.

Cilia (SIL-ē-ah; singular *cilium*) contain nine pairs of microtubules surrounding a central pair (Figure 4–8b). Cilia are anchored to a compact **basal body** situated just beneath the cell surface. In section, the organization of microtubules in the basal body resembles that of a centriole, but without the radial spokes. The exposed portion of the

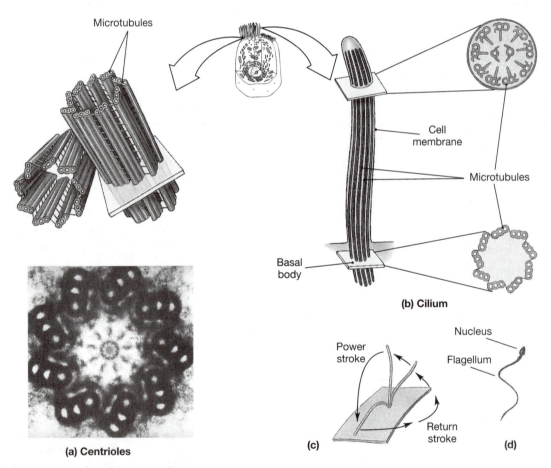

Microtubules

Cell membrane

Microtubules

Basal body

(b) Cilium

Nucleus

Power stroke

Flagellum

Return stroke

(c)

(d)

(a) Centrioles

Figure 4–8   Centrioles and Cilia.

(a) A centriole consists of nine microtubule triplets (known as a 9 + 0 array). The centrosome contains a pair of centrioles oriented at right angles to one another. **(b)** A cilium contains nine pairs of microtubules surrounding a central pair (9 + 2 array). The basal body to which the cilium is anchored has a structure similar to that of a centriole. **(c)** A single cilium swings forward and then returns to its original position. During the power stroke, the cilium is relatively stiff, but during the return stroke, it bends and moves parallel to the cell surface. **(d)** A sperm cell with its flagellum.

cilium is completely covered by the cell membrane. Cilia "beat" rhythmically, as depicted in Figure 4–8c, and their combined efforts move fluids or secretions across the cell surface. For example, cilia lining the respiratory tract beat in a synchronized manner to move sticky mucus and trapped dust particles toward the throat and away from delicate respiratory surfaces. If the cilia are damaged or immobilized by heavy smoking or some metabolic problem, the cleansing action is lost, and the irritants will no longer be removed. As a result, chronic respiratory infections develop.

Flagella (fla-JEL-ah; singular *flagellum*, Latin, whip) resemble cilia, but they are much larger and longer. Flagella move a cell through the surrounding fluid, rather than moving the fluid past a stationary cell. The sperm cell (Figure 4–8d) is the only human cell that has a flagellum, and the flagellum is used to move the cell along the female reproductive tract. If sperm flagella are paralyzed or otherwise abnormal, the individual will be sterile, because immobile sperm cannot reach and fertilize an egg.

Ribosomes

Ribosomes are intracellular factories that manufacture proteins, using information provided by the DNA of the nucleus. The number of ribosomes within a particular cell varies depending on the type of cell and its activities. For example, liver cells, which manufacture blood proteins, contain far more ribosomes than fat cells, which synthesize triglycerides.

Ribosomes are small, dense structures that cannot be seen clearly with the light microscope. In an electron micrograph, ribosomes appear as dense granules. A functional ribosome consists of two subunits that are normally separate and distinct (Figure 4–9). The subunits differ in size; one is a **small,** or *light,* **ribosomal subunit,** and the other is a **large,** or *heavy,* **ribosomal subunit.** These subunits contain special proteins and ribosomal RNA, one of the RNA types introduced in Chapter 3. Before protein synthesis can begin, a small and a large ribosomal subunit must join together with a strand of messenger RNA to create a functional ribosome.

There are two major types of functional ribosomes: free ribosomes and fixed ribosomes. **Free ribosomes** are scattered throughout the cytoplasm; the proteins they manufacture enter the cytosol. **Fixed ribosomes** are attached to the endoplasmic reticulum (ER), a membranous organelle inside the cell. Proteins manufactured by fixed ribosomes enter the ER, where they are modified.

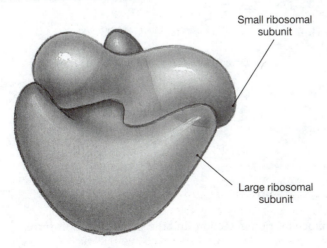

Small ribosomal subunit

Large ribosomal subunit

Figure 4–9   Ribosomes.
A diagrammatic view of the structure of an intact ribosome. The subunits are separate unless the ribosome is engaged in protein synthesis.

Mitochondria

Mitochondria (Mī-tō-KON-drē-ah; singular *mitochondrion;* Greek *mitos,* thread + *chondrion,* small granule) are the main energy-generating organelles of the cell. They are small organelles that can have a variety of shapes, from long and slender to short and fat. The number of mitochondria in a particular cell vary depending on its energy demands. Red blood cells have none, but mitochondria may account for 20 percent of the volume of an active liver cell.

Mitochondria have an unusual double membrane (Figure 4–10). An outer membrane surrounds the entire organelle, and a second, inner membrane contains numerous folds, called **cristae** (KRIS-tē; Latin *crista,* crest). Cristae increase the surface area exposed to the fluid contents, or matrix, of the mitochondrion. The matrix contains metabolic enzymes that perform the reactions that provide energy for cellular functions.

Most of the chemical reactions that release energy occur in the mitochondria, but most of the cellular activities that require energy occur in the surrounding cytoplasm. Cells must therefore store energy in a form that can be moved from place to place. Energy is stored and transferred in the form of high-energy bonds. Such a bond usually attaches a phosphate group (PO_4^{3-}) to a suitable molecule, creating a high-energy compound.

The most important high-energy compound is adenosine triphosphate, or ATP, discussed in Chapter 3. Living cells break the high-energy phosphate bond under controlled conditions, reconverting ATP to ADP and releasing energy for their use.

The Endoplasmic Reticulum

The **endoplasmic reticulum** (en-dō-plaz-mik re-TIK-ū-lum), or **ER,** is a network of intracellular membranes that is connected to the nuclear envelope surrounding the nucleus (Figure 4–11). The name comes from the Greek *endon,* inside and *plasma,* something formed, and Latin *reticulum,* a small net. The endoplasmic reticulum has four major functions:

1. **Synthesis:** Ribosomes associated with the ER membrane manufacture proteins, and enzymes of the ER membrane manufacture carbohydrates and lipids.

2. **Storage:** The ER can hold synthesized molecules or materials absorbed from the cytosol without affecting other cellular operations.

3. **Transport:** Materials can travel from place to place in the endoplasmic reticulum.

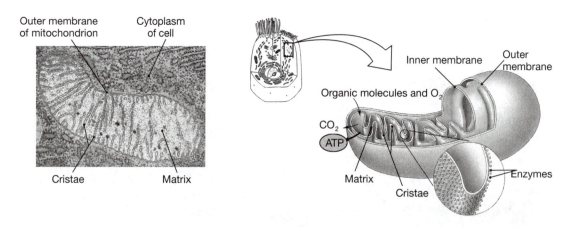

Figure 4–10 Mitochondria.
This electron micrograph shows a typical mitochondrion in section, and the sketch details its three-dimensional organization. (TEM × 46,332)

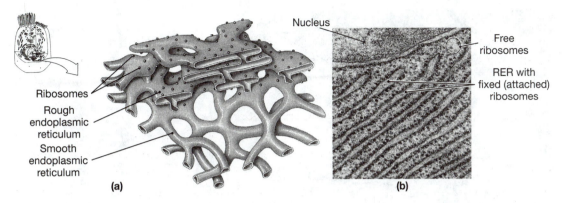

Figure 4–11   The Endoplasmic Reticulum.

(a) This diagrammatic sketch indicates the three-dimensional relationships between the rough and smooth endoplasmic reticula. **(b)** Rough endoplasmic reticulum and free ribosomes in the cytoplasm of a cell. (TEM × 73,600)

4. **Detoxification:** Drugs or toxins can be absorbed by the endoplasmic reticulum and neutralized by enzymes within the ER.

The endoplasmic reticulum forms hollow tubes, flattened sheets, and round chambers. The chambers are called **cisternae** (sis-TUR-nē; singular *cisterna*; Latin *cisterna*, a reservoir). There are two distinct types of endoplasmic reticulum: **smooth endoplasmic reticulum (SER)** and **rough endoplasmic reticulum (RER).**

There are no ribosomes associated with the smooth endoplasmic reticulum. The SER has a variety of functions that center around the synthesis of lipids and carbohydrates. Those functions include:

1. Synthesis of the phospholipids and cholesterol needed for maintenance and growth of the cell membrane, ER, nuclear membrane, and Golgi apparatus in all cells.
2. Synthesis of steroid hormones, such as androgens (male sex hormones) and estrogens (female sex hormones) in the reproductive organs and the steroid hormones of the adrenal gland.
3. Synthesis and storage of glycerides, especially triglycerides, in liver and fat cells.
4. Detoxification or inactivation of drugs in the SER of liver and kidney cells.
5. Synthesis and storage of glycogen in skeletal muscle and liver cells.
6. Removal and storage of calcium ions (Ca^{2+}) or larger molecules from the cytosol. Calcium ions are stored in the SER of skeletal muscle cells, neurons (nerve cells), and many other cell types.

The RER functions as a combination workshop and shipping depot. It is where many newly synthesized proteins undergo chemical modification and where they are packaged for export to their next destination, the Golgi apparatus. The outer surface of the rough endoplasmic reticulum contains fixed ribosomes. The ribosomes synthesize proteins, which enter the cisternae of the endoplasmic reticulum. Inside the ER the protein assumes its secondary or tertiary structure. Some of the proteins synthesized are enzymes that will function inside the ER. Other proteins are chemically modified within the ER by the attachment of carbohydrates, creating glycoproteins.

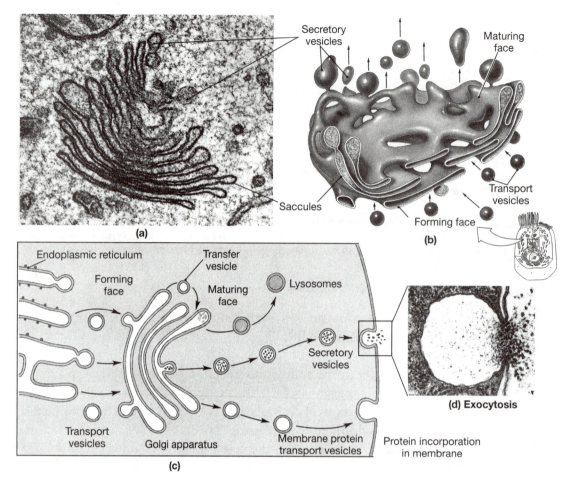

Figure 4–12 The Golgi Apparatus.

(a) A sectional view of the Golgi apparatus of an active secretory cell. (TEM × 57,660) **(b)** A three-dimensional view of the Golgi apparatus with a cut edge corresponding to part (a). **(c)** Transport vesicles carry the secretory product from the endoplasmic reticulum to the Golgi apparatus (simplified to clarify the relationships between the membranes). Transfer vesicles move membrane and materials between the Golgi saccules. At the maturing face, three functional categories of vesicles develop. Secretory vesicles carry the secretion from the Golgi to the cell surface, where exocytosis releases the contents into the extracellular fluid. Other vesicles add surface area and integral proteins to the cell membrane. Lysosomes, which remain in the cytoplasm, are vesicles filled with enzymes. **(d)** Exocytosis at the surface of a cell.

The Golgi Apparatus

The **Golgi** (GŌL-jē; Emilio Golgi, Italian anatomist) **apparatus** (Figure 4–12a) synthesizes and packages cellular secretions and plays a role in forming new cell membranes. A typical Golgi apparatus consists of five or six flattened membrane discs, called **saccules** (SAK-ūlz); a single cell may contain several sets, each resembling a stack of dinner plates. Most often these stacks lie near the nucleus of the cell.

Figure 4–12b, c diagrams the role of the Golgi apparatus in packaging secretions. Protein and glycoprotein synthesis occur in the RER, and transport vesicles then move these products to the Golgi apparatus. The transport vesicles fuse with the Golgi membrane, emptying their contents into the cisterna. Inside the Golgi, enzymes modify the arriving proteins and glycoproteins. For example, the carbohydrate structure of a glycoprotein may be changed, or a phosphate group, sugar, or fatty acid may be attached to a protein. Material moves from saccule to saccule by means of small transfer vesicles. When the product arrives at the last saccule in the series, vesicles form that carry materials away from the Golgi apparatus.

Three types of vesicles are produced at the Golgi apparatus:

- **Secretory vesicles: Secretory vesicles** are vesicles containing secretions that will be discharged from the cell. The glycoproteins that cover most cell surfaces are synthesized by the Golgi apparatus and released in this way.

- **New cell membrane components:** As vesicles produced at the Golgi apparatus fuse with the surface of the cell they are adding new lipids and proteins to the cell membrane. At the same time, other areas of the cell membrane are being removed. The Golgi apparatus can thus change the properties of the cell membrane over time. For example, new glycoprotein receptors can be added, making the cell more sensitive to a particular stimulus; alternatively, receptors can be removed, making the cell less sensitive. Such changes can profoundly alter the sensitivity and functions of the cell.

- **Packaging of intracellular enzymes:** A third class of vesicles produced at the Golgi apparatus never leaves the cytoplasm. These vesicles, called lysosomes, contain digestive enzymes. Their varied functions will be detailed in the next section.

Lysosomes

Lysosomes (LĪ-sō-sōmz; Greek *lyein*, loosen, release + *soma*, body) are vesicles filled with digestive enzymes. They are produced at the Golgi apparatus (Figure 4–12c). **Primary lysosomes** contain inactive enzymes (Figure 4–13). Activation occurs when the lysosome fuses with the membranes of damaged organelles, such as mitochondria or fragments of the endoplasmic reticulum. This fusion creates a **secondary lysosome,** which contains active enzymes. These enzymes then break down the lysosomal contents. Nutrients from the digested organelles reenter the cytosol. Molecules and parts of the organelles that cannot be recycled are eliminated from the cell.

Lysosomes also function in the defense against disease. Cells may remove bacteria, as well as liquids and organic debris, from their surroundings in vesicles formed at the cell surface. This process, called endocytosis, is described on page 169, and the role of lysosomes in receptor-mediated endocytosis is detailed in Figure 4–23, page 170. Lysosomes fuse with the vesicles created through endocytosis, and the digestive enzymes then break down the contents and release usable substances such as sugars or amino acids. In this way the cell both protects itself against pathogenic organisms and obtains valuable nutrients.

Figure 4–13 summarizes lysosomal functions. Lysosomes perform essential cleanup and recycling functions inside the cell. For example, when muscle cells are inactive, lysosomes gradually break down their contractile proteins; if the cells become active once again, this destruction ceases. This regulatory mechanism fails in a damaged or dead cell. Lysosomes then disintegrate, releasing active enzymes into the cytosol. These enzymes rapidly destroy the proteins and organelles of the cell, a process called **autolysis** (aw-TA-li-sis; Greek *autos,* self + *lyein,* release). We do not know how to control lysosomal activities or why the enclosed enzymes do not digest the lysosomal walls unless the cell is damaged.

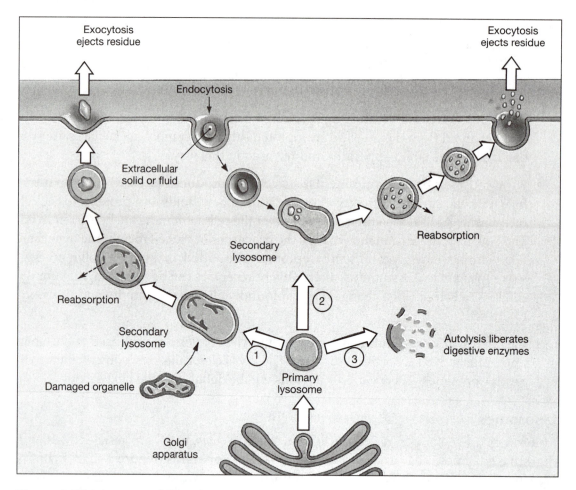

Figure 4–13 Lysosomal Functions.

Primary lysosomes, formed at the Golgi apparatus, contain inactive enzymes. Activation may occur under three basic conditions: (1) when the primary lysosome fuses with the membrane of another organelle, such as a mitochondrion; (2) when the primary lysosome fuses with an endocytic vesicle containing fluid or solid materials from outside the cell; or (3) in autolysis, when the lysosomal membrane breaks down after death of or injury to the cell.

Problems with lysosomal enzyme production cause more than 30 serious diseases affecting children. In these conditions, called **lysosomal storage diseases,** the lack of a specific lysosomal enzyme results in the buildup of waste products or debris normally removed and recycled by lysosomes. These individuals may die when vital cells, such as those of the heart, can no longer continue to function.

Peroxisomes

Peroxisomes are similar to lysosomes, but they are smaller and carry a different group of enzymes. In contrast to lysosomes, which are produced at the Golgi apparatus, peroxisomes probably originate at the RER. Peroxisomes absorb and neutralize toxins, such as alcohol or hydrogen peroxide (H_2O_2), that are absorbed from the interstitial fluid or generated by chemical reactions in the cytoplasm. Peroxisomes are most abundant in liver cells, which are responsible for removing and neutralizing toxins absorbed by the digestive tract. Peroxisomes protect all cells from the potentially damaging effects of free radicals produced during normal metabolic reactions. It has been suggested that the cumulative damage produced by free radicals inside and outside of our cells is a major factor in the aging process.

Membrane Flow

With the exception of the mitochondria, all of the membranous organelles in the cell are either interconnected or in communication through the movement of vesicles. The rough and smooth endoplasmic reticulum are continuous and connected to the nuclear envelope, the membrane that surrounds the nucleus. Transport vesicles connect the ER with the Golgi apparatus, and secretory vesicles link the Golgi apparatus with the cell membrane. Finally, vesicles forming at the exposed surface of the cell remove and recycle segments of the cell membrane. This continual movement and exchange is called **membrane flow.**

Membrane flow can be quite rapid. In an actively secreting cell, the Golgi membranes may undergo a complete turnover every 40 minutes. The membrane lost from the Golgi is added to the cell surface, and that addition is balanced by the formation of vesicles at the membrane surface. As a result, an area equal to the entire membrane surface may be replaced each hour.

Membrane flow is another example of the dynamic nature of cells; it provides a mechanism for cells to change the characteristics of their cell membranes—receptors, channels, anchors, and all—as they grow, mature, or respond to a specific environmental stimulus.

THE NUCLEUS

The **nucleus** is *the control center for cellular operations.* A single nucleus stores all of the information needed to control the synthesis of the 100,000 different proteins in the human body. By controlling what proteins are synthesized, and in what amounts, the nucleus determines the structural and functional characteristics of the cell. A cell without a nucleus could be compared to a car without a driver. However, a car can sit idle for years, but a cell without a nucleus will disintegrate within 3–4 months.

Most cells contain a single nucleus, but there are exceptions. For example, skeletal muscle cells have many nuclei, and mature red blood cells have none. Figure 4–14 details the structure of a typical nucleus. A **nuclear envelope** surrounds the nucleus and separates it from the cytosol. The nuclear envelope is a double membrane containing a narrow **perinuclear** (*peri-*, around) **space.** At several locations, the nuclear envelope is connected to the rough endoplasmic reticulum; this arrangement is diagrammed in Figure 4–4, p. 137.

The nucleus directs processes that take place in the cytosol and must in turn receive information about conditions and activities in the cytosol. Chemical communication between the nucleus and cytosol occurs through **nuclear pores.** These pores, which cover about 10 percent of the surface of the nucleus, are large enough to permit the movement of ions and small molecules, but they are they are too small for the passage of proteins or DNA. Proteins and other large molecules or groups of molecules that must enter or leave the nucleus do so by means of transport vesicles as described in the preceding section.

The term **nucleoplasm** (NOO-klē-ō-plazm) refers to the fluid contents of the nucleus. The nucleoplasm contains ions, enzymes, RNA and DNA nucleotides, proteins, small amounts of RNA, and DNA. The DNA strands form complex structures known as **chromosomes** (KRŌ-muh-sōmz; Greek *chroma*, color + *soma*, body). The nucleoplasm also contains a network of fine filaments, the **nuclear matrix,** that provides structural support and may be involved in the regulation of genetic activity.

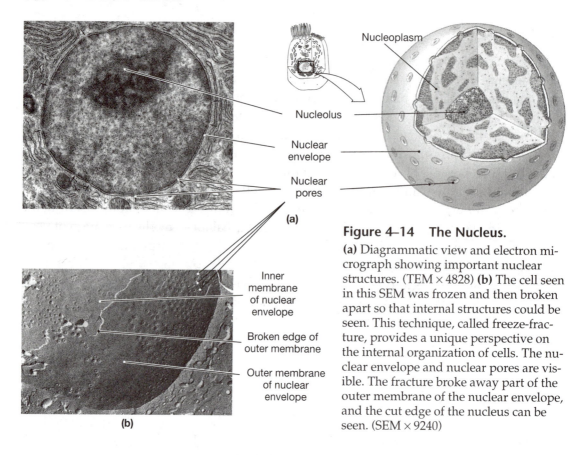

Nucleoplasm

Nucleolus

Nuclear envelope

Nuclear pores

Inner membrane of nuclear envelope

Broken edge of outer membrane

Outer membrane of nuclear envelope

(a)

(b)

Figure 4–14 The Nucleus.
(a) Diagrammatic view and electron micrograph showing important nuclear structures. (TEM × 4828) **(b)** The cell seen in this SEM was frozen and then broken apart so that internal structures could be seen. This technique, called freeze-fracture, provides a unique perspective on the internal organization of cells. The nuclear envelope and nuclear pores are visible. The fracture broke away part of the outer membrane of the nuclear envelope, and the cut edge of the nucleus can be seen. (SEM × 9240)

Most nuclei contain one to four dark-staining areas called **nucleoli** (noo-KLĒ-ō-lī; singular *nucleolus*) (Figure 4–14). Nucleoli are nuclear organelles that synthesize ribosomal RNA (rRNA, which was discussed in Chapter 3) and assemble the ribosomal subunits. A nucleolus contains structural proteins and enzymes as well as RNA, and it forms around a region of chromosomes that includes the DNA bearing the instructions for producing ribosomal proteins and RNA. Nucleoli are most prominent in cells that manufacture large amounts of proteins, such as liver cells and muscle cells, because these cells need large numbers of ribosomes.

Let's Review What You've Just Learned

► **Definitions**

In the space provided, write the term for each of the following definitions.

_____ **36.** An organelle containing rRNA and proteins that is essential in protein synthesis.

_____ **37.** A protein commonly found in thin microfilaments.

_____ **38.** The folds in the inner membrane of a mitochondrion.

_____ **39.** Slender protein strands that are usually less than 6 nm in diameter.

_____ **40.** The cytoplasm that surrounds centrioles.

_____ **41.** Masses of insoluble material found in the cytosol.

_____ **42.** Membrane-bound sacs containing secretions that will be discharged from a cell.

_____ **43.** A network of intracellular membranes that is connected to the membrane surrounding the nucleus.

_____ **44.** A protein commonly found in thick microfilaments.

_____ **45.** The globular protein that makes up microtubules.

_____ **46.** Small vesicles containing enzymes that can neutralize toxins and protect the cell against free radicals.

_____ **47.** Complex structures containing DNA and protein that are located in the cell nucleus.

_____ **48.** Small organelles that function in energy transformation.

_____ **49.** A ribosome that is bound to the surface of the endoplasmic reticulum.

_____ **50.** Organelles that are always in direct contact with the cytosol.

_____ **51.** Microscopic hollow tubes that form the primary components of the cytoskeleton.

_____ **52.** An organelle that consists of flattened membrane discs and is involved in the synthesis and packaging of cellular secretions.

_____ **53.** The membrane that separates the contents of the nucleus from the cytoplasm.

_____ **54.** A type of endoplasmic reticulum that functions in the synthesis of lipids and carbohydrates.

_____ **55.** The process whereby lysosomes release their enzymes and the enzymes rapidly destroy the proteins and organelles of the cell.

_____ **56.** The structure that anchors cilia to the cell membrane.

_____ **57.** Small, finger-shaped projections of a cell membrane.

_____ **58.** Vesicles filled with digestive enzymes.

_____ **59.** A collective term for organelles that are surrounded by a lipid membrane.

_____ **60.** Relatively massive bundles of myosin proteins up to 15 nm in diameter.

_____ **61.** A cylindrical structure composed of nine groups of short microtubules, in which each group consists of three microtubules.

_____ **62.** The flattened membrane discs that make up a Golgi apparatus.

_____ **63.** The continuous movement of new membrane to the cell surface and the exchange for old membrane.

_____ **64.** A nuclear organelle that synthesizes rRNA.

_____ **65.** Disease condition that results from the lack of a specific lysosomal enzyme.

_____ **66.** Ribosomes that are not attached to the surface of endoplasmic reticulum.

_____ **67.** The round chambers of the endoplasmic reticulum.

_____ **68.** A cylindrical organelle that consists of nine pairs of microtubules surrounding a central pair.

_____ **69.** Endoplasmic reticulum that has ribosomes bound to its surface.

_____ **70.** An organelle that contains the cell's genetic material, frequently referred to as the control center for cellular operations.

_____ **71.** An organelle that resembles a cilium but is much longer and functions in moving a cell through the surrounding fluid.

▶ Word Roots, Prefixes, Suffixes, and Combining Forms

In the space provided, list the boldfaced terms introduced in this section that contain the indicated word part.

Word Part	Meaning	Examples
neuro-	nerve	72. _____
endo-	inside	73. _____
myo-	muscle	74. _____
lys-	dissolve	75. _____
fil-	thread	76. _____
-some	body	77. _____
auto-	self	78. _____
chromo-	color	79. _____

▶ Labeling

Label the indicated structures on the following diagram of a generalized cell.

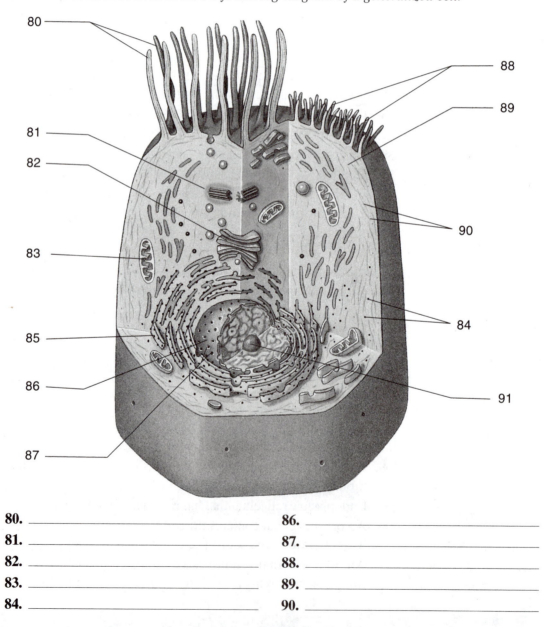

80. _____   86. _____

81. _____   87. _____

82. _____   88. _____

83. _____   89. _____

84. _____   90. _____

MEMBRANE PERMEABILITY

The cell membrane is a physical barrier that separates the inside of a cell from the surrounding extracellular fluid. Conditions inside and outside of the cell are very different, and those differences must be maintained to preserve homeostasis. Precisely which substances can enter or leave the cytoplasm is determined by the permeability of the cell membrane. If nothing could cross the cell membrane, it would be described as **impermeable.** If any substance at all could cross without difficulty, the membrane would be **freely permeable.** Cell membranes actually fall somewhere in between, and are thus said to be selectively permeable. A **selectively permeable membrane** permits the free passage of some materials and restricts the passage of others. The distinction may be on the basis of size, electrical charge, molecular shape, lipid solubility, or some combination of factors.

The permeability of a cell membrane varies depending on the organization and identity of membrane lipids and proteins. Passage across the membrane may be passive or active. **Passive processes** move ions or molecules across the cell membrane without any energy expenditure by the cell. **Active processes** require that the cell expend energy, usually in the form of ATP.

Transport mechanisms may also be categorized by the nature of the mechanism involved. The major categories are:

- **Diffusion,** which results from the random motion and collisions of ions and molecules. Diffusion is a passive process.

- **Filtration,** which occurs when hydrostatic (fluid) pressure forces fluid and solutes across a membrane barrier. Filtration is also a passive process.

- **Carrier-mediated transport,** which requires the presence of specialized integral membrane proteins. Carrier-mediated transport may be passive or active, depending on the substance transported and the nature of the transport mechanism.

- **Vesicular transport,** which involves the movement of materials within small membranous sacs, or **vesicles.** Vesicular transport is an active process.

Diffusion

Ions and molecules are in constant motion, colliding and bouncing off one another and off any obstacles in their paths. The random movement that occurs is called **diffusion.** One result of diffusion is that there will be a net movement of material from an area where its concentration is relatively high to an area where its concentration is relatively low. The difference between the high and low concentrations represents a **concentration gradient.** As some material moves from the area of high concentration to the area of low concentration, the concentration gradient decreases. If the system is allowed to reach equilibrium, the concentration gradient will be eliminated as the diffusing material becomes evenly distributed over all of the available area. After the gradient has been eliminated, diffusion continues, but there is no longer net movement in any particular direction. For convenience, we restrict use of the term *diffusion* to the directional movement that eliminates concentration gradients; this process is sometimes called **net diffusion.** Because diffusion spreads materials from a region of high concentration to one of relatively lower concentration, it is often described as proceeding "down a concentration gradient" or "downhill."

We have all experienced the effects of diffusion, which occurs in air as well as water. The smell of fresh flowers in a vase can sweeten the air in a large room, just as a drop of ink spreads to color an entire glass of water. In each case, you begin with an extremely high concentration of molecules in a very localized area. Consider dye dropped in a water glass (Step 1, Figure 4–15). Placing that drop in a large volume of clear water establishes a steep concentration gradient for the dye: The dye concentration is high at the drop and negligible everywhere else. As diffusion proceeds, the dye molecules spread through the solution (Step 2) until they are distributed evenly (Step 3).

Diffusion is important in body fluids because it tends to eliminate local concentration gradients. For example, an active cell generates carbon dioxide and absorbs oxygen. As a result, the extracellular fluid around the cell develops a relatively high concentration of carbon dioxide and a relatively low concentration of oxygen. Diffusion then distributes the carbon dioxide through the tissue and into the bloodstream. At the same time, oxygen diffuses out of the blood and into the tissue.

To be effective, the rate of diffusion of nutrients, waste products, and dissolved gases must be able to keep pace with the demands of active cells. Important factors that influence diffusion rates include:

1. **Distance:** Concentration gradients are eliminated quickly over short distances. The greater the distance, the longer the time required. In the human body, diffusion distances are usually small. For example, few living cells are farther than 125 μm from a blood vessel.

2. **Size of the gradient:** The larger the concentration gradient, the faster diffusion proceeds. When cells become more active, the intracellular concentration of oxygen declines. This decline increases the concentration gradient for oxygen between the inside of the cell (relatively low) and the interstitial fluid (relatively high). The rate of oxygen diffusion into the cell then increases.

3. **Size of the substance diffusing:** Ions and small organic molecules such as glucose diffuse faster than large proteins.

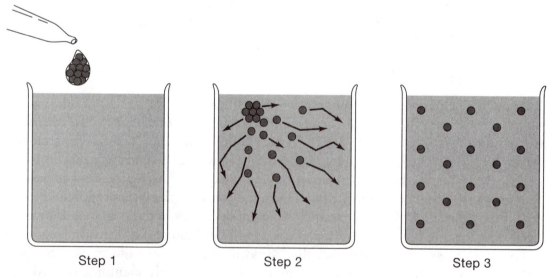

Figure 4–15   Diffusion.
Step 1: Placing an ink drop in a glass of water establishes a strong concentration gradient because there are many ink molecules in one location and none elsewhere. *Step 2:* As diffusion occurs, the ink molecules spread through the solution. *Step 3:* Eventually, diffusion eliminates the concentration gradient, and the ink molecules are distributed evenly. Molecular motion continues, but there is no directional movement.

Step 1   Step 2   Step 3

4. **Temperature:** The higher the temperature, the faster the diffusion rate. The human body maintains a temperature of around 37ºC, and diffusion proceeds much faster at this temperature than at normal environmental temperatures.

5. **Electrical forces:** For reasons that will be explored later, the interior of the cell membrane has a net negative charge relative to the exterior surface. Opposite charges (+ and –) are attracted to one another, whereas similar charges (+ and + or – and –) are repelled. The negative charge on the inside of the cell membrane will tend to pull positive ions into the cell and oppose the entry of negative ions. For example, when compared with the cytosol, interstitial fluid contains relatively high concentrations of sodium ions (Na^+) and chloride ions (Cl^-). The difference in ion concentrations between the cytosol and the interstitial fluid constitutes a chemical gradient for each ion. The difference in the electrical charge between the interior of the cell membrane (negative charge) and the exterior of the membrane (positive charge) constitutes an electrical gradient. Both the chemical gradient and the electrical gradient favor the diffusion of sodium ions (Na^+) from the interstitial fluid into the cell. In other words, sodium ions diffuse down their concentration gradient, and the positive sodium ions are attracted to the negative interior of the cell membrane. In the case of the chloride ion, even though the chemical gradient favors the diffusion of chloride ions from the interstitial fluid into the cell (from high concentration to low concentration), it is opposed by the electrical gradient (like charges repel each other). The opposition of the electrical gradient limits the number of chloride ions that will be able to diffuse into the cell. For any given ion, the net result of the chemical and electrical forces acting on a particular ion is called the **electrochemical gradient.**

Diffusion across Cell Membranes

In the extracellular fluids of the body, water and dissolved solutes diffuse freely. A cell membrane, however, acts as a barrier that selectively restricts diffusion: Some substances can pass through easily, whereas others cannot penetrate the membrane at all. There are only two ways for an ion or molecule to diffuse across a cell membrane: (1) pass through one of the membrane channels or (2) move across the lipid portion of the membrane (Figure 4–16). If a concentration gradient, or chemical gradient, for a particular ion or molecule exists, whether it moves across the cell membrane will depend on two major factors: its lipid solubility and its size relative to the sizes of the membrane channels.

1. **Lipid solubility:** Alcohol, fatty acids, and steroids can enter cells easily because they can diffuse through the lipid portions of the membrane by dissolving in it. Dissolved gases such as oxygen and carbon dioxide also enter and leave our cells by diffusion through the lipid bilayer.

2. **Size:** To diffuse into the cytoplasm, a water-soluble compound must pass through a membrane channel. These channels are very small, averaging about 0.8 nm in diameter. Water molecules can enter or exit freely, as can ions such as sodium, potassium, calcium, hydrogen, and chloride, but even a small organic molecule, such as glucose, is too big to fit through the channels.

Osmosis: A Special Case of Diffusion

As mentioned previously in the chapter, cell membranes are selectively permeable. That is, they allow some substances to pass through while restricting the passage of others. Cell membranes are generally permeable to water, but they are not always permeable to the solutes dissolved in water. As a result, when the movement of solutes along their

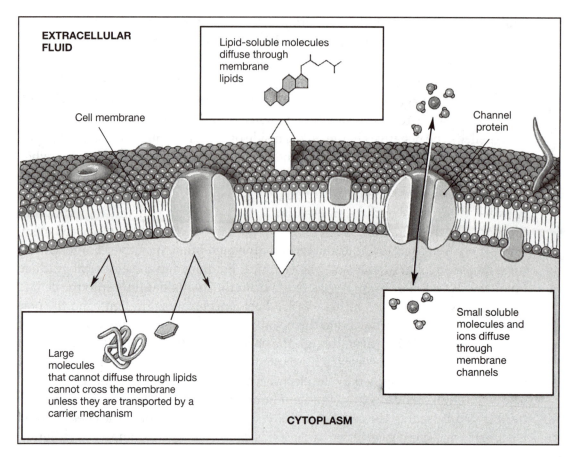

Figure 4–16   Diffusion across Cell Membranes.

Small ions and water-soluble molecules diffuse through membrane channels. Lipid-soluble molecules can cross the membrane by diffusing through the phospholipid bilayer. Large molecules that are not lipid-soluble, such as proteins and carbohydrates, cannot diffuse through the cell membrane.

concentration gradient is prevented by a selectively permeable barrier (such as a cell membrane), water will diffuse from one side of the barrier to another until the concentration of solutes on both sides is equal. The net diffusion of water across a membrane is so important that it is given a special name, **osmosis** (oz-MŌ-sis; Greek *osmos*, thrust).

Intracellular and extracellular fluids are solutions that contain a variety of dissolved materials. Each solute tends to diffuse as if it were the only material in solution. For example, the diffusion of sodium ions occurs in response to the existence of a concentration gradient for sodium. A change in the concentration of potassium ions will have no effect on the rate or direction of sodium ion diffusion. Some solutes diffuse into the cytoplasm, others diffuse out, and a few, such as proteins, are unable to cross the cell membrane at all. But if we ignore the individual identities and simply count solutes (molecules and ions), we find that the total concentration of dissolved molecules and ions on either side of the cell membrane stays the same.

This state of equilibrium persists because the entire cell membrane is freely permeable to water. Whenever a solute concentration gradient exists, there is also a concentration gradient for water. Because dissolved solute molecules occupy space that would otherwise be taken up by water molecules, the higher the solute concentration, the lower the water concentration. As a result, water molecules will tend to diffuse across a membrane toward the solution containing a higher solute concentration, because this direction follows the concentration gradient for water.

Three characteristics of osmosis should be remembered:

1. Osmosis is the diffusion of water molecules across a membrane.

2. Osmosis occurs across a selectively permeable membrane that is freely permeable to water but not freely permeable to solutes.

3. In osmosis, water will flow across a membrane toward the solution that has the highest concentration of solutes, because that is where the concentration of water is lowest.

Osmosis and Osmotic Pressure

Figure 4–17 diagrams the process of osmosis. Step 1 shows two solutions (A and B) that have different solute concentrations and are separated by a selectively permeable membrane. As osmosis occurs, water molecules cross the membrane until the solute concentrations in the two solutions are identical (Step 2a). Thus, the volume of solution B increases at the expense of solution A. The greater the initial difference in solute concentrations, the greater the movement of water (stronger osmotic flow). The **osmotic pressure** of a solution is the force generated by the diffusing water molecules that occurs as the result of differences in solute concentration. The greater the difference in solute concentrations, the greater the movement of water and the greater the osmotic pressure.

The osmotic pressure of a solution can be measured in several ways. For example, a strong enough opposing pressure can prevent the osmotic flow of water into the solution. Pushing against a fluid generates **hydrostatic (fluid) pressure;** in Step 2b, hydrostatic pressure opposes the osmotic pressure of solution B, and no net osmotic flow occurs.

Osmosis eliminates solute concentration differences much more quickly than one would predict on the basis of diffusion rates for other molecules. When water molecules cross a membrane they move in groups held together by hydrogen bonding. So, whereas solute molecules usually diffuse through membrane channels one at a time, water molecules move together in large numbers. This phenomenon is called **bulk flow.**

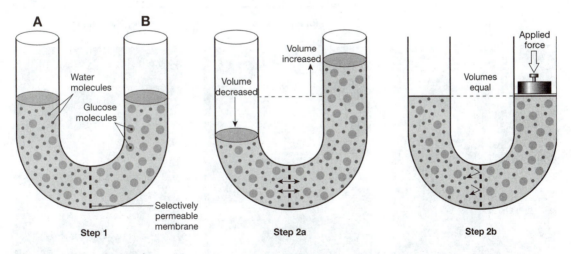

Figure 4–17   Osmosis.
Step 1: Two solutions containing different solute concentrations are separated by a selectively permeable membrane. Water molecules (small dots) begin to cross the membrane toward solution B, the solution with the higher concentration of solutes (larger circles). *Step 2a:* At equilibrium the solute concentrations on the two sides of the membrane are equal. The volume of solution B has increased at the expense of that of solution A. *Step 2b:* Osmosis can be prevented by resisting the volume change. The osmotic pressure of solution B is equal to the amount of applied force required to stop the flow of water.

Osmolarity and Tonicity

The total solute concentration in a solution is its **osmotic concentration,** or **osmolarity,** expressed in moles of solute per liter of solution. In a description of the effects of various osmotic solutions on living cells, the term **tonicity** (tō-NIS-eh-tē) is used instead of osmolarity. If a solution does not cause an osmotic flow of water into or out of a cell, it is called **isotonic** (Ī-sō-ton-ik; Greek *iso*, same + *tonos*, tension).

Figure 4–18a shows the appearance of a red blood cell immersed in an isotonic solution. A solution that has a lower osmotic concentration than the interior of the cell is called **hypotonic** (*hypo-*, below). When placed in such a solution, water will flow into the cell, and the red blood cell will swell up like a balloon (Figure 4–18b). Ultimately, it may rupture, releasing the intracellular contents. This event, known as **hemolysis** (hē-MOL-eh-sis); Latin *haemo-*, blood + *lysis*, dissolution), leaves an empty cell membrane known as a red blood cell "ghost." Red blood cell ghosts are often used for research on cell membrane structure.

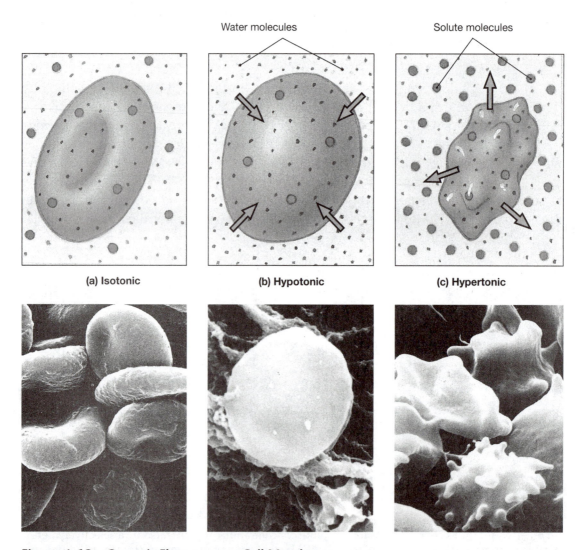

(a) Isotonic   **(b) Hypotonic**   **(c) Hypertonic**

Figure 4–18   Osmotic Flow across a Cell Membrane.
Arrows indicate the direction of osmotic water movement. **(a)** Because these red blood cells are immersed in an isotonic saline solution, no osmotic flow occurs, and the cells are normal in appearance. **(b)** Immersion in a hypotonic saline solution results in the osmotic flow of water into the cell. The swelling may continue until the cell membrane ruptures. **(c)** Exposure to a hypertonic solution results in the movement of water out of the cells. The red blood cells shrivel and become crenated. (SEM × 833)

A solution containing a higher osmotic concentration than the interior of the cell is called **hypertonic** (*hyper-*, above). A red blood cell placed in a hypertonic solution will lose water through osmosis. As water is lost, the cell shrivels and dehydrates. The shrinking of red blood cells, shown in Figure 4–18c, is called **crenation** (kre-NĀ-shen; Latin *crenatus*, notched).

It is often necessary to give patients large volumes of fluid after a severe blood loss or dehydration. One fluid often administered is a 0.9 percent (0.9 g/dl) solution of sodium chloride (NaCl). This solution, which approximates the normal osmotic concentration of the extracellular fluids, is called **normal saline.** It is used because sodium and chloride are the most abundant ions in the extracellular fluid. There is little net movement of either ion across cell membranes; thus, normal saline is essentially isotonic with respect to body cells. An alternative treatment involves the use of an isotonic solution containing dextran, a carbohydrate that cannot cross cell membranes.

Fluid Shifts

Minor fluctuations in intracellular and extracellular solute concentrations are eliminated in a matter of seconds by **fluid shifts,** the osmotic movement of water into or out of cells. It can take considerably longer for fluid shifts to compensate for systemwide changes in solute concentrations. For example, after you drink a large glass of pure water, it may take a half-hour for your intracellular and extracellular fluids to become isotonic again. Severe alterations in body water content, such as those occurring in dehydration, are extremely dangerous.

Filtration

In **filtration,** hydrostatic pressure forces water across a membrane, and solute molecules cross the membrane on the basis of their size. If the membrane pores are large enough, molecules of solute will be carried along with the water. We can see filtration in action in a coffee machine (Figure 4–19a). Gravity forces hot water through the filter, and the water carries with it a variety of dissolved compounds. The large coffee grounds never reach the pot because they cannot fit through the fine pores in the filter.

In the body, the heart pushes blood through the circulatory system and generates hydrostatic pressure. Filtration occurs across the walls of small blood vessels, pushing water and dissolved nutrients into the tissues of the body (Figure 4–19b). Filtration across specialized blood vessels in the kidneys is an essential step in the production of urine. When filtration occurs across these exceptionally permeable vessels, water moves by bulk flow. Because the filtration pores are very large, the clusters of water molecules carry dissolved ions with them. This action accelerates the filtration process.

Carrier-Mediated Transport

Carrier-mediated transport involves the activity of integral proteins that bind specific ions or organic substrates and facilitate their movement across the cell membrane. Two major examples of carrier-mediated transport are facilitated diffusion and active transport. All forms of carrier-mediated transport share several characteristics in common with enzymes:

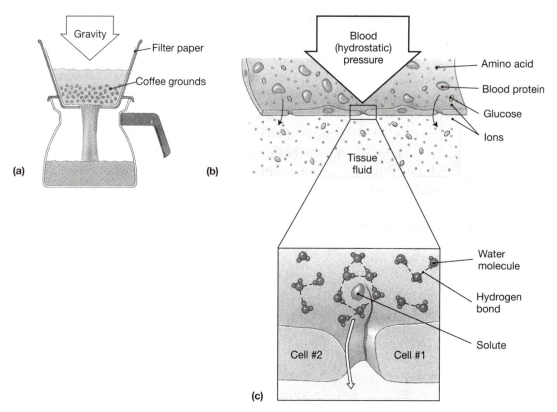

Figure 4–19 Filtration.
(a) In filtration, materials are removed from a solution on the basis of size. In a coffee maker, the paper filter keeps the coffee grounds trapped but lets smaller, dissolved molecules pass through. Gravity provides the hydrostatic pressure needed to force the coffee water through the filter. **(b)** In the most delicate blood vessels, blood pressure forces water and dissolved nutrients out of the bloodstream and into the interstitial fluid. Blood proteins are too large to pass through the openings between the cells that line the vessel. **(c)** Because adjacent water molecules are attracted to one another through the formation of hydrogen bonds, they cross a membrane in groups. Dissolved solutes small enough to fit through the pores will be carried along.

1. **Specificity:** Carrier proteins show *specificity.* That is, each carrier protein in the cell membrane is selective about what substances it will bind and transport. For example, the carrier protein that transports glucose will not transport many other simple sugars.

2. **Saturation:** The rate of transport into or out of a cell is limited by the availability of carrier proteins, just as enzymatic reaction rates are limited by enzyme concentrations. When all of the available carrier molecules are operating at maximum speed, the carrier system is said to be saturated. Because no more carrier proteins are available, and the existing ones cannot work any faster, the rate of transport cannot increase, regardless of the size of the concentration gradient.

3. **Regulation:** Carrier protein activity can be altered by the binding of other molecules, such as hormones. Hormones thus provide an important means of coordinating carrier protein activity throughout the body.

Facilitated Diffusion

Many essential nutrients, such as glucose and amino acids, are insoluble in lipids and too large to fit through membrane channels. These compounds can be passively transported across the membrane by carrier proteins in a process called **facilitated diffusion.**

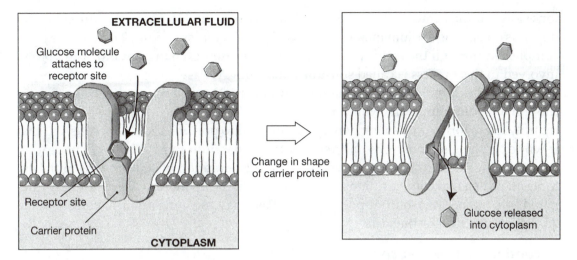

Figure 4–20   Carrier-Mediated Transport.
Facilitated diffusion. In this process an extracellular molecule, such as glucose, binds to a receptor site on a carrier protein. The binding alters the shape of the protein, which then releases the molecule to diffuse into the cytoplasm.

The molecule to be transported first binds to a receptor site on the protein. It is then moved to the inside of the cell membrane and released into the cytoplasm. The process is diagrammed in Figure 4–20.

As in the case of simple diffusion, no ATP is expended in facilitated diffusion, and the molecules move from an area of higher concentration to one of lower concentration. However, facilitated diffusion differs from ordinary diffusion because once the carrier proteins are saturated, the rate of transport cannot accelerate, regardless of further increases in the concentration gradient.

Active Transport

In **active transport** the high-energy bond in ATP (or another high-energy compound) provides the energy needed to move ions or molecules across a cell membrane. The process is complex, and specific enzymes must be present in addition to carrier proteins. Although it has an energy cost, active transport offers one great advantage: It does not depend on a concentration gradient. As a result, the cell can import or export specific materials regardless of their intracellular or extracellular concentrations.

All living cells contain carrier proteins called **ion pumps** that actively transport the cations sodium (Na^+), potassium (K^+), calcium (Ca^{2+}), and magnesium (Mg^{2+}) across their cell membranes. Specialized cells can transport additional ions such as iodide (I^-), chloride (Cl^-), and iron (Fe^{2+}). Many of these carrier proteins move a specific cation or anion in one direction only, either into or out of the cell. In a few instances, one carrier protein will move more than one ion at the same time. When a carrier protein moves one ion in one direction and a different ion in the opposite direction, the carrier protein is called an **exchange pump.** One such exchange pump is the sodium-potassium exchange pump.

Sodium-Potassium ATPase

Sodium and potassium ions are the principal cations in body fluids. Sodium ion concentrations in the extracellular fluids are high, and sodium ion concentrations in the cytoplasm are relatively low. The distribution of potassium in the body is just the opposite—low in the extracellular fluids and high in the cytoplasm. As a result, sodium ions slowly diffuse into a cell, and potassium ions leak out. Homeostasis within the cell depends on ejecting sodium ions and recapturing lost potassium ions. This balance is accomplished through the activity of a **sodium-potassium exchange pump.** The protein involved in this process is called **sodium-potassium ATPase.**

As indicated in Figure 4–21, the sodium-potassium exchange pump exchanges intracellular sodium for extracellular potassium. On the average, for each ATP molecule hydrolyzed to form ADP, enough energy is released to power the carrier protein so that it will eject three sodium ions and reclaim two potassium ions. When ATP is readily available, the rate of transport depends on the concentration of sodium ions in the cytoplasm. When that concentration rises, the pump becomes more active. The energy demands are impressive; sodium-potassium ATPase may consume up to 40 percent of the ATP produced by a resting cell.

Secondary Active Transport

In **secondary active transport,** the transport mechanism itself does not require energy, but the cell often needs to expend ATP at a later date to preserve homeostasis. Like facilitated transport, a secondary active transport mechanism moves a specific substance down a concentration gradient. However, unlike the proteins in facilitated transport, these carrier proteins can also move a second substance at the same time, without regard to its concentration gradient. In effect, the concentration gradient for one substance provides the driving force needed by the carrier protein, and the second substance gets a free ride. In **cotransport,** or **symport** (*sym-*, same), the carrier transports the two substances in the same direction, either into or out of the cell (Figure 4–22a). In **countertransport,** or **antiport** (*anti-*, against), one substance moves into the cell while the other moves out (Figure 4–22b).

The concentration gradient for sodium ions most often provides the driving force for cotransport mechanisms that move materials into the cell. For example, sodium-linked cotransport is important in the absorption of glucose and amino acids along the

Figure 4–21 The Sodium-Potassium Exchange Pump.

The sodium-potassium exchange pump is an example of an active transport system. For each ATP molecule converted to ADP, this protein, called sodium-potassium ATPase, carries three sodium ions (Na$^+$) out of the cell and two potassium ions (K$^+$) into the cell.

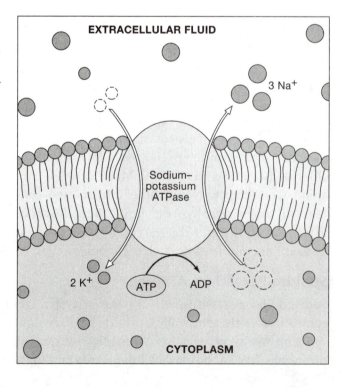

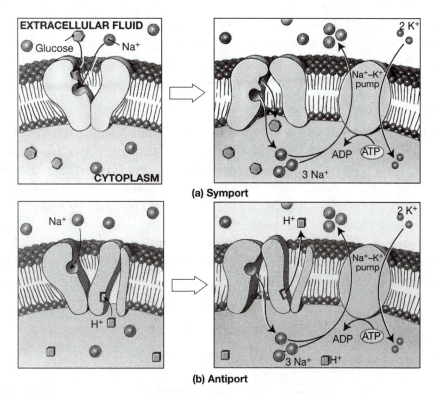

Figure 4–22   Secondary Active Transport.
(a) The transport of glucose by a carrier is an example of symport. Glucose transport by this carrier will occur only after the carrier has bound a sodium ion. In three cycles, three glucose molecules and three sodium ions move across the cell membrane. The sodium ions are then pumped out of the cell by the sodium-potassium exchange pump at a cost of one ATP. **(b)** Antiport is similar to symport except that the substance that is cotransported is moved in an opposite direction. An example would be the transport of hydrogen ions (H^+) at the kidneys. For each sodium ion that enters the cell, one hydrogen ion is transported out. As before, the cell must then pump the sodium ions across the cell membrane using the sodium-potassium exchange pump to maintain the normal intracellular concentration of sodium ions.

intestinal tract. Sodium ions are also involved with many countertransport mechanisms. Sodium-calcium countertransport is responsible for keeping intracellular calcium ion concentrations very low.

Although the transport activity proceeds without a direct energy expense, the cell must expend ATP to pump the arriving sodium ions out of the cell, via the sodium-potassium exchange pump.

Vesicular Transport

In **vesicular transport,** materials move into or out of the cell through the formation or breakdown of **vesicles,** small membranous sacs. Because large volumes of fluid and solutes are transported in this way, this process is also known as **bulk transport.** There are two major categories of vesicular transport, endocytosis and exocytosis.

Endocytosis

Endocytosis (EN-dō-sī-tō-sis) is the packaging of extracellular materials in a vesicle at the cell surface for importation into the cell. This process involves relatively large volumes of extracellular material. There are three major types of endocytosis: receptor-mediated endocytosis, pinocytosis, and phagocytosis. All three are active processes that require energy in the form of ATP.

All forms of endocytosis produce vesicles that move into the cytoplasm, where their contents remain isolated within the vesicle. Movement of materials from a vesicle into the surrounding cytoplasm may involve active transport, simple or facilitated diffusion, or the destruction of the vesicle membrane.

Receptor-Mediated Endocytosis

Receptor-mediated endocytosis involves the formation of small vesicles at the membrane surface. Receptor-mediated endocytosis is a selective process that produces vesicles that contain a specific target molecule in high concentrations. The process begins when materials in the extracellular fluid bind to receptors on the membrane surface (Figure 4–23). The receptor molecules are usually glycoproteins, and each has a specific target, or ligand, such as a transport protein or hormone.

Receptors bound to ligands cluster together, creating areas of cell membrane coated with ligands. The coated areas then fold inward to form grooves or pockets that pinch off to produce **coated vesicles.** Inside the cell, the coated vesicles fuse with lysosomes,

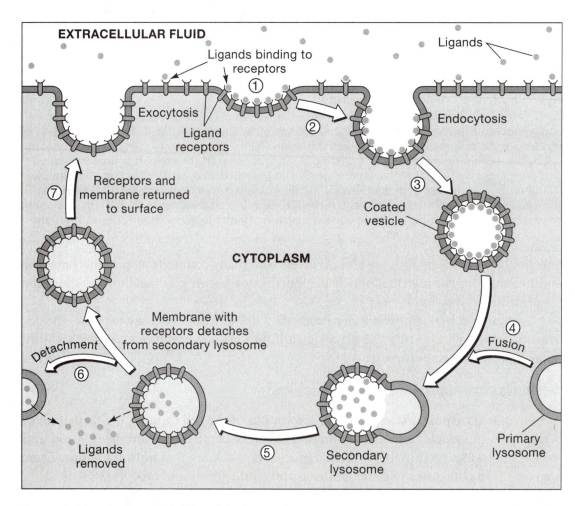

Figure 4–23   Receptor-Mediated Endocytosis.
In this process, (1) specific target molecules called ligands bind to receptors, generally glycoproteins, in the membrane surface. (2) Membrane areas coated with ligands pinch off to form (3) vesicles that (4) fuse with primary lysosomes. (5) The ligands are freed from the receptors and, if necessary, broken down by enzymes before diffusing or being transported into the surrounding cytoplasm. (6) The membrane containing the receptor molecules detaches from the membrane of the lysosome and (7) returns to the cell surface to bind additional ligands.

vesicles containing digestive enzymes. The fusion of a lysosome with another vesicle creates a secondary lysosome. Lysosomal enzymes then free the ligands, which enter the cytosol by diffusion or active transport, and the vesicle membrane pinches off and returns to the cell surface, its receptors ready to bind more ligands.

Many important substances, including cholesterol and iron ions (Fe^{2+}), are distributed through the body attached to special transport proteins. The proteins are too large to pass through membrane pores, but they can enter the cell through receptor-mediated endocytosis.

Pinocytosis

Pinocytosis (pi-nō-si-TŌ-sis), or "cell drinking," is the formation of small vesicles filled with extracellular fluid. This process is not as selective as receptor-mediated endocytosis because there are no receptors involved, and the goal appears to be the fluid contents in general, rather than specific bound ligands. In pinocytosis, a deep groove or pocket forms in the cell membrane and then pinches off. The SEM in Figure 4–24a gives a three-dimensional view of pinocytosis in action. The fate of a pinocytotic vesicle is the same as that of a vesicle formed through receptor-mediated endocytosis:

1. The vesicle usually fuses with a lysosome.

2. Lysosomal enzymes break down any organic molecules inside the vesicle.

3. Nutrients, such as lipids, sugars, or amino acids, enter the cytoplasm by diffusion or active transport.

4. The membrane of the pinocytotic vesicle then returns to the cell surface.

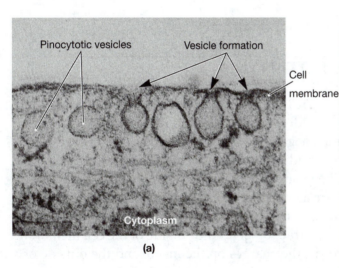

(a)

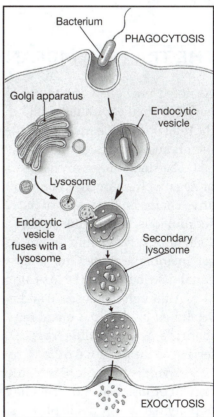

(b)

Figure 4–24   Pinocytosis and Phagocytosis.
(a) An electron micrograph showing pinocytosis at the bases of microvilli in a cell lining the intestinal tract. (b) Material brought into the cell through phagocytosis is enclosed in an endocytic vesicle and subsequently exposed to lysosomal enzymes. After absorption of nutrients from the vesicle, the residue is discharged through exocytosis.

Phagocytosis

Phagocytosis (fa-gō-sī-TŌ-sis), or "cell eating," produces vesicles containing solid objects that may be as large as the cell itself. This process is diagrammed in Figure 4–24b. Cytoplasmic extensions called **pseudopodia** (soo-dō-PŌ-dē-ah; Greek *pseudes*, false + *podos*, foot) surround the object, and their membranes fuse to form a vesicle. The vesicle may then fuse with a lysosome, whereupon its contents are digested by lysosomal enzymes.

Most cells display pinocytosis, but phagocytosis, especially the trapping of living or dead cells, is performed only by specialized cells, such as those of the immune system.

Exocytosis

Exocytosis (ek-sō-si-TŌ-sis) is the functional reverse of endocytosis. In this process, seen in Figures 4-12d (p. 152) and 4-24b, a vesicle created inside the cell fuses with the cell membrane and discharges its contents into the extracellular environment. The ejected material may be a secretory product, such as mucus, or waste products generated during the recycling of damaged organelles.

In a few specialized cells, endocytosis produces vesicles on one side of the cell that are discharged through exocytosis on the opposite side. This method of bulk transport is common in the cells that line capillaries, the most delicate blood vessels. These cells use a combination of pinocytosis and exocytosis to transfer fluid and solutes from the bloodstream into the surrounding tissues.

A Review of Membrane Permeability

Many different mechanisms can be moving materials into and out of the cell at any given moment. Before proceeding further, review and compare the mechanisms summarized in Table 4–4.

THE TRANSMEMBRANE POTENTIAL

As noted previously in this chapter (p. 161), the inside of a cell membrane has a slight negative charge with respect to the outside. It is important to remember, however, that the total positive charges equal the total negative charges both inside and outside the cell membrane. As a result, the interstitial fluid and the interior of a cell are electrically neutral. The slight negative charge on the inside of a cell membrane is due to the presence of negatively charged proteins that are associated with the membrane. This slight negative charge on the inside of the cell membrane attracts positively charged ions, such as sodium ions, to the outer surface. This attraction gives the outside of the cell membrane a slight positive charge. In other words, the charges on the inside and the outside of a cell membrane are not due to more or fewer ions on one side or the other but to the unequal distribution of the ions along the membrane.

Although the positive and negative charges are attracted to one another, they are separated by the lipid membrane. When positive and negative charges are held apart, there is a potential difference; we will use the term **transmembrane potential** when referring to the potential difference across a cell membrane.

A **volt** is the unit of measurement for potential difference (electrical potential energy). For instance, most cars have 12-volt batteries. The voltage indicates the amount of potential energy available for starting the engine and running the car's electrical systems. The transmembrane potentials of living cells are much smaller, averaging about

Table 4–4 Summary of Mechanisms Involved in Movement across Cell Membranes

Mechanism	Process	Factors Affecting Rate	Substances Involved (location)
Diffusion	Molecular movement of solutes; direction determined by relative concentrations	Size of gradient; size of molecule; charge; lipid solubility; temperature	Small inorganic ions; lipid-soluble materials (all cells)
Osmosis	Movement of water molecules toward solution containing relatively higher solute concentration; requires selectively permeable membrane	Concentration gradient; opposing osmotic or hydrostatic pressure	Water only (all cells)
Filtration	Movement of water, usually with solute, by hydrostatic pressure; requires filtration membrane	Amount of pressure; size of pores in filter	Water and small ions (blood vessels)
Carrier-Mediated Transport			
Facilitated diffusion	Carrier proteins passively transport solutes across a membrane down a concentration gradient	Size of gradient; temperature; and availability of carrier protein	Glucose and amino acids (all cells, but several different regulatory mechanisms exist)
Active transport	Carrier proteins actively transport solutes across a membrane regardless of any concentration gradients	Availability of carrier, substrate, and ATP	Na^+, K^+, Ca^{2+}, Mg^{2+} (all cells); other solutes by specialized cells
Secondary active transport	Carrier proteins passively transport 2 solutes, with one (normally Na^+) moving down its concentration gradient; the cell must later expend ATP to eject the Na^+	Availability of carrier, substrates, and ATP	Glucose and amino acids (specialized cells)
Vesicular Transport			
Endocytosis	Creation of membranous vesicles containing fluid or solid material	Stimulus and mechanics incompletely understood; requires ATP	Fluids, nutrients (all cells); debris, pathogens (specialized cells)
Exocytosis	Fusion of vesicles containing fluids and/or solids within the cell membrane	Stimulus and mechanics incompletely understood; requires ATP	Fluids, debris (all cells)

0.070 volts for a nerve cell membrane. This is usually reported as –70 mV, with **mV** indicating **millivolts** (thousandths of volt) and the minus sign signifying that the inside of the cell membrane is negative when compared with the outside.

The Significance of the Transmembrane Potential

If the lipid barrier separating charges were removed, the positive and negative charges would move together. The cell membrane thus acts as a dam across a river. A dam resists the water pressure building up on the upstream side; a cell membrane resists electrochemical forces that would otherwise drive ions into or out of the cell. Both the water retained behind a dam and the ions held on either side of the cell membrane contain potential energy.

The water behind a dam is like a book on a high shelf, and the membrane separating opposite charges is like a charged battery. People have designed many ways to make use of the potential energy stored behind a dam, and cells have ways of utilizing the potential energy across the cell membrane. For example, the sudden ion movements that occur when an ion channel opens or closes can function as an ON/OFF switch for a specific intracellular function. In other cases, a change in the transmembrane potential can by itself lead to the activation or inactivation of enzymes that trigger a response in the cell.

The Resting Potential

The **resting potential** is the transmembrane potential in an undisturbed cell. Each cell type has a characteristic resting potential between –10 mV and –100 mV. Examples include fat cells (–40 mV), thyroid cells (–50 mV), neurons (–70 mV), skeletal muscle cells (–85 mV), and cardiac muscle cells (–90 mV). The negativity of the normal resting potential primarily reflects the fact that the interior of the cell contains an abundance of negatively charged proteins, which cannot cross the cell membrane. The cell must expend energy to maintain the resting potential because leak channels permit the entry of sodium ions and the departure of potassium ions. Since the movement of positively charged sodium ions into a cell is matched by the movement of positively charge potassium ions out of the cell, there is no net change in the resting potential over time. However, over time the movement of sodium ions into the cell and potassium ions out of the cell change the concentration gradients that drive the diffusion of the two ions. The sodium-potassium exchange pump stabilizes the resting potential by ejecting sodium ions from the cytosol and reclaiming potassium ions from the extracellular fluid. Recall that the sodium-potassium pump exchanges three sodium ions for every two potassium ions. This unequal exchange helps to ensure that there will be more positive charges on the outside of the membrane than on the inside, thus helping to maintain the transmembrane potential. Figure 4–25 provides a diagrammatic view of a cell membrane at its resting potential.

Changes in the resting membrane potential and in transmembrane potentials play an important role in the transmission of nerve impulses in the nervous system and in the functioning of all types of muscle tissue.

✏️ Let's Review What You've Just Learned

▶ Definitions

In the space provided, write the term for each of the following definitions.

_____ 92. Cytoplasmic extensions that surround an object during the process of phagocytosis.

_____ 93. The movement of particles by random motion from an area of high concentration to an area of low concentration.

_____ 94. The ATP-dependent process of moving solutes across the cell membrane against their concentration gradients.

_____ 95. The effect of an osmotic solution on a living cell.

_____ 96. An isotonic solution that contains 0.9% NaCl.

_____ 97. A membranous sac in the cytoplasm of a cell.

_____ 98. The transmembrane potential of a normal cell under homeostatic conditions.

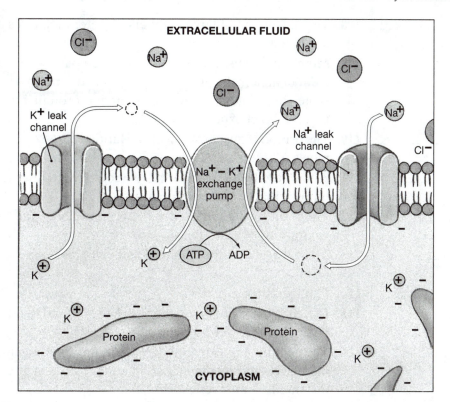

Figure 4–25   Ion Distribution across the Cell Membrane.
Potassium ions are continually leaking out of the cell through potassium leak channels, and sodium ions are entering through sodium leak channels. At the resting potential, three sodium ions enter the cell for every two potassium ions that leave the cell. These movements are counteracted by the activities of the sodium-potassium exchange pump, which removes three sodium ions from the cytoplasm in exchange for two potassium ions from the extracellular fluid (Figure 4–21). The net result is that the exchange pump maintains a stable ion distribution across the cell membrane.

_____ 99. The movement of water across a semipermeable membrane from an area of relatively low solute concentration to an area of relatively high solute concentration.

_____ 100. The process of cell shrinking that occurs when a cell is placed in a hypertonic solution.

_____ 101. Movement of a solution across a membrane whose pores restrict the passage of solute on the basis of size.

_____ 102. The introduction of fluids into the cytoplasm by enclosing them in membranous vesicles at the cell surface.

_____ 103. Passive movement of a substance across a cell membrane via a protein carrier.

_____ 104. The movement of relatively large volumes of extracellular material into the cytoplasm via the formation of membranous vesicles at the cell surface; includes pinocytosis and phagocytosis.

_____ 105. The breakdown of red blood cells that occurs when they are placed in a hypotonic solution.

_____ 106. A solution that has an osmolarity that does not result in water movement across the cell membrane.

_____ 107. The osmotic concentration of a solution expressed in moles solute per liter of water.

_____ **108.** The movement of large numbers of water molecules across a cell membrane.

_____ **109.** Membrane transport of a nutrient in company with the movement of an ion; the nutrient and the ion are transported in the same direction and require a carrier protein but do not involve direct expenditure of ATP.

_____ **110.** The osmotic concentration of a solution expressed in terms of moles of solute per liter of solution.

_____ **111.** A term used when comparing two solutions to refer to the solution with the higher osmolarity.

_____ **112.** The term for the difference between the high and low concentrations of a substance.

_____ **113.** The net result of the chemical and electrical forces acting on an ion.

_____ **114.** Fluid pressure.

_____ **115.** In a comparison of two solutions, the term used to refer to the one with the lower osmolarity.

_____ **116.** The engulfing of extracellular materials or pathogens; movement of extracellular materials into the cytoplasm by enclosure in a membranous vesicle.

_____ **117.** The force that must be applied to prevent the movement of water across a selectively permeable barrier by osmosis.

_____ **118.** The potential difference in millivolts measured across the cell membrane at any given time.

_____ **119.** Carrier proteins that actively transport ions across the cell membrane.

_____ **120.** A term describing a membrane that will allow only certain substances to pass through.

_____ **121.** Membrane transport of a substance in company with the movement of an ion; the substance and the ion are transported in opposite directions and require a carrier protein but do not involve direct expenditure of ATP.

_____ **122.** The ejection of cytoplasmic materials by fusion of a membranous sac with the cell membrane.

▶ **Word Roots, Prefixes, Suffixes, and Combining Forms**

In the space provided, list the boldfaced terms introduced in this section that contain the indicated word part.

Word Part	Meaning	Examples
phag-	to eat	**123.** _____
ex-	out	**124.** _____
hypo-	under	**125.** _____
trans-	across	**126.** _____
iso-	same	**127.** _____
hemo-	blood	**128.** _____
hyper-	above	**129.** _____
sym-	together	**130.** _____

pseudo-	false	**131.** _____
anti-	against	**132.** _____
ton-	tension	**133.** _____
per-	through	**134.** _____

▶ Completion

Complete each of the following statements.

135. _____ processes move ions or molecules across the cell membrane without any energy expenditure by the cell.

136. Diffusion moves molecules from an area of _____ concentration to an area of _____ concentration.

137. Five factors that influence the rate of diffusion are

    a. _____

    b. _____

    c. _____

    d. _____

    e. _____

138. Whether a substance moves across a cell membrane depends on two major factors: _____ and _____.

139. In osmosis, water will flow across a membrane toward the solution that has the _____ concentration of solutes.

140. The concentration of NaCl in a cell is approximately 0.9%. A solution of 5% salt would be _____ to a cell.

141. Carrier-mediated transport shares three characteristics with enzymes. They are

    a. _____

    b. _____

    c. _____

142. The unequal charge distribution across the cell membrane is the result of differences in the _____ of the membrane to different ions.

143. The transmembrane potential is a form of _____ energy.

☑ Self-Check Test

The following test will allow you to determine how well you have mastered the vocabulary and basic concepts of this chapter. It will also help you prepare for the type of questions you are likely to encounter on a test in an anatomy and physiology course. The self-check test will help you assess your understanding of the chapter material and will help you develop good test-taking skills.

The following questions test your ability to use vocabulary and to recall facts.

  1. The watery medium that surrounds a cell is known as

    a. cytosol

    b. protoplasm

    c. extracellular fluid

    d. cytoplasm

    e. a colloidal gel

2. Functions of the cell membrane include
   a. separation of the cytoplasm from the interstitial fluid
   b. regulation of exchange of materials with the environment
   c. sensitivity to changes in the interstitial fluid
   d. structural support
   e. all of the above

3. Each of the following is a function of membrane proteins except one. Identify the exception.
   a. bind to ligands
   b. regulate the passage of ions
   c. carrier molecules for various solutes
   d. anchors or stabilizers for the cell membrane
   e. energy transformation

4. Cell membranes are said to be
   a. impermeable
   b. freely permeable
   c. selectively permeable
   d. actively permeable
   e. none of the above

5. The movement of oxygen from an area of high concentration to an area of low concentration is an example of
   a. osmosis
   b. active transport
   c. diffusion
   d. facilitated transport
   e. filtration

6. The movement of water across a membrane from an area of relatively low solute concentration to an area of relatively high solute concentration is known as
   a. osmosis
   b. active transport
   c. diffusion
   d. facilitated transport
   e. filtration

7. The phenomenon of bulk flow refers to
   a. tonicity
   b. the mass movement of solute particles across a membrane
   c. the movement of groups of water molecules through a membrane at one time
   d. the active transport of substances against a concentration gradient
   e. the process of facilitated diffusion

8. A solution that contains a lower solute concentration than the cytoplasm of a cell is called
   a. merotonic
   b. hypertonic
   c. isotonic
   d. hypotonic
   e. none of the above

9. Each of the following is an example of a nonmembranous organelle except one. Identify the exception.

    a. lysosomes

    b. cilia

    c. centrioles

    d. ribosomes

    e. cytoskeleton

10. Proteins are synthesized by organelles called

    a. ribosomes

    b. microfilaments

    c. mitochondria

    d. Golgi apparatuses

    e. centrioles

11. The subunits of ribosomes are formed by

    a. the endoplasmic reticulum

    b. the Golgi apparatus

    c. lysosomes

    d. mitochondria

    e. nucleoli

12. Vesicles containing enzymes that neutralize toxins such as alcohol are

    a. lysosomes

    b. peroxisomes

    c. centrosomes

    d. endosomes

    e. toxisomes

13. The principal cations in our body fluids are

    a. sodium and potassium

    b. calcium and magnesium

    c. sodium and magnesium

    d. potassium and chloride

    e. sodium and chloride

14. A process that requires cellular energy to move a substance against its concentration gradient is called

    a. active transport

    b. passive transport

    c. facilitated diffusion

    d. osmosis

    e. diffusion

15. The process by which vesicles containing solid objects such as bacteria are formed on the surface of a cell for transport into the cell is called

    a. pinocytosis

    b. phagocytosis

    c. exocytosis

    d. receptor-mediated endocytosis

    e. emiocytosis

16. Compared with the outside surface, the inside of a resting cell membrane is
    a. positively charged
    b. negatively charged
    c. electrically charged
    d. continuously reversing its electrical charge
    e. positively charged whenever the sodium-potassium pump is active

17. Most of the ATP required to power cellular operations is produced in the
    a. ribosomes
    b. endoplasmic reticulum
    c. nucleus
    d. mitochondria
    e. Golgi apparatus

The following questions are more challenging and require you to synthesize the information that you have learned in this chapter.

18. Examination of a sample of glandular cells reveals an extensive network of smooth endoplasmic reticulum. Which of the following would be a possible product of these cells?
    a. digestive enzymes
    b. steroid hormones
    c. protein hormones
    d. transport proteins
    e. antibodies

19. If the permeability of the cell membrane to sodium ions increased
    a. more sodium ions would leave the cell
    b. the resting membrane potential would be less negative
    c. the resting membrane potential would be more negative
    d. the cell would lose potassium ions
    e. the cell would lose chloride ions

20. A molecule that blocks the channels in integral proteins in the cell membrane would interfere with
    a. cell recognition
    b. the movement of lipid-soluble molecules
    c. the ability of the cell membrane to change the transmembrane potential
    d. the ability of hormones to stimulate the cell
    e. the cell's ability to divide

☑Self-Assessment

If your score was

between 18 and 20, you are ready to proceed to the next chapter.

between 15 and 17, you have a good general idea of the chapter content, but you should review sections of the chapter that deal with items that you missed before proceeding to the next chapter.

less than 14, you have not mastered the chapter content well enough to proceed. Reread the chapter and rework the exercises. Then retake the self-check test. Repeat this process until you achieve a score that will allow you to continue.

Answers

1. cytosol
2. leak channels
3. somatic cells
4. micrometer
5. cytoskeleton
6. sperm
7. glycocalyx
8. cell
9. gated channel
10. cytology
11. cell membrane (or plasma membrane, plasmalemma)
12. integral proteins
13. cytoplasm
14. ligands
15. organelles
16. extracellular fluid (or interstitial fluid)
17. peripheral protein
18. ova
19. cytology, cytoplasm, cytosol, cytoskeleton
20. microscope, micrometer
21. glycocalyx
22. somatic
23. plasmalemma
24. ligand
25. phospholipids
26. scanning electron microscope
27. a. lubricate and protect the cell membrane
    b. anchor cell and participate in locomotion
    c. function as a receptor
    d. cell recognition
28. a. physical isolation
    b. regulation of exchange with the environment
    c. sensitivity
    d. structural support
29. a. cells are building blocks of all animals
    b. cells are produced by the division of pre-existing cells
    c. cells are the smallest units to perform vital physiological functions
    d. each cell maintains homeostasis at the cellular level

    e. homeostasis at higher levels of organization reflects the combined and coordinated activities of many cells

30. a. receptors
    b. channels
    c. carriers
    d. enzymes
    e. anchors
    f. identifiers
31. glycolipids
32. integral proteins
33. cholesterol
34. peripheral protein
35. integral protein with channel
36. ribosome
37. actin
38. cristae
39. microfilaments
40. centrosome
41. inclusions
42. secretory vesicles
43. endoplasmic reticulum
44. myosin
45. tubulin
46. peroxisomes
47. chromosomes
48. mitochondria
49. fixed ribosome
50. nonmembranous organelles
51. microtubules
52. Golgi apparatus
53. nuclear envelope
54. smooth endoplasmic reticulum
55. autolysis
56. basal body
57. microvilli
58. lysosomes
59. membranous organelles
60. thick filaments
61. centriole
62. saccules
63. membrane flow

64. nucleolus
65. lysosomal storage disease
66. free ribosomes
67. cisternae
68. cilium or flagellum
69. rough endoplasmic reticulum
70. nucleus
71. flagellum
72. neurofilament
73. endoplasmic reticulum
74. myosin
75. lysosome, autolysis
76. filament
77. ribosome, centrosome, chromosome
78. autolysis
79. chromosome
80. cilia
81. centriole
82. Golgi apparatus
83. mitochondrion
84. ribosomes
85. rough endoplasmic reticulum
86. nuclear envelope
87. nuclear pores
88. microvilli
89. microtubule
90. microfilament
91. nucleolus
92. pseudopodia
93. diffusion
94. active transport
95. tonicity
96. normal saline
97. vesicle
98. resting membrane potential
99. osmosis
100. crenation
101. filtration
102. pinocytosis
103. facilitated diffusion
104. endocytosis
105. hemolysis
106. isotonic
107. osmolarity
108. bulk flow
109. cotransport (or symport)

110. osmolarity
111. hypertonic
112. concentration gradient
113. electrochemical gradient
114. hydrostatic pressure
115. hypotonic
116. phagocytosis
117. osmotic pressure
118. transmembrane potential
119. ion pumps
120. selectively permeable
121. countertransport (or antiport)
122. exocytosis
123. phagocytosis
124. exocytosis
125. hypotonic
126. transmembrane potential
127. isotonic
128. hemolysis
129. hypertonic
130. symport
131. pseudopodia
132. antiport
133. tonicity, isotonic, hypertonic, hypotonic
134. permeability
135. Passive
136. high; low
137. a. distance
    b. size of the gradient
    c. size of the molecules
    d. temperature
    e. electrical forces
138. lipid solubility; size of the substance relative to the size of membrane channels
139. higher
140. hypertonic
141. a. specificity
    b. saturation
    c. regulation
142. permeability
143. potential

Answers to Self-Check Test

1. c 2. e 3. e 4. c 5. c 6. a 7. c 8. d 9. a 10. a 11. e 12. b 13. a 14. a 15. b 16. b 17. d 18. b 19. b 20. c

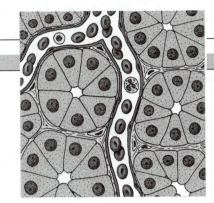

CHAPTER 5

Cellular Functions

Living cells are chemical factories. They break down organic molecules to obtain energy and molecular materials and use that energy and those materials to synthesize new molecules, grow, reproduce, and support a variety of other special functions that vary from cell to cell and tissue to tissue. To carry out these metabolic functions, our cells must have a reliable supply of raw materials, including oxygen, water, organic substrates, and mineral ions. Oxygen is absorbed at the lungs; the other items are obtained by absorption at the digestive tract. The cardiovascular system ensures prompt distribution to interstitial fluids throughout the body, where the absorbed materials become accessible to individual cells. The instructions for carrying out these processes are contained in molecules of the nucleic acid DNA. As cells divide this information is copied and passed along to each new cell. In this chapter we will examine three major areas of cellular function: (1) how cells obtain the energy they need to perform vital functions, (2) how genetic information determines the structural and functional properties of cells, and (3) how cells reproduce.

AN OVERVIEW OF CELLULAR METABOLISM

Figure 5–1 provides an overview of the ways cells use organic nutrients absorbed from the extracellular fluid (ECF). Simple sugars, amino acids, and lipids cross the cell membrane to join nutrients already in the cytoplasm. All of the cell's organic building blocks collectively form a nutrient pool.

Recall from Chapter 1 that the term *metabolism* is used to refer to all of the chemical reactions that occur within a living cell. Metabolic processes can be divided into two categories: catabolism and anabolism (see Chapter 2). In **catabolism,** molecules are broken down to form smaller molecules. **Anabolism** is the synthesis of new molecules from smaller components supplied by catabolism and the cell's environment.

Catabolism breaks down organic substrates, releasing energy that can be used to synthesize ATP or other high-energy compounds. Catabolism proceeds in a series of steps. In general, preliminary processing occurs in the cytosol, where enzymes break down large organic molecules into smaller fragments. For example, carbohydrates are broken down to short carbon chains, triglycerides are split into fatty acids and glycerol, and proteins are broken down to individual amino acids.

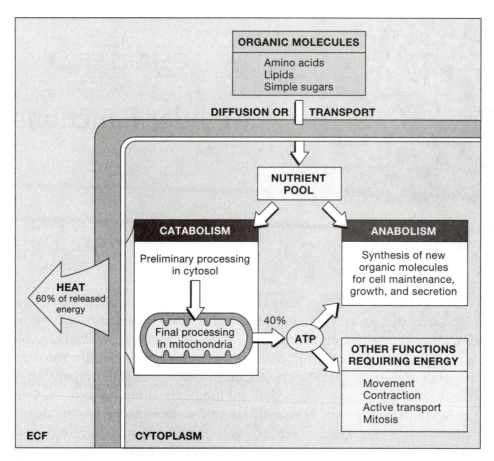

Figure 5–1   Aerobic Metabolism.
The cell obtains organic molecules from the extracellular fluid (ECF) and breaks them down to obtain ATP. Only about 40 percent of the energy released through catabolism is captured in ATP; the rest is radiated as heat. The ATP generated through catabolism provides energy for all vital cellular activities, including anabolism.

Relatively little ATP is produced during these preparatory steps. However, the simple molecules can be absorbed and processed by mitochondria, and the mitochondrial steps release significant amounts of energy. As mitochondrial enzymes break the covalent bonds that hold these molecules together, they capture roughly 40 percent of the energy released. The captured energy is used to convert ADP to ATP, and the rest escapes as heat that warms the interior of the cell and the surrounding tissues.

The ATP produced by mitochondria provides energy to support anabolism, the synthesis of new organic molecules, as well as other cell functions. Those additional functions, such as contraction, ciliary or cell movement, active transport, or cell division, vary from one cell to another. For example, muscle fibers need ATP to provide energy for contraction, and gland cells need ATP to synthesize and transport their secretions.

Anabolism is an uphill struggle that involves the formation of new chemical bonds. Cells synthesize new organic components for three basic reasons (Figure 5–2):

1. **To perform structural maintenance or repairs:** All cells must expend energy to perform ongoing maintenance and repairs, because most structures in the cell are temporary rather than permanent. Their removal and replacement are part of the process of metabolic turnover described in Chapter 3.

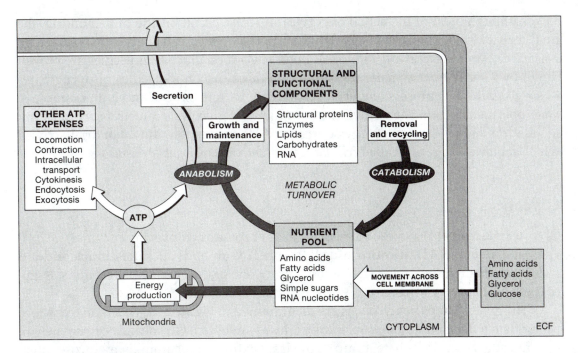

Figure 5–2   Metabolic Turnover and Cellular ATP Production.
Metabolic turnover is integrated into other cellular functions. Organic molecules released during metabolic turnover may be recycled by means of anabolic pathways and used to build other large molecules. They can also be broken down for energy production. Through catabolism, the cell must provide ATP for anabolism and for other cellular functions.

2. **To support growth:** Cells preparing for division enlarge and synthesize additional proteins and organelles.

3. **To produce secretions:** Secretory cells must synthesize their products and deliver them to the interstitial fluid.

The nutrient pool is the source for the substrates for both catabolism and anabolism. As you might expect, the cell tends to conserve the materials needed to build new compounds and breaks down the rest. The cell is continually replacing membranes, organelles, enzymes, and structural proteins. These anabolic activities require more amino acids than lipids and relatively few carbohydrates. In general, a cell with excess carbohydrates, lipids, and amino acids will break down carbohydrates first. Lipids are a second choice, and amino acids are seldom broken down. The next sections will detail the most important catabolic and anabolic reactions that occur within our cells.

CARBOHYDRATE METABOLISM

Most cells generate ATP and other high-energy compounds through the breakdown of carbohydrates, especially glucose. The complete reaction sequence can be summarized as:

$$C_6H_{12}O_6 + 6\,O_2 \longrightarrow 6\,CO_2 + 6\,H_2O$$

The breakdown occurs in a series of small steps, and several of the steps release sufficient energy to support the conversion of ADP to ATP. During the complete catabolism of glucose, a typical cell gains 36 ATP.

Although most of the actual energy production occurs inside mitochondria, the first steps take place in the cytosol. In this reaction sequence, called **glycolysis** (glī-KOL-i-sis; Greek *glykys*, sweet + *lysis*, dissolution), six-carbon glucose molecules are broken down by a series of enzymatic steps into two three-carbon molecules of **pyruvic** (pī-ROO-vik) **acid**. The process of glycolysis does not require oxygen and is an example of anaerobic metabolism. The pyruvic acid produced by glycolysis can be absorbed by mitochondria and used as an energy source for ATP production. Mitochondrial activity, which requires oxygen, is called *cellular respiration*, or *aerobic metabolism*.

Glycolysis

Glycolysis requires (1) glucose molecules, (2) appropriate cytoplasmic enzymes, (3) ATP and ADP, and (4) **NAD (nicotinamide** [NIK-uh-TIN-uh-mīd] **adenine dinucleotide**), a coenzyme that removes hydrogen atoms during one of the enzymatic reactions. If any of these participants is missing, glycolysis cannot take place.

The general steps in glycolysis are diagrammed in Figure 5–3. This is an overview, rather than a detailed description of the pathway involved. Glycolysis begins when an enzyme attaches a phosphate group to the last (sixth) carbon atom on a glucose molecule, creating **glucose-6-phosphate**. The process of attaching a phosphate group to an organic substrate such as glucose is called **phosphorylation**. Although this step "costs" the cell one ATP molecule, it has two important results: (1) It traps the glucose molecule within the cell, because phosphorylated glucose cannot cross the cell membrane, and (2) it prepares the glucose molecule for further biochemical reactions.

A second substrate phosphorylation occurs in the cytosol before the six-carbon chain is broken into two three-carbon fragments. Energy benefits begin to appear as these fragments are converted to pyruvic acid. Two of the steps release enough energy to generate ATP from ADP and inorganic phosphate (PO_4^{3-}, or P_i). In addition, two molecules of NAD pick up hydrogen atoms during the process and become **NADH** (this molecule is called reduced NAD). The overall reaction looks like this:

$$\text{glucose (6-carbon)} + 2\,\text{NAD} + 2\,\text{ATP} + 2\,\text{ADP} + 2\,P_i \longrightarrow$$

$$2\,\text{pyruvate (3-carbon)} + 4\,\text{ATP} + 2\,\text{NADH}$$

This reaction sequence provides a net gain of two ATP molecules for the cell for each glucose molecule converted to two pyruvic acids. A few highly specialized cells, such as red blood cells, lack mitochondria and derive all of their ATP through glycolysis. Skeletal muscle fibers rely on glycolysis for energy production during periods of active contraction, and most cells can survive for brief periods using the ATP provided by glycolysis. However, when oxygen is readily available, mitochondrial activity provides most of the ATP required by our cells.

ATP Production in the Mitochondria

Glycolysis yields an immediate net gain of two ATP molecules for the cell. However, a great deal of additional energy is still locked in the chemical bonds of pyruvic acid. The ability to capture that energy depends on the availability of oxygen. If oxygen supplies are adequate, mitochondria absorb the pyruvic acid molecules and break them down. The

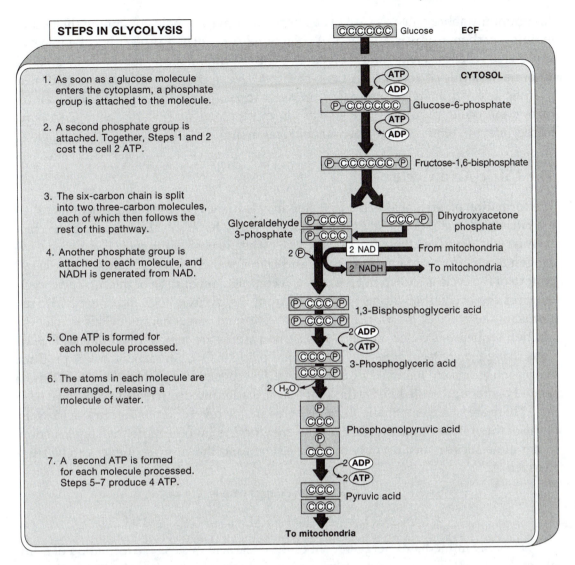

Figure 5–3 Glycolysis.

Glycolysis breaks down a six-carbon glucose molecule into two three-carbon molecules of pyruvic acid through a series of enzymatic steps. This diagram follows the fate of the carbon chain. There is a net gain of two ATP molecules for each glucose molecule converted to pyruvic acid. In addition, two molecules of the coenzyme NAD are converted to NADH. Once transferred to mitochondria, both the pyruvic acid and the NADH can still yield a great deal more energy. The further catabolism of pyruvic acid begins with its entry into a mitochondrion (see Figure 5–4).

hydrogen atoms are removed by coenzymes, and they will ultimately be the source of most of the energy gain for the cell. The carbon and oxygen atoms are removed and released as carbon dioxide, a process called **decarboxylation** (dē-kar-boks-i-LĀ-shun).

Recall from Chapter 4 that each mitochondrion has a double layer of membrane around it. The outer mitochondrial membrane contains large-diameter pores that are permeable to ions and small organic molecules such as pyruvic acid. The ions and molecules then enter the **intermembrane space** that separates the outer mitochondrial membrane from the inner mitochondrial membrane. The inner mitochondrial membrane contains a carrier protein that moves pyruvic acid into the mitochondrial matrix. Once inside the mitochondrion, a pyruvic acid molecule first loses one carbon atom in a complicated reaction involving NAD and an additional coenzyme called **coenzyme**

A, commonly abbreviated as **CoA**. The fragment of pyruvic acid containing the two remaining carbon atoms is attached to coenzyme A to form a molecule called acetyl-CoA. This reaction yields one molecule of carbon dioxide, one molecule of NADH, and one molecule of **acetyl-CoA** (as-e-til-CŌ-ā). Next, the two-carbon fragment from pyruvic acid is transferred from CoA to **oxaloacetic** (ok-SAL-ō-a-sē-tik) **acid**, a four-carbon molecule, producing the six-carbon molecule **citric** (SIT-rik) **acid**. CoA is released intact to bind another pyruvic acid fragment.

The Citric Acid Cycle

The formation of citric acid is the first step in a sequence of enzymatic reactions called the **citric acid cycle,** or *TCA cycle* (also known as the **Kreb's cycle** in honor of the biochemist who described these reactions in 1937). The purpose of the cycle is to remove hydrogen atoms from organic molecules and transfer them to coenzymes. The overall pattern of the cycle is shown in Figure 5–4. A complete revolution of the citric acid cycle removes the two carbon atoms introduced from the pyruvic acid and some hydrogen atoms. In the process, the four-carbon oxaloacetic acid is regenerated. (This is why the reaction sequence is called a cycle.) Two carbon atoms are removed in enzymatic reactions that generate two molecules of carbon dioxide (CO_2), a metabolic waste product. Hydrogen atoms are removed by coenzymes. The coenzymes involved are NAD and a related compound, called **FAD (flavin [FLĀ-vin] adenine dinucleotide)**.

There are seven enzymatic steps involved in one revolution of the citric acid cycle. Some of these steps require more than one enzyme and involve more than one reaction. Water molecules are tied up in two of those steps, and the entire sequence can be summarized as:

$$\text{acetyl-CoA} + 3\,\text{NAD} + \text{FAD} + \text{GDP} + P_i + 2\,H_2O \longrightarrow$$
$$\text{CoA} + 2\,CO_2 + 3\,\text{NADH} + \text{FADH}_2 + \text{GTP} + 2\,H^+$$

The only immediate energy benefit of the citric acid cycle is the formation of a single molecule of GTP (guanosine triphosphate, another high-energy compound introduced in Chapter 3). This is the equivalent of a molecule of ATP, because GTP + ADP → GDP + ATP. The formation of GTP from GDP in the citric acid cycle is an example of **substrate-level phosphorylation**. In this process, an enzyme uses the energy released by a chemical reaction to transfer a phosphate group to a suitable acceptor molecule.

Phosphorylation That Requires Oxygen

Oxidative phosphorylation (OK-si-dā-tiv fos-fōr-i-LĀ-shun) is the generation of ATP within mitochondria through a reaction sequence that requires coenzymes and consumes oxygen. This process produces over 90 percent of the ATP used by our cells. The foundation of this reaction sequence is very simple:

$$2\,H_2 + O_2 \longrightarrow 2\,H_2O$$

Living cells can easily obtain the ingredients for this reaction. Hydrogen is a component of all organic molecules, and oxygen is an atmospheric gas. The only problem is that the reaction releases a tremendous amount of energy all at once. In fact, this reaction releases so much energy that it is used to launch the space shuttle into orbit. Cells cannot handle energy explosions; energy release must be gradual, and this is the goal of

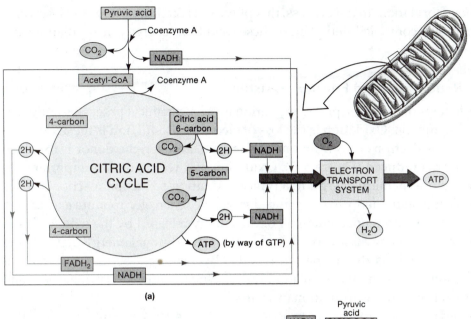

(a)

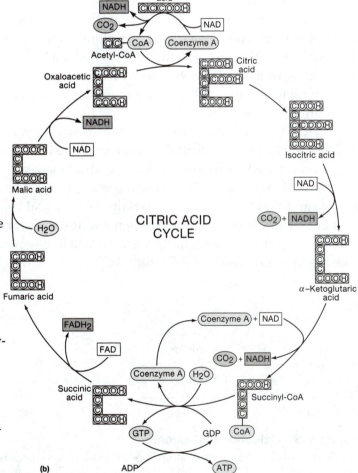

(b)

Figure 5–4   The Citric Acid Cycle.

The citric acid cycle completes the breakdown of organic molecules begun by glycolysis and other catabolic pathways. **(a)** An overview of the citric acid cycle and the distribution of carbon, hydrogen, and oxygen atoms. **(b)** A more complete diagrammatic view of the citric acid cycle, showing the fate of the carbon chains. The citric acid cycle begins with the transfer of an acetyl group from coenzyme A to oxaloacetic acid, a four-carbon molecule in the mitochondrial matrix. In a series of enzymatic reactions, two carbon atoms, together with oxygen atoms, are eliminated as carbon dioxide. One molecule of ATP is produced indirectly (via GTP) for each turn of the cycle, but much more ATP will ultimately be obtained from the hydrogen atoms that are removed by the coenzymes NAD and FAD.

oxidative phosphorylation. In the process, this powerful reaction proceeds in a series of small, enzymatically controlled steps. Under these conditions energy can be captured and ATP generated.

Oxidation, Reduction, and Energy Transfer

The enzymatic steps of oxidative phosphorylation involve chemical processes known as oxidation and reduction. **Oxidation** is the loss of electrons. **Reduction** is the acceptance of electrons. When electrons pass from one molecule to another, the donor is **oxidized** and the recipient is **reduced** (Figure 5–5). Oxidation and reduction are important because electrons store chemical energy. In a typical oxidation-reduction reaction, the oxidized molecule transfers energy to the reduced molecule when electrons are exchanged. The reduced molecule does not contain all of the energy released by the oxidized molecule, however. Some energy is always lost as heat, and additional energy may be used to perform work, such as the formation of ATP. By placing a series of oxidation-reduction reactions between hydrogen atoms and oxygen atoms, cells can harness and use the energy released in the formation of water.

Coenzymes play a key role in this process. A coenzyme acts as an intermediary that accepts electrons from one molecule and transfers them to another. In the citric acid cycle, NAD and FAD remove hydrogen atoms from organic substrates to become NADH (also written as NADH + H$^+$) and FADH$_2$ (reduced FAD). Each hydrogen atom contains an electron, as well as a proton, so when it accepts a hydrogen atom a coenzyme is reduced and gains energy. The donor molecule loses electrons and energy as it gives up its hydrogen atoms.

NADH and FADH$_2$ then transfer their hydrogen atoms to other coenzymes, such as **FMN (flavin mononucleotide)**, and **coenzyme Q (ubiquinone [ū-BIK-wi-nōn])**. These coenzymes are either free in the mitochondrial matrix (NAD) or bound to the inner mitochondrial membrane (FAD, FMN, coenzyme Q). The protons are subsequently released, and the electrons, which contain the chemical energy, enter a reaction sequence that ends with their transfer to oxygen and the formation of a water molecule (Figure 5–6). At several steps along the oxidation-reduction sequence, enough energy is released to support the synthesis of ATP from ADP.

Oxidation	Reduction	Oxidation	Reduction
$A \longrightarrow A^+ + e^-$	$B + e^- \longrightarrow B^-$	$AH \longrightarrow A + H$	$B + H \longrightarrow BH$
$A^+ \longrightarrow A^{2+} + e^-$	$B^+ + e^- \longrightarrow B$	$AH \longrightarrow A + H^+ + e^-$	$B + H^+ + e^- \longrightarrow BH$
$A^- \longrightarrow A + e^-$	$B^- + e^- \longrightarrow B^{2-}$		
(a)	(b)	(c)	(d)

Figure 5–5 Oxidation-Reduction.

(a) The loss of electrons from an atom is called oxidation. When a neutral atom is oxidized it gains a positive charge equal to the number of electrons lost. When a cation is oxidized it becomes more positive. When an anion is oxidized, it becomes less negative. **(b)** Electrons lost by one atom must be accepted by another. The gain of electrons is termed reduction. When a neutral atom is reduced it gains a negative charge equal to the number of electrons gained. When a cation is reduced, its positive charge decreases. When an anion is reduced, its negative charge increases. **(c)** In biological systems, electrons are transferred as part of a hydrogen atom, or in company with a proton (a hydrogen ion). Thus the oxidation of a molecule can result in the removal of a hydrogen atom. **(d)** Similarly, reduction can involve the gain of a hydrogen atom.

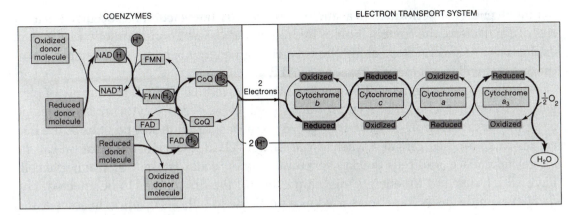

Figure 5–6   Oxidative Phosphorylation.
This diagram shows the steps in the transfer of hydrogen atoms through coenzymes and electrons along the electron transport chain.

The Electron Transport System

The **electron transport system (ETS)**, or **respiratory chain**, is a sequence of **metallo-proteins** (me-tal-o-PRŌ-tēn, a protein that contains a metal ion as part of its molecule) called **cytochromes** (SĪ-tō-krōmz; *cyto-*, cell + *chroma*, color). Each cytochrome has two components: a protein and a pigment. The protein, embedded in the inner mitochondrial membrane, surrounds the pigment complex, which contains a metal ion, either iron (Fe^{3+}) or copper (Cu^{2+}). There are four cytochromes: b, c, a, and a_3.

Figure 5–6 summarizes the major steps in oxidative phosphorylation. These steps are:

Step 1: A coenzyme strips a pair of hydrogen atoms from a substrate molecule. As we have seen, different coenzymes are used for different substrate molecules. During glycolysis, which occurs in the cytoplasm, NAD is reduced, producing NADH, and within mitochondria both NAD and FAD are reduced through reactions of the citric acid cycle.

Step 2: NADH and $FADH_2$ deliver hydrogen atoms to coenzymes embedded in the inner mitochondrial membrane. It is the electrons that carry the energy, and the protons (H^+) that accompany them will be released before the electrons are transferred to the electron transport system. As indicated in Figure 5–6, the path taken to the ETS differs depending on whether the donor is NADH or $FADH_2$.

Step 3: Electrons are passed along the electron transport system, losing energy in a series of small steps. The sequence is cytochrome b to c to a to a_3.

Step 4: At the end of the electron transport system an oxygen atom accepts the electrons, creating an oxide ion (O^{2-}). This ion has a very strong affinity for hydrogen ions (H^+); it quickly combines with two hydrogen ions in the mitochondrial matrix, forming a molecule of water.

Notice that this reaction sequence started with the removal of two hydrogen atoms from a substrate molecule, and it ended with the formation of water from two hydrogen ions and one oxide anion. This is the reaction that we described initially and that released too much energy if performed in a single step. Because the reaction has occurred in a series of small steps, the combination of hydrogen and oxygen occurs quietly rather than explosively. At several steps along the way, enough energy is released to establish conditions that will result in the formation of ATP.

Cells obtain oxygen by diffusion from the extracellular fluid. If the supply of oxygen is cut off, mitochondrial ATP production will cease because cytochrome a_3 has no acceptor for the electrons it has to transfer. With the last reaction stopped, the entire ETS comes to a halt, like cars at a washed-out bridge. Oxidative phosphorylation can no longer take place, and cells quickly succumb to energy starvation. Because nerve cells have a high demand for energy, the brain is one of the first organs to be affected. Hydrogen cyanide gas is sometimes used as a pesticide to kill rats or mice; in some states where capital punishment is legal, it is used to execute criminals. The cyanide ion (CN^-) binds to cytochrome a_3 and prevents the transfer of electrons to oxygen. As a result, cells die from energy starvation.

ENERGY YIELD OF GLYCOLYSIS AND CELLULAR RESPIRATION

The complete reaction pathway that begins with glucose and ends with carbon dioxide and water is for most cells the primary method of generating ATP. Figure 5–7 summarizes the entire process from an energy standpoint.

- **Glycolysis:** During glycolysis, the cell gains two molecules of ATP directly for each glucose molecule broken down to pyruvic acid. Two molecules of NADH are also produced. In most cells, the NADH passes electrons to FAD using an intermediary in the intermembrane space. This sequence of events generates NAD and $FADH_2$. The transfer of electrons from $FADH_2$ to CoQ and the electron transport system will ultimately provide an additional two ATP.

- **The citric acid cycle:** The two pyruvic acid molecules derived from each glucose molecule are fully broken down in mitochondria. Two revolutions of the citric acid cycle, each yielding a molecule of ATP, provide a total gain of two more molecules of ATP.

- **The electron transport system:** Both the citric acid cycle itself and the step leading into it (formation of acetyl-CoA from pyruvic acid) produce additional molecules of reduced coenzymes (NADH and $FADH_2$). Each revolution of the citric acid cycle generates three molecules of NADH and one molecule of $FADH_2$. Through the ETS, each molecule of NADH yields three molecules of ATP and one of water; the $FADH_2$ yields two molecules of ATP and one of water. These coenzymes feed electrons into the electron transport chain, with a total yield of an additional 32 molecules of ATP.

Summing up, for each glucose molecule processed the cell gains 36 molecules of ATP. All but two of them are produced by the mitochondria.

Heart muscle cells and liver cells are able to gain an additional two ATP for each glucose molecule broken down. This gain is accomplished by increasing the energy yield from the NADH generated during glycolysis from four ATP to six ATP. In these cells, each NADH passes electrons to an intermediary that crosses the inner mitochondrial mem-

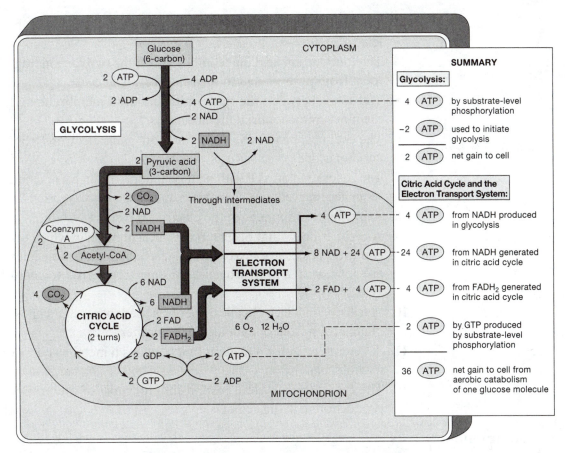

Figure 5–7   A Summary of the Energy Yield of Aerobic Metabolism.
For each glucose molecule broken down via glycolysis, only two molecules of ATP (net) are produced. The citric acid cycle generates an additional two ATP molecules from the GTP. However, glycolysis, the formation of acetyl-CoA, and the citric acid cycle all yield molecules of reduced coenzymes (NADH and/or $FADH_2$). Many additional ATP molecules are produced when electrons from these coenzymes pass through the electron transport system. Each of the eight NADH molecules produced inside the mitochondrion yields three ATP molecules. In most cells, each of the two NADH molecules produced in glycolysis provides only two ATP molecules, the same amount gained from each of the two $FADH_2$ molecules generated within the mitochondrion.

brane and generates NADH in the mitochondrial matrix. The subsequent transfer of electrons to FMN, CoQ, and the ETS results in the production of six ATP, just as if the two NADH molecules had been generated in the citric acid cycle.

Let's Review What You've Just Learned

► Definitions

In the space provided, write the term for each of the following definitions.

_____ **1.** The chemical process by which an atom loses electrons.

_____ **2.** The breakdown of a glucose molecule into two molecules of pyruvic acid, with a net gain of two ATP molecules.

_____ 3. The removal of a molecule of carbon dioxide from an organic acid.

_____ 4. The four-carbon acid that combines with the two carbon fragment from pyruvic acid to start the citric acid cycle.

_____ 5. The space between the outer mitochondrial membrane and the inner mitochondrial membrane.

_____ 6. The chemical process by which an atom gains electrons from another atom.

_____ 7. The generation of ATP within mitochondria through a reaction sequence that requires coenzymes and consumes oxygen.

_____ 8. A pigment component of the electron transport system.

_____ 9. A cyclic process that occurs in the mitochondria in which organic molecules are broken down, carbon dioxide molecules are generated, and hydrogen atoms are transferred to coenzymes.

_____ 10. A reaction in which chemical energy is used to transfer a phosphate group from one molecule to another.

_____ 11. A general term for a protein that contains a metal as part of its molecule.

_____ 12. The cytochrome system responsible for most of the energy production in living cells.

▶ **Completion**

Complete the following summary of energy yields for glycolysis (questions 13–15) and the citric acid cycle and electron transport system (questions 16–20).

Glycolysis

_____ 13. ATP by substrate-level phosphorylation

_____ 14. ATP to initiate glycolysis

_____ 15. ATP net gain from glycolysis

Citric Acid Cycle and the ETS

_____ 16. ATP from NADH produced in glycolysis

_____ 17. ATP from NADH generated in the citric acid cycle

_____ 18. ATP from $FADH_2$ generated in citric acid cycle

_____ 19. ATP by way of GTP produced by substrate-level phosphorylation

_____ 20. ATP net gain to cell from aerobic catabolism of one glucose molecule

OTHER CATABOLIC PATHWAYS

Aerobic metabolism is relatively efficient and capable of generating large amounts of ATP. It is the cornerstone for normal cellular metabolism, but it has one obvious limitation: The cell must have adequate supplies of both oxygen and glucose. Low glucose

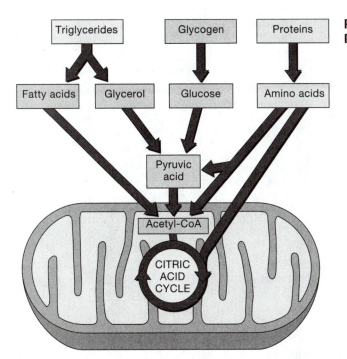

Figure 5–8   Alternative Catabolic Pathways.

concentrations have a much smaller effect on most cells than do low oxygen supplies, because the cells can break down other nutrients to provide substrates for the citric acid cycle, as shown in Figure 5–8. Many cells can switch from one nutrient source to another as the need arises. For example, many cells can shift from glucose-based to lipid-based ATP production when necessary. Skeletal muscles catabolize glucose when actively contracting, but they utilize fatty acids when at rest.

Cells break down proteins for energy only when lipids or carbohydrates are unavailable, primarily because proteins make up the enzymes and organelles that the cell needs to survive. Nucleic acids are present only in small amounts, and they are seldom catabolized for energy, even when the cell is dying of acute starvation. This restraint makes sense, because it is the DNA in the nucleus that determines all of the structural and functional characteristics of the cell. We will consider the catabolism of other compounds in later sections as we discuss lipid, protein, and nucleic acid metabolism.

CARBOHYDRATE SYNTHESIS

The synthesis of glucose from nonglucose precursors is called **gluconeogenesis** (gloo-kō-nē-ō-JEN-e-sis). Because some of the steps in glycolysis are not reversible, carbohydrate synthesis involves a different set of regulatory enzymes, and carbohydrate breakdown and synthesis are independently regulated. Pyruvic acid or other three-carbon molecules can be used as starting materials. As indicated in Figure 5–9, this reaction sequence enables a cell to create glucose molecules from other carbohydrates, glycerol, or some amino acids. However, acetyl-CoA cannot be used to make glucose because the step that removes carbon dioxide (*a decarboxylation step*) between pyruvic acid and acetyl-CoA cannot be reversed. Fatty acids and many amino acids cannot be converted to glucose because their catabolic pathways, described in later sections, produce acetyl-CoA.

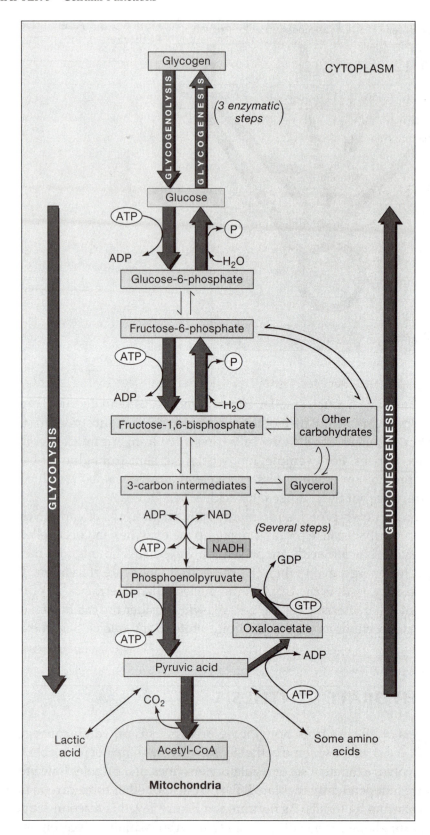

Figure 5–9   Carbohydrate Synthesis.
A flow chart of the pathways for glycolysis and gluconeogenesis. Many of the reactions are freely reversible, but separate regulatory enzymes control the key steps. Some amino acids, carbohydrates other than glucose, and glycerol can be converted to glucose. Notice that the enzymatic reaction that converts pyruvic acid to acetyl-CoA cannot be reversed.

Glucose molecules created by gluconeogenesis can be used to manufacture other simple sugars, complex carbohydrates, proteoglycans, or nucleic acids. In the liver and in skeletal muscle, glucose molecules are stored as glycogen. The process of glycogen formation is known as **glycogenesis** (glī-kō-JEN-e-sis). Glycogen is an important energy reserve that can be broken down when the cell cannot obtain enough glucose from the interstitial fluid. Although glycogen molecules are large, glycogen reserves take up very little space because they form compact, insoluble granules.

LIPID METABOLISM

Lipid molecules, like carbohydrates, contain carbon, hydrogen, and oxygen, but these atoms are present in different proportions (see Chapter 3). Because triglycerides are the most abundant lipid in the body, our discussion will focus on pathways for triglyceride breakdown and synthesis.

Lipid Catabolism

During lipid catabolism, or **lipolysis** (lī-POL-i-sis), lipids are broken down into pieces that can be converted to pyruvic acid or channeled directly into the citric acid cycle.

A triglyceride is first split into its component parts through hydrolysis. This step yields one molecule of glycerol and three fatty acid molecules. Glycerol enters the citric acid cycle after enzymes in the cytosol convert it to pyruvic acid. The catabolism of fatty acids involves a completely different set of enzymes.

Beta-oxidation

Fatty acid molecules are broken down into two-carbon fragments by means of a sequence of reactions known as **beta-oxidation**. This process occurs inside mitochondria, so the carbon chains can enter the citric acid cycle immediately. Figure 5–10 diagrams the process of beta-oxidation. Each step generates molecules of acetyl-CoA, $FADH_2$, and NADH and leaves a shorter carbon chain bound to coenzyme A.

Beta-oxidation provides substantial energy benefits. For each two-carbon fragment removed from the fatty acid, the cell gains 12 ATP from the processing of acetyl-CoA in the citric acid cycle, plus five ATP from the NADH and $FADH_2$. The cell can therefore gain 144 ATP from the breakdown of an 18-carbon fatty acid molecule. This is almost 1.5 times the energy obtained by the complete breakdown of three six-carbon glucose molecules. The catabolism of other lipids follows similar patterns, usually ending with the formation of acetyl-CoA.

Lipids and Energy Production

Lipids are important as an energy reserve because they can provide large amounts of ATP. Because they are insoluble, lipids can be stored in compact droplets in the cytosol. This ability saves space, but when the lipid droplets are large it is difficult for water-soluble enzymes to get at them. Lipid reserves are therefore more difficult to access than are carbohydrate reserves. In addition, most lipids are processed inside mitochondria, and mitochondrial activity is limited by the availability of oxygen. The net result is that lipids cannot provide large amounts of ATP in a short amount of time. Cells with modest energy demands, however, can shift to lipid-based energy production when glucose

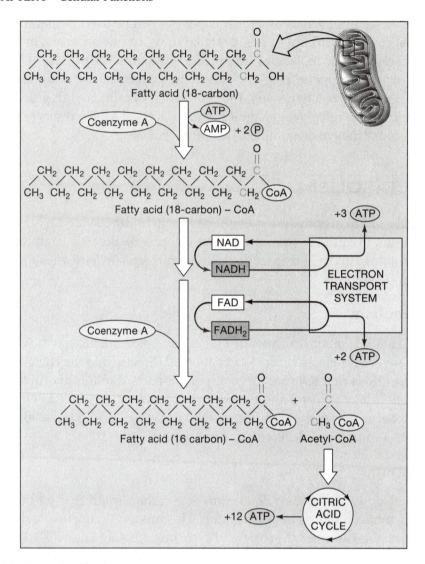

Figure 5–10 Beta-Oxidation.
During beta-oxidation, the carbon chains of fatty acids are broken down to yield molecules of acetyl-CoA, which can be used in the citric acid cycle. The reaction also donates hydrogen atoms to coenzymes that deliver them to the electron transport system.

supplies are limited. Skeletal muscle fibers normally cycle between lipid and carbohydrate metabolism. At rest, when energy demands are low, they break down fatty acids. When active, and energy demands are both large and immediate, skeletal muscle fibers shift to metabolizing glucose.

Lipid Synthesis

The synthesis of lipids is known as **lipogenesis** (lī-pō-JEN-e- sis). Figure 5–11 shows the major pathways of lipogenesis. Glycerol synthesis reverses the steps of glycolysis; the synthesis of most other lipids begins with acetyl-CoA. Lipogenesis can use almost any organic substrate because lipids, amino acids, and carbohydrates can be converted to acetyl-CoA.

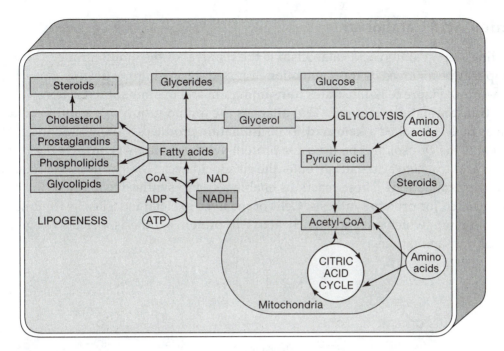

Figure 5–11   Lipid Synthesis.
Pathways of lipid synthesis begin with acetyl-CoA. Molecules of acetyl-CoA can be strung together in the cytosol, yielding fatty acids. Those fatty acids can be used to synthesize glycerides or other lipid molecules. Lipids can be synthesized from amino acids or carbohydrates by using acetyl-CoA as an intermediate.

Fatty acid synthesis involves a reaction sequence quite distinct from that of beta-oxidation. Our cells cannot build every fatty acid they can break down. **Linoleic acid** and **linolenic acid**, both 18-carbon, polyunsaturated fatty acids, cannot be synthesized at all. These are called **essential fatty acids** because they must be included in the diet. They are synthesized by plants, and cases of essential fatty acid deficiency are usually limited to hospitalized individuals receiving nutrients in an intravenous solution. A diet poor in linoleic acid slows growth and alters the appearance of the skin. These fatty acids are also needed to synthesize prostaglandins and some of the phospholipids incorporated in cell membranes throughout the body.

PROTEIN METABOLISM

There are roughly 100,000 proteins in the human body, with varied forms, functions, and structures. All contain varying combinations of the same 20+ amino acids that were introduced in Chapter 3. Under normal conditions, there is a continual turnover of cellular proteins. Peptide bonds are broken, and the free amino acids are used to manufacture new proteins. This recycling occurs in the cytosol.

If other energy sources are inadequate, mitochondria can break down amino acids in the citric acid cycle to generate ATP. Not all amino acids enter the citric acid cycle at the same point, so the ATP benefits vary. However, the average yield is comparable to that of carbohydrate catabolism.

Amino Acid Catabolism

The first step in amino acid catabolism is the removal of the amino group. The amino group may be removed by transamination (trans-am-i-NĀ-shun) or deamination (dē-am-i-NĀ-shun). Figure 5–12 illustrates transamination and deamination reactions.

Transamination (Figure 5–12a) attaches the amino group of an amino acid to a similar molecule called a **keto acid**. Transamination produces a "new" amino acid that can enter the cytosol and be used for protein synthesis. It also converts the original amino acid to a keto acid that can enter the citric acid cycle. Many different tissues perform transaminations. These reactions enable a cell to synthesize many of the amino acids needed for protein synthesis. Cells of the liver, skeletal muscles, heart, lung, kidney, and brain, which are particularly active in protein synthesis, perform large numbers of transaminations.

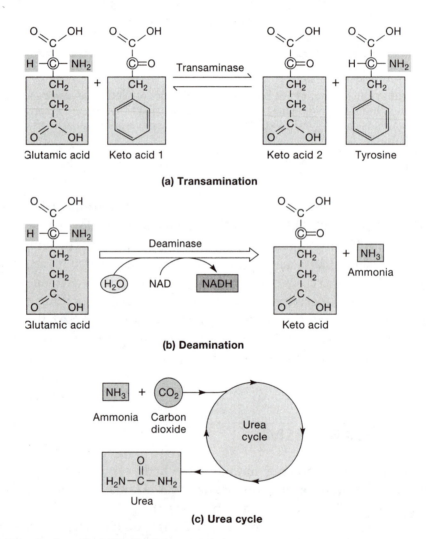

(a) Transamination

(b) Deamination

(c) Urea cycle

Figure 5–12 Amino Acid Catabolism.
(a) During transamination, an enzyme removes the amino group (-NH$_2$) from one molecule and attaches it to a keto acid. **(b)** During deamination, an enzyme strips the amino group and a hydrogen atom from an amino acid and produces a keto acid and ammonia. **(c)** The urea cycle takes two metabolic waste products, carbon dioxide and ammonia, and produces a molecule of urea. Urea is a relatively harmless, soluble compound that is excreted in the urine.

Deamination (Figure 5–12b) is performed in preparing an amino acid for breakdown in the citric acid cycle. Deamination is the removal of an amino group in a reaction that generates an ammonia molecule. Ammonia molecules are highly toxic, even in low concentrations. The liver, the primary site of deamination, has the enzymes needed to deal with the problem of ammonia generation. Liver cells take the ammonia and convert it to **urea**, a relatively harmless, water-soluble compound that is excreted in the urine. The **urea cycle** is the reaction sequence involved (Figure 5–12c).

When glucose supplies are low and lipid reserves are inadequate, liver cells break down internal proteins and absorb additional amino acids from the blood. The amino acids are deaminated, and the carbon chains are broken down to provide ATP.

There are several inherited metabolic disorders that result from an inability to produce specific enzymes involved with amino acid metabolism. **Phenylketonuria** (fēn-il-kē-tō-NOO-rē-uh), or **PKU**, is an example. Individuals with PKU cannot convert the amino acid phenylalanine to the amino acid tyrosine because of a defect in the enzyme required for the conversion (phenylalanine hydroxylase). This reaction is an essential step in the synthesis of molecules necessary for proper body function. If PKU is not detected in infancy, development of the nervous system is inhibited and severe brain damage results.

Proteins and Energy Production

Several factors make protein catabolism an impractical source of quick energy:

1. Proteins are more difficult to break apart than are complex carbohydrates or lipids.

2. One of the byproducts, ammonia, is a toxin that can damage cells.

3. Proteins form the most important structural and functional components of any cell. Extensive protein catabolism therefore threatens homeostasis at the cellular and systems levels.

NUCLEIC ACID METABOLISM

Living cells contain both DNA and RNA. DNA is absolutely essential to the long-term survival of the cell. As a result, the DNA in the nucleus is never catabolized for energy, even if the cell is dying of starvation. The RNA in the cell is involved with protein synthesis, and RNA molecules are broken down and replaced on a regular basis.

RNA Catabolism

In breaking down a strand of RNA, the bonds between nucleotides are broken, and the molecule is disassembled into individual nucleotides. These nucleotides are usually recycled into new nucleic acids. However, they can be catabolized to simple sugars and nitrogen bases. The sugars can enter the glycolytic pathways. Pyrimidines (cytosine and uracil) are converted to acetyl-CoA and metabolized in the citric acid cycle.

RNA AND ENERGY PRODUCTION

RNA catabolism makes a relatively insignificant contribution to the total energy budget of the cell. Proteins account for 15 to 30 percent of the weight of the cell, and much more energy can be provided through the catabolism of nonessential proteins. Even when RNA is broken down, only the sugars and pyrimidines provide energy. The purines (adenine and guanine) cannot be catabolized at all. Instead they are deaminated and excreted as uric acid. **Uric acid** is another relatively nontoxic waste product, but it differs from urea in that it is far less soluble. Urea and uric acid are called **nitrogenous wastes** because they contain nitrogen atoms.

Normal plasma uric acid concentrations average 2.7–7.4 mg/dl, depending on sex and age. When plasma concentrations exceed 7.4 mg/dl, **hyperuricemia** (hī-per-ū-ri-SĒ-mē-ah) exists. This condition may affect 18 percent of the U.S. population. At these concentrations body fluids are saturated with uric acid. Although symptoms may not appear at once, uric acid crystals may begin to form in body fluids. The condition that then develops is called **gout**.

Let's Review What You've Just Learned

► **Definitions**

In the space provided, write the term for each of the following definitions.

_____ 21. A waste product of protein metabolism that is formed in the liver.

_____ 22. The catabolism of lipids.

_____ 23. The removal of an amino group from an amino acid.

_____ 24. The synthesis of glycogen.

_____ 25. An elevated level of uric acid in the blood.

_____ 26. Polyunsaturated fatty acids that cannot be synthesized by the body and must be included in the diet.

_____ 27. The synthesis of lipids.

_____ 28. The molecule that remains after the deamination or transamination of an amino acid.

_____ 29. A disorder characterized by the formation of uric acid crystals in body fluids.

_____ 30. The synthesis of glucose from lipid or protein precursors.

_____ 31. A waste product of purine catabolism.

_____ 32. The process of fatty acid catabolism that produces acetyl-CoA.

_____ 33. The transfer of an amino group from an amino acid to another organic molecule.

_____ 34. A genetic disorder characterized by the inability to convert the amino acid phenylalanine into the amino acid tyrosine.

_____ 35. A general term for metabolic waste products that contain the element nitrogen.

▶ **Word Roots, Prefixes, Suffixes, and Combining Forms**

In the space provided, list the boldfaced terms introduced in this section that contain the indicated word part.

Word Part	Meaning	Examples
-emia	in the blood	**36.** _____
-lysis	to dissolve	**37.** _____
-uria	in the urine	**38.** _____
glyco-	sugar	**39.** _____
trans-	across	**40.** _____
lipo-	fat	**41.** _____
neo-	new	**42.** _____
-genesis	birth	**43.** _____
de-	away	**44.** _____

▶ **Completion**

Complete each of the following statements.

45. Two essential fatty acids are _____ and _____.

46. For aerobic metabolism to occur, a cell must have adequate supplies of _____ and _____.

47. The glycerol produced by the catabolism of triglycerides is converted to _____ before entering the energy pathways.

48. For each two-carbon fragment removed from a fatty acid in the process of beta-oxidation, the cell gains _____ ATP.

49. Lipid reserves are more difficult to access than carbohydrate reserves, because lipids are _____.

50. When RNA is catabolized, only the _____ and _____ in the molecule provide energy.

51. Proteins are an impractical source of quick energy because

    a. _____

    b. _____

    c. _____

DNA AND INFORMATION STORAGE

The basic structure of nucleic acids was described in Chapter 3. Chapter 4 considered the organization of the nucleus, the organelle that contains the cell's DNA. The DNA of the nucleus controls the cell by directing the synthesis of specific proteins. Proteins make up 15–30 percent of the weight of each cell, and through control of protein synthesis virtually every aspect of cell structure and function can be regulated. There are two levels of control involved, one direct and the other indirect.

    1. The DNA of the nucleus has direct control over the synthesis and structure of proteins, such as cytoskeletal components, membrane proteins (including receptors), and secretory products. By issuing appropriate orders, the nucleus can alter the internal structure of the cell, its sensitivity to substances in the extracellular environment, or its secretory functions to meet changing circumstances.

2. The DNA of the nucleus has indirect control over all other aspects of cellular metabolism because it regulates the synthesis of enzymes. By ordering the production of appropriate enzymes, the nucleus can regulate all of the metabolic activities and functions of the cell. For example, the nucleus can accelerate the rate of glycolysis by increasing the number of glycolytic enzymes in the cytoplasm.

Chromosome Structure

It is the DNA in the nucleus that stores the vital information, and the DNA is found in complex structures called **chromosomes**. Each chromosome contains DNA strands bound to special proteins called **histones**. The DNA strands are coiled around the histones, and the histones help package the DNA in a small space. The interactions between the DNA and the histones help determine what information is available.

At intervals, the DNA strands wind around the histones, forming a complex known as a **nucleosome**. The entire chain of nucleosomes may coil around other histones. The degree of coiling determines whether the chromosome is long and thin or short and fat. Chromosomes in a dividing cell are very tightly coiled, so they can be seen clearly as separate structures in light or electron micrographs. In cells that are not dividing, the chromosomes are loosely coiled, forming a tangle of fine filaments known as **chromatin** that give the nucleus a clumped, grainy appearance.

Human somatic cell nuclei contain 23 pairs of chromosomes; one member of each pair is derived from our mother and one from our father. The structure of a typical chromosome is diagrammed in Figure 5–13.

Figure 5–13 Chromosome Structure.
DNA strands are coiled around histones to form nucleosomes. Nucleosomes form coils that may be very tight or rather loose. In cells that are not dividing, the DNA is loosely coiled, forming a tangled network known as chromatin. When the coiling becomes tighter, as it does in preparation for cell division, the DNA becomes visible as distinct structures called chromosomes.

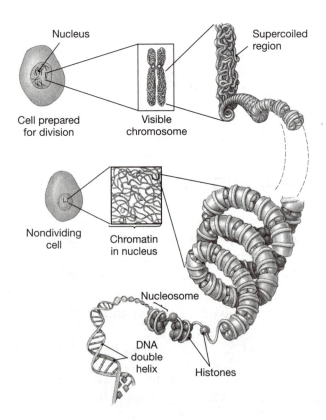

The Genetic Code

The **genetic code** is the method of information storage within the DNA strands of the nucleus. An appreciation of the genetic code has given us the opportunity to determine how cells build proteins and how various structural and functional characteristics are inherited from generation to generation. We are now beginning to experiment with the manipulation of the genetic information in human cells, and the techniques may revolutionize the treatment of a variety of serious diseases.

Recall from Chapter 3 that a single DNA molecule consists of a pair of nucleotide strands held together by hydrogen bonding between complementary nitrogenous bases. Those nitrogenous bases are adenine, A; thymine, T; cytosine, C; and guanine, G. Information is stored in the sequence of nitrogenous bases along the length of the DNA strands.

The genetic code is called a *triplet code* because a sequence of three nitrogenous bases can specify the identity of a single amino acid. Each **gene** consists of all the "triplets" needed to produce a specific peptide chain. The number of triplets in a gene varies, depending on the size of the peptide represented. A relatively short peptide chain might require fewer than a hundred triplets, whereas the instructions for building a large protein might involve a thousand or more.

Each gene also contains segments responsible for regulating its activity. In effect, these are triplets that say "do (or do not) read this message," "message starts here," and "message ends here." The "read me," "don't read me," and "start here" signals form a special control segment at the start of each gene.

Every nucleated somatic cell in the human body carries the same 46 chromosomes and identical DNA segments. However, all of the DNA in the nucleus does not code for proteins, and a significant percentage of DNA segments have no known function. Some of the "useless" segments contain the same nucleotide sequence repeated over and over. The number of segments and the number of repetitions vary from individual to individual. The pattern of these repeating DNA segments is called a **DNA fingerprint**. The chances of any two individuals, other than identical twins, having the same pattern of repeating segments (DNA fingerprint) is less than one in 9 billion. In other words, it is extremely unlikely that you will ever encounter someone else who has the same pattern of repeating nucleotide sequences that is present in your DNA.

Individual identification can therefore be made on the basis of a pattern of DNA analysis, just as it can on the basis of a fingerprint. Skin scrapings, blood, semen, hair, or other tissues can be used as a sample source. Information from DNA fingerprinting has already been used to convict or acquit persons accused of violent crimes, such as rape or murder.

GENE ACTIVATION AND PROTEIN SYNTHESIS

Each DNA strand contains thousands of individual genes. The DNA containing these genes is normally tightly coiled, and specialized proteins bound to the control segments prevent their activation. Before a specific gene is activated, the DNA containing the genes must unwind, enzymes must temporarily disrupt the weak bonds between the nitrogen bases, and the protein guarding the control segment must be detached. The enzyme **RNA polymerase** then binds to the initial segment of the gene.

The events that follow can be divided into two stages:

1. **Transcription:** RNA polymerase uses the genetic information to assemble a strand of mRNA.

2. **Translation:** Ribosomes use the information carried by the mRNA strand to assemble functional proteins.

Transcription

Activated genes do not leave the nucleus, nor do they lose their connections with other genes along the length of the DNA strand. Instead, a messenger carries the instructions from the nucleus to the cytoplasm. The carrier is a single strand of **messenger RNA (mRNA)**. The process of mRNA formation is called transcription, because the mRNA is "taking notes" from the gene. The two DNA strands of a gene are mirror images. The one containing the triplets that will be transcribed is called the **template strand**; the other is called the **coding strand**. Figure 5–14 details the process of transcription.

Step 1: Once the DNA strands have separated, and the control segment has been exposed, transcription can begin. The key event is the attachment of RNA-polymerase to the control segment of the template strand. RNA polymerase

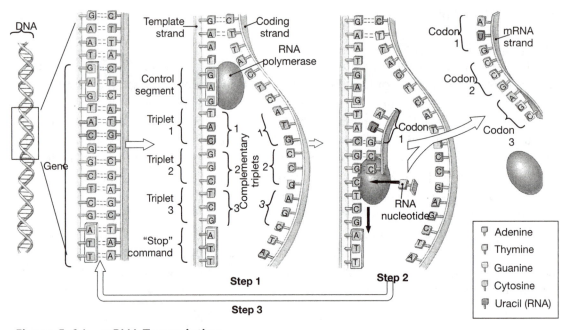

Figure 5–14   mRNA Transcription.
This diagram shows a small portion of a single DNA molecule, containing a single gene available for transcription. **Step 1:** The two DNA strands separate, and RNA polymerase binds to the control segment of the gene. **Step 2:** The RNA polymerase moves from one nucleotide to another along the length of the template strand. At each site, complementary RNA nucleotides form hydrogen bonds with the DNA nucleotides of the template strand. The RNA polymerase then strings the arriving nucleotides together into a strand of mRNA. **Step 3:** Upon reaching the stop signal at the end of the gene, the RNA polymerase and the mRNA strand detach, and the two DNA strands reassociate.

promotes hydrogen bonding between the nitrogenous bases of the gene and complementary nucleotides in the nucleoplasm. The nucleotides involved are those characteristic of RNA, not DNA; RNA polymerase may attach adenine, guanine, cytosine, or uracil, but never thymine. Thus, wherever an A occurs in the DNA strand, the polymerase will attach a U rather than a T.

Step 2: Only a small portion of the gene interacts with RNA polymerase at any one time as the enzyme travels down its length. As it moves from triplet to triplet, the RNA polymerase collects additional nucleotides and attaches them to the growing chain. In this way it assembles a complete strand of mRNA.

Step 3: At the "stop here" command, the enzyme and the mRNA strand detach. The complementary DNA strands now reassociate.

Each gene includes a number of noncoding regions that do not contain information needed to build a functional protein. As a result, the mRNA strand assembled during transcription, called **pre-mRNA**, must be "edited" before it leaves the nucleus to direct protein synthesis. In this **RNA processing**, the noncoding regions, called **introns**, are snipped out by specific enzymes, and the remaining segments, or **exons**, are spliced together. This process creates a much shorter, functional strand of mRNA, which then enters the cytoplasm through one of the nuclear pores.

Translation

Translation is the construction of a functional polypeptide using the information provided by an mRNA strand. A **codon** (KŌ-don) is a sequence of three nitrogenous bases along an mRNA strand. Each codon specifies a particular amino acid. Codons contain nitrogenous bases that are complementary to those of the triplets of the template strand. For example, if the triplet on the DNA strand is T-C-G, the corresponding codon on the mRNA will be A-G-C. Every amino acid has at least one unique and specific codon, and most have more than one; Table 5–1 lists representative examples of codons and the amino acids they specify. During translation, the sequence of codons will determine the sequence of amino acids in the polypeptide. The amino acids are provided by another form of RNA, **transfer RNA**

Table 5–1	Examples of the Triplet Code			
Second Position				
Coding strand	Template strand	mRNA codon	tRNA anticodon	Amino acid
TTT	AAA	UUU	AAA	Phenylalanine
TTA	AAT	UUA	AAU	Leucine
TGT	ACA	UGU	ACA	Cysteine
GTT	CAA	GUU	CAA	Valine
CCC	GGG	CCC	GGG	Proline
GCC	CGG	GCC	CGG	Alanine

(tRNA) (Figure 5–15). Each tRNA delivers an amino acid of a specific type. There are more than 20 different kinds of transfer RNA, at least one for each of the amino acids used in protein synthesis.

At one place in its structure each tRNA molecule has a trio of nitrogenous bases, known as an **anticodon**, that is complementary to the three bases in one of the codons. The anticodon varies depending on the type of amino acid the tRNA carries. For example, a tRNA with the anticodon GGG always carries the amino acid proline, whereas a tRNA with the anticodon GCC carries alanine.

During translation, each codon along the mRNA strand will bind to a complementary anticodon on a tRNA molecule. So if the mRNA has the codons (CCC)-(CGG)-(CCC) it will bind to tRNAs with anticodons (GGG)-(GCC)-(GGG). The amino acid sequence of the peptide chain created is determined by the sequence of the codons on the mRNA. So in this case the amino acid sequence in the peptide would be proline-alanine-proline.

Translation proceeds in three steps: (1) initiation, which begins the process; (2) elongation, which produces the peptide chain; and (3) termination, which completes the process and releases the completed peptide. These steps are diagrammed in Figure 5–16.

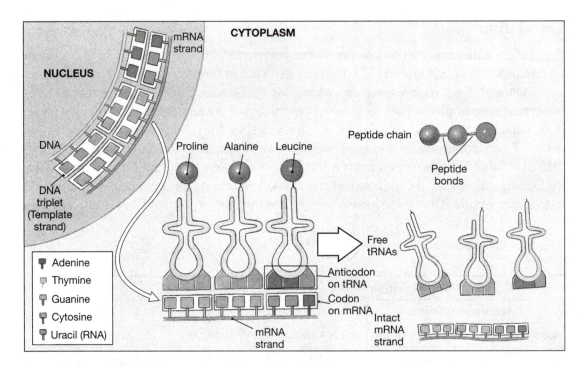

Figure 5–15   An Overview of Protein Synthesis.
An mRNA strand assembled during transcription contains codons that are complementary to triplets on one of the DNA strands (the template strand). The mRNA then detaches from the DNA strand and enters the cytoplasm. Molecules of tRNA contain anticodons that are complementary to the mRNA codons. During translation, different amino acids are delivered to the mRNA strand by tRNAs with appropriate anticodons; examples are indicated in Table 5-1. The sequence of amino acids in the completed peptide will reflect the sequence of tRNA arrival. The tRNAs arrive one after the other, and the peptide chain grows one amino acid at a time. Figure 5–16 shows the sequence of events.

Initiation

Step 1: Initiation begins as the mRNA strand binds to a small ribosomal subunit. The first tRNA to arrive bears an anticodon sequence of U-A-C; this tRNA carries the amino acid methionine. (This amino acid will ultimately be removed from the finished protein.) The anticodon sequence will bind to the first codon of the mRNA strand, or initiator codon, which always has the base sequence A-U-G.

Step 2: When this binding occurs, a large ribosomal subunit joins the complex to create a complete ribosome. The mRNA strand nestles in the gap between the small and large subunits.

Elongation

Step 3: A second tRNA now arrives at the adjacent site of the ribosome, and its anticodon binds to the next codon of the mRNA strand.

Step 4: Enzymes of the large ribosomal subunit then break the linkage between the tRNA molecule and its amino acid. At the same time, they attach the amino acid to its neighbor by means of a peptide bond. The ribosome then moves one codon down the mRNA strand.

Step 5: The cycle is then repeated with the arrival of another molecule of tRNA. The tRNA already stripped of its amino acid drifts away. It will soon bind to another amino acid and be ready to participate in protein synthesis at a later date.

Termination

Step 6: Elongation continues, adding amino acids to the growing polypeptide chain, until the ribosome reaches the "stop here" signal, or terminator codon, at the end of the mRNA strand. The ribosomal subunits now detach, leaving an intact strand of mRNA and a completed polypeptide.

Translation proceeds swiftly, producing a typical protein in around 20 seconds. The mRNA strand remains intact, and it can interact with other ribosomes to create additional copies of the same peptide chain. The process does not continue indefinitely, however, because mRNA strands are broken down and the nucleotides are recycled after a few minutes, or at most a few hours.

Polyribosomes

During translation, only two mRNA codons are being "read" by a ribosome at any one time, although the entire strand may contain thousands of codons. As a result, a single mRNA strand can be bound to several ribosomes. Each ribosome reads a different part of the same message and ends up constructing the same protein as all the other ribosomes. The effect is similar to a line of people at a buffet lunch; each person will assemble the same meal, but always a step behind the person ahead. A series of ribosomes attached to the same mRNA strand is called a **polyribosome** (Figure 5–17). Polyribosome formation greatly increases the rate of protein synthesis.

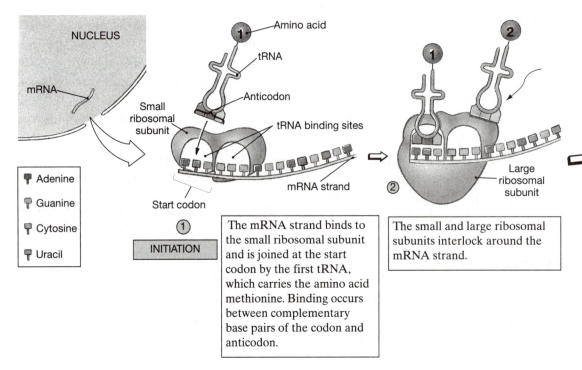

Figure 5–16   The Process of Translation.

MUTATIONS

Mutations are permanent alterations in a cell's DNA that affect the nucleotide sequence of one or more genes. The simplest is a **point mutation**, a change in a single nucleotide that affects one codon. The triplet code has some flexibility because several different codons can signal the same amino acid. But a point mutation that produces a codon that specifies a different amino acid will change the structure of the completed protein. A single change in the amino acid sequence of a structural protein or enzyme can prove fatal. Several cancers and two blood disorders, thalassemia and sickle-cell anemia, result from variations in a single nucleotide.

More than 100 inherited disorders have been traced to abnormalities in enzyme or protein structure that reflect alterations in nucleotide sequence. More elaborate mutations can affect multiple codons within a gene, several adjacent genes, or the structure of one or more chromosomes.

Because mutations most often occur during DNA replication, they are most likely to involve cells undergoing cell division. A single cell, a group of cells, or an entire individual may be affected. The latter will be the case if the changes occur during the formation of sex cells or early in development. For example, a mutation affecting the DNA of an individual's gametes (sperm or ova) will be inherited by that individual's children. Our current understanding of genetic structure is opening the possibility for diagnosing and correcting some of these problems.

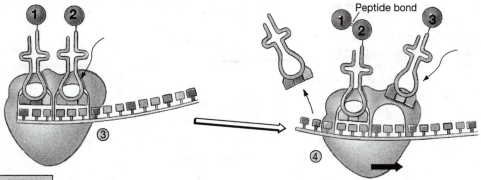

ELONGATION

A second tRNA arrives at the adjacent site of the ribosome. The anticodon of the second tRNA binds to the next mRNA codon.

The first amino acid is detached from its tRNA and is joined to the second amino acid by a peptide bond. The ribosome moves one codon farther along the mRNA strand; the first tRNA detaches as another tRNA arrives.

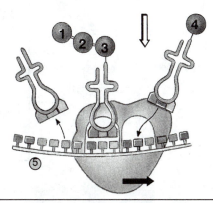

This cycle is repeated as the ribosome moves along the length of the mRNA strand, binds new tRNAs, and incorporates their amino acids into the polypeptide chain.

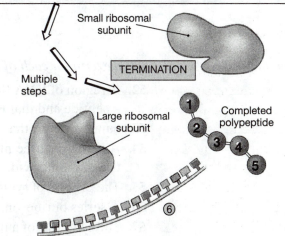

Elongation continues until the stop codon is reached; the components then separate.

Figure 5–17 Polyribosomes.
Each polyribosome consists of one strand of mRNA that is being read simultaneously by a number of ribosomes. In this way a single strand of mRNA can produce many polypeptide molecules in a short time.

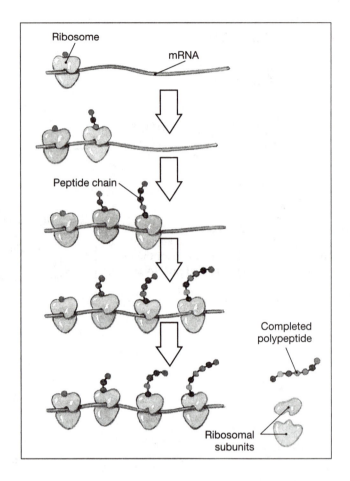

 Let's Review What You've Just Learned

▶ **Definitions**

In the space provided, write the term for each of the following definitions.

_____ 52. A region of RNA that does not contain coding sequences for a peptide and that is removed during RNA processing.

_____ 53. Small proteins that bind to the DNA in chromosomes.

_____ 54. A series of three nucleotides in mRNA that specifies a particular amino acid.

_____ 55. The process of synthesizing mRNA from DNA.

_____ 56. A series of ribosomes attached to the same mRNA.

_____ 57. The synthesis of a polypeptide as directed by an mRNA on a ribosome.

_____ 58. The relationship between the codons and their role in protein synthesis.

_____ 59. A type of RNA molecule that carries amino acids to ribosomes to be incorporated into polypeptide chains.

_____ 60. The process by which introns are removed from a molecule of pre-mRNA.

_____ **61.** The enzyme necessary for transcribing mRNA from DNA.

_____ **62.** The complex formed when a molecule of DNA is wrapped around a group of four histones.

_____ **63.** A permanent alteration in a cell's DNA.

_____ **64.** The coding regions of a pre-mRNA molecule that are spliced together to form a functional molecule of mRNA.

_____ **65.** The region of a tRNA molecule that contains a sequence of three nucleotides that is complementary to a codon on a molecule of mRNA.

_____ **66.** The loosely coiled tangle of fine chromosome filaments found in the nuclei of cells that are not dividing.

_____ **67.** A type of RNA molecule that contains a sequence of codons that dictates the sequence of amino acids in a polypeptide.

_____ **68.** The type of mutation that occurs when a single nucleotide in a codon is changed.

_____ **69.** The pattern formed by the number and size of repetitious, noncoding DNA segments.

_____ **70.** The "unedited" molecule of mRNA that is transcribed from DNA.

_____ **71.** The segment of a DNA molecule that contains all of the triplets needed to produce a specific peptide chain.

► Completion

Complete each of the following statements by filling in the appropriate word or phrase in the space provided.

72. The key event in the process of transcription is the attachment of _____ to the gene.

73. When an A (adenine) nucleotide appears in a gene it specifies a _____ nucleotide in the mRNA.

74. Initiation of the translation process occurs when an mRNA strand binds to a _____.

75. The start codon always has the nucleotide sequence _____.

76. A tRNA locates its specific place on the mRNA because it contains an _____ that is complementary to a codon in mRNA.

77. During the elongation part of translation, a ribosome will move down the mRNA one _____ at a time.

78. During translation, elongation continues until the ribosome reaches a _____.

THE CELL LIFE CYCLE

Between fertilization and physical maturity a human being goes from a single cell to roughly 75 trillion cells. This amazing increase in size and complexity involves a form of cellular reproduction called **cell division**. The division of a single cell produces a pair of **daughter cells**, each half the size of the original. These cells will grow until each reaches the size of the original cell, when they will usually divide in turn.

Even when development has been completed, cell division continues to be essential to survival. Although cells are highly adaptable, they can be damaged by physical wear and tear, toxic chemicals, temperature changes, or other environmental hazards. In addition, cells, like individuals, are subject to aging. The life span of a cell varies from hours to decades, depending on the type of cell and the environmental stresses involved. Many cells appear to be "programmed" to self-destruct after a certain period of time. Their destruction results from the activation of specific "suicide genes" in the nucleus. The genetically controlled death of cells is called **apoptosis** (ap-op-TŌ-sis; Greek *apos*, away from + *ptosis*, fall). One gene involved in regulation of this process has been identified. This gene, called bcl-2, appears to prevent apoptosis and keep a cell alive and functional. If something interferes with the function of this gene, the cell self-destructs.

Because a typical cell does not live nearly as long as a typical person, cell populations must be maintained over time by cell division. Central to cell reproduction is the accurate duplication of the cell's genetic material and its distribution to the two new daughter cells formed by division. This process is called **mitosis** (mī-TŌ-sis). Mitosis occurs during the division of somatic cells. Somatic cells include all of the cells in the body other than the sex cells, which give rise to sperm or ova. Production of sperm and ova involves a distinct process, **meiosis** (mī-Ō-sis), that will be described in Chapter 7.

Figure 5–18 presents the life cycle of a typical cell in greater detail. That life cycle includes a relatively brief period of mitosis followed by an interphase period of variable duration.

Interphase

Most cells spend only a small part of their time actively engaged in cell division. Somatic cells spend the majority of their functional lives in a state known as **interphase**. During interphase a cell performs all of its normal functions plus, if necessary, making preparations for cell division. Interphase can be divided into the G_0, G_1, S, and G_2 phases.

Figure 5–18   The Cell Life Cycle.

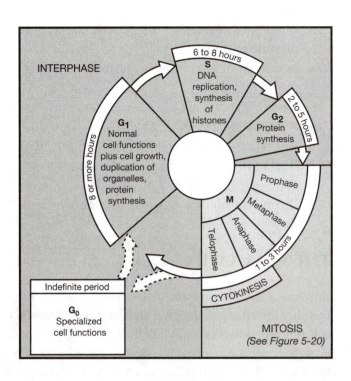

The G_0 Phase

An interphase cell in the G_0 **phase** is not preparing for mitosis but is performing all other normal cell functions. Some mature cells, such as skeletal muscle cells and many nerve cells, remain in G_0 indefinitely and may never undergo cell division. In contrast, cells known as stem cells, which divide repeatedly with very brief interphase periods, have eliminated the G_0 phase.

The G_1 Phase

A cell that is going to divide first enters the G_1 **phase**. In this phase the cell manufactures enough cytoskeletal elements, centrioles, endoplasmic reticulum, ribosomes, Golgi membranes, and cytosol to make two functional cells. During this time the mitochondria also divide, producing enough for two cells. In cells dividing at top speed, G_1 may last as little as 8–12 hours. Such cells pour all of their energy into mitosis, and all other activities cease. If G_1 lasts for days, weeks, or months, preparation for mitosis occurs as the cells perform their normal functions.

The S Phase and DNA Replication

When the activities of G_1 have been completed the cell enters the **S phase**. Over the next 6–8 hours the cell duplicates its chromosomes. In this process, it copies its DNA and combines it with histones and other proteins in the nucleus.

Throughout the life of a cell, the DNA strands in the nucleus remain intact. DNA synthesis, or **DNA replication**, occurs in cells preparing to undergo mitosis or meiosis. The goal of replication is to copy the genetic information in the nucleus so that one set of chromosomes can be given to each of the two daughter cells produced.

As you already know, a DNA molecule consists of a pair of DNA strands held together by hydrogen bonding between complementary nitrogenous bases. Figure 5–19 diagrams the process of DNA replication. It begins when enzymes disrupt the weak bonds between the nitrogenous bases and the strands unwind. As they do so, molecules of the enzyme **DNA polymerase** bind to the exposed nitrogenousbases. This enzyme promotes bonding between the nitrogenous bases of the DNA strand and complementary DNA nucleotides dissolved in the nucleoplasm.

Many molecules of DNA polymerase work simultaneously along the DNA strands. The two DNA strands are oriented in opposite directions (Figure 3–17, p. 123), and DNA polymerase can work in only one direction. On one strand, DNA polymerase moves forward as the original strands unwind, producing an intact complementary DNA strand (Figure 5–19). On the other strand, DNA polymerase works away from the point of unwinding, creating short nucleotide chains that must be linked together by enzymes called **ligases** (LĪ-gās-ez; Latin *ligare*, to tie). The final result is a pair of identical DNA molecules.

The G_2 Phase

Once DNA replication has been completed, there is a brief (2–5 hours) G_2 **phase** devoted to last-minute protein synthesis. The cell then enters the **M phase**, and mitosis begins.

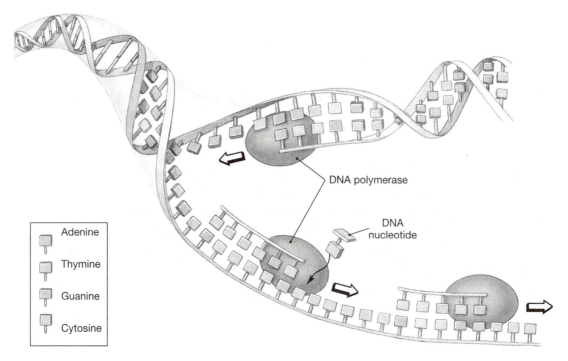

☐	Adenine
☐	Thymine
☐	Guanine
☐	Cytosine

Figure 5–19   DNA Replication.
In replication, the DNA strands unwind, and DNA polymerase begins attaching complementary DNA nucleotides along each strand. This process produces two identical copies of the original DNA molecule.

MITOSIS

Mitosis is a process that separates the duplicated chromosomes of the original cell into two identical nuclei. Mitosis specifically refers to the division and duplication of the nucleus of the cell. Separation of the cytoplasm to form two separate and distinct cells involves a separate but related process known as **cytokinesis** (sī-tō-ki-NĒ-sis; Greek *kytos*, vessel + *kinein*, to move).

Figure 5–20 summarizes the four stages of mitosis: prophase, metaphase, anaphase, and telophase.

Stage 1: Prophase

Prophase (PRŌ-fāz; *pro*, before) begins when the chromosomes coil so tightly that they become visible as individual structures. As a result of DNA replication during the S phase, there are now two copies of each chromosome. Each copy, called a **chromatid** (KRŌ-ma-tid), is connected to its duplicate at a single point, the **centromere** (SEN-trō-mēr).

As the chromosomes appear, the two pairs of centrioles move toward opposite poles of the nucleus. An array of microtubules, called **spindle fibers**, extend between the centriole pairs. Smaller microtubules, called **astral rays**, radiate into the surrounding cytoplasm. Prophase ends with the disappearance of the nuclear envelope.

Stage 2: Metaphase

Metaphase (MET-a-fāz; *meta*, after) begins after the disintegration of the nuclear envelope. The spindle fibers now enter the nuclear region, and the chromosomes (composed of two chromatids) become attached to spindle fibers called **chromosomal microtubules**.

Once attachment has been completed, the chromosomes are moved to a narrow central zone called the **metaphase plate**. Metaphase ends when all of the chromosomes are aligned in the plane of the metaphase plate.

Stage 3: Anaphase

Anaphase (AN-uh-fāz; *ana*, apart) begins when the chromatids separate. At this point the structures are no longer chromatids but **daughter chromosomes**. The two daughter chromosomes are now pulled toward opposite ends of the cell along the chromosomal microtubules. Anaphase ends when the daughter chromsomes arrive near the centrioles at opposite ends of the cell.

Stage 4: Telophase

During **telophase** (TEL-ō-fāz; *telo*, end) the cell prepares to return to the interphase state. The nuclear envelope forms, the nuclei enlarge, and the chromosomes gradually uncoil. Once the chromosomes have relaxed and the find filaments of chromatin become visible, nucleoli reappear and the nuclei resemble those of interphase cells. This marks the end of the process of mitosis.

CYTOKINESIS

As you have just learned, mitosis is the separation of chromosomal material into two identical nuclei. The separation of the cytoplasm into two different daughter cells involves the process of cytokinesis. Cytokinesis usually begins in late anaphase. As the daughter chromosomes near the ends of the spindle apparatus, the cytoplasm constricts along the plane of the metaphase plate. This process continues throughout telophase and is usually completed sometime after the nuclear envelope has reformed. The completion of cytokinesis marks the end of the process of cell division.

THE MITOTIC RATE

The preparations for cell division that occur between G_1 and the end of the S phase are difficult to recognize in a light micrograph. However, the start of mitosis is easy to recognize, because the chromosomes become condensed and highly visible. The frequency of cell division can thus be estimated by the number of cells in mitosis at any given time. As a result, the term **mitotic rate** is often used when discussing rates of cell division. In general, the longer the life expectancy of a cell type, the slower the mitotic rate. Relatively long-lived cells, such as muscle cells and nerve cells, either never divide or do so only under special circumstances. Other cells, such as those covering the surface of the skin or the lining of the digestive tract, are subject to attack by chemicals, pathogens, and abrasion. They survive only for days or even hours. Special cells called **stem cells** maintain these cell populations through repeated cycles of cell division.

Stem cells are relatively unspecialized, and their only function is the production of daughter cells. Each time a stem cell divides, one of the daughter cells develops functional specializations while the other prepares for further divisions. The rate of stem cell division can vary, depending on the tissue and the demand for new cells. In heavily abraded skin, stem cells may divide more than once a day, but stem cells in adult connective tissues may remain inactive for years.

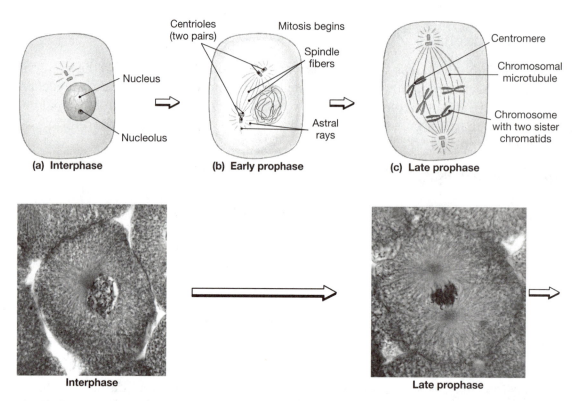

Figure 5–20   Interphase and Mitosis.
(a)–(f) Diagrammatic views. Photos (below) × 581.

ENERGETICS AND CELL DIVISION

Dividing cells use an unusually large amount of energy. For example, they must synthesize new organic materials and move organelles and chromosomes within the cell. All of these processes require ATP in substantial amounts. Cells that do not have adequate energy sources cannot divide, and in starvation normal cell growth and maintenance grind to a halt. For this reason, prolonged starvation stunts growth, slows wound healing, lowers resistance to disease, thins the skin, and changes the lining of the digestive tract. The same changes are seen in the late stages of many cancers, because the cancer cells are "stealing" the nutrients that would otherwise be used to support normal cell growth and maintenance.

THE REGULATION OF THE CELL LIFE CYCLE

Mitotic rates are usually well controlled, and in normal tissues the rates of cell division balance cell loss or destruction. The rates are genetically controlled, and many different stimuli may be responsible for activating genes that promote cell division. The most important of these stimuli appear to be extracellular compounds, usually peptides, that stimulate the division of specific cell types. These compounds include several hormones and a variety of growth factors. Table 5–2 lists several of these stimulatory compounds

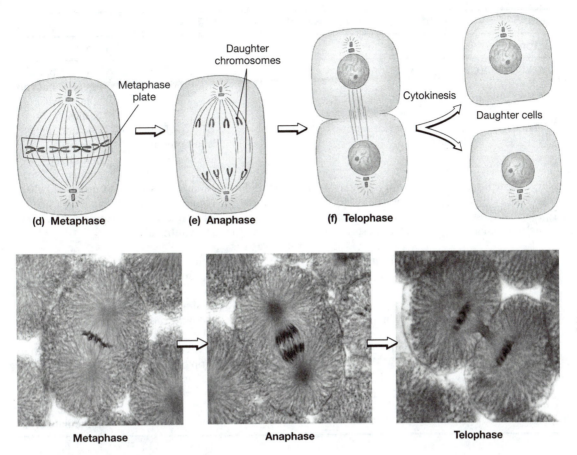

(d) Metaphase (e) Anaphase (f) Telophase

Metaphase Anaphase Telophase

Figure 5–20 (continued).

and their target tissues. Each of these compounds appears to exert its effects by binding to receptors on the cell membrane. This binding initiates a series of biochemical events that ultimately trigger cell division. The effects of these stimulatory factors may be opposed by a poorly understood class of peptides called **chalones** (KĀ-lōnz, Greek *chalan*, to slacken).

Genetic mechanisms for inhibiting cell division have recently been identified. The genes involved are known as **repressor genes**. One gene, called p53, controls a protein that resides in the nucleus and activates genes that direct the production of growth-inhibiting factors inside the cell. Roughly half of all cancers are associated with abnormal forms of the p53 gene.

Cell Division and Cancer

When the balance between cell division and growth and cell death breaks down, a tissue begins to enlarge. A **tumor**, or **neoplasm**, is a mass or swelling produced by the abnormal cell growth and division. In a **benign tumor** the cells remain within a connective tissue capsule. Such a tumor seldom threatens an individual's life. Surgery can usually remove the tumor if its size or position disturbs tissue formation.

Cells in a **malignant tumor** are no longer responding to normal control mechanisms. These cells spread into the surrounding tissues, a process called **invasion**. The cancer cells may also spread to other tissues and organs. This dispersion is called **metastasis**

Table 5–2 Representative Chemical Factors Affecting Cell Division

Factor	Source	Effect	Target
Growth hormone	Anterior pituitary gland	Stimulation of growth, cell division, differentiation	All cells, especially in epithelial and connective tissues
Prolactin	Anterior pituitary gland	Stimulation of growth, cell division, development	Gland and duct cells of mammary glands
Nerve growth factor (NGF)	Salivary glands; other sources suspected	Stimulation of neural tissue repair and development	Neurons and glial cells
Epidermal growth factor (EGF)	Duodenal glands; other sources suspected	Stimulation of stem cell divisions and epithelial repairs	Epidermis of skin
Fibroblast growth factor (FGF)	Unknown	Division and differentiation of fibroblasts and related cells	Connective tissues
Erythropoietin	Kidneys (primary source)	Stimulation of stem cell divisions and maturation of red blood cells	Bone marrow
Thymosins and related compounds	Thymus	Stimulation of division and differentiation of lymphocytes (especially T cells)	Thymus and other lymphoid tissues and organs
Chalones	Many tissues	Inhibition of cell division	Cells in the immediate area

(me-TAS-ta-sis; Greek *meta*, after + *stasis*, standing). Metastasis is dangerous and difficult to control. Once in a new location, the metastatic cells produce secondary tumors.

The term **cancer** refers to an illness characterized by malignant cells. Cancer cells gradually lose their resemblance to normal cells. They change size and shape, often becoming unusually large or abnormally small. Organ function begins to deteriorate as the number of cancer cells increases. The cancer cells may not perform their original functions at all, or they may perform normal functions in an unusual way. For example, endocrine cancer cells may produce normal hormones but in abnormally large amounts. Cancer cells compete for space and nutrients with normal cells. They do not use energy very efficiently, and they grow and multiply at the expense of normal tissues. These features account for the starved appearance of many patients in the late stages of cancer.

CELL DIVERSITY AND DIFFERENTIATION

Liver cells, fat cells, and neurons contain the same chromosomes and genes, but in each case a different set of genes has been turned off. In other words, liver cells differ from other cells because they have different genes available for transcription.

When a gene is "turned off," the cell loses the ability to create a particular protein and thus to perform any functions involving that protein. Each time another gene switches off, the cell's functional abilities become more restricted. This specialization process is called **differentiation** (dif-ur-en-shē-Ā-shun).

Fertilization produces a single cell with all of its genetic potential intact. There follows a period of repeated cell division, and differentiation begins as the number of cells increases. Differentiation produces specialized cells with limited capabilities. These cells form organized collections known as tissues, each with discrete functional roles. The next chapter examines the structure and function of tissues and considers the role of tissue interactions in the maintenance of homeostatsis.

Let's Review What You've Just Learned

▶ **Definitions**

In the space provided, write the term for each of the following definitions.

_____ **79.** The two copies of a duplicated chromosome that are connected to a centromere.

_____ **80.** A process in cell division in which chromosomes in the cell are duplicated and evenly distributed between two daughter cells.

_____ **81.** A tumor or mass of abnormal tissue.

_____ **82.** The initial phase of mitosis, characterized by the appearance of chromosomes, breakdown of the nuclear membrane, and formation of the spindle apparatus.

_____ **83.** A class of peptides that act to oppose the stimulatory effects of growth factors.

_____ **84.** The phase in the life cycle of a cell that follows DNA replication and during which protein synthesis occurs.

_____ **85.** The spread of malignant cells from one organ to another.

_____ **86.** The cells produced as a result of cell division.

_____ **87.** A stage in mitosis during which the chromosomes line up along the equatorial plate of the cell.

_____ **88.** The gradual appearance of characteristic cellular specializations during development, as the result of gene activation or repression.

_____ **89.** Localized region where two chromatids remain connected after chromosome replication; site of spindle fiber attachment.

_____ **90.** The process by which the DNA in new chromosomes is synthesized.

_____ **91.** The phase in a cell life cycle during which mitosis takes place.

_____ **92.** Special cells that maintain cell populations through repeated cycles of cell division.

_____ **93.** A tumor composed of cells that usually remain in a connective tissue capsule.

_____ **94.** Genes that code for peptides that inhibit cell division.

_____ **95.** The genetically controlled death of cells.

_____ 96. A phase in the cell life cycle during which the cell is performing normal cell functions but is not preparing for mitosis.

_____ 97. An enzyme that promotes bonding between the nitrogenous bases of a DNA strand and complementary DNA nucleotides dissolved in the nucleoplasm.

_____ 98. The cytoplasmic movement that separates one cell into two daughter cells during cell division.

_____ 99. The stage of mitosis in which the paired chromatids separate and move toward opposite poles.

_____ 100. An illness characterized by malignant cells.

_____ 101. The stage in the life cycle of a cell during which the chromosomes are uncoiled and all normal cellular functions except mitosis are under way.

_____ 102. The phase in a cell's life cycle during which DNA is replicated.

_____ 103. Enzymes that function to link small nucleotide chains together.

_____ 104. Spindle fibers that attach to chromatids during metaphase of mitosis.

_____ 105. The final stage of mitosis.

_____ 106. The common name for a neoplasm.

_____ 107. The phase in a cell's life cycle during which it manufactures enough materials, organelles, and cytosol to make two functional cells.

_____ 108. Microtubules that extend from the centrioles during mitosis.

_____ 109. A narrow central zone in the cell where chromosomes align during metaphase of mitosis.

_____ 110. The frequency of cell division.

_____ 111. A tumor that does not respond to normal cellular control mechanisms and spreads to surrounding tissue.

_____ 112. Small microtubules that radiate from centrioles into the surrounding cytoplasm.

▶ Word Roots, Prefixes, Suffixes, and Combining Forms

In the space provided, list the boldfaced terms introduced in this section that contain the indicated word part.

Word Part	Meaning	Examples
-ptosis	falling away	113. _____
telo-	end	114. _____
pro-	before	115. _____
centro-	in the middle	116. _____
meta-	after	117. _____
chrom-	color	118. _____
inter-	between	119. _____
ana-	back	120. _____
liga-	to bind	121. _____
cyto-	cell	122. _____
neo-	new	123. _____
mal-	bad	124. _____

► **Labeling**

Label the stages of mitosis shown on the following diagrams.

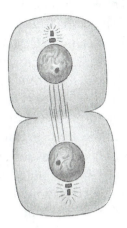

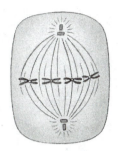 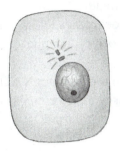 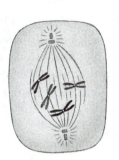

125. _____ **126.** _____ **127.** _____

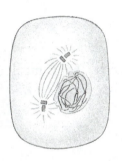 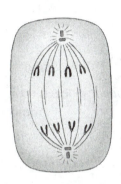

128. _____ **129.** _____ **130.** _____

☑ Self-Check Test

The following test will allow you to determine how well you have mastered the vocabulary and basic concepts of this chapter. It will also help you prepare for the type of questions you are likely to encounter on a test in an anatomy and physiology course. The self-check test will help you assess your understanding of the chapter material and will help you develop good test-taking skills.

The following questions test your ability to use vocabulary and to recall facts.

1. During glycolysis
   a. a molecule of glucose is converted into two molecules of pyruvic acid
   b. six molecules of ATP are produced
   c. carbon dioxide is produced
   d. NADH molecules attach to the cytochromes
   e. more energy is used than is released
2. Inside a mitochondrion, each pyruvic acid molecule
   a. forms a molecule of citric acid
   b. loses a carbon atom
   c. attaches to NAD

    d. directly enters the electron transport system

    e. is phosphorylated

3. The citric acid cycle

    a. begins with the formation of a molecule of citric acid

    b. directly produces most of the ATP from the catabolism of glucose

    c. does not form any carbon dioxide

    d. contains enzymes called cytochromes

    e. forms acetyl-CoA from glucose-6-phosphate

4. In the electron transport chain

    a. coenzymes receive hydrogen atoms from NADH and $FADH_2$

    b. reduced molecules gain energy at the expense of oxidized molecules

    c. ATP is formed

    d. oxidative phosphorylation takes place

    e. all of the above

5. The carbon dioxide of respiration is formed during

    a. glycolysis

    b. the citric acid cycle

    c. electron transport

    d. the formation of pyruvic acid

    e. the formation of water

6. In the process of cellular respiration, each molecule of glucose that is metabolized yields enough energy to form _____ molecules of ATP.

    a. 2

    b. 4

    c. 30

    d. 36

    e. 64

7. During lipolysis

    a. triglycerides are converted into molecules of acetyl-CoA

    b. triglycerides are broken down into glycerol and fatty acids

    c. lipids are converted into glucose molecules

    d. lipids are formed from excess carbohydrates

    e. lipids are metabolized to yield ATP

8. The largest metabolic reserves for the average adult are stored as

    a. carbohydrates

    b. proteins

    c. amino acids

    d. triglycerides

    e. fatty acids

9. In transamination, the amino group of an amino acid is

    a. converted to ammonia

    b. converted to urea

    c. transferred to a keto acid

    d. transferred to a molecule in the glycolytic pathway

    e. transferred to acetyl-CoA

10. The process of deamination produces

    a. keto acids

    b. urea

    c. ammonia

    d. acetyl-CoA

    e. B vitamins

11. A codon is

    a. a gene that codes for a specific polypeptide

    b. a sequence of three nucleotides that codes for a specific amino acid

    c. a group of chromosomes that codes for a specific polypeptide

    d. a complementary base pair found on DNA that codes for amino acids

    e. the part of a ribosome that binds to mRNA

12. The process of forming messenger RNA is called

    a. replication

    b. transcription

    c. translation

    d. ribolation

    e. protein synthesis

13. Amino acids are carried to ribosomes by

    a. chromosomes

    b. rRNA molecules

    c. tRNA molecules

    d. mRNA molecules

    e. cDNA molecules

14. The stage in a cell's life cycle in which the cell performs its normal functions and prepares for division is called

    a. prophase

    b. metaphase

    c. telophase

    d. interphase

    e. anaphase

15. A cell duplicates its chromosomes during the

    a. G_0 phase

    b. G_1 phase

    c. G_2 phase

    d. M phase

    e. S phase

16. During the process of mitosis, chromatids separate into daughter chromosomes during

    a. prophase

    b. metaphase

    c. interphase

    d. telophase

    e. anaphase

17. When genes are "turned off," the cell loses its ability to synthesize certain proteins. The process of specialization that results is called

    a. adaptation

    b. differentiation

    c. structural integration

    d. cellular activation

    e. apoptosis

The following questions are more challenging and require you to synthesize the information that you have learned in this chapter.

18. In oxidative phosphorylation, energy for the synthesis of ATP is provided by the
   a. splitting of oxygen molecules
   b. breaking of the covalent bonds in glucose
   c. movement of hydrogen ions through channels in the respiratory enzymes
   d. combination of two atoms of hydrogen and one atom of oxygen to form water
   e. oxidation of acetyl-CoA

19. Catabolism of protein is not a practical source of quick energy because
   a. proteins are more difficult to break apart than lipids
   b. the energy yield from protein is less than the yield from lipids
   c. one of the byproducts of protein catabolism is a toxin
   d. extensive destruction of protein would threaten homeostasis at the cellular and organismal levels
   e. all of the above

20. The mRNA sequence that is complementary to the sequence ATC on DNA is
   a. ATC
   b. TAG
   c. UAG
   d. AUG
   e. AUC

☑ Self-Assessment

If your score was

between 18 and 20, you are ready to proceed to the next chapter.

between 15 and 17, you have a good general idea of the chapter content, but you should review sections of the chapter that deal with items that you missed before proceeding to the next chapter.

less than 14, you have not mastered the chapter content well enough to proceed. Reread the chapter and rework the exercises. Then retake the self check test. Repeat this process until you achieve a score that will allow you to continue.

Answers

1.	oxidation	**13.**	4
2.	glycolysis	**14.**	−2
3.	decarboxylation	**15.**	2
4.	oxaloacetic acid	**16.**	4
5.	intermembrane space	**17.**	24
6.	reduction	**18.**	4
7.	oxidative phosphorylation	**19.**	2
8.	cytochrome	**20.**	36
9.	TCA (citric acid cycle or Kreb's) cycle	**21.**	urea
10.	phosphorylation	**22.**	lipolysis
11.	metalloprotein	**23.**	deamination
12.	electron transport system (ETS), or respiratory chain	**24.**	glycogenesis
		25.	hyperuricemia

26. essential fatty acid
27. lipogenesis
28. alpha-ketoacid
29. gout
30. gluconeogenesis
31. uric acid
32. beta-oxidation
33. transamination
34. phenylketonuria
35. nitrogenous waste
36. hyperuricemia
37. lipolysis
38. phenylketonuria
39. glycogenesis
40. transamination
41. lipolysis, lipogenesis
42. gluconeogenesis
43. gluconeogenesis, lipogenesis, glycogenesis
44. deamination
45. linoleic acid; linolenic acid
46. oxygen; glucose
47. pyruvic acid
48. 12
49. insoluble
50. sugars; pyrimidines
51. a. Proteins are more difficult to break apart than complex carbohydrates or lipids.
    b. One of the products, ammonia, is a toxin.
    c. Proteins form the most important structural and functional components of any cell.
52. intron
53. histones
54. codon
55. transcription
56. polyribosome
57. translation
58. genetic code
59. tRNA
60. RNA processing
61. RNA polymerase
62. nucleosome
63. mutation
64. exons
65. anticodon
66. chromatin
67. mRNA
68. point mutation
69. DNA fingerprint
70. pre-mRNA
71. gene
72. RNA polymerase
73. U (uracil)
74. small ribosomal subunit
75. AUG
76. anticodon
77. codon
78. stop codon

79. chromatids
80. mitosis
87. neoplasm
81. prophase
83. chalones
84. G_2 phase
85. metastasis
86. daughter cells
87. metaphase
88. differentiation
89. centromere
90. replication
91. M phase
92. stem cells
93. benign tumor
94. repressor genes
95. apoptosis
96. G_0 phase
97. DNA polymerase
98. cytokinesis
99. anaphase
100. cancer
101. interphase
102. S phase
103. ligases
104. chromosomal microtubules
105. telophase
106. tumor
107. G_1 phase
108. spindle fibers
109. metaphase plate
110. mitotic rate
111. malignant tumor
112. astral rays
113. apoptosis
114. telophase
115. prophase
116. centromere
117. metaphase
118. chromatid
119. interphase
120. anaphase
121. ligase
122. cytokinesis
123. neoplasm
124. malignant tumor
125. metaphase
126. interphase
127. telophase
128. prophase (early)
129. anaphase
130. prophase (late)

Answers to Self-Check Test

1. a 2. b 3. a 4. e 5. b 6. d 7. b 8. d 9. c 10. c 11. b 12. b
13. c 14. d 15. e 16. e 17. b 18. c 19. e 20. c

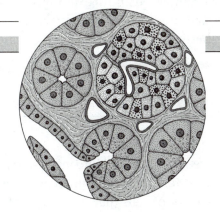

CHAPTER 6

Tissues

Sophisticated scanning procedures can provide images of the intact body, but they often do not tell the whole story. For example, an abnormal growth seen in an X-ray may be a relatively harmless tumor or a deadly cancer. Determining which is the case requires examination of a small sample of the tissue involved. Such vital diagnostic decisions are often made while surgery is in progress, and proper treatment depends on recognizing the differences between normal and abnormal cells and tissues. This chapter introduces the structure and function of normal tissues. These tissues, in various combinations, form all of the organs and organ systems in the human body.

AN OVERVIEW OF TISSUES

No single cell contains the metabolic machinery and organelles needed to perform all the many functions of the human body. Instead, during development, characteristic cellular specializations develop as genes are turned on or off, a process known as **differentiation.** Through the process of differentiation each cell develops a characteristic set of structural features and a limited number of functions. These structures and functions can be quite distinct from those of nearby cells. Nevertheless, cells in a given location all work together. A detailed examination of the body reveals a number of patterns at the cellular level. Although there are trillions of cells in the human body, there are only about 200 types of cells. These cell types combine to form **tissues,** collections of specialized cells and cell products that perform a relatively limited number of functions. There are four basic tissue types: epithelial tissue, connective tissue, muscle tissue, and neural tissue.

- **Epithelial tissue** covers exposed surfaces and lines internal passageways and chambers.
- **Connective tissue** fills internal spaces, provides structural support for other tissues, and stores energy reserves.
- **Muscle tissue** contracts to perform specific movements and in the process generates heat that warms the body.
- **Neural tissue** carries information from one part of the body to another in the form of electrical impulses.

Histology is *the study of tissues*, and such a study provides beautiful examples of the interplay between form and function. This chapter will discuss the characteristics of each major tissue type, focusing on the relationship between cellular organization and tissue function.

EPITHELIAL TISSUE

Epithelial tissue includes the *epithelia* that cover exposed surfaces and line internal passageways and chambers and *glands*, secretory structures derived from epithelial tissue. An **epithelium** (e-pi-THĒ-lē-um; plural *epithelia*) is a layer of cells that forms a barrier with specific properties. Epithelia cover every exposed body surface. The surface of the skin is a good example, but epithelia also line the digestive, respiratory, reproductive, and urinary tracts—passageways that communicate with the outside world. Epithelia also line internal cavities and passageways, such as the chest cavity; fluid-filled chambers in the brain, eye, and inner ear; and the inner surfaces of blood vessels and the heart.

Important characteristics of epithelia include:

- Epithelia consist mainly of cells, rather than extracellular materials.
- An epithelium may consist of a single layer of cells (a **simple epithelium**) or multiple layers (a **stratified epithelium**).
- Although firmly attached to underlying connective tissues, an epithelium always has a free surface exposed to the external environment or to some internal chamber or passageway.
- There are no blood vessels in epithelia. Because of this **avascular** (ā-VAS-kū-lar; Greek *a-*, without + Latin *vasculum*, little vessel) condition, epithelial cells must obtain nutrients by diffusion or absorption from deeper tissues or from their exposed surfaces.
- The mitotic rate in epithelia can be very high, especially in situations in which the epithelial cells are exposed to harsh physical or chemical environments.

Functions of Epithelial Tissue

Epithelial tissues perform essential functions that can be summarized as follows:

1. **Provide physical protection:** Epithelia protect exposed and internal surfaces from abrasion, dehydration, and destruction by chemical or biological agents.
2. **Control permeability:** Any substance that enters or leaves the body has to cross an epithelium. Some epithelia are relatively impermeable, whereas others are easily crossed by compounds as large as proteins. Many epithelia contain the molecular "machinery" needed for selective absorption or secretion. The epithelial barrier can be regulated and modified in response to various stimuli. For example, hormones can affect the transport of ions and nutrients through epithelial cells. Even physical stress can alter the structure and properties of epithelia; think of the calluses that form on your hands when you do rough work for a period of time.
3. **Provide sensations:** Most epithelia are extensively innervated by sensory nerves. Specialized epithelial cells can detect changes in the environment they encounter and convey information about such changes to the nervous system. For example,

touch receptors in the deepest epithelial layers of the skin respond to pressure by stimulating adjacent sensory nerves. A **neuroepithelium** is an epithelium containing sensory cells providing sensations of smell, taste, sight, equilibrium, or hearing.

4. **Produce specialized secretions:** Epithelial cells that produce secretions are called **gland cells.** Individual gland cells are often scattered among other cell types in an epithelium. In a glandular epithelium, most or all of the epithelial cells produce secretions.

Specializations of Epithelial Cells

Epithelial cells have several specializations that distinguish them from other body cells. Many epithelial cells are specialized for (1) the production of secretions, (2) the movement of fluids over the epithelial surface, or (3) the movement of fluids through the epithelium itself. These specialized epithelial cells usually show a definite polarity along the axis that extends from the basement membrane to the exposed surface of the epithelium. In other words, the organelles are distributed unevenly along this axis. The actual arrangement varies depending on the function of the individual cells. The cells shown in Figure 6–1a show a common type of polarity. Most epithelial cells have microvilli on their exposed surfaces; there may be just a few, or the entire surface may be covered by them. Microvilli are especially abundant on epithelial surfaces where absorption and secretion take place, such as along portions of the digestive and urinary tracts. The epithelial cells in these locations are transport specialists, and a cell with microvilli has at least 20 times the surface area of a cell without them. Microvilli are shown

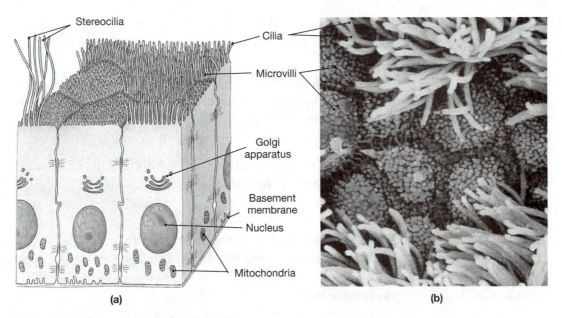

(a) (b)

Figure 6–1 Polarity of Epithelial Cells.

(a) Many epithelial cells differ in internal organization along an axis between the free surface (here, the top) and the basement membrane. In many cases, the free surface bears microvilli; in some cases, the surface may have cilia or (very rarely) stereocilia. (All three would not normally be found on the same group of cells but are depicted here for purposes of illustration.) In some epithelia, such as the lining of the kidney tubules, mitochondria are concentrated near the base of the cell, probably to provide energy for the cell's transport activities. **(b)** Micrograph showing the surface of a ciliated epithelium that lines most of the respiratory tract. The small bristly areas are microvilli on the exposed surfaces of mucus-producing cells that are scattered among the ciliated epithelial cells. (SEM × 15,200)

in Figure 6–1b. **Stereocilia** are very long microvilli (up to 250 μm) that are incapable of movement. Stereocilia are found in two places only: (1) along portions of the male reproductive tract and (2) on receptor cells of the inner ear.

Figure 6–1b shows the surface of a **ciliated epithelium.** A typical ciliated cell contains about 250 cilia that beat in a coordinated fashion. Substances are moved over the epithelial surface by the synchronized beating of the cilia, as if on a continuously moving escalator. For example, the ciliated epithelium that lines the respiratory tract moves mucus up from the lungs and toward the throat. The mucus traps particulate matter and pathogens and carries them away from more delicate surfaces deeper in the lungs. Injury to the cilia or to the epithelial cells in general can stop ciliary movement and block the protective flow of mucus. This is one effect of smoking.

Maintaining the Integrity of the Epithelium

Three factors are involved in maintaining the physical integrity of an epithelium: (1) intercellular connections, (2) attachment to the basement membrane, and (3) replacement of damaged epithelial cells.

Intercellular Connections

Cells in epithelia are firmly attached to one another, and the epithelium as a unit is attached to extracellular fibers of the underlying connective tissues. Because epithelial cells are specialists in intercellular connection, we will consider the topic at this time. However, many other cells in the body form permanent or temporary bonds to other cells or extracellular materials.

Intercellular connections may involve extensive areas of opposing cell membranes, or they may be concentrated at specialized attachment sites called cell junctions.

- Large areas of opposing cell membranes may be interconnected by binding between transmembrane proteins called **cell adhesion molecules,** or **CAMs.** For example, CAMs on the attached base of an epithelium lock them onto the underlying basement membrane. Different tissues frequently have different cell adhesion molecules.

- There are four types of specialized **cell junctions,** connections between cells: gap junctions, tight junctions, intermediate junctions, and desmosomes.

Gap Junctions

At a **gap junction** (Figure 6–2a) two cells are held together by an interlocking of membrane proteins. Because these are channel proteins, the result is a narrow passageway that lets small molecules and ions pass from cell to cell. Gap junctions are most common in cardiac muscle and smooth muscle tissue.

Tight Junctions

At a **tight junction,** shown in Figure 6–2b, there is a partial fusion of the lipid portions of the two cell membranes. Because the membranes are fused together, tight junctions are the strongest intercellular connections. In addition to providing mechanical strength, tight junctions block the passage of water or solutes between the cells. Tight junctions, which are found near the exposed surfaces of cells lining the digestive tract, keep enzymes, acids, and wastes from damaging delicate underlying tissues.

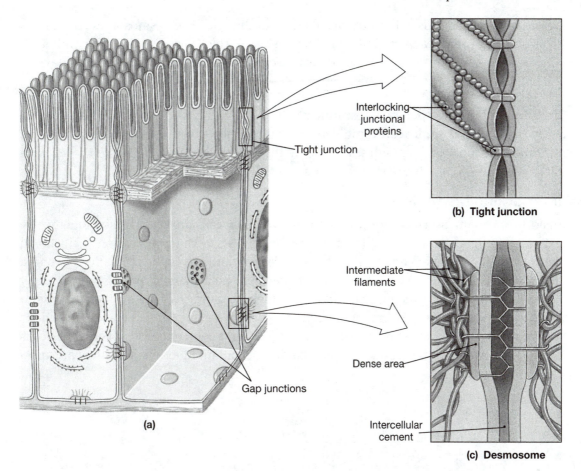

(b) Tight junction

(c) Desmosome

Figure 6–2   Cell Attachements.
(a) Diagrammatic view of an epithelial cell, showing the major types of intercellular connections.
(b) A tight junction is formed by the fusion of the outer layers of two cell membranes. Bands of tight
junctions encircle the apical portion of cuboidal and columnar epithelial cells, preventing the diffusion of fluids and solutes between the cells. **(c)** A desmosome has a more organized network of intermediate filaments. Desmosomes attach one cell to another or attach a cell to extracellular
structures, such as the protein fibers in connective tissues. A continuous belt of desmosomes lies
deep to the tight junctions.

Intermediate Junctions

At an **intermediate junction** the opposing cell membranes, while remaining distinct,
are held together by a thick layer of proteoglycans. This proteoglycan layer is called **intercellular cement;** the primary component is the polysaccharide **hyaluronic** (hī-uh-
loo-RON-ik) **acid.** The cytoplasm at an intermediate junction contains a dense network
of microfilaments that anchor the junction to the cytoskeleton. This arrangement adds
strength and helps stabilize the shape of the cell.

Desmosomes

At **desmosomes** (DEZ-mō-sōmz; Greek *desmos*, band or bond + *soma*, body) there is a
very thin proteoglycan layer between the opposing cell membranes, reinforced by a network of intermediate filaments that lock the two cells together (Figure 6–2c). Desmosomes are very strong and can resist stretching and twisting. These connections are most

abundant between cells in the superficial layers of the skin. The desmosomes create links so strong that even dead skin cells are usually shed in thick sheets, rather than individually. Desmosomes are also found in cardiac muscle tissue, interconnecting the muscle cells.

Junctional Complexes

Cells lining the digestive tract, respiratory tract, or other passageways are held together by **junctional complexes.** A single junctional complex consists of a tight junction, an intermediate junction, and a desmosome, with the tight junction closest to the cell surface. Figure 6–3a details the structure of a typical junctional complex.

Interlocking Membranes

In addition to junctional complexes, adjacent epithelial cells are often locked together by extensive folding of opposing cell membranes (Figure 6–3c). The combination of junctional complexes, intercellular cement, and physical interlocking gives the epithelium strength and stability. The extensive connections between cells hold them together and may deny access to chemicals or pathogens that may cover their free surfaces. If the epithelium is damaged or the connections are broken, infection can easily occur. For this reason, infections are a serious risk after a severe burn or abrasion. The tight interconnection of epithelial cells has one noteworthy disadvantage: Epithelia do not contain blood vessels (they are avas-

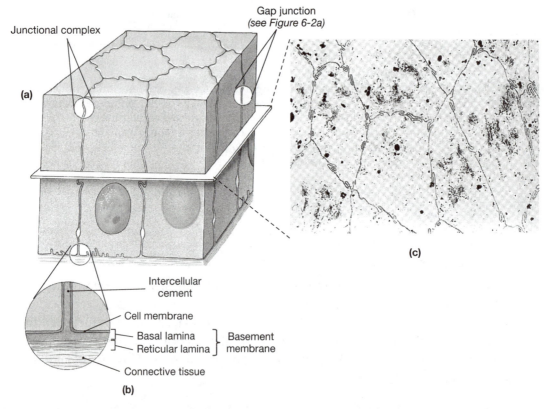

Figure 6–3   Organization of Epithelia.

(a) The relative positions of epithelial cells are maintained through extensive junctional complexes and intercellular cement. **(b)** At their inner surfaces, epithelia are attached to a basement membrane that forms the boundary between the epithelial cells and the underlying connective tissue. **(c)** In addition, adjacent cell membranes are often interlocked. The micrograph indicates the degree of such interlocking between columnar epithelial cells. (TEM × 3042)

cular), and the interconnections that tie cells together also slow or stop diffusion between cells. In epithelia containing many layers of cells, tight junctions often create a network of narrow passageways that branch throughout the epithelium. These canals provide a route for the distribution of nutrients throughout the epithelium.

The Basement Membrane

Epithelial cells not only hold onto one another, they also remain firmly connected to the rest of the body. The inner surface of each epithelium is attached to a special two-part **basement membrane** (Figure 6–3b). The layer closest to the epithelium is called the **basal lamina** (LA-mi-na; Latin *lamina*, plate). The basal lamina provides a barrier that restricts the movement of proteins and other large molecules from the underlying connective tissue into the epithelium. The deeper portion of the basement membrane is the **reticular** (re-TIK-ū-lar); Latin *reticulum*, small net) **lamina.** The reticular lamina gives the basement membrane its strength. Attachments between the fibers of the basal lamina and those of the reticular lamina hold the two together.

Epithelial Maintenance and Repair

An epithelium must continually repair and renew itself. Epithelial cells lead hard lives, for they may be exposed to disruptive enzymes, toxic chemicals, pathogenic bacteria, or mechanical abrasion. Under severe conditions, such as those encountered inside the small intestine, an epithelial cell may survive for just a day or two before it is lost or destroyed. The only way the epithelium can maintain its structure over time is through the continual division of stem cells. These stem cells, also known as **germinative** (JUR-min-uh-tiv) **cells,** are usually found in the deepest layers of the epithelium, close to the basement membrane.

Classification of Epithelia

Epithelia are classified according to the number of cell layers and the shape of the exposed cells. The classification scheme recognizes two types of layering—simple and stratified—and three cell shapes—squamous, cuboidal, and columnar. The shape classification is based on the appearance of the cell when seen in a section that is perpendicular to the epithelial surface and the basement membrane.

If there is only a single layer of cells covering the basement membrane, the epithelium is termed **simple epithelium.** Simple epithelia are relatively thin, and because all the cells have the same polarity, the nuclei form a row above the basement membrane. Because they are so thin, simple epithelia are also relatively fragile. A single layer of cells cannot provide much mechanical protection, and simple epithelia are found only in protected areas inside the body. They line internal compartments and passageways, including the ventral body cavities, the chambers of the heart, and all blood vessels.

Simple epithelia are also characteristic of regions where secretion or absorption occurs, such as the lining of the intestines and the gas-exchange surfaces of the lungs. In those places, the thinness of simple epithelia is an advantage, for it speeds the passage of materials across the epithelial barrier.

A **stratified epithelium** has several layers of cells above the basement membrane. Stratified epithelia are usually found in areas subject to mechanical or chemical stresses, such as the surface of the skin and the lining of the mouth. Combining the two basic epithelial layouts (simple and stratified) and the three possible cell shapes (squamous, cuboidal, and columnar) enables one to describe almost every epithelium in the body. In most stratified epithelia, the shapes of the cells change as they approach the exposed surface. As a result, the classification scheme for stratified epithelia is based only on the appearance of the cells in the superficial layer.

Squamous Epithelium

In a **squamous epithelium** (SKWĀ-mus; Latin *squamas*, scale) the cells are thin, flat, and somewhat irregular in shape, like puzzle pieces (Figure 6–4a). In a sectional view, the nucleus occupies the thickest portion of each cell; from the surface, the cells look like fried eggs laid side by side. A simple squamous epithelium is the most delicate type of epithelium in the body. This type of epithelium is found in protected regions where absorption takes place or where a slick, slippery surface reduces friction. Examples include the respiratory exchange surfaces of the lungs, the lining of the ventral body cavities, and the inner surfaces of the cardiovascular system.

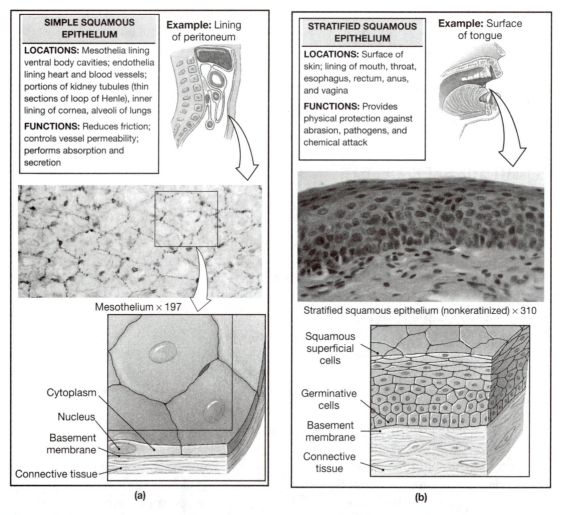

SIMPLE SQUAMOUS EPITHELIUM

LOCATIONS: Mesothelia lining ventral body cavities; endothelia lining heart and blood vessels; portions of kidney tubules (thin sections of loop of Henle), inner lining of cornea, alveoli of lungs

FUNCTIONS: Reduces friction; controls vessel permeability; performs absorption and secretion

Example: Lining of peritoneum

Mesothelium × 197

Cytoplasm
Nucleus
Basement membrane
Connective tissue

(a)

STRATIFIED SQUAMOUS EPITHELIUM

LOCATIONS: Surface of skin; lining of mouth, throat, esophagus, rectum, anus, and vagina

FUNCTIONS: Provides physical protection against abrasion, pathogens, and chemical attack

Example: Surface of tongue

Stratified squamous epithelium (nonkeratinized) × 310

Squamous superficial cells
Germinative cells
Basement membrane
Connective tissue

(b)

Figure 6–4 Squamous Epithelia.

(a) A superficial view of the simple squamous epithelium (mesothelium) that lines the peritoneal cavity. The three-dimensional drawing shows the epithelium in superficial and sectional view.
(b) Sectional and diagrammatic views of the stratified epithelium that covers the tongue.

Special names have been given to simple squamous epithelia that line chambers and passageways that do not communicate with the outside world. The simple squamous epithelium that lines the ventral body cavities is known as a **mesothelium** (mez-ō-THĒ-lē-um; Greek *mesos*, middle + *thele*, nipple). The pleura, peritoneum, and pericardium each contain a superficial layer of mesothelium. The simple squamous epithelium lining the heart and all blood vessels is called an **endothelium** (en-dō-THĒ-lē-um).

A **stratified squamous epithelium** (Figure 6–4b) is usually found where mechanical stresses are severe. Note how the cells form a series of layers, like the layers in a sheet of plywood. The surface of the skin and the lining of the mouth, esophagus, and anus are areas where this epithelial type provides protection from physical and chemical attack.

Cuboidal Epithelia

The cells of a **cuboidal epithelium** resemble little hexagonal boxes; they appear square in typical sectional views. The nuclei are near the center of each cell, with the distance between adjacent nuclei roughly equal to the height of the epithelium. A simple cuboidal epithelium provides limited protection and occurs in regions where secretion or absorption takes place. Such an epithelium lines portions of the kidney tubules, as seen in Figure 6–5a. In the pancreas and salivary glands, simple cuboidal epithelia secrete enzymes and buffers and line the ducts that discharge those secretions. The thyroid gland contains chambers, called *thyroid follicles,* that are lined by a cuboidal secretory epithelium. Thyroid hormones accumulate within the follicles before being released into the bloodstream.

Stratified cuboidal epithelia are almost always composed of just two layers of cuboidal cells. They are relatively rare in the human body. They can be found in the secretory portion of sweat glands and along the ducts of sweat glands (Figure 6–5b), as well as in the larger ducts of the mammary glands.

Transitional Epithelium

A **transitional epithelium,** shown in Figure 6–5c, is unusual because, unlike most epithelia, it tolerates considerable stretching. It is called *transitional* because the appearance of the epithelium changes as the stretching occurs. A transitional epithelium is found in regions of the urinary system, such as the urinary bladder, where large changes in volume occur. In an empty urinary bladder (Figure 6–5c) the epithelium seems to have many layers, and the outermost cells are typically plump cuboidal cells. The layered appearance results from overcrowding; the actual structure of the epithelium can be seen in the full urinary bladder, when the pressure of the urine has stretched the lining to its natural thickness.

Columnar Epithelia

Columnar epithelial cells are also hexagonal in cross section, but they are taller and more slender than cuboidal epithelial cells. The nuclei are crowded into a narrow band close to the basement membrane, and the height of the epithelium is several times the distance between two nuclei (Figure 6–6a). A **simple columnar epithelium** is often encountered where absorption or secretion is under way, such as inside the small intestine. Inside the stomach and large intestine, the secretions of simple columnar epithelia provide protection from chemical stresses.

Portions of the respiratory tract contain a columnar epithelium that includes several different cell types with varying shapes and functions. Because the cell nuclei are situated at varying distances from the surface, the epithelium appears to be layered, or

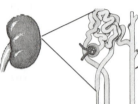

SIMPLE CUBOIDAL EPITHELIUM

LOCATIONS: Glands, ducts, portions of kidney tubules, thyroid gland
FUNCTIONS: Limited protection, secretion and/or absorption

Example:
Convoluted tubule of kidney

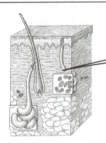

STRATIFIED CUBOIDAL EPITHELIUM

LOCATIONS: Lining of some ducts (rare)
FUNCTIONS: Protection, secretion, absorption

Example:
Duct of sweat gland

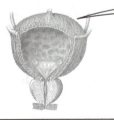

TRANSITIONAL EPITHELIUM

LOCATIONS: Urinary bladder, renal pelvis, ureters
FUNCTIONS: Permit expansion and recoil after stretching

Example:
Lining of urinary bladder

Figure 6–5   Cuboidal Epithelia.
(a) A section through the cuboidal epithelia cells of a kidney tubule. **(b)** Sectional view of the stratified cuboidal epithelium lining of a sweat gland duct in the skin. **(c)** At left, the lining of the empty urinary bladder, showing transitional epithelium in the relaxed state. At right, the lining of the full bladder, showing the effects of stretching on the appearance of cells in the epithelium. (LM × 408)

stratified. But it is not truly stratified, because all of the epithelial cells contact the basement membrane. Because it looks stratified but is not, it is known as a **pseudostratified** (soo-dō-STRAT-i-fīd; Greek *pseudes*, false) **columnar epithelium** (Figure 6–6b). Pseudostratified columnar epithelial cells always possess cilia. This type of epithelium lines most of the nasal cavity, the trachea (windpipe), bronchi, and portions of the male reproductive tract.

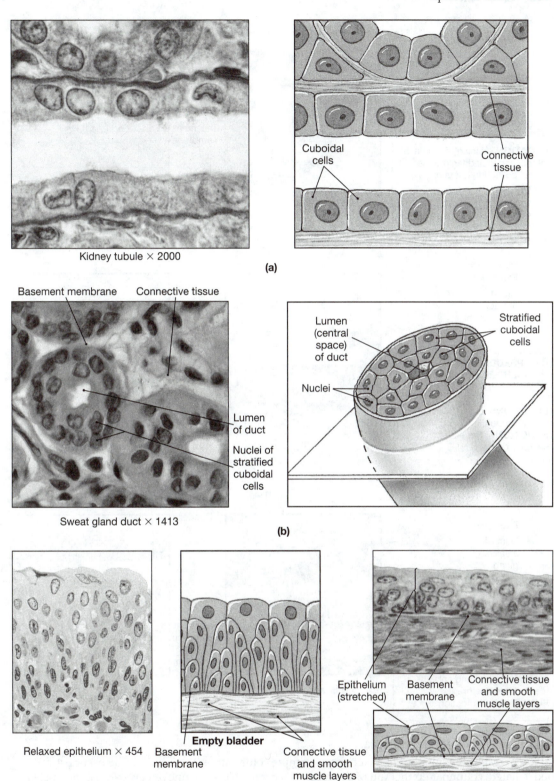

Kidney tubule × 2000

Cuboidal cells

Connective tissue

(a)

Basement membrane   Connective tissue

Lumen of duct

Nuclei of stratified cuboidal cells

Sweat gland duct × 1413

Lumen (central space) of duct

Stratified cuboidal cells

Nuclei

(b)

Relaxed epithelium × 454   Basement membrane

Empty bladder

Basement membrane

Connective tissue and smooth muscle layers

Epithelium (stretched)   Basement membrane   Connective tissue and smooth muscle layers

Full bladder

(c)

Stratified columnar epithelia are relatively rare, providing protection along portions of the pharynx, urethra, and anus, as well as along a few large excretory ducts. The epithelium may have only two layers (Figure 6–6c) or more than two layers; when more than two layers exist, only the superficial cells are columnar.

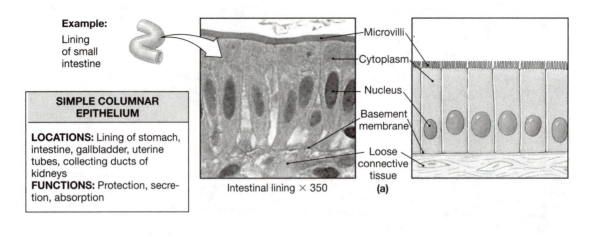

Example:
Lining
of small
intestine

**SIMPLE COLUMNAR
EPITHELIUM**

LOCATIONS: Lining of stomach,
intestine, gallbladder, uterine
tubes, collecting ducts of
kidneys
FUNCTIONS: Protection, secretion, absorption

Microvilli
Cytoplasm
Nucleus
Basement
membrane
Loose
connective
tissue

Intestinal lining × 350   **(a)**

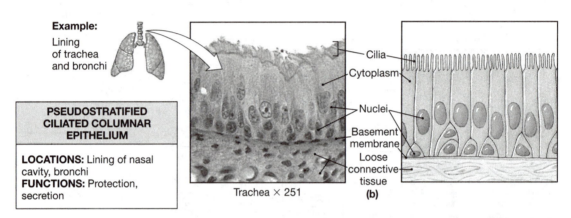

Example:
Lining
of trachea
and bronchi

**PSEUDOSTRATIFIED
CILIATED COLUMNAR
EPITHELIUM**

LOCATIONS: Lining of nasal
cavity, bronchi
FUNCTIONS: Protection,
secretion

Cilia
Cytoplasm
Nuclei
Basement
membrane
Loose
connective
tissue

Trachea × 251   **(b)**

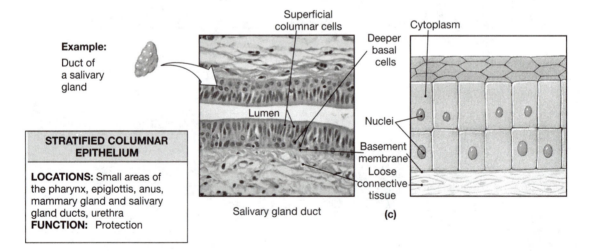

Superficial
columnar cells

Deeper
basal
cells

Cytoplasm

Example:
Duct of
a salivary
gland

Lumen

Nuclei

**STRATIFIED COLUMNAR
EPITHELIUM**

LOCATIONS: Small areas of
the pharynx, epiglottis, anus,
mammary gland and salivary
gland ducts, urethra
FUNCTION: Protection

Basement
membrane
Loose
connective
tissue

Salivary gland duct   **(c)**

Figure 6–6   Columnar Epithelia.
(a) Micrograph showing the characteristics of simple columnar epithelium. **(b)** The pseudostratified, ciliated, columnar epithelium of the respiratory tract. Note the uneven layering of the nuclei.
(c) A stratified columnar epithelium occurs along some large ducts, such as this salivary gland duct.
Note the thickness of the epithelium and the location and orientation of the nuclei.

WHAT SHED EPITHELIAL CELLS CAN TELL US

Exfoliative cytology (eks-FŌ-lē-a-tiv; Latin *ex*, from + *folium*, leaf) is the study of cells
shed or collected from epithelial surfaces. The cells may be examined for a variety of
reasons, including checking for cellular changes that indicate cancer formation and iden-

tifying the pathogens involved in an infection. The cells are collected by sampling the fluids that cover the epithelia lining the respiratory, digestive, urinary, or reproductive tract or by removing fluid from one of the ventral body cavities. The sampling procedure is often called a **Pap test,** named after George Papanicolaou. Probably the most familiar Pap test is the test for cervical cancer, which involves scraping a small number of cells from the tip of the *cervix*, a portion of the uterus that projects into the vagina.

Amniocentesis is another important test that relies on exfoliative cytology. In this procedure, shed epithelial cells are collected from a sample of amniotic fluid, the fluid that surrounds and protects a developing fetus. Examination of these cells can determine if the fetus has a genetic abnormality, such as Down syndrome.

GLANDS AND GLAND CELLS

Many epithelia contain gland cells that produce secretions. In general, glands and gland cells are classified as endocrine or exocrine according to the final distribution of their secretions.

Endocrine Glands

Endocrine (EN-dō-krin; Greek *endon,* inside + *krinein,* to separate) **glands** produce secretions that remain inside the body. These glands release their secretions into the surrounding interstitial fluid. Because there are no endocrine ducts, endocrine glands are often called ductless glands. From the interstitial fluids, these secretions, called **hormones,** enter the circulation for distribution throughout the body. Hormones regulate or coordinate the activities of other cells that may reside in the same tissue or in other tissues and organs.

Endocrine cells may be part of an epithelial surface, such as the lining of the digestive tract, or they may be separate, as in the pancreas, thyroid gland, thymus, and pituitary gland.

Exocrine Glands

Exocrine (EK-sō-krin; Greek *exos,* outside + *krinein,* to separate) **glands** produce secretions that are discharged onto epithelial surfaces. Most exocrine glands release their secretions into tubular passageways, called **ducts,** that empty onto the surface of the skin or onto an epithelial surface lining one of the internal passageways that communicates with the exterior. There are many kinds of exocrine secretions, all performing a variety of functions. Only a few complex glands produce both exocrine and endocrine secretions. For example, the pancreas contains endocrine cells that secrete hormones as well as exocrine cells that produce digestive enzymes and buffers. Exocrine glands may be classified by their mode of secretion, the type of secretion, and the structure of the gland.

Modes of Secretion

A glandular epithelial cell may use one of three methods to release its secretions: merocrine secretion, apocrine secretion, or holocrine secretion. In **merocrine** (MER-ō-krin; Greek *meros,* part + *krinein,* to separate) **secretion,** the product is released through exocytosis (Figure 6–7a). This is the most common mode of secretion. One merocrine secretion, called **mucus,** is an effective lubricant, protective barrier, and a sticky trap for foreign particles and microorganisms. The mucous secretions of merocrine glands coat the passageways of the digestive and respiratory tracts. In the skin, **merocrine sweat glands** produce the watery perspiration that helps cool the body on a hot day.

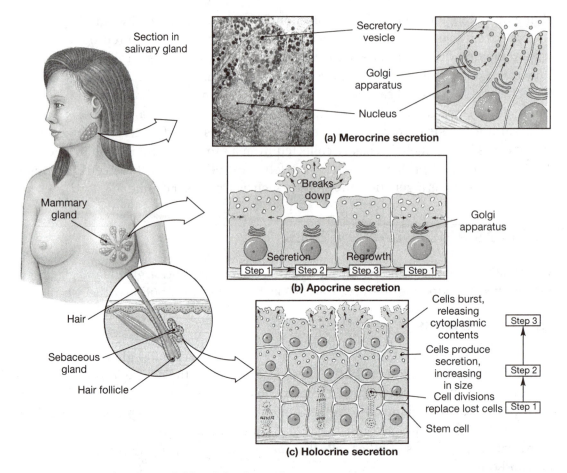

Figure 6–7 Mechanisms of Glandular Secretion.
(a) In merocrine secretion, secretory vesicles are discharged at the surface of the gland cell through exocytosis. **(b)** Apocrine secretion involves the loss of apical cytoplasm. Inclusions, secretory vesicles, and other cytoplasmic components are shed in the process. The gland cell then undergoes a period of growth and repair before it releases additional secretions. **(c)** Holocrine secretion occurs as superficial gland cells burst. Continued secretion involves the replacement of these cells through the mitotic divisions of underlying stem cells.

Apocrine (ĀP-ō-krin; Greek *apo-*, away from + *krinein*, to separate) **secretion** involves the loss of cytoplasm as well as the secretory product (Figure 6–7b). The outermost portion of the cytoplasm becomes packed with secretory vesicles before it is shed. Milk production in the female mammary glands involves a combination of merocrine and apocrine secretion.

Merocrine and apocrine secretions leave a cell intact and able to continue secreting. **Holocrine** (HŌ-lō-krin; Greek *holos*, entire + *krinein*, to separate) **secretion** destroys the gland cell. During holocrine secretion, the entire cell becomes packed with secretory products and then bursts apart (Figure 6–7c). The secretion is released, but the cell dies. Further secretion depends on gland cells' being replaced by the division of stem cells. Sebaceous glands, associated with hair follicles, produce an oily hair coating by means of holocrine secretion.

Type of Secretion

Exocrine glands may be categorized according to the nature of the secretion produced:

- **Serous glands** secrete a watery solution that usually contains enzymes.

- **Mucous glands** secrete *mucins*, glycoproteins that absorb water and form mucus, a slippery lubricant.

- **Mixed exocrine glands** contain more than one type of gland cell and may produce two different exocrine secretions, one serous and the other mucous. The submandibular gland, one of the salivary glands, is an example of a mixed exocrine gland.

Gland Structure

In epithelia that contain scattered gland cells, the individual secretory cells are called **unicellular glands. Multicellular glands** include glandular epithelia and groups of gland cells that produce exocrine or endocrine secretions.

The only examples of **unicellular exocrine glands** in the body are goblet cells. **Goblet cells,** which secrete mucins, are scattered among other epithelial cells (Figure 6–8). For example, the pseudostratified columnar epithelium that lines the trachea and the columnar epithelium of the small and large intestines contain an abundance of goblet cells.

The simplest **multicellular exocrine gland** is called a **secretory sheet.** In a secretory sheet, glandular cells dominate the epithelium lining an organ and release their secretions into the organ. The mucin-secreting cells that line the stomach are an example. Their continual secretion protects the stomach from the acids and enzymes it contains. Most other multicellular glands are found in pockets set back from the epithelial surface; their secretory products travel through one or more ducts to reach the epithelial surface. Examples include the salivary glands, which produce mucins and digestive enzymes.

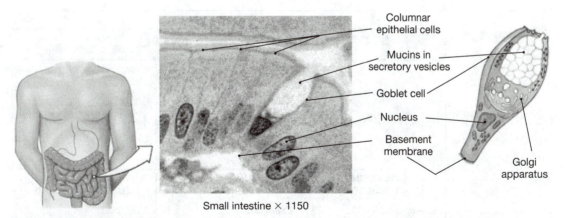

Columnar
epithelial cells

Mucins in
secretory vesicles

Goblet cell

Nucleus

Basement
membrane

Golgi
apparatus

Small intestine × 1150

Figure 6–8   Goblet Cells.

Goblet cells are unicellular exocrine glands. These secretory cells are often scattered among the simple or pseudostratfied columnar epithelial cells of the digestive and respiratory tracts. The micrograph shows a goblet cell in the intestinal epithelium (simple columnar type).

Multicellular exocrine glands may be complex in structure. Three characteristics are used to describe the organization of a multicellular gland: (1) the shape of the secretory portion of the gland, (2) the branching pattern of the duct, and (3) the relationship between the ducts and the glandular areas.

1. Glands whose glandular cells form tubes are called **tubular;** those that form blind pockets are called **alveolar** (al-VĒ-ō-lar; Latin, *alveolus*, small basin), or *acinar* (Ā-si-nar; Latin *acinus*, berry). Glands whose gland cells form both tubes and pockets are called **tubuloacinar** (too-bū-lō-ĀS-i-nar).

2. A gland is called **branched** if several glandular areas (tubular or acinar) share a common duct. Note that the term *branched* always refers to the glandular areas not to the duct.

3. A gland is called **simple** if there is a single duct that does not divide on its way to the gland cells. The gland is called **compound** if the duct divides repeatedly.

Figure 6–9 diagrams this method of classification based on gland structure.

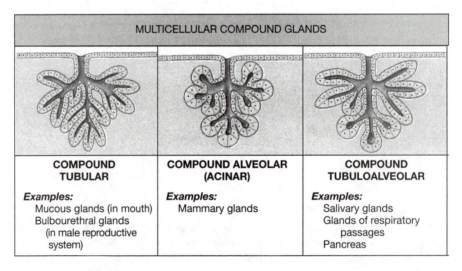

Figure 6–9   A Structural Classification of Exocrine Glands.

Let's Review What You've Just Learned

► **Definitions**

In the space provided, list the boldface terms included in this section that contain the indicated word part.

_____ **1.** A term meaning no blood vessels.

_____ **2.** The biological discipline that deals with the study of tissues.

_____ **3.** The type of secretion in which the secretory product is released from the cell by exocytosis.

_____ **4.** Glands that produce secretions that are discharged onto epithelial surfaces.

_____ **5.** The term that describes a gland that has a single duct.

_____ **6.** A union between two cells where the cells are held together by interlocking channel proteins.

_____ **7.** The simple squamous epithelium that lines the ventral body cavities.

_____ **8.** Structures similar to microvilli that are very long and incapable of movement.

_____ **9.** A collection of cells and cell products that perform a relatively limited number of similar functions.

_____ **10.** A type of secretion in which the secretory cells become filled with product and rupture.

_____ **11.** Transmembrane proteins that connect adjacent cells together.

_____ **12.** An epithelium that consists of only a single layer of cells.

_____ **13.** The layer of the basement membrane that is closest to the epithelium.

_____ **14.** A thin layer of proteoglycans reinforced by intermediate filaments that functions in connecting one cell to another.

_____ **15.** Stem cells that through continuous division maintain the structure of an epithelium.

_____ **16.** A layer of cells that forms a barrier with specific properties.

_____ **17.** Glands that secrete a watery solution that usually contains enzymes.

_____ **18.** Unicellular exocrine glands that secrete mucus.

_____ **19.** The layer of the basement membrane that contains bundles of coarse protein fibers that give the basement membrane strength.

_____ **20.** The study of cells shed or collected from epithelial surfaces.

_____ **21.** The type of tissue that fills internal spaces, provides structural support for other tissues, and stores energy reserves.

_____ **22.** The type of epithelium that consists of several layers of cells above the basement membrane.

_____ **23.** A cell junction in which opposing cell membranes are held together by a thick layer of proteoglycans.

_____ **24.** A type of epithelial cell in which the height is several times the distance between two nuclei.

_____ **25.** A gland that contains more than one type of gland cell and may produce two different exocrine secretions.

_____ **26.** Glands that release their secretions into the surrounding interstitial fluid.

_____ **27.** A type of secretion that involves the loss of cytoplasm as well as the secretory product from the secreting cell.

_____ **28.** Tissue that can contract to perform specific movements.

_____ **29.** An epithelium that contains sensory cells.

_____ **30.** The cell junction formed by the partial fusion of the lipid portions of two cell membranes.

_____ **31.** The two-part membrane that is attached to the inner surface of an epithelium.

_____ **32.** The simple squamous epithelium that lines the heart and all blood vessels.

_____ **33.** The procedure in which shed epithelial cells are collected from a sample of amniotic fluid.

_____ **34.** A general term for the secretion produced by an endocrine gland.

_____ **35.** Tubular passageways that carry the secretions of exocrine glands to the epithelial surface.

_____ **36.** A gland whose glandular cells form blind pockets.

_____ **37.** A tissue that can carry information from one part of the body to another in the form of electrical impulses.

_____ **38.** A type of epithelium in which the cells are thin, flat, and somewhat irregular in shape.

_____ **39.** A term for the proteoglycan layers that contain primarily hyaluronic acid and function to hold cells together.

_____ **40.** A cell-to-cell connection that consists of a tight junction, intermediate junction, and a desmosome.

_____ **41.** The type of tissue that covers exposed surfaces, lines internal passageways and chambers, and forms glands.

_____ **42.** A type of epithelium that can tolerate considerable stretching and that changes in appearance as the stretching occurs.

_____ **43.** A sampling procedure in which some epithelial cells are collected from an organ for analysis.

_____ **44.** A merocrine secretion that serves as a lubricant, protective barrier, and sticky trap for foreign material and microorganisms.

_____ **45.** A gland that has a duct that divides repeatedly.

▶ **Word Roots, Prefixes, Suffixes, and Combining Forms**

In the space provided, list the boldface terms included in this section that contain the indicated word part.

Word Part	Meaning	Examples
pseudo-	false	46. _____
mero-	part	47. _____
epi-	on	48. _____
histo-	tissue	49. _____
holo-	entire	50. _____
desmo-	band	51. _____
stereo-	involving three dimensions	52. _____
a-	without	53. _____
reticul-	network	54. _____
-centesis	puncture	55. _____
apo-	from	56. _____
-crine	to separate	57. _____

▶ **Completion**

Complete the following table by filling in the blank with the appropriate tissue or example.

	Tissue Type	Example Organ or Structure
58.		lining of the small intestine
59.	transitional epithelium	
60.	simple cuboidal epithelium	
61.		lining of the trachea
62.		epidermis of skin
63.	simple squamous epithelium	
64.		lining of sweat gland ducts

► **Labeling**

Label each of the following types of epithelial tissue.

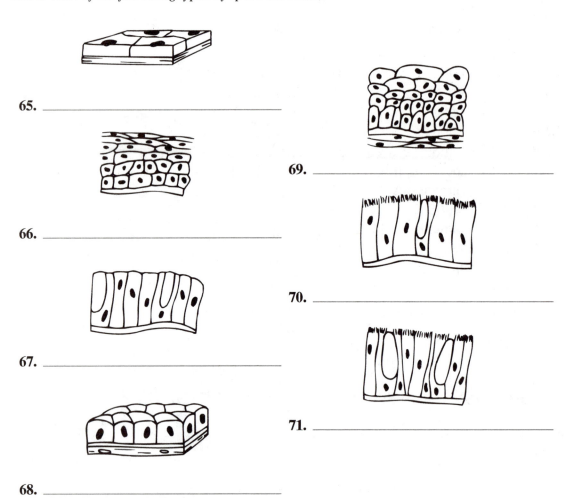

65. _____

66. _____

67. _____

68. _____

69. _____

70. _____

71. _____

Label each of the following types of gland.

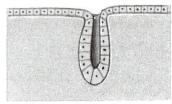

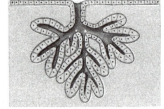

72. _____

73. _____

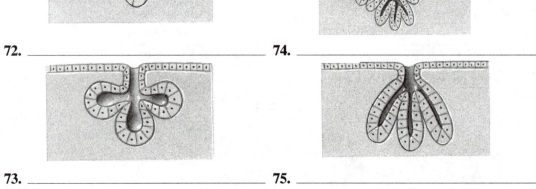

74. _____

75. _____

CONNECTIVE TISSUES

Connective tissues include bone, fat, and blood tissues that are quite different in appearance and function. Nevertheless, all connective tissues have three basic components: (1) specialized cells, (2) extracellular protein fibers, and (3) a fluid known as the **ground substance.** The extracellular fibers and ground substance make up the **matrix,** the material that surrounds the cells. Whereas epithelial tissue consists almost entirely of cells, the extracellular matrix typically accounts for most of the volume of connective tissues.

Connective tissues are found throughout the body but are never exposed to the environment outside the body. Most connective tissues are highly vascular and contain sensory receptors that provide pain, pressure, temperature, and other sensations.

Connective tissues have six main functions; they:

1. Establish a structural framework for the body.

2. Transport fluids and dissolved materials from one region of the body to another.

3. Provide protection for delicate organs.

4. Support, surround, and interconnect other tissue types.

5. Store energy reserves, especially in the form of lipids.

6. Defend the body from invasion by microorganisms.

HOW CONNECTIVE TISSUES ARE CLASSIFIED

Connective tissue can be classified into three categories: (1) connective tissue proper, (2) fluid connective tissues, and (3) supporting connective tissues.

1. **Connective tissue proper** refers to connective tissues with many types of cells and extracellular fibers in a syrupy ground substance. These connective tissues differ in terms of the number of cell types they contain and the relative properties and proportions of fibers and ground substance. Adipose (fat) tissue and tendons are both connective tissue proper, but they have very different structural and functional characteristics. Connective tissue proper is divided into loose connective tissues and dense connective tissues on the basis of the relative proportions of cells, fibers, and ground substance.

2. **Fluid connective tissues** have a distinctive population of cells suspended in a watery matrix that contains dissolved proteins. There are two fluid connective tissues, blood and lymph.

3. **Supporting connective tissues** are of two types, cartilage and bone. These tissues have a less diverse cell population than connective tissue proper and a matrix that contains closely packed fibers. The matrix of cartilage is a gel whose characteristics vary depending on the predominant fiber type. The matrix of bone is said to be **calcified** because it contains mineral deposits, primarily calcium salts. These minerals give the bone strength and rigidity.

CONNECTIVE TISSUE PROPER

Connective tissue proper contains extracellular fibers, a viscous ground substance, and a varied cell population. Some of these cells are involved with local maintenance, repair, and energy storage. These cells include fibroblasts, fixed macrophages, adipocytes, mesenchymal cells, and, in a few locations, melanocytes. Other cells are responsible for the defense and repair of damaged tissues. These cells include free macrophages, mast cells, lymphocytes, plasma cells, and microphages.

The number of cells and cell types within a tissue at any given moment varies depending on local conditions. Refer to Figure 6–10a as we describe the cells and fibers of connective tissue proper.

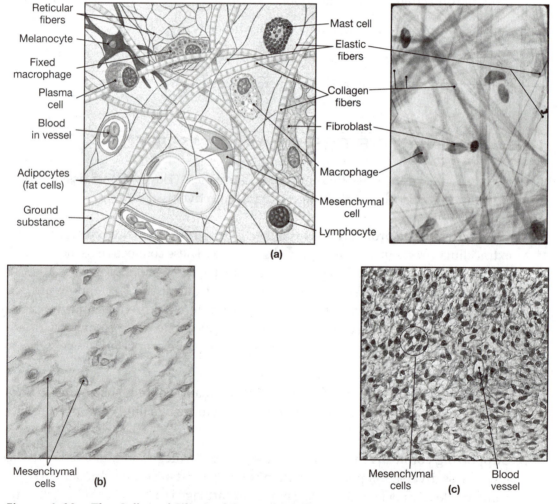

(a)

(b)

(c)

Figure 6–10   The Cells and Fibers of Connective Tissue Proper.

(a) A summary of the cell types and fibers of connective tissue proper. (LM × 384) **(b)** Mesenchyme, the first connective tissue to appear in the embryo. (LM × 136) **(c)** Mucous connective tissue. This sample was taken from the umbilical cord of a fetus. Mucous connective tissue in this location is also known as *Wharton's jelly*. (LM × 136)

The Cells Found in Connective Tissue Proper

The major cell types of connective tissue proper include the following:

- **Fibroblasts** (FĪ-brō-blasts) are the most abundant fixed cells in connective tissue proper. These slender or star-shaped cells are responsible for the production and maintenance of the connective tissue fibers. Each fibroblast manufactures and secretes protein subunits that interact to form large extracellular fibers. In addition, fibroblasts secrete hyaluronic acid, a proteoglycan that gives the ground substance its syrupy consistency.

- **Fixed macrophages** (MAK-rō-fāj-ez; Greek *makros,* large + *phagein,* to eat) are large cells that are scattered among the fibers. These cells engulf damaged cells and **pathogens** (PATH-uh-jen; Greek *pathos,* disease + *genes,* born), disease-causing organisms, that enter the tissue. Although fixed macrophages are not abundant, they play an important role in mobilizing the body's defenses. When stimulated they release chemicals that activate the immune system and attract large numbers of wandering cells involved in tissue defense.

- **Adipocytes** (AD-i-pō-sīts) are also known as fat cells, or *adipose cells.* A typical adipocyte contains a single, enormous lipid droplet. The nucleus and other organelles are squeezed to one side, making the cell in section resemble a class ring. The number of fat cells varies from one type of connective tissue to another, from one region of the body to another, and from individual to individual.

- **Mesenchymal cells** are stem cells that are present in many connective tissues. These cells respond to local injury or infection by dividing to produce daughter cells that differentiate into fibroblasts, macrophages, or other connective tissue cells.

- **Melanocytes** (me-LAN-o-sīts) synthesize and store a brown pigment, **melanin** (ME-la-nin), that gives the tissue a dark color. Melanocytes are common in the epithelium of the skin, where they play a major role in determining skin color. However, melanocytes are also abundant in connective tissues of the eye, and they are present in the dermis of the skin, although there are regional, individual, and racial differences in the number present.

- **Free macrophages** wander throughout the body. When an infection occurs, these phagocytic cells are drawn to the affected area. In effect, the few fixed macrophages in a tissue provide a "front-line" defense that will be reinforced by the arrival of free macrophages and other specialized cells in massive numbers.

- **Mast cells** are small, mobile connective tissue cells often found near blood vessels. The cytoplasm of a mast cell is filled with granules of **histamine** (HIS-ta-mēn) and **heparin** (HEP-a-rin). These chemicals, released after injury or infection, stimulate local inflammation. Histamine and heparin granules are also found in **basophils,** white blood cells that enter damaged tissues and exaggerate the inflammation process.

- **Lymphocytes** (LIM-fō-sīts), like free macrophages, migrate throughout the body. Their numbers increase markedly wherever tissue damage occurs, and some of the lymphocytes may then develop into **plasma cells.** Plasma cells are responsible for the production of **antibodies,** proteins involved in defending the body against disease.

- **Microphages** are phagocytic blood cells that move through connective tissues in small numbers. When an infection or injury occurs, chemicals released by fixed macrophages and mast cells attract them in large numbers.

Connective Tissue Fibers

Three basic types of fibers are found in connective tissue: collagen fibers, reticular fibers, and elastic fibers. All three types of fibers are formed by fibroblasts.

1. **Collagen fibers** are long, straight, and unbranched. These are the most common fibers in connective tissue proper. Each collagen fiber consists of a bundle of fibrous protein subunits wound together like the strands of a rope. Like a rope, a collagen fiber is flexible, but it is stronger than steel when pulled from either end. Tendons, which connect skeletal muscles to bones, consist almost entirely of collagen fibers. Typical ligaments are similar to tendons, but they connect one bone to another. Tendons and ligaments can withstand tremendous forces; uncontrolled muscle contractions or skeletal movements are more likely to break a bone than snap a tendon or ligament.

2. **Reticular** (re-TIK-ū-lar) **fibers** contain the same protein subunits as collagen fibers but they are arranged in a different way. These fibers are thinner than collagen fibers, and form a branching, interwoven framework that is tough but flexible. Because they form a network, rather than running in the same direction, reticular fibers can resist forces applied from many different directions. This arrangement stabilizes the relative positions of an organ's cells, blood vessels, and other structures despite changing body positions and the pull of gravity.

3. **Elastic fibers** contain the protein **elastin.** Elastic fibers are branched and wavy, and after stretching they will return to their original length. Elastic ligaments are dominated by elastic fibers. They are relatively rare but have important functions, such as interconnecting the vertebrae (bones that make up the backbone).

Ground Substance

Ground substance fills the spaces between cells and surrounds the connective tissue fibers (Figure 6–10a). Ground substance in normal connective tissue proper is clear and colorless. It often has a consistency similar to maple syrup because of the presence of proteoglycans and glycoproteins. The ground substance is dense enough that bacteria have trouble moving through it (imagine swimming in molasses). This density slows the spread of pathogens through the tissue and makes them easier for phagocytes to catch. Some bacteria secrete the enzyme **hyaluronidase** (hī-uh-loo-RON-i-dās), which breaks down hyaluronic acid. These bacteria are dangerous because they can spread rapidly by liquefying the ground substance and dissolving the intercellular cement that holds epithelial cells together.

Embryonic Connective Tissues

Mesenchyme (MEZ-en-kīm), or *embryonic connective tissue,* is the first connective tissue to appear in the developing embryo. Mesenchyme contains star-shaped cells that are separated by a matrix that contains very fine protein filaments. This connective tissue (Figure 6–10b) gives rise to all other forms of connective tissue, including fluid connective tissues, cartilage, and bone. **Mucous connective tissue** (Figure 6–10c) is a loose connective tissue found in many portions of the embryo, including the umbilical cord. Neither form of connective tissue is found in the adult. However, many adult connective tissues contain scattered mesenchymal cells that can assist in tissue repairs after injury.

Loose Connective Tissues

Loose connective tissue, or **areolar** (a-RĒ-ō-lar; Latin *areolas,* little area) **tissue,** is the "packing material" of the body. It fills spaces between organs, provides cushioning, and supports epithelia. Loose connective tissue also surrounds and supports blood vessels and nerves, stores lipids, and provides a route for the diffusion of materials.

Typical loose connective tissue (Figure 6–10a) is the least specialized connective tissue in the adult body. This tissue contains all of the cells and fibers found in any connective tissue proper. Loose connective tissue has an open framework, and ground substance accounts for most of its volume. This syrupy fluid cushions shocks, and, because the fibers are loosely organized, loose connective tissue can distort without damage. The presence of elastic fibers makes it fairly resilient, so this tissue returns to its original shape after external forces are relieved.

Loose connective tissue forms a layer that separates the skin from deeper structures. In addition to providing padding, the elastic properties of this layer allow a considerable amount of independent movement. Thus, pinching the skin of the arm does not affect the underlying muscle. Conversely, contractions of the underlying muscles do not pull against the skin; as the muscle bulges, the loose connective tissue stretches. Because this tissue has an extensive circulatory supply, drugs are typically injected into the loose connective tissue layer under the skin.

In addition to delivering oxygen and nutrients and removing carbon dioxide and waste products, the capillaries in loose connective tissue carry wandering cells to and from the tissue. Epithelia usually cover a layer of loose connective tissue, and fibroblasts are responsible for maintaining the reticular lamina of the basement membrane. The epithelial cells rely on diffusion across that membrane, and the capillaries in the underlying connective tissue provide the necessary oxygen and nutrients.

There are two variations on loose connective tissue that are relatively common, adipose tissue and reticular tissue.

Adipose Tissue

The distinction between loose connective tissue and fat, or **adipose** (AD-i-pōs) **tissue,** is usually somewhat arbitrary. Adipocytes account for most of the volume of adipose tissue (Figure 6–11a) but only a fraction of the volume of loose connective tissue. Adipose tissue provides padding, cushions shocks, acts as an insulator to slow heat loss through the skin, and serves as packing or filler around structures. Adipose tissue is common under the skin of the groin, sides, buttocks, and breasts. It fills the bony sockets behind the eyes, surrounds the kidneys, and dominates extensive areas of loose connective tissue in the pericardial and abdominal cavities.

Brown Fat

In infants and young children, the adipose tissue between the shoulder blades, around the neck, and possibly elsewhere in the upper body is different from most of the adipose tissue in the adult. It has a rich blood supply, and the individual adipocytes contain numerous mitochondria. Together these characteristics give the tissue a deep, rich color responsible for the name brown fat. When stimulated by the nervous system, lipid breakdown accelerates; the cells do not capture the energy released, and it radiates into the surrounding tissues as heat. This heat warms the circulating blood, which distributes it

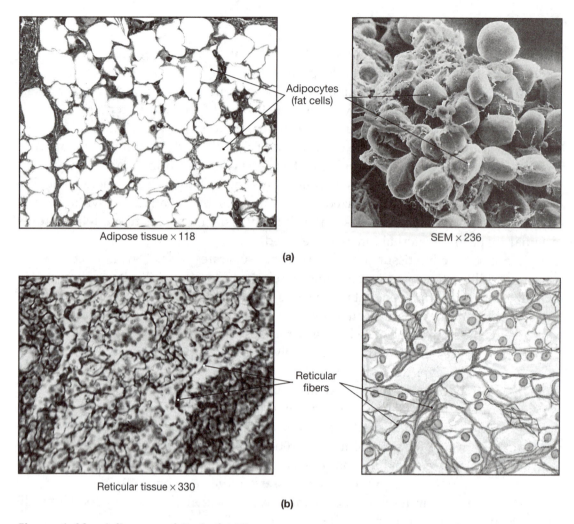

Adipocytes (fat cells)

Adipose tissue × 118

SEM × 236

(a)

Reticular fibers

Reticular tissue × 330

(b)

Figure 6–11   Adipose and Reticular Tissues.
(a) Adipose tissue is a loose connective tissue that is dominated by adipocytes. In standard histological prepartions, the tissue looks empty because the lipids in the fat cells dissolve in the alcohol used in tissue processing. **(b)** Reticular tissue has an open framework of reticular fibers. These fibers are usually difficult to see because of the large numbers of cells around them.

throughout the body. In this way, an infant can accelerate metabolic heat generation by 100 percent very quickly. There is little if any brown fat in the adult; with increased body size, skeletal muscle mass, and insulation, shivering is significantly more effective in elevating body temperature.

Adipose Tissue and Weight Loss

Adipocytes are metabolically active cells; their lipids are continually being broken down and replaced. When nutrients are scarce, adipocytes deflate like collapsing balloons. This deflation is what occurs during a weight-loss program. Because the cells are not killed, but are merely reduced in size, the lost weight can easily be regained in the same areas of the body.

Adipocytes in the adult are incapable of dividing, and the number of fat cells in peripheral tissues is established in the first few weeks of a newborn's life, perhaps in response to the amount of fats in the diet. However, this is not the end of the story, because loose connective tissues also contain mesenchymal cells. If circulating lipid levels are chronically elevated, the mesenchymal cells will divide, giving rise to cells that differentiate into fat cells. As a result, areas of loose connective tissue can become adipose tissue in times of nutritional plenty, even in the adult. In the procedure known as **liposuction** (LĪ-pō-suk-shen), unwanted adipose tissue is surgically removed. Because adipose tissue can regenerate through differentiation of mesenchymal cells, liposuction provides only a temporary solution to the problem.

Reticular Tissue

Reticular tissue is found in organs such as the spleen and liver, where reticular fibers create a complex three-dimensional network, or **stroma,** that supports the functional cells of these organs. This fibrous framework is also found in the lymph nodes and bone marrow (Figure 6–11b). Fixed macrophages and fibroblasts are associated with the reticular fibers, but these cells are seldom visible because the organs are dominated by specialized cells with other functions.

Dense Connective Tissues

Most of the volume of dense connective tissues is occupied by fibers. Dense connective tissues are often called **collagenous** (kō-LA-jin-us) **tissues** because collagen fibers are the dominant fiber type. Two types of dense connective tissues are found in the body: (1) dense regular connective tissue and (2) dense irregular connective tissue.

Dense Regular Connective Tissue

In **dense regular connective tissue** the collagen fibers are arranged parallel to each other, packed tightly, and aligned with the forces applied to the tissue. Four major locations of this tissue type are tendons, aponeuroses, elastic tissue, and ligaments.

1. **Tendons** (Figure 6–12a) are cords of dense regular connective tissue that attach skeletal muscles to bones. The collagen fibers run along the long axis of the tendon and transfer the pull of the contracting muscle to the bone. Large numbers of fibroblasts are found between the collagen fibers.

2. **Aponeuroses** (ap-ō-noo-RŌ-sēz) are collagenous sheets or ribbons that resemble flat, broad tendons. Aponeuroses may cover the surface of a muscle and assist in attaching superficial muscles to another muscle or separate structure.

3. **Elastic tissue** contains large numbers of elastic fibers. Because elastic fibers outnumber collagen fibers, the tissue has a springy, resilient nature. This ability to stretch and rebound allows it to tolerate cycles of expansion and contraction. Elastic tissue often underlies transitional epithelia; it is also found in the walls of blood vessels and surrounds the respiratory passageways.

4. **Ligaments** (LIG-a-ments) resemble tendons, but they connect one bone to another. Ligaments often contain significant numbers of elastic fibers as well as collagen fibers, and they can tolerate a modest amount of stretching. An even higher proportion of elastic fibers is found in elastic ligaments, which resemble tough rubber bands. Although uncommon elsewhere, elastic ligaments along the spinal column are very important in stabilizing the positions of the vertebrae (Figure 6–12b).

**DENSE REGULAR
CONNECTIVE TISSUE**

LOCATIONS: Between skeletal
muscles and skeleton (tendons and
aponeuroses); between bones
(ligaments); covering skeletal
muscles (deep fasciae)
FUNCTIONS: Provides firm
attachment; conducts pull of
muscles; reduces friction between
muscles; stabilizes relative
positions of bones

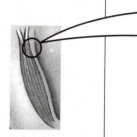

Example:
Tendon

**ELASTIC
LIGAMENTS**

LOCATION: Between vertebrae of
the spinal column (ligamentum flava
and ligamentum nuchae)
FUNCTIONS: Stabilizes positions of
vertebrae; cushions shocks

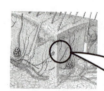

Example:
Elastic ligament

**Figure 6–12 Dense Connective
Tissues.**
(a) The dense regular connective tissue in a tendon. Notice the densely
packed, parallel bundles of collagen
fibers. The fibroblast nuclei can be
seen flattened between the bundles.
(b) An elastic ligament from between
the vertebrae of the spinal column.
The bundles are fatter than those of a
tendon or ligament composed of collagen. **(c)** The deep dermis of the skin
contains a thick layer of dense irregular connective tissue.

**DENSE IRREGULAR
CONNECTIVE TISSUE**

LOCATIONS: Capsules
of visceral organs; periostea
and perichondria; nerve and
muscle sheaths; dermis
FUNCTIONS: Provides strength to
resist forces applied from many
directions; helps prevent over-
expansion of organs such as the
urinary bladder

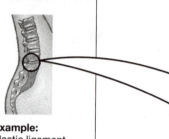

Example:
Deep dermis
of skin

Dense Irregular Connective Tissue

The fibers in **dense irregular connective tissue** form an interwoven meshwork and do
not show any consistent pattern (Figure 6–12c). These tissues provide strength and support to areas subjected to stresses from many directions. A layer of dense irregular connective tissue gives skin its strength; a piece of cured leather (animal skin) provides an

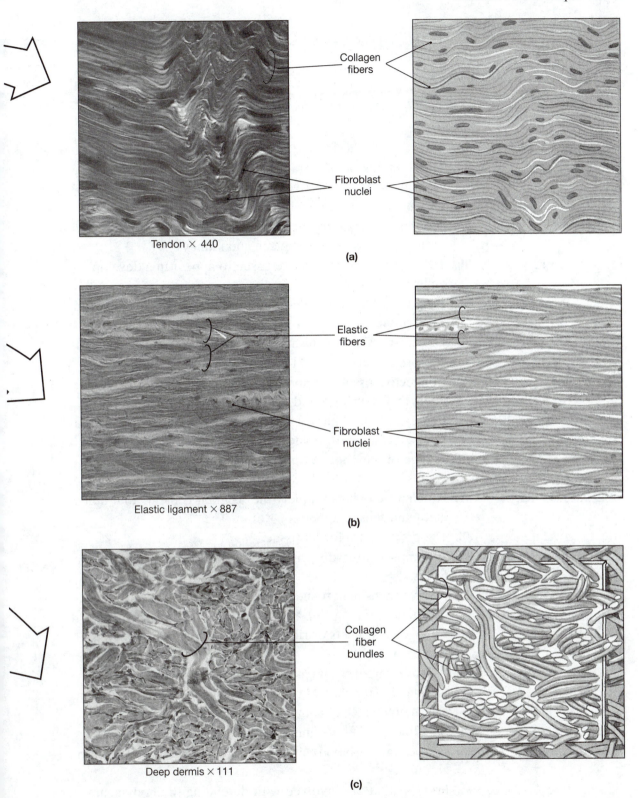

Collagen fibers

Fibroblast nuclei

Tendon × 440

(a)

Elastic fibers

Fibroblast nuclei

Elastic ligament × 887

(b)

Collagen fiber bundles

Deep dermis × 111

(c)

excellent illustration of the interwoven nature of this tissue. Dense irregular connective tissue also forms a thick fibrous layer, called a **capsule,** that surrounds internal organs such as the liver, kidneys, and spleen and encloses the cavities of joints.

Let's Review What You've Just Learned

▶ **Definitions**

In the space provided, list the boldface terms included in this section that contain the indicated word part.

_____ 76. Cells that synthesize and store the pigment melanin.

_____ 77. The combination of extracellular fibers and ground substance that surrounds connective tissue cells.

_____ 78. Dense connective tissue that connects bone to bone.

_____ 79. A layer of dense irregular connective tissue that surrounds some organs such as the spleen and kidneys.

_____ 80. The first type of connective tissue to appear in a developing embryo.

_____ 81. Phagocytic blood cells that move through connective tissue in small numbers.

_____ 82. Disease-causing organisms.

_____ 83. The proper term for a fat cell.

_____ 84. Connective tissues composed of many cells and extracellular fibers in a syrupy ground substance.

_____ 85. Large, stationary, phagocytic cells found scattered among the fibers of connective tissues.

_____ 86. A type of lymphocyte that produces molecules called antibodies.

_____ 87. An enzyme that can liquefy the "cellular cement" that holds epithelial cells together.

_____ 88. The proper term for fat tissue.

_____ 89. A complex three-dimensional network formed by reticular fibers.

_____ 90. A springy, resilient tissue that contains large numbers of elastic fibers.

_____ 91. Collagenous sheets or ribbons that resemble flat, broad tendons.

_____ 92. A brown pigment that gives tissues a dark color.

_____ 93. Slender or star-shaped cells responsible for the production and maintenance of connective tissue fibers.

_____ 94. The fluid portion of connective tissue's extracellular matrix.

_____ 95. A type of white blood cell that contains histamine and heparin granules.

_____ 96. Proteins that are involved with defending the body against disease.

_____ 97. A loose connective tissue found in many parts of an embryo.

_____ 98. The surgical removal of unwanted adipose tissue.

_____ 99. A type of connective tissue in which fibers form an interwoven meshwork that does not show any consistent pattern.

_____ **100.** Another term for the loose connective tissue that fills the spaces between organs and supports epithelia.

_____ **101.** Fibers that are thinner than collagen fibers and form a tough yet flexible interwoven meshwork.

_____ **102.** Small mobile connective tissue cells that contain granules of histamine and heparin.

_____ **103.** Connective tissues composed of a distinctive population of cells suspended in a watery matrix containing dissolved proteins.

_____ **104.** Stem cells that are present in many connective tissues.

_____ **105.** Long, straight, unbranched fibers that are the most common found in connective tissue proper.

_____ **106.** Cords of dense regular connective tissue that attach skeletal muscles to bones.

_____ **107.** Connective tissue fibers that after being stretched will return to their original length.

_____ **108.** A general term for the large phagocytic cells that wander throughout the body.

_____ **109.** The type of connective tissue represented by cartilage and bone.

_____ **110.** The term for connective tissue matrix that contains deposits of calcium salts.

_____ **111.** Tissues in which collagen is the dominant fiber type.

▶ Word Roots, Prefixes, Suffixes, and Combining Forms

In the space provided, list the boldface terms included in this section that contain the indicated word part.

Word Part	Meaning	Examples
-blast	precursor	**112.** _____
patho-	disease	**113.** _____
reticul-	network	**114.** _____
adip-	fat	**115.** _____
lipo-	fat	**116.** _____
hyal-	clear	**117.** _____
anti-	against	**118.** _____
micr-	small	**119.** _____
-cyte	cell	**120.** _____
phag-	to eat	**121.** _____
melan-	black	**122.** _____

► **Labeling**

Label each of the following types of connective tissue.

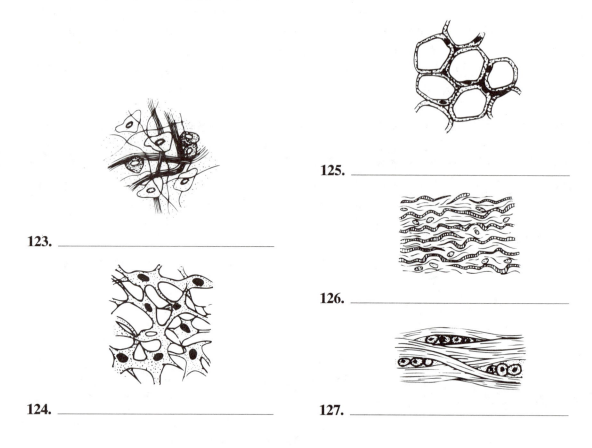

123. _____

124. _____

125. _____

126. _____

127. _____

FLUID CONNECTIVE TISSUES

Blood and **lymph** (limf) are connective tissues that contain distinctive collections of cells in a fluid matrix. The watery matrix of blood and lymph contains many different types of suspended proteins that do not form insoluble fibers under normal conditions.

Blood contains blood cells and fragments of cells, collectively known as **formed elements** (Figure 6–13). A single cell type, the **red blood cell,** or **erythrocyte** (e-RITH-rō-sīt; Greek *erythros*, red + *kytos*, container), accounts for almost half of the volume of blood. Red blood cells are responsible for the transport of oxygen and, to a lesser degree, carbon

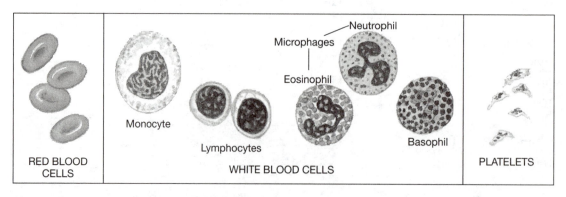

Figure 6–13   Formed Elements of the Blood.

dioxide in the blood. The watery ground substance, called **plasma** (PLAZ-ma), also contains small numbers of white blood cells, or **leukocytes** (LOO-kō-sīts; Greek *leukos,* white + *kytos,* container). White blood cells include phagocytic microphages (**neutrophils** [NOO-truh-philz) and **eosinophils** [ē-ō-SIN-uh-filz]), basophils, lymphocytes, and macrophages called **monocytes.** The white blood cells are important components of the immune system, which protects the body from infection and disease. Tiny, membrane-wrapped packets of cytoplasm, called **platelets,** contain enzymes and special proteins. Platelets function in the clotting response, which seals breaks in the endothelial lining.

Plasma is one of the three major subdivisions of the body's **extracellular fluid** (fluid that is not contained in cells), which also includes interstitial fluid and lymph. Plasma is normally confined to the vessels of the cardiovascular system, and the contractions of the heart keep it in constant motion. **Arteries** carry blood away from the heart toward fine, thin-walled vessels called **capillaries. Veins** drain the capillaries and return blood to the heart, completing the circuit. In tissues, filtration moves water and small solutes out of the capillaries and into the **interstitial** (in-ter-STISH-ul) **fluid** that bathes the cells of the body. The major difference between plasma and interstitial fluid is that plasma contains large numbers of suspended proteins.

Lymph forms as interstitial fluid enters small passageways, or **lymphatics** (lim-FAT-iks), which return it to the cardiovascular system. Along the way, cells of the immune system monitor the composition of the lymph and respond to signs of injury or infection. The number of cells in lymph may vary, but ordinarily 99 percent of them are lymphocytes, and the rest are wandering macrophages or microphages.

SUPPORTING CONNECTIVE TISSUES

Cartilage and bone are called supporting connective tissues because they provide a strong framework that supports the rest of the body. In these connective tissues the matrix contains numerous fibers and, in some cases, deposits of insoluble calcium salts.

Cartilage

The matrix of **cartilage** is a firm gel that contains proteoglycans called **chondroitin** (kon-DROY-tin; Greek *chondros,* cartilage) **sulfates.** Cartilage cells, or **chondrocytes** (KON-drō-sīts), are the only cells found within the matrix. These cells live in small pockets known as **lacunae** (la-KOO-nē; Latin *lacus,* lake). The physical properties of cartilage depend on the type and abundance of extracellular fibers, as well as the proteoglycan content.

Cartilage is avascular, and all nutrient and waste product exchange must occur by diffusion through the matrix. Blood vessels do not grow into cartilage because chondrocytes produce a chemical that discourages their formation. This chemical has been named **antiangiogenesis** (an-tē-an-jē-ō-JEN-eh-sis; Greek *anti-,* against + *angeion,* vessel + *genesis,* origination) **factor.** There is now interest in this compound as a potential anticancer agent. Cancers enlarge rapidly because blood vessels usually grow into areas where cells are crowded and active, improving nutrient and oxygen delivery. This growth could theoretically be prevented by antiangiogenesis factor, but the quantities produced in normal human cartilage are extremely small.

A cartilage is usually set apart from surrounding tissues by a fibrous **perichondrium** (per-i-KON-drē-um; Greek *peri-,* around + *chondros,* cartilage). The perichondrium contains two distinct layers, an outer, fibrous region of dense irregular connective tissue and an inner, cellular layer. The fibrous layer provides mechanical support and protection and

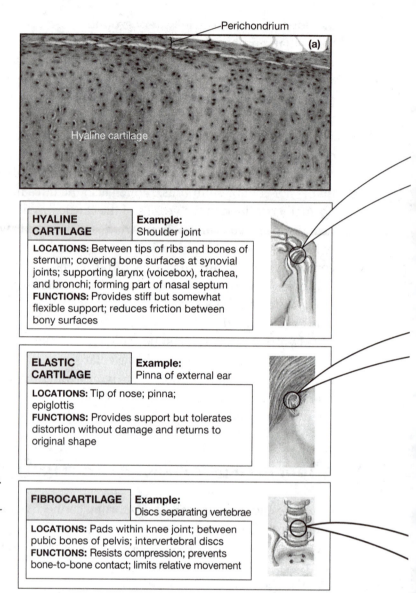

Figure 6–14   The Perichondrium and Types of Cartilage.

(a) A perichondrium separates cartilage from other tissues. (b) Hyaline cartilage. Note the translucent matrix and the absence of prominent fibers. (c) Elastic cartilage. The closely packed elastic fibers are visible between the chondrocytes. (d) Fibrocartilage. The collagen fibers are extremely dense, and the chondrocytes are relatively far apart.

attaches the cartilage to other structures. The cellular layer is important to the growth and maintenance of the cartilage.

Types of Cartilage

Three major types of cartilage are found in the body: (1) hyaline cartilage, (2) elastic cartilage, and (3) fibrocartilage.

1. **Hyaline** (HĪ-a-lin; Greek *hyalos*, glass) **cartilage** is the most common type of cartilage. The matrix of hyaline cartilage contains closely packed collagen fibers, making it tough but somewhat flexible. Because the fibers do not stain well, they are not always apparent in light microscopy (Figure 6–14a). Examples of this type of cartilage in the adult body include (1) the connections between the ribs and the ster-

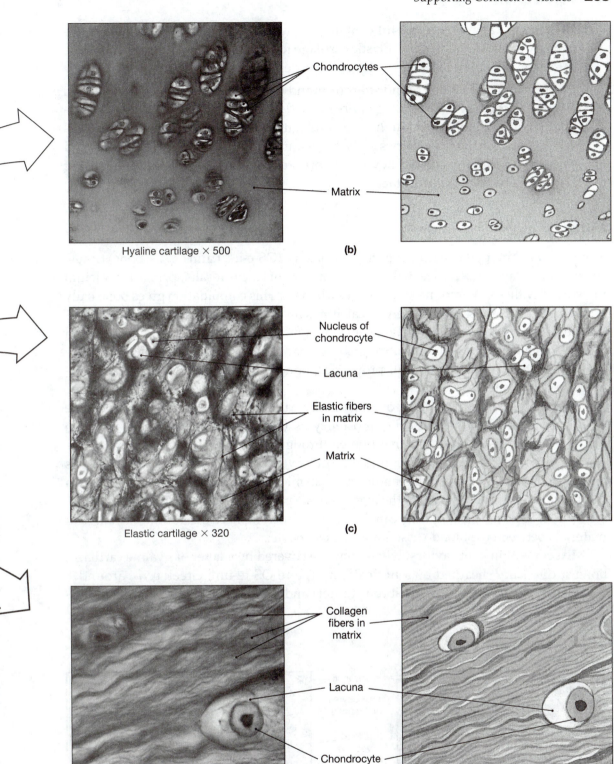

Hyaline cartilage × 500 **(b)**

Chondrocytes

Matrix

Elastic cartilage × 320 **(c)**

Nucleus of chondrocyte

Lacuna

Elastic fibers in matrix

Matrix

Fibrocartilage × 750 **(d)**

Collagen fibers in matrix

Lacuna

Chondrocyte

num, (2) the supporting cartilages along the conducting passageways of the respiratory tract, and (3) the cartilages covering articular surfaces within some joints, such as the elbow or knee.

2. **Elastic cartilage** (Figure 6–14b) contains numerous elastic fibers that make it extremely resilient and flexible. Elastic cartilage forms the external flap (pinna) of the outer ear, the epiglottis, and the tip of the nose.

3. **Fibrocartilage** has little ground substance, and the matrix is dominated by collagen fibers (Figure 6–14c). The collagen fibers are densely interwoven, making this tissue extremely durable and tough. Fibrocartilaginous pads lie between the spinal vertebrae, between the pubic bones of the pelvis, and around or within a few joints and tendons. In these positions they resist compression, absorb shocks, and prevent damaging bone-to-bone contact.

Bone

Roughly one-third of the matrix of **bone,** or **osseous** (OS-ē-us; Latin *osseus,* bone) **tissue,** consists of collagen fibers. The balance is a mixture of calcium salts, primarily calcium phosphate with lesser amounts of calcium carbonate. This combination gives bone truly remarkable properties. By themselves, calcium salts are strong but rather brittle. Collagen fibers are weaker but relatively flexible. In bone, the minerals are organized around the collagen fibers. The result is a strong, somewhat flexible combination that is very resistant to shattering. In its overall properties, bone can compete with the best steel-reinforced concrete.

The general organization of osseous tissue can be seen in Figure 6–15. Lacunae within the matrix contain bone cells, or **osteocytes** (OS-tē-ō-sīts). The lacunae are often organized around blood vessels that branch through the bony matrix. Although diffusion cannot occur through the calcium salts, osteocytes communicate with blood vessels and with one another through slender cytoplasmic extensions. These extensions run through long, slender passages in the matrix. These passageways, called **canaliculi** (kan-a-LIK-ū-lē; Latin *canaliculus,* little canal), form a branching network for the exchange of materials between the blood vessels and the osteocytes.

Except within joint cavities, where they are covered by a layer of hyaline cartilage, bone surfaces are sheathed by a **periosteum** (pe-rē-OS-tē-um; Greek *peri-,* around + Latin *osseus,* bone) composed of fibrous (outer) and cellular (inner) layers. The perios-

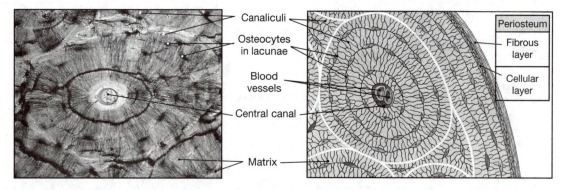

Figure 6–15 Bone.
The osteocytes in bone are generally organized in groups around a central space that contains blood vessels. Bone dust produced during grinding fills the lacunae and the central canal, making them appear dark. (LM × 362)

teum assists in the attachment of a bone to surrounding tissues and to associated tendons and ligaments. The cellular layer functions in bone growth and participates in repairs after an injury. Unlike cartilage, bone undergoes extensive remodeling on a regular basis, and complete repairs can be made even after severe damage has occurred. Bones also respond to the stresses placed upon them, growing thicker and stronger with exercise and thin and brittle with inactivity. Table 6–1 summarizes the similarities and differences between cartilage and bone.

Table 6–1 A Comparison of Cartilage and Bone

Characteristic	Cartilage	Bone
Structural Features		
Cells	Chondrocytes in lacunae	Osteocytes in lacunae
Ground substance	Chonodroitin sulfate (in proteoglycan) and water	A small volume of liquid surrounding insoluble crystals of calcium phosphate and calcium carbonate
Fibers	Collagen, elastic, and reticular fibers (proportions vary)	Collagen fibers predominate
Vascularity	None	Extensive
Covering	Perichondrium, two-part	Periosteum, two-part
Strength	Limited: bends easily but hard to break	Strong: resists distortion until breaking point
Metabolic Features		
Oxygen demands	Relatively low	Relatively high
Nutrient delivery	By diffusion through matrix	By diffusion through cytoplasm and fluid in canaliculi
Repair capabilities	Limited ability	Extensive ability

✎ Let's Review What You've Just Learned

▶ Definitions

In the space provided, list the boldface terms included in this section that contain the indicated word part.

_____ **128.** A type of blood cell responsible for the transport of oxygen.

_____ **129.** The proper term for a cartilage cell.

_____ **130.** A type of cartilage that has a matrix containing little ground substance and large amounts of collagen fibers.

_____ **131.** Vessels that carry blood away from the heart.

_____ **132.** Formed elements of blood that are tiny, membrane-wrapped packets of cytoplasm containing enzymes and special proteins.

_____ **133.** The watery ground substance of blood.

_____ **134.** The proper term for bone tissue.

_____ **135.** A fibrous tissue that separates cartilage from surrounding tissues.

_____ **136.** The collective term for the cells and cell fragments found in blood.

_____ **137.** Passageways that return lymph to the circulatory system.

_____ **138.** Blood vessels that carry blood towards the heart.

_____ **139.** A bone cell.

_____ **140.** Small pockets found in cartilage and osseous tissue.

_____ **141.** Thin-walled vessels that connect arteries to veins.

_____ **142.** The fluid connective tissue found in lymphatic vessels.

_____ **143.** Body fluid that is not located within cells.

_____ **144.** Slender passageways in the matrix of bone that form a branching network for the exchange of materials between osteocytes and the blood.

_____ **145.** A type of cartilage that is extremely resilient and flexible.

_____ **146.** The proper term for white blood cells.

_____ **147.** The fibrous covering of osseous tissue.

_____ **148.** A type of leukocyte that functions as a macrophage.

_____ **149.** A special type of proteoglycan found in the matrix of cartilage.

_____ **150.** The fluid that bathes the cells of the body.

_____ **151.** A type of cartilage containing closely packed collagen fibers.

_____ **152.** A chemical that prevents the formation of blood vessels in a tissue.

▶ **Word Roots, Prefixes, Suffixes, and Combining Forms**

In the space provided, list the boldface terms included in this section that contain the indicated word part.

Word Part	Meaning	Examples
peri-	around	**153.** _____
-phil	love	**154.** _____
inter-	between	**155.** _____
neutr-	neutral	**156.** _____
chondro-	cartilage	**157.** _____
extra-	outside of	**158.** _____
osteo-	bone	**159.** _____
angio-	vessel	**160.** _____
erythro-	red	**161.** _____
leuko-	white	**162.** _____

▶ **Labeling**

Label each of the following types of connective tissue.

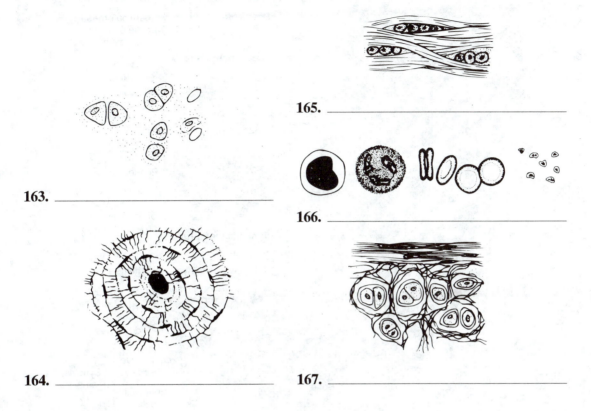

163. _____

164. _____

165. _____

166. _____

167. _____

MEMBRANES

Epithelia and connective tissues combine to form coverings called membranes that protect other structures and tissues in the body. There are four such membranes: (1) mucous membranes, (2) serous membranes, (3) the cutaneous membrane (skin), and (4) synovial membranes.

Mucous Membranes

Mucous membranes line cavities that communicate with the exterior, including the digestive, respiratory, reproductive, and urinary tracts (Figure 6–16a). The epithelial surfaces are kept moist at all times; they may be lubricated by mucus produced by goblet cells or multicellular glands or by exposure to fluids such as urine or semen. The loose connective tissue component of a mucous membrane is called the **lamina** (LAM-i-na) **propria** (PRŌ-prē-a).

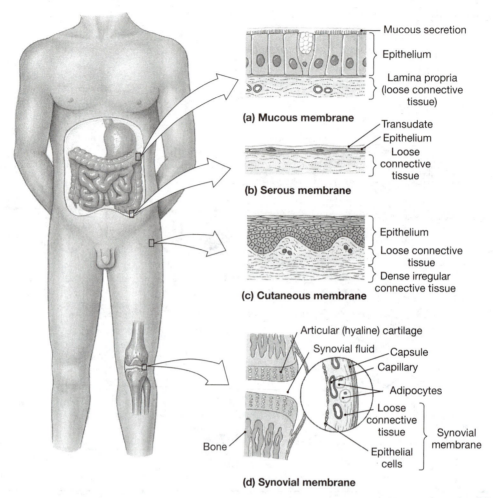

(a) Mucous membrane

Mucous secretion
Epithelium
Lamina propria (loose connective tissue)

(b) Serous membrane

Transudate
Epithelium
Loose connective tissue

(c) Cutaneous membrane

Epithelium
Loose connective tissue
Dense irregular connective tissue

(d) Synovial membrane

Articular (hyaline) cartilage
Synovial fluid
Capsule
Capillary
Adipocytes
Loose connective tissue
Epithelial cells
Synovial membrane
Bone

Figure 6–16   Membranes.
(a) Mucous membranes are coated with the secretions of mucous glands. Mucous membranes line the digestive, respiratory, urinary, and reproductive tracts. **(b)** Serous membranes line the ventral body cavities (the peritoneal, pleural, and pericardial cavities). **(c)** The cutaneous membrane, or skin, covers the outer surface of the body. **(d)** Synovial membranes line joint cavities and produce the fluid within the joint.

The epithelial portion of many mucous membranes is a simple epithelium that performs absorptive or secretory functions, such as the simple columnar epithelium of the digestive tract. However, other types of epithelia may be involved. For example, a stratified squamous epithelium is part of the mucous membrane of the mouth, and the mucous membrane along most of the urinary tract has a transitional epithelium.

Serous Membranes

Serous (SĒR-us) **membranes** line the sealed, internal cavities of the body. There are three serous membranes, each consisting of a mesothelium supported by loose connective tissue (see Figure 6–16b). These membranes were introduced in Chapter 1 (p. 41): (1) the pleura lines the pleural cavities and covers the lungs; (2) the peritoneum lines the peritoneal cavity and covers the surfaces of the enclosed organs; and (3) the pericardium lines the pericardial cavity and covers the heart. Serous membranes are very thin, and they are firmly attached to the body wall and to the organs they cover. When you are look-ing at an organ, such as the heart or stomach, you are really seeing the tissues of the organ through a transparent serous membrane.

The surfaces of the serous membranes covering an organ and lining the wall of the cavity around the organ are in close contact at all times. Minimizing friction between these two surfaces is the primary function of serous membranes. Because the mesothelia are very thin, serous membranes are relatively permeable, and tissue fluids diffuse onto the exposed surface, keeping it moist and slippery.

The fluid formed on the surfaces of a serous membrane is called a **transudate** (TRANS-ū-dāt; Latin *trans*, across + *sudare*, to sweat). Specific transudates are called pleur-al fluid, peritoneal fluid, or pericardial fluid, depending on their source. In normal healthy individuals the total volume of transudate is extremely small, just enough to prevent fric-tion between the walls of the cavities and the surfaces of internal organs. But after an in-jury or in certain disease states, the volume of transudate may increase dramatically, complicating existing medical problems or producing new ones.

The Cutaneous Membrane

The **cutaneous** (kū-TĀ-nē-us) **membrane** of the skin covers the surface of the body. It con-sists of a stratified squamous epithelium and a layer of loose connective tissue (Figure 6–16c) that is reinforced by underlying dense connective tissue. In contrast to serous or mucous membranes, the cutaneous membrane is thick, relatively waterproof, and usually dry.

Synovial Membranes

A **synovial** (sīn-Ō-vē-al) **membrane** consists of extensive areas of loose connective tissue bounded by a superficial layer of squamous or cuboidal cells (Figure 6–16d). Although usually called an epithelium, it differs from other epithelia in two respects: (1) There is no basement membrane, and (2) the cellular layer is incomplete, and gaps exist between adjacent cells. Some of the lining cells are phagocytic and others are secretory. The secretory cells regulate the composition of the synovial fluid within a joint cavity.

THE CONNECTIVE TISSUE FRAMEWORK OF THE BODY

Connective tissues create the internal framework of the body. Layers of connective tissue connect the organs within the dorsal and ventral body cavities with the rest of the body. These layers (1) provide strength and stability, (2) maintain the relative positions of inter-nal organs, and (3) provide a route for the distribution of blood vessels, lymphatics, and nerves. The connective tissue layers and wrappings can be divided into three major com-ponents: the superficial fascia, the deep fascia, and the subserous fascia. The functional anatomy of these layers is illustrated in Figure 6–17.

- The **superficial fascia** (FĀSH-uh; Latin *fascias*, band), or **subcutaneous** (sub-kū-TĀ-nē-us; Latin *sub*, below + *cutis*, skin) **layer,** is also termed the **hypodermis** (hī-pō-DER-mis; Greek *hypo*, below + *derma*, skin). This layer of loose connective tissue separates the skin from underlying tissues and organs. It provides insulation and padding and lets the skin or underlying structures move independently.

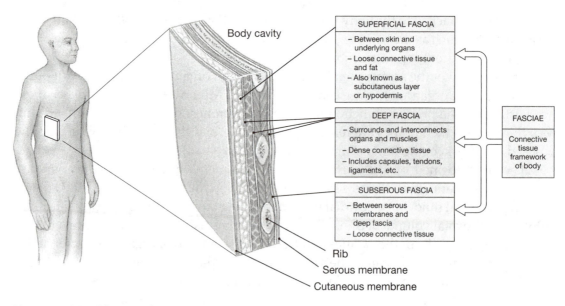

Figure 6–17   The Fasciae.
The relationship of connective tissue elements in the body.

- The **deep fascia** consists of dense connective tissue. The fiber organization resembles that of plywood: All the fibers in an individual layer run in the same direction, but the orientation of the fibers changes from one layer to another. This arrangement helps the tissue resist forces applied from many different directions. The tough capsules that surround most organs, including the kidneys and the organs in the thoracic and peritoneal cavities, are components of the deep fascia. The perichondrium around cartilages, the periosteum around bones, the ligaments that connect bones, and the connective tissues of muscle, including tendons and aponeuroses, are all part of the deep fascia. The dense connective tissue components are interwoven; for example, the deep fascia around a muscle blends into the tendon, whose fibers intermingle with those of the periosteum. This arrangement creates a strong, fibrous network for the body and ties structural elements together.

- The **subserous fascia** is a layer of loose connective tissue that lies between the deep fascia and the serous membranes that line body cavities. Because this layer separates the serous membranes from the deep fascia, movements of muscles or muscular organs do not severely distort the delicate lining.

MUSCLE TISSUE

Muscle tissue is specialized for contraction. Individual muscle cells are relatively long and slender; as a result they are usually called muscle fibers. Muscle fibers possess organelles and properties distinct from those of other cells. They are capable of powerful contractions that shorten the fiber along its longitudinal axis. Because they are different from "typical" cells the term **sarcoplasm** (SAHR-kō-plazm) is used to refer to the cytoplasm of a muscle fiber, and one refers to the **sarcolemma** (sar-kō-LEM-uh) rather than the cell membrane.

Three types of muscle tissue are found in the body: (1) skeletal, (2) cardiac, and (3) smooth. The contraction mechanism is similar in all three, but they differ in their internal organization.

Skeletal Muscle Tissue

Skeletal muscle tissue contains very large muscle fibers. Skeletal muscle fibers are unusual because they may be a foot or more in length, and each cell is multinucleated, containing hundreds of nuclei. Nuclei lie just under the surface of the sarcolemma (Figure 6–18a). Skeletal muscle fibers are incapable of dividing, but new muscle fibers can be produced through the division of **satellite cells,** mesenchymal cells that persist in adult skeletal muscle tissue. As a result, skeletal muscle tissue can at least partially repair itself after an injury.

Because the actin and myosin filaments are arranged in organized groups, skeletal muscle fibers appear to have a banded or striated appearance. Skeletal muscle fibers will not usually contract unless stimulated by nerves, and the nervous system provides voluntary control over their activities. Thus, skeletal muscle is called **striated voluntary muscle.**

Skeletal muscle tissue is tied together by loose connective tissue. The collagen and elastic fibers surrounding each cell and group of cells blend into those of a tendon or aponeurosis that conducts the force of contraction, usually to a bone of the skeleton. When the muscle tissue contracts, it pulls on the bone, and the bone moves.

Cardiac Muscle Tissue

Cardiac muscle tissue is found only in the heart. A typical cardiac muscle cell, also known as a **cardiocyte,** or **cardiac myocyte,** is smaller than a skeletal muscle fiber. A cardiac muscle cell usually has one centrally placed nucleus, although it may (rarely) have as many as three nuclei. The prominent striations visible in Figure 6–18b resemble those of skeletal muscle because the actin and myosin filaments are arranged the same way in both fiber types.

Cardiac muscle cells form extensive connections with one another. The connections occur at specialized regions known as **intercalated** (in-TUR-kuh-lā-tid) **discs.** As a result, cardiac muscle tissue consists of a branching network of interconnected muscle cells. The interconnections help channel the forces of contraction and coordinate the activities of individual cardiac muscle cells. Like skeletal muscle fibers, cardiac muscle cells are incapable of dividing, and because this tissue lacks satellite cells, cardiac muscle tissue damaged by injury or disease cannot regenerate.

Cardiac muscle cells do not rely on nerve activity to start a contraction. Instead, specialized cardiac muscle cells, called **pacemaker cells,** establish a regular rate of contraction. Although the nervous system can alter the rate of pacemaker activity, it does not provide voluntary control over individual cardiac muscle cells. Therefore, cardiac muscle is called **striated involuntary muscle.**

Smooth Muscle Tissue

Smooth muscle tissue can be found in the walls of blood vessels; around hollow organs such as the urinary bladder; and in layers around the respiratory, circulatory, digestive, and reproductive tracts. A smooth muscle cell is small with tapering ends, containing

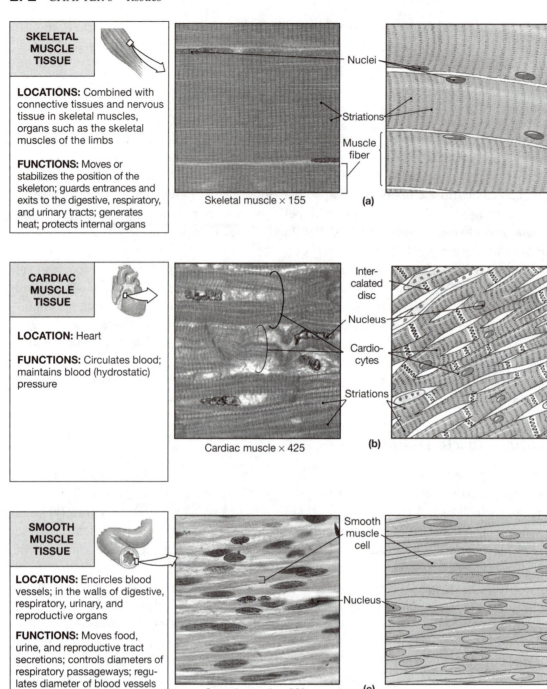

SKELETAL MUSCLE TISSUE

LOCATIONS: Combined with connective tissues and nervous tissue in skeletal muscles, organs such as the skeletal muscles of the limbs

FUNCTIONS: Moves or stabilizes the position of the skeleton; guards entrances and exits to the digestive, respiratory, and urinary tracts; generates heat; protects internal organs

Skeletal muscle × 155

Nuclei

Striations

Muscle fiber

(a)

CARDIAC MUSCLE TISSUE

LOCATION: Heart

FUNCTIONS: Circulates blood; maintains blood (hydrostatic) pressure

Cardiac muscle × 425

Inter-calated disc

Nucleus

Cardio-cytes

Striations

(b)

SMOOTH MUSCLE TISSUE

LOCATIONS: Encircles blood vessels; in the walls of digestive, respiratory, urinary, and reproductive organs

FUNCTIONS: Moves food, urine, and reproductive tract secretions; controls diameters of respiratory passageways; regulates diameter of blood vessels and thereby contributes to regulation of tissue blood flow

Smooth muscle × 330

Smooth muscle cell

Nucleus

(c)

Figure 6–18   Muscle Tissue.

(a) Skeletal muscle fibers are large, have multiple, peripherally located nuclei, and exhibit a prominent banding pattern and an unbranched arrangement. **(b)** Cardiac muscle cells differ from skeletal muscle fibers in three major ways: size (cardiac muscle cells are smaller), organization (cardiac muscle cells branch), and number and locations of nuclei (a typical cardiac muscle cell has one centrally placed nucleus). Both contain actin and myosin filaments in an organized array that produces striations. **(c)** Smooth muscle cells are small and spindle-shaped, with a central nucleus. They do not branch, and there are no striations.

a single oval nucleus (Figure 6–18c). Smooth muscle cells can divide, and smooth muscle tissue can regenerate after an injury. The actin and myosin filaments in smooth muscle cells are organized differently from those of skeletal and cardiac muscle, and there are no striations. Smooth muscle cells may contract on their own, or their contractions may be triggered by nerve cell activity. When areas of smooth muscle are innervated, the nerve activity is involuntarily controlled. Because the nervous system usually does not provide voluntary control over smooth muscle contractions, smooth muscle is known as **nonstriated involuntary muscle.**

NEURAL TISSUE

Neural (NOO-rul) **tissue,** also known as **nervous tissue** or **nerve tissue,** is specialized for the conduction of electrical impulses from one region of the body to another. Most of the neural tissue in the body (98 percent) is concentrated in the brain and spinal cord, the control centers for the nervous system. Neural tissue contains two basic types of cells: **nerve cells,** or **neurons** (NOO-rons), and several different kinds of supporting cells, collectively called **neuroglia** (noo-RŌ-glē-ah; Greek *neuron,* nerve + *glia,* glue). Our conscious and unconscious thought processes reflect the communication between neurons in the brain. Neuron communication involves the transmission of electrical impulses that are changes in the transmembrane potential. Information is conveyed by the frequency and pattern of impulse generation. Neuroglia have different functions, such as to provide a supporting framework for neural tissue and to play a role in providing nutrients to neurons.

Neurons are the longest cells in the body; many reach a meter in length. Most neurons are incapable of dividing under normal circumstances, and they have a very limited ability to repair themselves after injury. A typical neuron has a cell body, or **soma,** that contains a large prominent nucleus (Figure 6–19). Extending from the soma are various

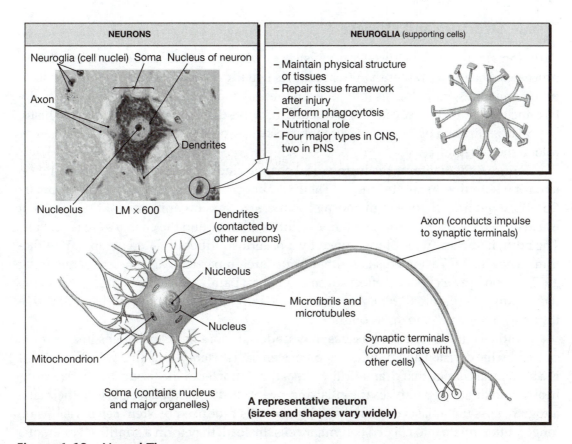

Figure 6–19   Neural Tissue.

branching processes termed **dendrites** (DEN-drīts; Greek *dendron,* a tree) and a single **axon.** Dendrites receive incoming messages; axons conduct outgoing messages. Because axons are often very long and slender, they are also called **nerve fibers.**

TISSUE INJURIES AND AGING

Tissues in the body are not isolated; they combine to form organs with diverse functions. Any injury to the body affects several different tissue types simultaneously, and these tissues must respond in a coordinated manner to preserve homeostasis.

Inflammation and Regeneration

The restoration of homeostasis after a tissue injury involves two related processes. First, the area is isolated while damaged cells, tissue components, and any dangerous microorganisms are cleaned up. This phase, which coordinates the activities of several different tissues, is called **inflammation,** or the **inflammatory response.** Inflammation begins immediately after an injury and produces several familiar sensations, including swelling, redness, and pain. An **infection** involves inflammation resulting from the presence of pathogens, such as bacteria.

Second, the damaged tissues are replaced or repaired to restore normal function. This repair process is called **regeneration.** Inflammation and regeneration are controlled at the tissue level. The two phases overlap; isolation establishes a framework that guides the cells responsible for reconstruction, and repairs are under way well before cleanup operations have ended.

Tissue Structure and Disease

Pathologists (pa-THO-lō-jists) are physicians who specialize in the study of disease processes. Diagnosis, rather than treatment, is usually the main focus of their activities. In their analyses, pathologists integrate anatomical and histological observations to determine the nature and severity of a disease. Because disease processes affect the histological organization of tissues and organs, tissue samples, or **biopsies,** often play a key role in their diagnoses.

Figure 6–20 diagrams the histological changes induced by one relatively common irritating stimulus, cigarette smoke. The first abnormality to be observed is **dysplasia** (dis-PLĀ-zē-uh), a change in the normal shape, size, and organization of tissue cells. It is usually a response to chronic irritation or inflammation, and the changes are reversible. The normal trachea (windpipe) is lined by a pseudostratified, ciliated columnar epithelium. The cilia move a mucus layer that traps foreign particles and moistens incoming air. The drying and chemical effects of smoking first paralyze the cilia, halting the movement of mucus (Figure 6–20a). As mucus builds up, the individual coughs to dislodge it (the well-known "smoker's cough").

Epithelia and connective tissues may undergo more radical changes in structure, caused by the division and differentiation of stem cells. **Metaplasia** (me-tuh-PLĀ-zē-uh) is a structural change that dramatically alters the character of the tissue. In our example, heavy smoking first paralyzes the cilia, and over time the epithelial cells lose their cilia altogether. As metaplasia occurs, the epithelial cells produced by stem cell divisions no longer differentiate into ciliated columnar cells. Instead, they form a stratified squamous epithelium that provides a greater resistance to drying and chemical irritation (Figure

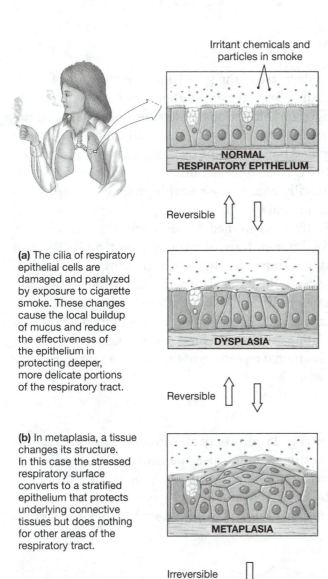

Irritant chemicals and particles in smoke

NORMAL RESPIRATORY EPITHELIUM

Reversible

DYSPLASIA

Reversible

METAPLASIA

Irreversible

ANAPLASIA

(a) The cilia of respiratory epithelial cells are damaged and paralyzed by exposure to cigarette smoke. These changes cause the local buildup of mucus and reduce the effectiveness of the epithelium in protecting deeper, more delicate portions of the respiratory tract.

(b) In metaplasia, a tissue changes its structure. In this case the stressed respiratory surface converts to a stratified epithelium that protects underlying connective tissues but does nothing for other areas of the respiratory tract.

(c) In anaplasia, the tissue cells become tumor cells; anaplasia produces a cancerous tumor.

Figure 6–20   Changes in a Tissue under Stress.

(a) The cilia of respiratory epithelial cells are damaged and paralyzed by exposure to cigarette smoke. These changes cause the local buildup of mucus and reduce the effectiveness of the epithelium in protecting deeper, more delicate portions of the respiratory tract. **(b)** In metaplasia, a tissue changes in structure. In this case, the stressed respiratory surface converts to a stratified epithelium that protects underlying connective tissues but does nothing to other areas of the respiratory tract. **(c)** In anaplasia, the tissue cells become tumor cells; anaplasia produces cancer.

6–20b). This epithelium protects the underlying tissues more effectively, but it completely eliminates the moisturization and cleaning properties of the epithelium. The cigarette smoke will now have an even greater effect on more-delicate portions of the respiratory tract. Fortunately, metaplasia is reversible, and the epithelium gradually returns to normal once the individual quits smoking.

During **anaplasia** (a-nuh-PLĀ-zē-uh), tissue organization breaks down. Tissue cells change size and shape, often becoming unusually large or abnormally small. In anaplasia (Figure 6–20c), which occurs in smokers developing one form of lung cancer, the cells divide more frequently, but not all divisions proceed in the normal way, and many of the tumor cells have abnormal chromosomes. Unlike dysplasia and metaplasia, anaplasia is irreversible.

Aging and Tissue Repair

Tissues change with age, and there is a decrease in the speed and effectiveness of tissue repairs. In general, repair and maintenance activities throughout the body slow down, and a combination of hormonal changes and alterations in lifestyle affect the structure and chemical composition of many tissues. Epithelia get thinner, and connective tissues more fragile. Individuals bruise easily, and bones become brittle; joint pains and broken bones are common complaints. Because cardiac muscle cells and neurons cannot be replaced, cumulative damage can eventually cause major health problems such as cardiovascular disease or deterioration in mental function.

Some of these changes are genetically programmed. For example, the chondrocytes of older individuals produce a slightly different form of proteoglycan than do those of younger people. The difference probably accounts for the observed changes in the thickness and resilience of cartilage. In other cases, the tissue degeneration may be temporarily slowed or even reversed. The age-related reduction in bone strength in women, a condition called **osteoporosis,** often results from a combination of inactivity, low dietary calcium levels, and a reduction in circulating estrogens (female sex hormones). A program of exercise, calcium supplements, and hormonal replacement therapies can usually maintain normal bone structure for many years.

Aging and Cancer Incidence

Cancer rates increase with age, and roughly 25 percent of all Americans develop cancer at some point in their lives. It has been estimated that 70–80 percent of these cases result from chemical exposure, environmental factors, or some combination of the two, and 40 percent of these cancers are caused by cigarette smoke. Each year, more than 500,000 Americans are killed by cancer, making this Public Health Enemy Number 2, second only to heart disease.

SUMMARY

This chapter has introduced the four basic tissue types found in the human body. In terms of their contribution to total body weight, muscle tissue is most important (around 50 percent), followed by connective tissues (45 percent), epithelium and glands (3 percent), and neural tissue (2 percent). In combination, these tissues form all of the organs and systems discussed in the next three chapters.

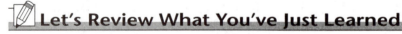

Let's Review What You've Just Learned

▶ **Definitions**

In the space provided, write the term for each of the following definitions.

_____ **168.** A heart muscle cell.

_____ **169.** The type of membrane lining cavities that communicate with the outside of the body.

_____ **170.** The fluid formed on the surface of a serous membrane.

_____ **171.** The cytoplasm of a muscle fiber.

_____ **172.** The body of a neuron.

_____ **173.** A change in the normal shape, size, and organization of tissue cells.

_____ **174.** Mesenchymal cells found in adult skeletal muscle.

_____ **175.** The membrane that covers the surface of the body.

_____ **176.** Muscle tissue that contains very large, striated muscle fibers.

_____ **177.** The supporting cells found in neural tissue.

_____ **178.** The branching processes that extend from the soma of a neuron and receive information from other cells.

_____ **179.** The extensive connections found between cardiac muscle cells.

_____ **180.** The loose connective tissue component of a mucous membrane.

_____ **181.** The layer of loose connective tissue that separates the skin from underlying tissues and organs.

_____ **182.** A structural change that dramatically alters the character of a tissue.

_____ **183.** Specialized cardiocytes that set the rate of contraction of cardiac muscle tissue.

_____ **184.** The membrane that surrounds a skeletal muscle fiber.

_____ **185.** Membranes that line the sealed, internal cavities of the body.

_____ **186.** A layer of loose connective tissue that lies between the deep fascia and serous membranes.

_____ **187.** Tissue that is specialized for the conduction of electrical impulses from one region of the body to another.

_____ **188.** Physicians who specialize in the study of disease processes.

_____ **189.** The replacement and repair of damaged tissue to restore normal function.

_____ **190.** A type of muscle tissue that is found only in the heart.

_____ **191.** Tissue that is specialized for contraction.

_____ **192.** A membrane that lines joint capsules.

_____ **193.** A dense connective tissue that consists of layers of fibers and that surrounds most of the body's internal organs.

_____ **194.** Muscle tissue that is composed of spindle-shaped cells and that is found in the walls of internal organs.

_____ **195.** A single process that extends from the soma of a neuron and carries information to other cells.

_____ **196.** The first phase of tissue response to injury, during which damaged cells, tissue components, and dangerous microorganisms are cleaned up.

_____ **197.** The removal of a small sample of tissue for pathological analysis.

_____ **198.** A cell found in neural tissue that is specialized for intercellular communication.

► Word Roots, Prefixes, Suffixes, and Combining Forms

In the space provided, list the boldface terms included in this section that contain the indicated word part.

Word Part	Meaning	Examples
dys-	painful	199. _____
neuro-	nerve	200. _____
sarco-	flesh	201. _____
osteo-	bone	202. _____
dendr-	tree	203. _____
cardio-	heart	204. _____
-lemma	husk	205. _____
cut-	skin	206. _____
derm-	skin	207. _____
-glia	glue	208. _____
-plasia	formation	209. _____

► Labeling

Label each of the following types of tissue.

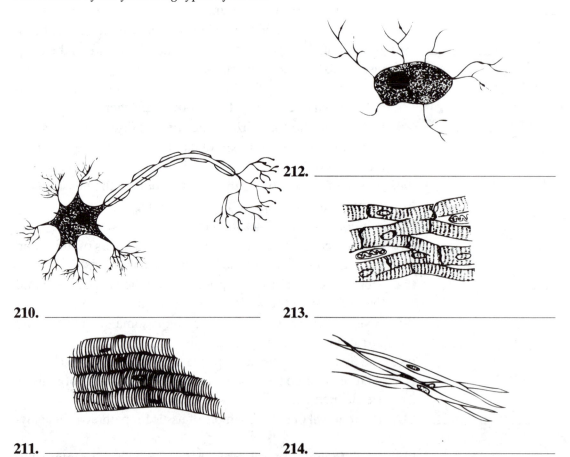

212. _____

210. _____

213. _____

211. _____

214. _____

☑ Self-Check Test

The following test will allow you to determine how well you have mastered the vocabulary and basic concepts of this chapter. It will also help you prepare for the type of questions you are likely to encounter on a test in an anatomy and physiology course. The self-check test will help you assess your understanding of the chapter material and will help you develop good test-taking skills. The following questions test your ability to use vocabulary and recall facts.

1. Tissue that is specialized for contraction is
   a. loose connective tissue
   b. dense connective tissue
   c. epithelial tissue
   d. nerve tissue
   e. muscle tissue

2. The type of epithelium that is found lining internal body cavities and blood vessels is
   a. simple squamous epithelium
   b. stratified squamous epithelium
   c. simple cuboidal epithelium
   d. stratified cuboidal epithelium
   e. transitional epithelium

3. You would find pseudostratified columnar epithelium lining the
   a. trachea
   b. urinary bladder
   c. secretory portions of the pancreas
   d. surface of the skin
   e. stomach

4. The fibrous components of connective tissue are produced by
   a. fibroblasts
   b. macrophages
   c. adipocytes
   d. mast cells
   e. melanocytes

5. Chondrocytes
   a. form bone
   b. store fat
   c. form cartilage
   d. form loose connective tissue
   e. form dense connective tissue

6. Glands that secrete hormones into the blood or tissue fluids are
   a. endocrine glands
   b. mixed glands
   c. exocrine glands
   d. merocrine glands
   e. holocrine glands

7. The cell that accounts for almost half the volume of blood is the
   a. leukocyte
   b. monocyte
   c. lymphocyte
   d. erythrocyte
   e. platelet

8. Which of the following lines cavities that communicate with the exterior of the body?
   a. synovial membrane
   b. serous membrane
   c. cutaneous membrane
   d. peritoneal membrane
   e. mucous membrane

9. The muscle tissue that shows no striations is
   a. skeletal muscle
   b. cardiac muscle
   c. smooth muscle
   d. voluntary muscle
   e. multinucleated muscle

10. Each of the following is a part of a neuron except one. Identify the exception.
    a. soma
    b. dendrite
    c. axon
    d. nerve fiber
    e. sarcolemma

11. Which of the following terms refers to a reversible change in the normal shape, size, and organization of tissue cells?
    a. metaplasia
    b. metastasis
    c. dysplasia
    d. anaplasia
    e. inflammation

12. Which of the following is a layer of glycoproteins and a network of fine protein filaments that prevents the movement of proteins and other large molecules from the connective tissue to the epithelium?
    a. desmosomes
    b. the basal lamina
    c. the reticular lamina
    d. areolar tissue
    e. tight junctions

13. Which of the following is an example of a unicellular exocrine gland?
    a. mammary gland
    b. sweat gland
    c. goblet cell
    d. pancreas
    e. salivary gland

14. Cells that remove damaged cells or pathogens from connective tissue are
   a. fibroblasts
   b. fixed macrophages
   c. adipocytes
   d. mast cells
   e. melanocytes

15. Each of the following is an example of dense connective tissue except one. Identify the exception.
   a. tendon
   b. aponeurosis
   c. ligament
   d. areolar tissue
   e. elastic tissue

16. Osseous tissue is better known as
   a. cartilage
   b. fat
   c. tendon
   d. bone
   e. ligament

17. Which of the following terms refers to the dense connective tissue that forms the capsules surrounding many organs?
   a. superficial fascia
   b. hypodermis
   c. deep fascia
   d. subserous fascia
   e. subcutaneous layer

The following questions are more challenging and require you to synthesize the information that you have learned in this chapter.

18. Examination of a tissue sample reveals groups of cells united by junctional complexes and interlocking membranes. The cells have one free surface and lack blood vessels. The tissue is most likely
   a. muscle tissue
   b. neural tissue
   c. epithelial tissue
   d. connective tissue
   e. adipose tissue

19. Microscopic examination of a tissue reveals an open framework of fibers with a large volume of fluid ground substance and elastic fibers. This tissue would most likely have come from the
   a. inner wall of a blood vessel
   b. lungs
   c. spleen
   d. tissue that separates skin from underlying muscle
   e. bony socket of the eye

20. Why does damaged cartilage heal slowly?
    a. Chondrocytes cannot be replaced if killed, and other cell types must take their place.
    b. Cartilage is avascular, so nutrients and other molecules must diffuse to the site of injury.
    c. Damaged cartilage becomes calcified, thus blocking the movement of materials required for healing.
    d. Chondrocytes divide more slowly than other cell types, delaying the healing process.
    e. Damaged collagen cannot be quickly replaced, thus the healing process is slower.

☑ Self-Assessment

If your score was

between 18 and 20, you are ready to proceed to the next chapter.

between 15 and 17, you have a good general idea of the chapter content, but you should review sections of the chapter that deal with items that you missed before proceeding to the next chapter.

less than 14, you have not mastered the chapter content well enough to proceed. Reread the chapter and rework the exercises. Then retake the self-check test. Repeat this process until you achieve a score that will allow you to continue.

Answers

1. avascular
2. histology
3. merocrine secretion
4. exocrine glands
5. simple
6. gap junction
7. mesothelium
8. stereocilia
9. tissue
10. holocrine secretion
11. cell adhesion molecules (CAMs)
12. simple epithelium
13. basal lamina
14. desmosome
15. germinative cells
16. epithelium
17. serous glands
18. goblet cells
19. reticular lamina
20. exfoliative cytology
21. connective tissue
22. stratified epithelium
23. intermediate junction
24. columnar epithelial cell
25. mixed gland
26. endocrine glands
27. apocrine secretion
28. muscle tissue
29. neuroepithelium

30. tight junction
31. basement membrane
32. endothelium
33. amniocentesis
34. hormone
35. ducts
36. alveolar gland
37. neural tissue
38. squamous epithelium
39. cellular cement
40. a junctional complex
41. epithelial tissue
42. transitional epithelium
43. Pap test
44. mucins, which mix with water to form mucus
45. compound gland
46. pseudostratified
47. merocrine
48. epithelium
49. histology
50. holocrine
51. desmosome
52. stereocilia
53. avascular
54. reticular lamina
55. amniocentesis
56. apocrine
57. merocrine, holocrine, apocrine
58. simple columnar epithelium

59. urinary bladder, renal pelvis, ureters
60. glands, ducts, portions of kidney tubules
61. pseudostratified columnar epithelium
62. stratified squamous epithelium
63. respiratory exchange surface, lining of ventral body cavities, and lining of blood vessels
64. stratified cuboidal epithelium
65. simple squamous epithelium
66. stratified squamous epithelium
67. simple columnar epithelium
68. simple cuboidal epithelium
69. transitional epithelium
70. simple ciliated columnar epithelium
71. pseudostratified columnar epithelium
72. simple tubular gland
73. simple branched alveolar gland
74. compound tubular gland
75. simple branched tubular gland
76. melanocytes
77. matrix
78. ligament
79. capsule
80. mesenchyme
81. microphages
82. pathogens
83. adipocyte
84. connective tissue proper
85. fixed macrophages
86. plasma cell
87. hyaluronidase
88. adipose tissue
89. stroma
90. elastic tissue
91. aponeurosis
92. melanin
93. fibroblasts
94. ground substance
95. basophil
96. antibodies
97. mucous connective tissue
98. liposuction
99. dense irregular connective tissue
100. areolar tissue
101. reticular fibers
102. mast cells
103. fluid connective tissue
104. mesenchymal cells
105. collagen
106. tendons
107. elastic fibers
108. free macrophages
109. supporting connective tissue
110. calcified
111. collagenous tissue
112. fibroblast
113. pathogen
114. reticular fiber, reticular tissue
115. adipocyte, adipose tissue
116. liposuction
117. hyaluronidase
118. antibodies
119. microphage
120. melanocyte, lymphocyte, adipocyte
121. microphage, macrophage
122. melanin, melanocyte
123. loose connective tissue (areolar tissue)
124. reticular tissue
125. adipose tissue
126. dense regular connective tissue (tendon)
127. dense regular connective tissue (ligament)
128. red blood cell, or erythrocyte
129. chondrocyte
130. fibrocartilage
131. arteries
132. platelets
133. plasma
134. osseous tissue
135. perichondrium
136. formed elements
137. lymphatic vessels
138. veins
139. osteocyte
140. lacunae
141. capillaries
142. lymph
143. extracellular fluid
144. canaliculi
145. elastic cartilage
146. leukocytes
147. periosteum
148. monocyte
149. chondroitin sulfate
150. interstitial fluid
151. hyaline cartilage
152. antiangiogenesis factor
153. periosteum, perichondrium
154. neutrophil, eosinophil
155. interstitial fluid
156. neutrophil
157. chondrocyte, perichondrium, chondroitin sulfate
158. extracellular fluid
159. osteocyte, periosteum
160. antiangiogenesis factor
161. erythrocyte
162. leukocyte
163. hyaline cartilage
164. bone (osseous tissue)
165. fibrocartilage
166. blood (fluid connective tissue)
167. elastic cartilage
168. cardiocyte (myocardiocyte)
169. mucous membrane
170. transudate
171. sarcoplasm
172. soma
173. dysplasia
174. satellite cells
175. cutaneous membrane
176. skeletal muscle tissue
177. neuroglia
178. dendrite

179. intercalated discs
180. lamina propria
181. superficial fascia (subcutaneous layer or hypodermis)
182. metaplasia
183. pacemaker cells
184. sarcolemma
185. serous membranes
186. subserous fascia
187. neural tissue (nervous tissue)
188. pathologists
189. regeneration
190. cardiac muscle tissue
191. muscle tissue
192. synovial membrane
193. deep fascia
194. smooth muscle tissue
195. axon
196. inflammation (inflammatory response)
197. biopsy
198. neuron
199. dysplasia
200. neuron, neural tissue, neuroglia
201. sarcolemma, sarcoplasm
202. osteoporosis
203. dendrite
204. cardiocyte
205. sarcolemma
206. cutaneous tissue, subcutaneous layer
207. hypodermis
208. neuroglia
209. anaplasia, metaplasia, dysplasia
210. neuron
211. skeletal muscle tissue
212. neuroglia
213. cardiac muscle tissue
214. smooth muscle tissue

Answers to Self-Check Test

1. e 2. a 3. a 4. a 5. c 6. a 7. d 8. e 9. c 10. e 11. c 12. b 13. c 14. b 15. d 16. d 17. c 18. c 19. d 20. b

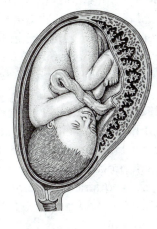

CHAPTER 7

Development and Inheritance

The process of development is the gradual modification of anatomical structures during the period from conception to maturity. The changes are truly remarkable; what begins as a single cell slightly larger than the period at the end of this sentence becomes an individual whose body contains trillions of cells organized into tissues, organs, and organ systems. The creation of different cell types during development is called differentiation. The basic mechanism involved was introduced in Chapter 6: Differentiation occurs through selective changes in genetic activity. As development proceeds, some genes are turned off and others are turned on. The identities of these genes vary from one cell type to another.

A basic understanding of development and genetics provides a framework that greatly enhances the understanding of anatomical structure and physiological processes. In addition, many of the mechanisms of development and growth are similar to those responsible for the repair of injuries, and many, if not all, diseases have a genetic component. This chapter will focus on major aspects of development and genetics and consider highlights of those processes rather than describe the events in great detail. Few topics in the biological sciences hold such fascination, and fewer still confront the investigator with so dazzling an array of technological, moral, and logistical challenges.

AN OVERVIEW OF TOPICS IN DEVELOPMENT

Development involves (1) the division and differentiation of cells and (2) changes in genetic activity that produce and modify anatomical structures. Development begins at fertilization, or **conception**, and can be divided into periods characterized by specific anatomical changes. **Embryological** (em-brē-ō-LOJ-i-kul) **development** comprises those events that occur during the first 2 months after fertilization. The study of these events is called **embryology** (em-brē-OL-ō-jē). **Fetal** (FĒ-tul) **development** begins at the start of the ninth week and continues up to the time of birth. Embryological and fetal development are sometimes referred to collectively as **prenatal** (prē-NĀ-tul) **development**. **Postnatal** (post-NĀ-tul) **development** commences at birth and continues to maturity, when another process, **senescence** (se-NES-ense; Latin *senescere*, to grow old), or aging, begins.

Although all human beings go through the same developmental stages, their differences in genetic makeup produce distinctive individual characteristics. **Inheritance** refers to the transfer of genetically determined characteristics from generation to generation. **Genetics** is the study of the mechanisms responsible for inheritance. This chapter considers basic genetics as it applies to the appearance of inherited characteristics such as sex, hair color, and various diseases.

We will begin our overview of development with a discussion of gamete (sperm and ova) formation, or **gametogenesis** (ga-mē-tō-JEN-e-sis). Although development actually begins at fertilization, the production of functional gametes establishes important guidelines for future development. With this background, we will proceed to a description of fertilization and zygote formation. We will then follow the sequence of events under way during prenatal and postnatal development, adolescence, and maturity. We will conclude our survey with an overview of basic genetic principles.

MEIOSIS AND GAMETOGENESIS

Meiosis (mī-Ō-sis) is *a special form of cell division involved in gamete production*. It differs significantly from mitosis (introduced in Chapter 5) in terms of the events that take place in the nucleus. Mitosis is part of the process of somatic cell division, which produces two daughter cells, each containing 23 pairs of chromosomes (46 chromosomes total). Each pair consists of one chromosome provided by the male parent and another provided by the female parent at the time of fertilization. Because somatic cells contain both members of each chromosome pair, they are called **diploid** (DIP-loyd; Greek *diploos*, double) cells. If a gamete resembled somatic cells, at fertilization the fusion of an egg with a sperm would produce a cell containing 92 chromosomes. The next generation would contain 184, the one after that 368 and so on. This multiplication of chromosomes would hardly be practical. Even ignoring the potential problems arising from excess copies of every gene, the extra chromosomes would take up space needed for organelles, such as mitochondria and endoplasmic reticulum, and other components of cytoplasm. These problems are avoided because gametes are formed by meiosis rather than mitosis. Meiosis involves a pair of divisions and produces four cells, each of which contains 23 individual chromosomes, that are called **haploid** (HAP-loyd; Greek *haploeides*, single) cells. Gametes are therefore different from ordinary somatic cells because they contain only half the normal number of chromosomes.

In gametogenesis, the chromosome pairs of somatic stem cells are separated by meiosis and the subsequent cell divisions produce haploid gametes (Figure 7–1). The events in the nucleus are the same whether you consider the formation of sperm (**spermatogenesis** [spur-ma-tō-JEN-e-sis]), or ova (**oogenesis** [ō-ō-JEN-e-sis]). During the interphase period preceding meiosis, all of the chromosomes within the nucleus duplicate themselves as if the cell were about to undergo mitosis. As prophase (prophase I) of the first meiotic division, **meiosis I**, arrives, the chromosomes condense and become visible. As in mitosis, each chromosome consists of two duplicate chromatids (see Chapter 5). The corresponding paternal and maternal chromosomes now come together, an event known as **synapsis** (sin-AP-sis). Synapsis produces 23 pairs of chromosomes, each member of the pair consisting of two identical chromatids. A matched set of four chromatids

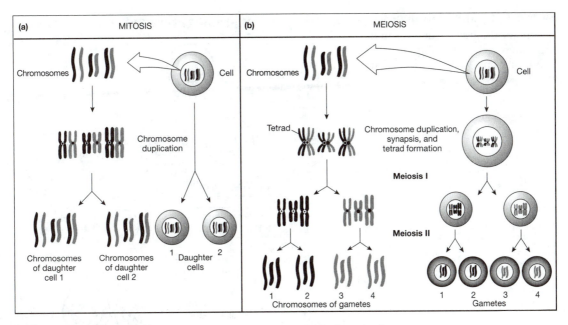

Figure 7–1 Chromosomal Events during Mitosis and Meiosis.
(a) Steps in mitosis. (See Figure 5–20.) (b) Steps in meiosis.

is called a **tetrad** (TET-rad; Greek, *tetras*, four). Some exchange of genetic material can occur between the chromatids at this stage of meiosis. This exchange, called **crossing-over**, increases genetic variation among offspring; it will be detailed later in the chapter.

As metaphase I begins, the nuclear envelope disappears and the tetrads line up along the metaphase plate. At the end of metaphase I the chromosomes forming the tetrads separate. This phase is a major difference between mitosis and meiosis: In mitosis, each daughter cell receives one of the two copies of every chromosome, maternal and paternal, whereas in meiosis each daughter cell receives both copies of either the maternal chromosome or the paternal chromosome from each tetrad.

As anaphase proceeds, the maternal and paternal chromosomes are randomly distributed. As a result, telophase I ends with the formation of two daughter cells containing unique combinations of maternal and paternal chromosomes. Each daughter cell contains 23 chromosomes, and each chromosome still contains two duplicate chromatids. Because the first meiotic division reduces the number of chromosomes from 46 to 23, it is called a **reductional division**.

The interphase separating meiosis I and II is generally brief. The daughter cells produced by the first meiotic division proceed into prophase II without further growth or DNA replication. The completion of metaphase II, anaphase II, and telophase II produces four cells, each containing 23 chromosomes. Because the chromosome number has not changed, meiosis II represents an **equational division**.

Spermatogenesis

Spermatogenesis involves three integrated processes: mitosis, meiosis, and spermiogenesis. The process begins with stem cells called **spermatogonia** (sper-mat-ō-GŌ-nē-uh; singular, *spermatogonium*) which are located in tubular structures called

Figure 7–2 Spermatogenesis.
Schematic diagram of meiosis in the
seminiferous tubules, showing the distribution of only a few chromosomes.

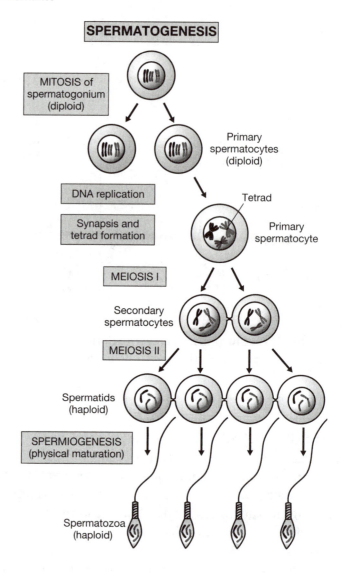

SPERMATOGENESIS

MITOSIS of
spermatogonium
(diploid)

Primary
spermatocytes
(diploid)

DNA replication

Synapsis and
tetrad formation

Tetrad

Primary
spermatocyte

MEIOSIS I

Secondary
spermatocytes

MEIOSIS II

Spermatids
(haploid)

SPERMIOGENESIS
(physical maturation)

Spermatozoa
(haploid)

seminiferous (sem-i-NIF-ur-us) **tubules** located in the testes (Figure 7–2). These cells
undergo mitosis and cell division throughout adult life. Each time one of these cells divides, one of the daughter cells remains as an undifferentiated stem cell, while the other
differentiates into a **primary spermatocyte** (sper-MA-tō-sīt) that prepares to begin
meiosis. The daughter cells produced by the first meiotic division (meiosis I) are called
secondary spermatocytes. The completion of the second meiotic division (meiosis II)
produces four **spermatids** (SPER-muh-tidz), each containing 23 chromosomes. For
each primary spermatocyte that enters meiosis, four spermatids are produced. Because
cytokinesis is not completed in meiosis I or meiosis II, the four spermatids initially remain interconnected by cytoplasmic bridges. These connections assist in the transfer of
nutrients and hormonal messages between the cells, thus helping to ensure that the
cells develop in synchrony.

Spermatids are small, relatively unspecialized cells. In the process of **spermiogenesis** (spur-mē-ō-JEN-e-sis), spermatids differentiate into physically mature **spermatozoa** (spur-ma-tō-ZŌ-uh; singular *spermatozoon*). Spermatozoa are among the most highly
specialized cells in the body, and spermiogenesis involves major changes in the internal
and external structure of the spermatid.

Oogenesis

Ovum production, or oogenesis (Figure 7–3), begins before birth, accelerates at puberty, and ends at menopause. Between puberty and menopause, oogenesis occurs on a regular basis, as part of the ovarian cycle.

Unlike the situation in the male gonads, the stem cells or **oogonia** (ō-ō-GŌ-nē-uh), of the female complete their mitotic divisions before birth. Between the third and seventh months of fetal development, the daughter cells, or **primary oocytes** (Ō-ō-sīts), prepare to undergo meiosis. They proceed as far as prophase I of meiosis, but at that time the process comes to a halt. The primary oocytes then remain in a state of suspended development until puberty. At that time, rising levels of specific hormones start the

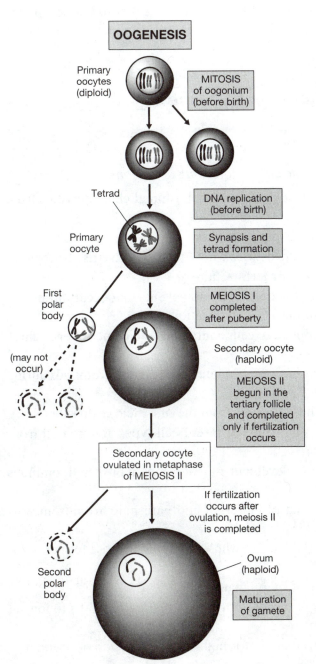

Figure 7–3   Oogenesis.

In oogenesis, a single primary oocyte produces an ovum and two or three nonfunctional polar bodies. Compare with Figure 7–2.

ovarian cycle, and in each cycle thereafter some of the primary oocytes will be stimulated to undergo further development. Not all of the primary oocytes produced in development survive until puberty. There are roughly 2 million primary oocytes in the ovaries at birth; by the time of puberty that number has declined to around 400,000. The rest of the primary oocytes along with their support cells degenerate, a process called **atresia** (a-TRĒ-zē-a).

Although the nuclear events under way during meiosis in the ovary are the same as those in the testes, the process differs in two important details:

1. The cytoplasm of the primary oocyte is not evenly distributed during the two meiotic divisions. Oogenesis produces one functional ovum, which contains most of the original cytoplasm, and three nonfunctional polar bodies that later disintegrate.

2. The ovary releases a **secondary oocyte** rather than a mature ovum. The secondary oocyte is suspended in metaphase of meiosis II, and meiosis will not be completed until fertilization occurs.

Let's Review What You've Just Learned

▶ **Definitions**

In the space provided, write the term for each of the following definitions.

_____ 1. The transfer of genetically determined characteristics from one generation to another.

_____ 2. The process of sperm formation.

_____ 3. Stem cells in the ovaries whose divisions give rise to oocytes.

_____ 4. Another term for fertilization.

_____ 5. The study of the developmental events that occur during the first two months after fertilization.

_____ 6. The term applied to cells containing two copies of each chromosome.

_____ 7. The exchange of genetic material between chromatids during prophase I of meiosis.

_____ 8. The egg cell that results from the first meiotic division.

_____ 9. The process by which different cell types are created from stem cells.

_____ 10. The process of development that begins at birth and continues to maturity.

_____ 11. The combining of maternal and paternal chromosomes to form tetrads during meiosis.

_____ 12. Stem cells in the testes whose divisions give rise to spermatocytes.

_____ 13. The process of sperm maturation.

_____ 14. The events that occur during the first two months following fertilization.

_____ 15. Meiotic cells that are formed from the division of oogonia.

_____ 16. A special form of cell division involved in gamete production.

_____ **17.** The sperm cells that result from the second meiotic division.

_____ **18.** The process by which primary oocytes and their support cells degenerate.

_____ **19.** The term for mature sperm cells.

_____ **20.** The study of the mechanisms responsible for inheritance.

_____ **21.** A cell division in which the number of chromosomes is reduced to one half the original number.

_____ **22.** The cells that are formed at the end of the first meiotic division in males.

_____ **23.** The term for a cell that contains only one copy of each chromosome.

_____ **24.** A collective term for embryological and fetal development.

_____ **25.** Tubular structures in the testes that are the site of sperm production.

_____ **26.** The matched set of four chromatids that is formed during prophase I of meiosis.

_____ **27.** The general term for a process in which gametes are formed.

_____ **28.** The process of aging.

_____ **29.** A type of cell division that produces daughter cells with the same number of chromosomes as the parent cell.

_____ **30.** The development that occurs between the beginning of the ninth week and birth.

_____ **31.** Meiotic cells that are formed from divisions of spermatogonia.

_____ **32.** The process of producing ova.

► Word Roots, Prefixes, Suffixes, and Combining Forms

In the space provided, list the boldfaced terms introduced in this section that contain the indicated word part.

Word Part	Meaning	Examples
oo-	egg	**33.** _____
tetra-	four	**34.** _____
-cyte	cell	**35.** _____
nata-	birth	**36.** _____
fer-	to carry	**37.** _____

► Completion

Complete the following table by filling in the blank with the phase of meiosis or description.

	Phase of Meiosis	Description
38.		Tetrads line up along the equatorial plate.
39.	anaphase I	
40.	prophase I	
41.		Chromatids separate and become chromosomes.
42.		Haploid nuclei are formed.
43.	metaphase II	

► **Labeling**

Label the cells in this diagram of spermatogenesis.

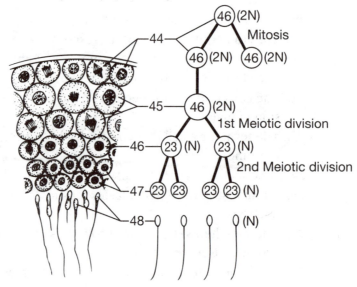

44. _____   47. _____

45. _____   48. _____

46. _____

Label the cells in this diagram of oogenesis.

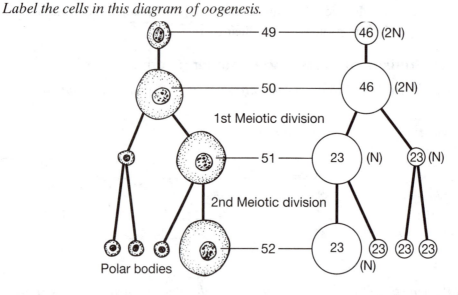

49. _____   51. _____

50. _____   52. _____

FERTILIZATION

Fertilization involves the fusion of two haploid gametes, producing a **zygote** (ZĪ-gōt; Greek *zygotos*, yoked) containing the normal somatic number of chromosomes (46 in humans). The functional roles and contributions of the spermatozoon and the ovum are very different. The spermatozoon simply delivers the paternal chromosomes to the site of fertilization. It is the ovum that must provide all of the nourishment and genetic programming to support the embryonic development for nearly a week after conception. The volume of the ovum is therefore much greater than that of the spermatozoon. At the time of fertilization, the diameter of the ovum is more than twice the entire length of the spermatozoon. The relationship between the egg and sperm volumes is even more striking, on the order of 2000:1.

The sperm arriving in the vagina are already motile, but they cannot fertilize an egg until they have undergone **capacitation** (ka-pas-i-TĀ-shun), a process in which the spermatozoon is activated so that it can fertilize an ovum. It appears that a substance secreted by the male reproductive tract prevents capacitation while spermatozoa are within the male. However, the precise mechanism of capacitation within the female reproductive tract remains uncertain.

Normal fertilization occurs in a structure called the **uterine tube**, usually within a day of ovulation. Over this period of time, the oocyte has traveled a few centimeters, but the spermatozoa must cover the distance between the vagina and the egg. Since an individual spermatozoon can propel itself at speeds of only about 12.5 cm (5 in.) per hour, it should be several hours before any spermatozoa arrive in the vicinity of the egg. The actual passage of time, however, ranges from 2 hours to as little as 30 minutes. Contractions of the uterine musculature and ciliary currents in the uterine tubes have been suggested as likely mechanisms for accelerating the movement of spermatozoa from the vagina to the fertilization site.

Even with this transport assistance, this is not an easy trip. Of the roughly 200 million spermatozoa introduced into the vagina in a typical ejaculation, only around 10,000 enter the uterine tube, and fewer than 100 actually reach the vicinity of the egg. Large numbers of spermatozoa are required for successful fertilization because of the condition of the oocyte at ovulation.

The Oocyte at Ovulation

Ovulation occurs before the oocyte is completely mature: The secondary oocyte leaving the follicle (a specialized structure in which the ovum develops) is in metaphase of the second meiotic division. The cell's metabolic operations have been discontinued, and the oocyte drifts in a sort of suspended animation, awaiting the stimulus for further development. If fertilization does not occur, the oocyte disintegrates without completing meiosis.

Fertilization is complicated by the fact that when it leaves the ovary, the oocyte is surrounded by a layer of cells called the **corona** (co-RŌ-nuh; Latin *corona*, crown) **radiata** (rā-dē-AH-ta; Latin *radiata*, radiant). The events that follow are diagrammed in Figure 7–4. The cells of the corona radiata protect the secondary oocyte as it passes from the ovary into the uterine tube. Although the physical process of fertilization requires only a single sperm in contact with the oocyte membrane, that spermatozoon must first penetrate the corona radiata. The sperm cell contains hyaluronidase, an enzyme that breaks down the intercellular cement between adjacent cells of the corona. At least a hundred spermatozoa must release hyaluronidase before the connections between the cells break down enough to permit fertilization.

No matter how many spermatozoa slip through the gap between cells, normally only a single spermatozoon will accomplish fertilization and activate the oocyte. When that spermatozoon contacts the secondary oocyte, the plasma membranes of the two cells fuse, and the sperm enters the **ooplasm** (Ō-ō-plazm), or cytoplasm of the oocyte. This event alters the chemical environment inside the oocyte, and **oocyte activation** occurs.

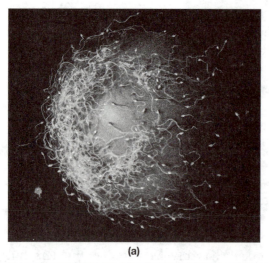

(a)

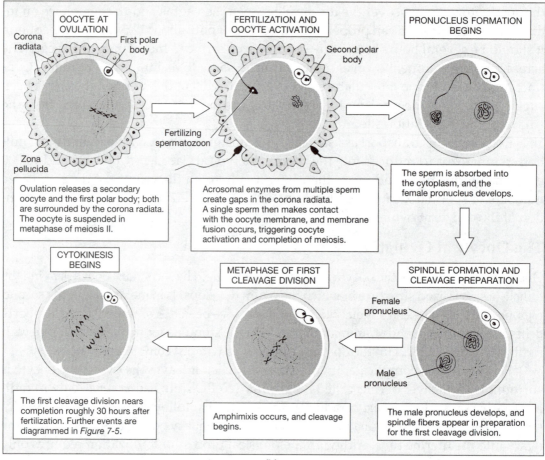

(b)

Figure 7–4 Fertilization.

Fertilization and the preparations for cleavage.

Oocyte Activation

Activation involves a series of changes in the metabolic activity of the oocyte. The most dramatic changes are:

1. The metabolic rate of the oocyte increases rapidly, and meiosis II is completed.

2. Vesicles just beneath the surface of the oocyte fuse with the cell membrane and discharge their contents through exocytosis. This process, called a **cortical reaction**, is responsible for preventing penetration by more than one sperm, a condition known as **polyspermy** (POL-ē-spur-mē). If the oocyte cortical reaction is abnormal, and polyspermy does occur, the zygote will die.

Pronucleus Formation and Amphimixis

After oocyte activation and the completion of meiosis, the nuclear material remaining within the ovum reorganizes as the **female pronucleus**. While these changes are under way, the nucleus of the spermatozoon swells, becoming the **male pronucleus**. The male pronucleus then migrates toward the center of the cell, and the two pronuclei fuse in a process called **amphimixis** (am-fi-MIK-sis). Fertilization is now complete, with the formation of a zygote containing the normal complement of 46 chromosomes.

Induction and the Regulation of Development

During prenatal development, a single cell forms a 3–4 kg infant that in postnatal development grows through adolescence and maturity toward old age and eventual death. One of the most fascinating aspects of development is its apparent order and simplicity. A continuity exists at all levels and at all times. Nothing leaps into existence, unannounced and without apparent precursors: Differentiation and increasing structural complexity occur hand in hand.

Differentiation involves different changes in the genetic activity of different cells. Chapter 4 considered the exchange of information between the nucleus and cytoplasm in a cell. Activity in the nucleus varies in response to chemical messages arriving from the surrounding cytoplasm. In turn, ongoing nuclear activity will alter conditions within the cytoplasm by directing the synthesis of specific proteins. In this way, the nucleus can affect enzyme activity, cell structure, and membrane properties.

In development, differences in the cytoplasmic composition of individual cells trigger alterations in genetic activity. These changes in turn lead to further changes in the cytoplasm, and the process continues in a sequential fashion. But if all the cells of the embryo are derived from cell divisions of a zygote, how do the cytoplasmic differences originate? What sets this process in motion? The important first step occurs before fertilization while the oocyte is in the ovary.

Before ovulation, the growing oocyte accepts amino acids, nucleotides, and glucose as well as more-complex materials such as phospholipids, mRNAs, and proteins from the surrounding cells. Because these cells are not all manufacturing and delivering the same nutrients and instructions to the oocyte, the contents of the oocyte cytoplasm are not evenly distributed. After fertilization, subsequent divisions subdivide the cytoplasm of the zygote into ever smaller cells that differ from one another in their cytoplasmic composition. These differences alter genetic activity, creating cell lines with increasingly diverse fates.

As development proceeds, some of these cells will release chemical substances, such as RNAs, polypeptides, and small proteins, that affect the differentiation of other embryonic cells. This type of chemical interplay between developing cells is called **induction** (in-DUK-shun). Induction can work over very short distances, as when two different cell types are in direct contact. It may also operate over longer distances, with the inducing chemicals functioning as hormones.

This type of regulation, which involves an integrated series of interacting steps, can control very complex processes. The mechanism is not without risk, however, and the appearance of an abnormal or inappropriate inducer can throw the entire development plan off course.

Let's Review What You've Just Learned

► **Definitions**

In the space provided, write the term for each of the following definitions.

_____ **53.** The process in which the male and female pronuclei fuse.

_____ **54.** The cytoplasm of an ovum.

_____ **55.** Fertilization of an egg by more than one spermatozoon.

_____ **56.** The cell produced by the fusion of two haploid gametes.

_____ **57.** The site where fertilization normally takes place.

_____ **58.** The reorganized nuclear material of an egg cell after activation.

_____ **59.** The process by which one cell affects the development of another by means of chemical stimuli.

_____ **60.** The process in which gametes fuse to form a diploid cell.

_____ **61.** The layer of cells that surrounds the secondary oocyte at the time of ovulation.

_____ **62.** A swollen male nucleus within the cytoplasm of an egg cell.

_____ **63.** A reaction involving the egg cell membrane that results in blocking sperm from penetrating the membrane.

_____ **64.** A process that occurs in the female reproductive tract whereby a sperm cell is rendered capable of fertilizing an ovum.

_____ **65.** The process that occurs immediately after fertilization during which the metabolic rate of the ovum increases and chemical changes involving the membrane block other sperm cells from penetrating.

► **Word Roots, Prefixes, Suffixes, and Combining Forms**

In the space provided, list the boldfaced terms introduced in this section that contain the indicated word part.

Word Part	Meaning	Examples
poly-	many	**66.** _____
zyg-	yoked	**67.** _____
pro-	before	**68.** _____
coron-	crown	**69.** _____
amphi-	both	**70.** _____

PRENATAL DEVELOPMENT

The time spent in prenatal development is known as the period of **gestation** (jes-TĀ-shun; Latin *gestare*, to carry). For convenience, the gestation period is usually considered as three integrated **trimesters**, each 3 months in duration:

- The **first trimester** is the period of embryonic and early fetal development. During this period the rudiments of all the major organ systems appear.

- In the **second trimester** the organs and organ systems complete most of their development. The body proportions change, and by the end of the second trimester the fetus looks distinctively human.

- The **third trimester** is characterized by rapid fetal growth. Early in the third trimester most of the major organ systems become fully functional, and an infant born 1 month or even 2 months prematurely has a reasonable chance of survival.

THE FIRST TRIMESTER

At the moment of conception, the fertilized ovum is a single cell with a diameter of around 0.135 mm (0.005 in.). In the first month, its weight increases by a factor of 140,000. By the end of the first trimester (twelfth developmental week) the fetus is almost 75 mm (3 in.) long and weighs perhaps 14 g (0.5 oz). Many important and complex developmental events occur during the first trimester. We will focus on four general processes: cleavage, implantation, placentation, and embryogenesis.

1. **Cleavage** (KLĒV-ij) is a sequence of cell divisions that begins immediately after fertilization and ends at the first contact with the uterine wall. Over this period the zygote becomes a **pre-embryo** that develops into a multicellular complex known as a **blastocyst** (BLAS-tō-sist; Greek *blastos*, germ + *kystis*, bladder).

2. **Implantation** begins with the attachment of the blastocyst to the lining of the uterus and continues as the blastocyst invades the maternal tissues. During the time implantation is under way, other important events take place that set the stage for the formation of vital embryonic structures.

3. **Placentation** (plas-en-TĀ-shun) occurs as blood vessels form around the periphery of the blastocyst and the placenta appears. The **placenta** is a vital link between maternal and embryonic systems that will support the fetus during the second and third trimesters.

4. **Embryogenesis** (em-brē-ō-JEN-e-sis) is the formation of a viable embryo. This process establishes the foundations for all major organ systems.

These processes are both complex and vital to the survival of the embryo. Perhaps because the events in the first trimester are so complex, this is the most dangerous period in prenatal life. Only about 40 percent of conceptions produce embryos that survive the first trimester. For this reason pregnant women are usually warned to take great care to avoid drugs or other disruptive stresses during the first trimester, in the hopes of preventing an error in the delicate processes under way.

Cleavage and Blastocyst Formation

Cleavage (Figure 7–5) is a series of cell divisions that subdivides the cytoplasm of the zygote. The first cleavage division produces a pre-embryo consisting of two identical cells. After 3 days of cleavage, the pre-embryo is a solid ball of cells, resembling a mulberry. This stage is called the **morula** (MOR-ū-la; Latin *morula*, mulberry). The morula usually reaches the uterus on day 4. Over the next 2 days, the cells of the morula form a hollow ball, the blastocyst, with an inner cavity known as the **blastocoele** (BLAS-tō-sēl; Greek *blastos*, germ + *koilia*, cavity). The cells are no longer identical in size and shape. The outer layer

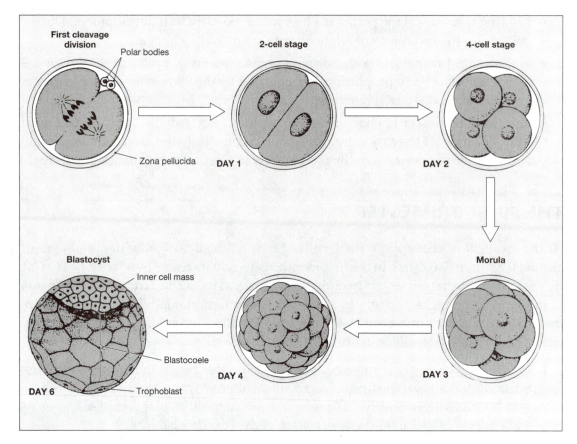

Figure 7–5   Cleavage and Blastocyst Formation.

of cells, which separates the outside world from the blastocoele, is called the **trophoblast** (TRŌ-fō-blast; *trophe*, nourish + *blastos*, germ). The function of this layer is implied by the name. These cells will be responsible for providing food to the developing embryo. A second group of cells, the **inner cell mass**, lies clustered at one end of the blastocyst. These cells are exposed to the blastocoele but insulated from contact with the outside environment by the trophoblast. In time, the inner cell mass will form the embryo.

Implantation

At fertilization the zygote is still 4 days away from the uterus. The events previously discussed occur as the pre-embryo travels through the uterine tube to the uterus. During this time, the pre-embryo is moved by the ciliary currents and muscle contractions of the uterine tube. The pre-embryo arrives in the uterine cavity as a morula, and over the next 2–3 days blastocyst formation occurs. Over this period the cells are gaining nutrients from the fluid within the uterine cavity. This fluid, rich in glycogen, is secreted by glands in the uterine lining. When fully formed, the blastocyst contacts the uterine lining and implantation occurs. Stages in the implantation process are illustrated in Figure 7–6.

Implantation begins as the surface of the blastocyst closest to the inner cell mass touches and adheres to the uterine lining (see day 7, Figure 7–6). At the point of contact the trophoblast cells divide rapidly, making the trophoblast several layers thick. Near the uterine wall, the cell membranes separating the trophoblast cells disappear, creating a layer of cytoplasm containing multiple nuclei (day 8). This outer layer is called the **syncytial** (sin-SISH-al) **trophoblast**, or **syncytiotrophoblast** (sin-sish-ē-ō-TRŌ-fō-blast).

Figure 7–6 Stages in the Implantation Process.

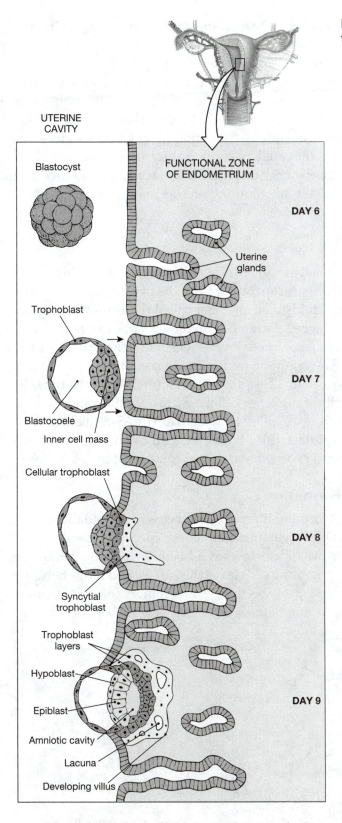

The syncytial trophoblast erodes a path through the uterine epithelium by secreting the enzyme hyaluronidase. This enzyme dissolves the intercellular cement between adjacent epithelial cells, just as the hyaluronidase released by spermatozoa dissolves the connections between cells of the corona radiata. At first, this erosion creates a gap in the uterine lining, but the migration and divisions of epithelial cells soon repair the surface.

When the repairs are completed, the blastocyst loses contact with the uterine cavity, and development occurs entirely within the uterine lining.

As implantation proceeds, the syncytial trophoblast continues to enlarge and spread into the surrounding tissue. The digestion of glands in the uterine lining releases nutrients that are absorbed by the syncytial trophoblast and distributed by diffusion across the underlying cellular trophoblast to the inner cell mass. These nutrients provide the energy needed to support the early stages of embryo formation. Trophoblastic extensions grow around uterine capillaries and, as the capillary walls are destroyed, maternal blood begins to percolate through trophoblastic channels known as **lacunae**. Fingerlike villi extend away from the trophoblast into the surrounding uterine lining, and these extensions gradually increase in size and complexity.

Formation of the Blastodisc

In the early blastocyst stage the inner cell mass has little visible organization. Yet by the time of implantation, the inner cell mass is separating from the trophoblast. The separation gradually increases, creating a fluid-filled chamber called the **amniotic** (am-nē-OT-ik) **cavity**. The trophoblast will later be separated from the amniotic cavity by layers of cells that originate at the inner cell mass. These layers, which line the amniotic cavity, form the **amnion** (AM-nē-on). The amniotic cavity can be seen in day 9 of Figure 7–6, and additional details from days 10 to 12 are shown in Figure 7–7. At the time the amniotic cavity first appears, the cells of the inner cell mass are organized into an oval sheet that is two cell layers thick. This oval, called a **blastodisc** (BLAS-tō-disk), initially consists of an epithelial layer, or **epiblast** (EP-i-blast), facing the amniotic cavity and an underlying **hypoblast** (HĪ-pō-blast) exposed to the fluid contents of the blastocoele.

Gastrulation and Germ Layer Formation

A few days later, a third layer begins forming through the process of **gastrulation** (gas-troo-LĀ-shun) (day 12, Figure 7–7). During gastrulation, cells in specific areas of the epiblast move toward the center of the blastodisc, toward a line known as the **primitive streak**. At the primitive streak these migrating cells leave the surface and move between the epiblast and hypoblast. This movement creates three distinct embryonic layers, called **primary germ layers**, with markedly different fates. Once gastrulation begins, the layer

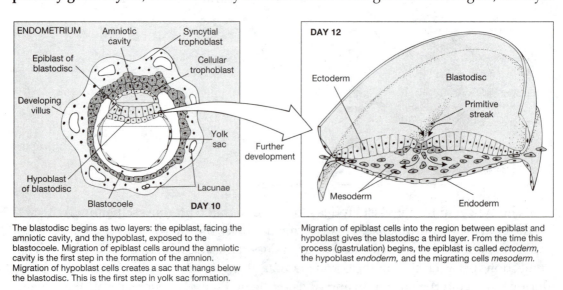

The blastodisc begins as two layers: the epiblast, facing the amniotic cavity, and the hypoblast, exposed to the blastocoele. Migration of epiblast cells around the amniotic cavity is the first step in the formation of the amnion. Migration of hypoblast cells creates a sac that hangs below the blastodisc. This is the first step in yolk sac formation.

Migration of epiblast cells into the region between epiblast and hypoblast gives the blastodisc a third layer. From the time this process (gastrulation) begins, the epiblast is called *ectoderm*, the hypoblast *endoderm*, and the migrating cells *mesoderm*.

Figure 7–7 Blastodisc Organization and Gastrulation.

remaining in contact with the amniotic cavity is called the **ectoderm** (EK-tō-durm), the hypoblast is known as the **endoderm** (EN-dō-durm), and the intervening, poorly organized layer is the **mesoderm** (MEZ-ō-durm). Table 7–1 contains a listing of the contributions each germ layer makes to the various body systems.

The Formation of Extraembryonic Membranes

Germ layers also participate in the formation of four **extraembryonic** (eks-truh-em-brē-ON-ik) **membranes**: the yolk sac (endoderm and mesoderm), the amnion (ectoderm and mesoderm), the allantois (endoderm and mesoderm), and the chorion (mesoderm and trophoblast). Although these membranes support embryonic and fetal development, they leave few traces of their existence in adult systems. Figure 7–8 shows representative stages in the development of the extraembryonic membranes.

- **The yolk sac:** The first of the extraembryonic membranes to appear is the **yolk sac**. The yolk sac begins as the hypoblast cells spread out around the outer edges of the blastocoele to form a complete pouch suspended below the blastodisc. This pouch is already visible 10 days after fertilization (Figure 7–7). As gastrulation proceeds, mesodermal cells migrate around this pouch and complete the formation of the yolk sac (Figure 7–8). Blood vessels soon appear within the mesoderm, and the yolk sac becomes an important site of blood cell formation.

- **The amnion:** The ectodermal layer also undergoes an expansion, and ectodermal cells spread over the inner surface of the amniotic cavity. Mesodermal cells soon follow, creating a second, outer layer (Figure 7–8). This combination of mesoderm and

---

Table 7–1 The Fates of the Primary Germ Layers

Ectodermal Contributions

Integumentary system: epidermis, hair follicles and hairs, nails and glands communicating with the skin (apocrine and merocrine sweat glands, mammary glands, and sebaceous glands)

Skeletal system: pharyngeal cartilages and their derivatives in the adult (portion of sphenoid bone, the auditory ossicles, the styloid processes of the temporal bones, the cornu and superior rim of the hyoid bone)

Nervous system: all neural tissue, including brain and spinal cord

Endocrine system: pituitary gland and adrenal medullae

Respiratory system: mucous epithelium of nasal passageways

Digestive system: mucous epithelium of mouth and anus, salivary glands

Mesodermal Contributions

Skeletal system: all components except some pharyngeal derivatives

Muscular system: all components

Endocrine system: adrenal cortex, endocrine tissues of heart, kidneys, and gonads

Cardiovascular system: all components, including bone marrow

Lymphatic system: all components

Urinary system: the kidneys, including the nephrons and the initial portions of the collecting system

Reproductive system: the gonads and the adjacent portions of the duct systems

Miscellaneous: the lining of the body cavities (thoracic, pericardial, and peritoneal) and the connective tissues that support all organ systems

Endodermal Contributions

Endocrine system: thymus, thyroid, and pancreas

Respiratory system: respiratory epithelium (except nasal passageways) and associated mucous glands

Digestive system: mucous epithelium (except mouth and anus), exocrine glands (except salivary glands), liver, and pancreas

Urinary system: urinary bladder and distal portions of the duct system

Reproductive system: distal portions of the duct system, stem cells that produce gametes

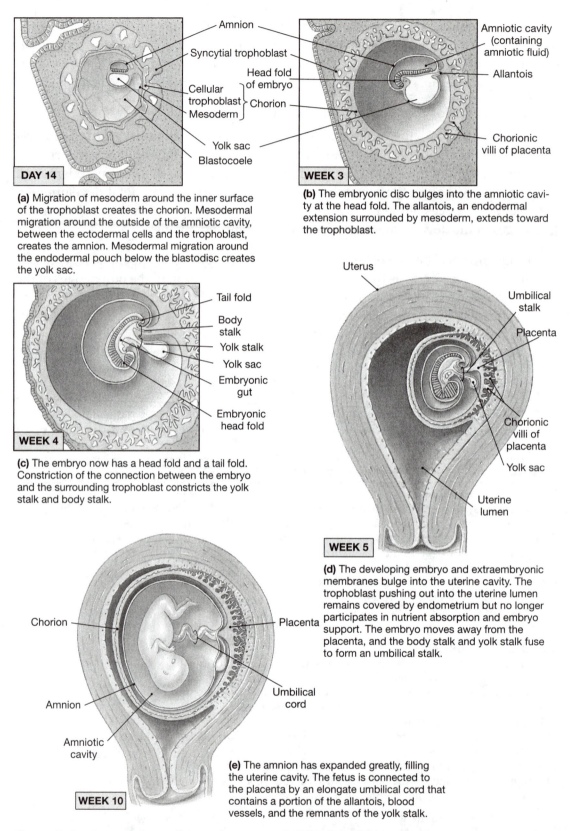

(a) Migration of mesoderm around the inner surface of the trophoblast creates the chorion. Mesodermal migration around the outside of the amniotic cavity, between the ectodermal cells and the trophoblast, creates the amnion. Mesodermal migration around the endodermal pouch below the blastodisc creates the yolk sac.

(b) The embryonic disc bulges into the amniotic cavity at the head fold. The allantois, an endodermal extension surrounded by mesoderm, extends toward the trophoblast.

(c) The embryo now has a head fold and a tail fold. Constriction of the connection between the embryo and the surrounding trophoblast constricts the yolk stalk and body stalk.

(d) The developing embryo and extraembryonic membranes bulge into the uterine cavity. The trophoblast pushing out into the uterine lumen remains covered by endometrium but no longer participates in nutrient absorption and embryo support. The embryo moves away from the placenta, and the body stalk and yolk stalk fuse to form an umbilical stalk.

(e) The amnion has expanded greatly, filling the uterine cavity. The fetus is connected to the placenta by an elongate umbilical cord that contains a portion of the allantois, blood vessels, and the remnants of the yolk stalk.

Figure 7–8 **Extraembryonic Membranes and Placenta Formation.**

ectoderm is the amnion. As development proceeds, this membrane continues to expand, increasing the size of the amniotic cavity. The amnion encloses **amniotic fluid** that surrounds and cushions the developing embryo or fetus (Figure 7–8).

- **The allantois:** The third extraembryonic membrane begins as an outpocketing of the endoderm near the base of the yolk sac (Figure 7–8b). This sac of endoderm and mesoderm is the **allantois** (a-LAN-tō-is). The base of the allantois later gives rise to the urinary bladder.

- **The chorion:** The mesoderm associated with the allantois spreads until it extends completely around the inside, forming a mesodermal layer underneath the trophoblast. This combination of mesoderm and trophoblast is the **chorion** (KŌR-ē-on) (Figure 7–8b). When implantation first occurs, the nutrients absorbed by the trophoblast can easily reach the blastodisc by simple diffusion. But as the embryo and the trophoblastic complex enlarge, the distance between the two increases, and diffusion alone can no longer keep pace with the demands of the developing embryo. Blood vessels now begin to develop within the mesoderm of the chorion, creating a rapid-transit system linking the embryo with the trophoblast.

The appearance of blood vessels in the chorion is the first step in the creation of a functional placenta. By the third week of development (Figures 7–8b and 7–9), the mesoderm extends along the core of each of the trophoblastic villi, forming **chorionic villi** in contact with maternal tissues. These villi continue to enlarge and branch, creating an intricate network within the lining of the uterus. Embryonic blood vessels develop within each of the villi, and circulation through those chorionic vessels begins early in the third week of development, when the heart starts beating.

As the chorionic villi enlarge, more maternal blood vessels are eroded, and maternal blood slowly percolates through lacunae lined by the syncytial trophoblast. Chorionic blood vessels pass close by, and exchange between the embryonic and maternal circulations occurs by diffusion across the syncytial and cellular trophoblast layers.

Placentation

At first the entire blastocyst is surrounded by chorionic villi. The chorion continues to enlarge, expanding like a balloon within the uterine lining, and by the fourth week the embryo, amnion, and yolk sac are suspended within an expansive, fluid-filled chamber (Figure 7–8c). The connection between embryo and chorion, known as the **body stalk**, contains the distal portions of the allantois and blood vessels carrying blood to and from the placenta. The narrow connection between the endoderm of the embryo and the yolk sac is called the **yolk stalk**.

As the end of the first trimester approaches, the fetus moves farther away from the placenta (Figure 7–8d, e). It remains connected by the **umbilical** (um-BIL-i-kul) **cord**, or **umbilical stalk**, which contains the allantois, the placental blood vessels, and the yolk stalk.

Figure 7–9a diagrams circulation at the placenta near the end of the first trimester. Blood flows to the placenta through the paired **umbilical arteries** and returns in a single **umbilical vein**. The chorionic villi (Figure 7–9b) provide the surface area for active and passive exchange between the fetal and maternal bloodstreams. The placenta places a considerable demand on the maternal cardiovascular system, and blood flow to the uterus and placenta is extensive. If the placenta is torn or otherwise damaged, the consequences may prove fatal for both fetus and mother.

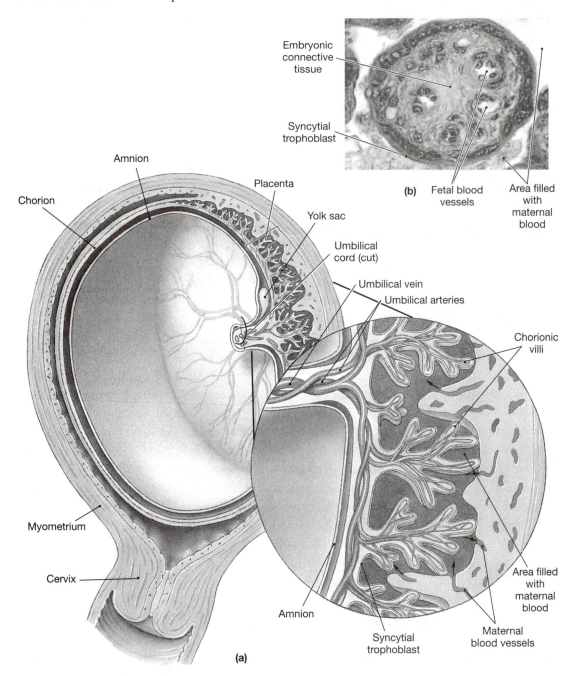

Figure 7–9   A Three-Dimensional View of Placental Structure.

For clarity, the uterus is shown after the embryo has been removed and the umbilical cord cut. Arrows indicate the direction of blood flow. Blood flows into the placenta through ruptured maternal blood arteries. It then flows around chorionic villi, which contain fetal blood vessels. Fetal blood arrives over paired umbilical arteries and leaves through a single umbilical vein. Maternal blood reenters the venous system of the mother through the broken walls of small uterine veins. Note that no actual mixing of maternal and fetal blood occurs.

Embryogenesis

Shortly after gastrulation begins, folding and differential growth of the embryonic disc produce a bulge that projects into the amniotic cavity (Figure 7–8b). This projection is known as the **head fold**, and similar movements lead to the formation of a **tail fold**

(Figure 7–8c). The embryo is now physically as well as developmentally separated from the blastodisc and the extraembryonic membranes. The definitive orientation of the embryo can now be seen, complete with dorsal and ventral surfaces and left and right sides.

These changes in proportions and appearance that occur between the fourth developmental week and the end of the first trimester are visually summarized in Figure 7–10. The first trimester is a critical period for development because events in the first 12 weeks establish the basis for organ formation, a process called **organogenesis** (or-ga-nō-JEN-e-sis).

THE SECOND AND THIRD TRIMESTERS

By the start of the second trimester (Figure 7–10c,d) the basic components of all the major organ systems have formed. Over the next 3 months, the fetus will grow to a weight of around 0.64 kg (1.4 lb). During this period, the fetus, encircled by the amnion, grows faster than the surrounding placenta. Figure 7–11 shows a 4-month fetus as viewed with a fiber-optic endoscope and a 6-month fetus as seen in ultrasound.

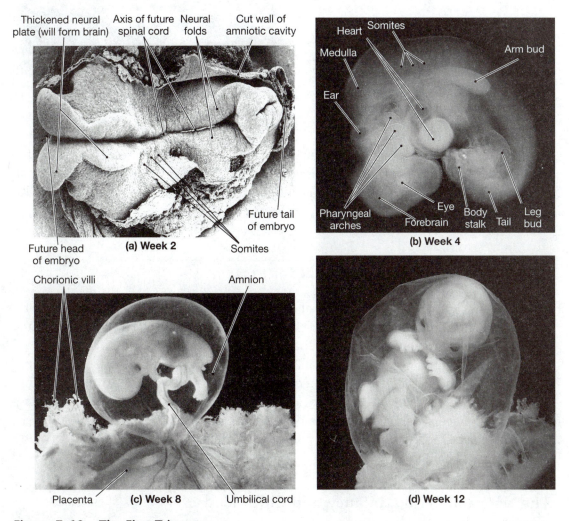

Figure 7–10   The First Trimester

(a) SEM of the superior surface of a monkey embryo after 2 weeks of development. A human embryo at this stage would look essentially the same. **(b–d)** Fiber-optic views of human embryos at 4, 8 and 12 weeks.

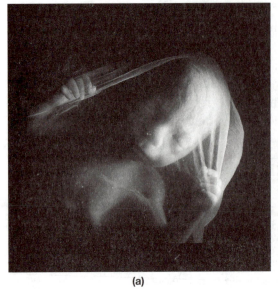

(a)

Figure 7–11   The Second and Third Trimesters.
A 4-month fetus, as seen through a fiber-optic endoscope. **(b)** Head of a 6-month fetus, as seen through ultrasound.

(b)

During the third trimester, the organ systems develop and most become ready to fulfill their normal functions. The rate of growth starts to decrease, but in absolute terms this trimester sees the largest weight gain. In 3 months the fetus puts on around 2.6 kg (5.7 lb), reaching a full-term weight of somewhere near 3.2 kg (7 lb).

POSTNATAL DEVELOPMENT

Developmental processes do not cease at delivery, for the newborn infant has few of the anatomical, functional, or physiological characteristics of the mature adult. In the course of postnatal development every individual passes through a number of **life stages**, each typified by a distinctive combination of characteristics and abilities. These stages are a familiar part of human experience. You could probably identify the features and functions associated with infancy, childhood, adolescence, and maturity. Although each stage has distinctive features, the transitions between them are gradual and the boundaries often indistinct. Once maturity has arrived, development ends, and the process of aging, or senescence, begins.

The Neonatal Period, Infancy, and Childhood

The **neonatal period** extends from the moment of birth to 1 month thereafter. **Infancy** then continues to 2 years of age, and **childhood** lasts until puberty commences. Two major events are under way during these developmental stages:

1. The major organ systems other than those associated with reproduction become fully operational and gradually acquire the functional characteristics of adult structures.

2. The individual grows rapidly, and there are significant changes in body proportions.

Pediatrics is a medical specialty focusing on postnatal development from infancy through adolescence. Because infants and young children cannot clearly describe the problems they are experiencing, pediatricians and parents must be skilled observers. A number of standardized testing procedures are used to assess an individual's developmental progress relative to normal values.

The Neonatal Period

A variety of physiological and anatomical alterations occur as the fetus completes the transition to the status of a newborn infant, or **neonate** (NĒ-ō-nāte). Before delivery, dissolved gases, nutrients, waste products, hormones, and antibodies were transferred across the placenta. At birth, the newborn infant must become relatively self-sufficient, with the processes of respiration, digestion, and excretion performed by its own specialized organs and organ systems. The transition from fetus to neonate may be summarized as follows:

1. The lungs at birth are collapsed and filled with fluid. Filling them with air involves a massive and powerful inspiratory movement.

2. When the lungs expand, the pattern of cardiovascular circulation changes because of alterations in blood pressure and flow rates.

3. Typical heart rates of 120–140 beats per minute and respiratory rates of 30 breaths per minute in neonates are considerably higher than those of adults.

4. Before birth, the digestive system remains relatively inactive, although it does accumulate a mixture of secretions, mucus, and epithelial cells. This collection of debris is excreted in the first few days of life. Over that period the newborn infant begins to nurse.

5. As waste products build up in the arterial blood they are filtered into the urine at the kidneys. The kidneys of neonates cannot concentrate urine to any significant degree. As a result, urinary water losses are high, and fluid requirements of neonates are much greater than those of adults.

6. The neonate has little ability to control body temperature, particularly in the first few days after delivery. As the infant grows larger and increases the thickness of its insulating subcutaneous adipose "blanket," its metabolic rate also rises. Daily and even hourly alterations in body temperature continue throughout childhood.

Throughout the neonatal period the newborn is dependent on nutrients contained in the milk secreted by the maternal mammary glands.

Infancy and Childhood

The most rapid growth occurs during prenatal development, and after delivery the relative rate of growth continues to decline. Postnatal growth during infancy and childhood occurs under the direction of circulating hormones. These hormones affect each

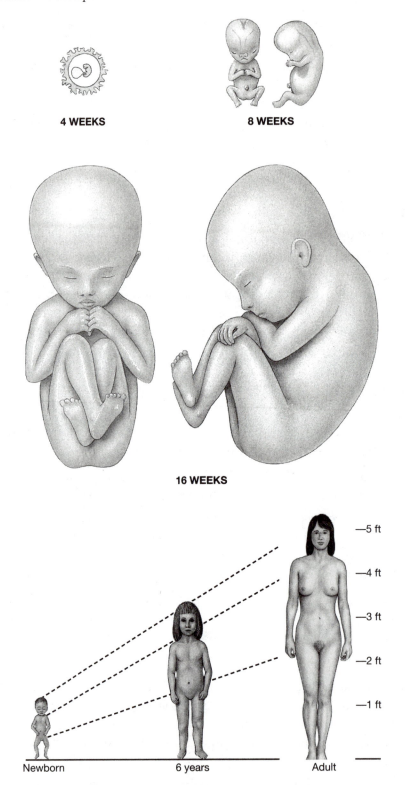

4 WEEKS

8 WEEKS

16 WEEKS

Newborn   6 years   Adult

—5 ft

—4 ft

—3 ft

—2 ft

—1 ft

Figure 7–12   Growth and Changes in Body Form.
The views at 4, 8, and 16 weeks are presented at actual size. Notice the changes in body form and proportions as development proceeds. These changes do not stop at birth. For example, the head, which contains the brain and sense organs, is relatively large at birth.

tissue and organ in specific ways, depending on the sensitivities of the individual cells. As a result, growth does not occur uniformly, and the body proportions gradually change (Figure 7–12).

Adolescence and Maturity

Adolescence begins at puberty, when sexual maturation takes place. Under the influence of several hormones, the ovaries in females and the testes in males initiate gametogenesis and the production of male or female sex hormones that stimulate the appearance of secondary sexual characteristics (anatomical changes indicative of each sex, such as development of the genitalia and body hair distribution) and behaviors.

In the years that follow, the continued background secretion of sex hormones maintains these sexual characteristics. In addition, the combination of sex hormones and other hormones leads to a sudden acceleration in the growth rate. The timing of the increase in size varies between the sexes, corresponding to different ages at the onset of puberty. In girls, the growth rate is maximum between ages 10 and 13, whereas boys grow most rapidly between ages 12 and 15. Growth continues at a slower pace until ages 18–21.

The boundary between adolescence and maturity is very hazy, for it has physical, emotional, behavioral, and legal aspects. Maturity is often associated with the end of growth in the late teens or early twenties. Although growth normally ceases at maturity, physiological changes continue. These changes are part of the process of senescence, or aging. Aging reduces the efficiency and capabilities of the individual, and even in the absence of other factors senescence will ultimately lead to death.

Table 7–2 summarizes the age-related changes that occur in the body's systems. Taken together, these alterations reduce the functional abilities of the individual. They also affect homeostatic mechanisms. As a result, the elderly are less able to make homeostatic adjustments in response to internal or environmental stresses than are younger persons. As immune function deteriorates, the risks of contracting a variety of bacterial or viral diseases are proportionately increased. This deterioration leads to drastic physiological alterations that affect all internal systems. Death finally occurs when some combination of stresses cannot be countered by existing homeostatic mechanisms.

Physicians attempt to forestall death by adjusting homeostatic mechanisms or removing the sources of stress. **Geriatrics** (jer-ē-AT-ricks; Greek *gerios*, old age) is a medical specialty concerned with the mechanics of the aging process, and physicians trained in geriatrics are known as **geriatricians** (jer-ē-uh-TRISH-unz). Problems commonly encountered by geriatricians include infections, cancers, heart disease, strokes, arthritis, and anemia; these conditions can be directly related to the age-induced changes in vital systems.

Table 7–2   Effects of Aging on Organ Systems

The characteristic physical and functional alterations that are part of the aging process affect all organ systems. Examples include:

- A loss of elasticity in the skin that produces sagging and wrinkling
- A decline in the rate of bone deposition, leading to weak bones, and degenerative changes in joints that make them less mobile
- Reductions in muscular strength and ability
- Impairment of coordination, memory, and intellectual function
- Reductions in the production of and sensitivity to circulating hormones
- Appearance of cardiovascular problems and a reduction in blood flow that can affect a variety of vital organs
- Reduced sensitivity and responsiveness of the immune system, leading to problems with infection and cancer
- Reduced elasticity in the lungs, leading to decreased respiratory function
- Decreased smooth muscle activity and muscle tone along the digestive tract
- Decreased peristalsis and muscle tone in the urinary system, coupled with a reduction in the rate of urine production
- Functional impairment of the reproductive system, which eventually becomes inactive

✎ Let's Review What You've Just Learned

▶ **Definitions**

In the space provided, write the term for each of the following definitions.

_____ 71. The group of cells in the blastocyst that will form the embryo.

_____ 72. The developmental process that results in the formation of germ layers.

_____ 73. The fluid-filled chamber that surrounds the developing embryo as it grows and becomes a fetus.

_____ 74. The germ layer formed from the hypoblast.

_____ 75. A pouch containing nutrients that is suspended below the blastodisc; it is the first extraembryonic membrane to form.

_____ 76. The process of forming a viable embryo.

_____ 77. The sequence of cell divisions that begins immediately after fertilization.

_____ 78. Blood vessels in the umbilical cord that carry blood from the fetus to the placenta.

_____ 79. The period of time spent in prenatal development.

_____ 80. A solid mass of cells formed from the zygote after approximately three days of cleavage.

_____ 81. The outer layer of the blastocyst.

_____ 82. The extraembryonic membrane that is a sac composed of endoderm and mesoderm.

_____ 83. The structure that connects the fetus to the placenta.

_____ 84. An oval sheet two cell layers thick that is formed from the inner cell mass.

_____ 85. A special organ in females that develops only during pregnancy and functions as a link between maternal and embryonic, and later fetal, systems.

_____ 86. One of the three divisions of the gestation period.

_____ 87. The layer of the blastodisc that faces the amniotic cavity.

_____ 88. The germ layer that develops from the epiblast.

_____ 89. The extraembryonic membrane enclosing the fluid-filled cavity that surrounds the fetus.

_____ 90. The connection between the embryo and the chorion.

_____ 91. The line formed in the center of the blastodisc where cells leave the surface and migrate between the epiblast and the hypoblast.

_____ 92. The process by which the blastocyst attaches to and then invades the uterine lining.

_____ 93. The cavity inside of the blastocyst.

_____ 94. The germ layer that forms in the space between the endoderm and ectoderm.

_____ 95. The fluid that fills the amniotic cavity.

_____   **96.** The blood vessel in the umbilical cord that carries blood from the placenta to the fetus.

_____   **97.** The medical specialty focusing on postnatal development from infancy through adolescence.

_____   **98.** The process of organ formation.

_____   **99.** A hollow ball of cells that forms from the morula.

_____   **100.** The process of forming a placenta.

_____   **101.** The structure that connects the embryo to the yolk sac.

_____   **102.** A medical specialty concerned with the mechanics of the aging process.

_____   **103.** The layer of the blastodisc exposed to the fluid contents of the blastocoele.

_____   **104.** Channels in the trophoblast that contain maternal blood.

_____   **105.** The outer layer of the trophoblast consisting of a mass of mult-inucleate cytoplasm.

_____   **106.** Fingerlike extensions of mesoderm that are in contact with maternal tissues.

_____   **107.** Membranes derived from the germ layers that function in support of embryonic and fetal development.

_____   **108.** The extraembryonic membrane formed from the combination of mesoderm and trophoblast.

► Word Roots, Prefixes, Suffixes, and Combining Forms

In the space provided, list the boldfaced terms introduced in this section that contain the indicated word part.

Word Part	Meaning		Examples
blast-	precursor	**109.**	_____
epi-	on	**110.**	_____
gest-	to bear	**111.**	_____
neo-	new	**112.**	_____
tri-	three	**113.**	_____
tropho-	nutrition	**114.**	_____
geri-	old	**115.**	_____
-coel	cavity	**116.**	_____
hypo-	under	**117.**	_____
meso-	middle	**118.**	_____
pedia-	child	**119.**	_____
extra-	outside of	**120.**	_____
-derm	skin	**121.**	_____
-genesis	give birth	**122.**	_____
syn-	together	**123.**	_____
ecto-	outside	**124.**	_____
endo-	inside	**125.**	_____

▶ **Completion**

Complete the following table by filling in the blank with a description of the main events occurring during each trimester.

	Trimester	Main Events
126.	First trimester	
127.	Second trimester	
128.	Third trimester	

▶ **Labeling**

Label the numbered structures and processes on the following diagram of development.

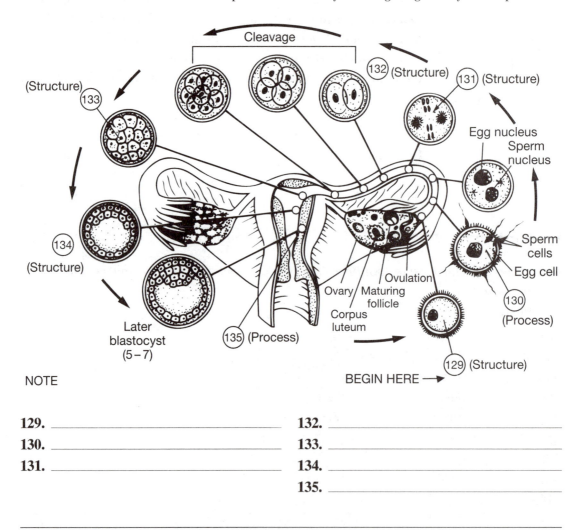

NOTE

BEGIN HERE ➤

129. _____		**132.** _____	
130. _____		**133.** _____	
131. _____		**134.** _____	
		135. _____	

GENETICS AND INHERITANCE

Every somatic cell in the body carries copies of the original 46 chromosomes present in the zygote. Those chromosomes and their component genes represent the individual's **genotype** (JĒN-ō-tīp), or hereditary makeup. Through development and differentiation, the instructions contained within the genotype are expressed in many different ways. No single living cell or tissue makes use of all the information and instructions contained within the genotype. For example, in muscle fibers the genes important for the formation of excitable membranes and contractile proteins are active, whereas a different set of genes controlling specific enzyme and hormone production is operating in the cells of the pancreas. Collectively, however, the instructions contained within the genotype determine the anatomical and physiological characteristics of each individual. Those characteristics are known as the individual's **phenotype** (FĒN-ō-tīp).

Your genotype is derived from the genotypes of your parents, but not in a simple way. You are not an exact copy of either parent, nor are you an easily identifiable mixture of their characteristics. Our discussion of genetics will begin with the basic patterns of inheritance and their implications.

Genes and Chromosomes

Chromosome structure and the functions of genes were introduced in Chapter 5. Chromosomes contain DNA, and genes are functional segments of DNA. Each gene carries the information needed to direct the synthesis of a specific polypeptide.

Every somatic cell contains 23 pairs of chromosomes. One member of each pair was contributed by the spermatozoon at fertilization and the other by the ovum. The members of each pair are known as **homologous** (hō-MOL-o-gus; Greek *homologos*, in agreement) **chromosomes**. Twenty-two of those pairs are known as **autosomal** (aw-tō-SŌ-mul; Greek *autos*, self + *soma*, body) **chromosomes**. Most of the genes on these chromosomes affect somatic characteristics, such as hair color, skin pigmentation, and the size and shape of bones. The chromosomes of the twenty-third pair are called the **sex chromosomes** because they differ in the two sexes. Figure 7–13 shows the chromosomes of a normal male individual.

Autosomal Chromosomes

The two chromosomes in an autosomal pair have the same structure and carry genes that affect the same traits. If one member of the pair contains three genes in a row, with number 1 determining hair characteristics, number 2 blood type, and number 3 a specific

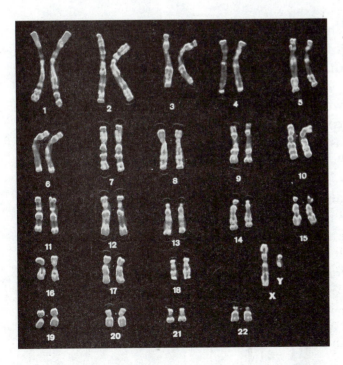

Figure 7–13   Human Chromosomes.
The 23 pairs of somatic-cell chromosomes of a normal male.

stomach enzyme, the other chromosome will carry genes affecting the same traits and in the same sequence. The various forms of any one gene are called **alleles** (a-LĒLZ; Greek *allelon*, one another). It is these alternate forms that determine the effect of the gene on the individual's phenotype. If both chromosomes of a homologous pair carry the same allele of a particular gene, the individual is **homozygous** (hō-mō-ZĪ-gus; Greek *homozygos*, matching) for that trait. For example, if an individual receives an allele for curly hair from the spermatozoon and one for curly hair from the ovum, the individual will be homozygous for curly hair.

Because the chromosomes of a homologous pair have different origins, one paternal and the other maternal, they do not necessarily carry the same alleles. When an individual has two different alleles of the same gene, the individual is **heterozygous** (het-er-ō-ZĪ-gus: Greek *heterozygos*, not matching) for that trait. If an individual is heterozygous for a particular trait, the phenotype will be determined by the interactions between the corresponding alleles.

- If an allele is **dominant** it will be expressed in the phenotype regardless of any conflicting instructions carried by the other allele.

- If an allele is **recessive**, it will be expressed in the phenotype only if it is present on both chromosomes of a homologous pair. For example, the albino condition is characterized by an inability to synthesize a yellow-brown pigment called melanin. The presence of one normal allele will result in normal skin, hair, and eye coloration. Two recessive alleles must be present to produce an albino individual.

An individual who receives two dominant alleles for a given trait is said to be **homozygous dominant**. An individual who receives two recessive alleles for a particular trait is said to be **homozygous recessive**. Usually about 80 percent of an individual's genotype consists of homozygous alleles.

Predicting Inheritance

In **simple inheritance** phenotypic characters are determined by interactions between a single pair of alleles. Some examples are included in Table 7–3. If you restrict attention to these alleles it is possible to predict the characteristics of individuals on the basis of those of their parents.

The gametes involved in fertilization each contribute a single allele for a given trait. That allele must be one of the two contained by all cells in the parental body. Consider, for example, the condition known as albinism, which we will abbreviate with the letter A. Dominant alleles are traditionally indicated by capitalized abbreviations, and recessives are abbreviated in lower case letters. Since albinism is a recessive characteristic, the allele for albinism would be a and the allele for normal pigmentation would be A. We might ask what kinds of offspring would be expected from an albino mother and a normally-pigmented father. Because albinism is a recessive, the maternal genotype would be abbreviated aa. No matter which of her ova gets fertilized, it will carry the recessive a allele. The father has normal coloration, a dominant trait. He may therefore be homozygous (AA) or heterozygous (Aa) for this trait, since both will give rise to the same phenotype. A homozygous father will produce sperm that all carry the A allele. A

Table 7–3 The Inheritance of Selected Phenotypic Characters

DOMINANT TRAITS
One allele determines phenotype; the other is suppressed:
>   lack of freckles
>   brachydactyly (short fingers)
>   ability to taste phenylthiocarbamate (PTC)
>   free earlobes
>   curly hair
>   ability to roll the tongue into a U shape
>   color vision

Both dominant alleles may be expressed (codominance):
>   presence of A or B antigens on red blood cell membranes
>   particular structure of serum proteins (albumins, transferrins)

Two alleles produce intermediate traits (incomplete dominance):
>   hemoglobin A and hemoglobin S production

RECESSIVE TRAITS
>   albinism
>   freckles
>   normal digits
>   inability to taste phenylthiocarbamete (PTC)
>   attached earlobes
>   straight hair
>   red hair
>   lack of A or B surface antigens (Type O blood)
>   inability to roll the tongue into a U shape

X-LINKED TRAITS
>   color blindness
>   hemophilia

POLYGENIC TRAITS
>   eye color
>   hair colors other than red
>   skin color

Note: For a listing of inherited clinical conditions, see Table 7–4.

heterozygous father, however, will produce two different kinds of sperm: Fifty percent (one half) will carry the dominant allele A and the other fifty percent (one half) will carry the recessive allele a.

We can use a simple box diagram known as a Punnett square to help us predict the genotypes of the children from this couple as well as the probability that a particular genotype will occur. In the sample Punnett square shown in Figure 7–14, the maternal alleles are listed along the horizontal axis and the paternal ones along the vertical axis. (It really doesn't matter which axis represents the mother and which the father as long as it's clearly indicated.) The possible genotypes of the offspring are indicated in the boxes by bringing the letters down from the top and across from the side such that each box receives two letters, one from the father and one from the mother. (This represents the maternal and paternal contribution of genes to their offspring.) Figure 7–14a considers the possible offspring of an albino (aa) mother and a normal father who is homozygous dominant (AA). As you can see, all of the children are heterozygous and have the genotype Aa, so all will have normal coloration (normal phenotype). Compare these results with those of Figure 7–14b, for a heterozygous father (Aa) and an albino mother (aa). The heterozygous individual produces two types of gametes, those carrying the A allele and

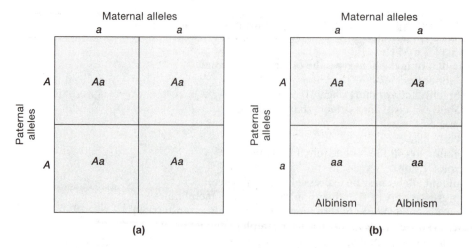

Figure 7–14   Predicting Phenotypic Characteristics by Using Punnett Squares.
(a) All the offspring of a homozygous dominant father *(AA)* and a homozygous recessive mother *(aa)* will be heterozygous *(Aa)* for that trait. Their phenotype will be the same as that of the father. **(b)** The offspring of a heterozygous father and a homozygous recessive mother will be either heterozygous or homozygous for the recessive trait. In this example, half the offspring will have normal skin coloration, and the other half will be albinos.

those carrying the a allele, and the egg may be fertilized by either one. As a result, there is a 50 percent probability that a child of such parents will inherit the genotype Aa and so have normal coloration. The probability of inheriting the genotype aa, and thus having the albino phenotype, is also 50 percent.

A Punnett square can also be used in reverse, to draw conclusions about the identity and genotype of a parent. For example, a man with the genotype AA cannot be the father of an albino child (aa) (refer back to Figure 7–14a).

The frequency of appearance of an inherited disorder, or genetic disease, resulting from simple inheritance can also be predicted using a Punnett square. Although genetic disorders tend to be rare in terms of overall numbers, more than 1200 different inherited conditions have been identified that reflect the presence of one or two abnormal alleles for a single gene. A partial listing is included in Table 7–4.

Sex Chromosomes

Unlike autosomal chromosomes, the sex chromosomes are not necessarily identical in appearance and gene content. There are two different sex chromosomes, an **X chromosome** and a **Y chromosome**. The Y chromosomes are considerably smaller than X chromosomes and contain fewer genes, but among those genes are dominant alleles that specify that an individual with that chromosome will be a male. The normal male sex chromosome complement is XY. Females do not have a Y chromosome, and their sex chromosome pair is XX.

The ova produced by a woman will always carry an X chromosome, whereas sperm may carry an X or a Y chromosome. Thus, if you make a Punnett square you can show that the male:female sex ratio in the offspring should be 1:1 (50 percent males and 50 percent females). Actual birth statistics differ slightly from that prediction, with 106 males born for every 100 females. It has been suggested that more males are born because the sperm carrying the Y chromosome can reach the oocyte first, because they do not have to carry the extra weight of the larger X chromosome.

In addition to its role in determining gender, the X chromosome also carries genes that affect somatic structures. These characteristics are called **X-linked**. (Genes that are located on a specific chromosome are said to be linked to that chromosome.) The inheritance of characteristics regulated by these genes differs slightly from the pattern of inheritance we just examined involving autosomal chromosomes. This difference is due to the fact that normal males have only one X chromosome and must express whatever alleles are present on that chromosome in their phenotype.

The inheritance of red-green color blindness exemplifies the differences between sex-linked and autosomal inheritance. Red-green color blindness is a relatively common disorder caused by a recessive allele on the X chromosome. Normal color vision is determined by the presence of a dominant allele, C. Since a woman has two X chromosomes, she can be either homozygous dominant (CC) or heterozygous (Cc) and still have normal color vision. She will be color-blind only if she carries two recessive alleles, cc. But a male has only one X chromosome, so whatever that chromosome carries will determine whether he has normal color vision or is color-blind. A Punnett square for this X-linked trait, as in Figure 7–15, reveals that the sons produced by a father with normal vision and a mother with normal vision who is heterozygous will have a 50 percent chance of being color-blind, while the daughters will all have normal color vision.

A number of clinical disorders are X-linked traits, including certain forms of hemophilia, diabetes insipidus, and muscular dystrophy. In several instances, advances in molecular genetic techniques have permitted the localization of the specific genes on the X chromosome. This technique provides a relatively direct method of screening for the presence of a particular condition before the symptoms appear and even before birth.

Interactions between Alleles

Not every allele can be neatly characterized as dominant or recessive. For some genes, there can be more than two dominant alleles. If an individual receives two different alleles that are both dominant, the resulting phenotype will depend on how the two dominant genes interact.

- In **suppression** one allele suppresses the other, and the phenotype is the same as if the second allele were recessive.

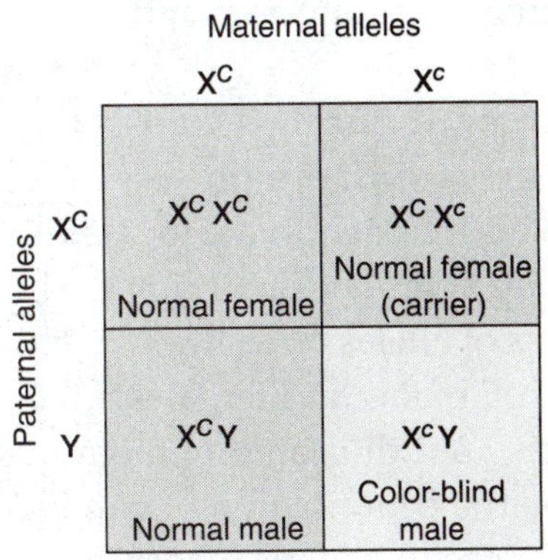

Figure 7–15 **X-Linked Inheritance.**

Maternal alleles	X^C	X^c
X^C	$X^C X^C$ Normal female	$X^C X^c$ Normal female (carrier)
Y	$X^C Y$ Normal male	$X^c Y$ Color-blind male

Paternal alleles

- In **codominance** both alleles are fully expressed and the one pair of alleles produces two distinct characteristics in the phenotype. For example, there are two dominant alleles and one recessive allele for the gene that controls a person's A, B, or O blood type. One dominant allele specifies type A blood, and the other type B blood. When a person receives both alleles (one for A and one for B), both are expressed and the individual has type AB blood.

- In **complementary gene action** or **incomplete dominance** the two dominant alleles interact to produce a phenotype different from that resulting from either allele by itself.

Polygenic Inheritance

Unfortunately, most human traits are not the result of simple inheritance (as you can see by looking at Table 7–3). Most human characteristics are the product of multiple genes and complex gene interactions.

Polygenic inheritance involves interactions among the alleles of several different genes. Because multiple genes are involved, the frequency of a trait's occurrence cannot easily be predicted using a simple Punnett square. Several common phenotypic characters including height, skin color, hair color, and eye color are polygenic traits in humans. Several important adult disorders, including hypertension and coronary artery disease, fall into this category as well.

Many of the developmental disorders responsible for fetal mortalities and congenital malformations result from multiple genetic interactions. In these cases, the particular genetic composition of the individual does not by itself determine the onset of the disease. Instead, the conditions regulated by these genes establish a susceptibility to particular environmental influences. This means that not every individual with the genetic tendency for a particular condition will actually develop it. It is therefore difficult to track polygenic conditions through successive generations. However, because many inherited polygenic conditions are likely but not guaranteed to occur, steps can be taken to prevent a crisis. For example, hypertension (high blood pressure) may be prevented or reduced by controlling diet and fluid volume, and coronary artery disease may be prevented by lowering serum cholesterol concentrations.

Sources of Individual Variation

You are not a copy of either parent, nor are you a 50:50 mixture of their characteristics. One reason was noted earlier in the chapter: During meiosis, maternal and paternal chromosomes are randomly assorted, so each gamete contains a unique blend of maternal and paternal chromosomes.

In addition, parts of chromosomes can become rearranged during synapsis (Figure 7–16). When tetrads are formed, adjacent chromatids may overlap, a process called crossing-over. Under these conditions, they may break and reattach in a process that switches a portion of one chromatid for the corresponding segment on another. This process results in **genetic recombination**, new combinations of alleles on a chromosome. Genetic recombination, which occurs during meiosis in both males and females, greatly increases the range of possible variation among gametes, and thus among members of successive generations, whose genotypes are formed by the combination of gametes in fertilization. It can also complicate the tracing of inheritance of genetic disorders.

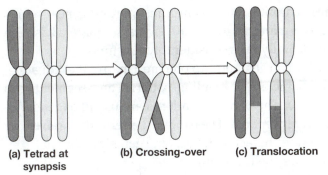

Figure 7–16 Genetic Recombination.
(a) Synapsis, with the formation of a tetrad during meiosis. **(b)** Crossing-over of homologous portions of two chromosomes. **(c)** The breakage and exchange of corresponding sections on the two chromosomes in part (b).

(a) Tetrad at synapsis **(b) Crossing-over** **(c) Translocation**

Variations at the level of the individual gene may also appear as a result of mutations. **Spontaneous mutations** are the result of random errors in the DNA replication process. Such incidents are relatively common. At least 10 percent of fertilizations produce zygotes with abnormal chromosomes, and because spontaneous mutations usually fail to produce visible defects, the actual number of mutations must be far larger. Many of the changes may have no effect on phenotype, and each of us has unique, individual characteristics. Given the complexity of the interactions between genotype and phenotype, some degree of individual variation is inevitable.

Zygotes with more significant abnormalities usually produce embryos that die before completing development, and only about 0.5 percent of newborn infants show chromosomal abnormalities resulting from spontaneous mutations. Individuals with **chromosomal abnormalities** have damaged, broken, missing, or extra copies of chromosomes. Chromosomal abnormalities produce a variety of serious clinical conditions, in addition to contributing to prenatal mortality. Few individuals with chromosomal abnormalities survive to full term. The high mortality rate and severity of the problems reflect the fact that large numbers of genes have been added or deleted.

Chromosomal abnormalities can be detected by **karyotyping** (KAR-ē-ō-tīp-ing; Greek *karyon*, kernel + *typos*, mark), a technique that is used to examine chromosomes. First, a cell sample is obtained from an individual, and the cells are grown in tissue culture. After several rounds of cell division, a chemical is added to stop mitosis in the cells. Cells that have been arrested in metaphase are located with the aid of a microscope, and the metaphase chromosomes are photographed. The pictures of all the chromosomes are cut out of the photograph and arranged on a sheet of paper from largest to smallest and according to their structural characteristics. This final product is called a **karyotype** (KAR-ē-ō-tīp). A normal human karyotype is shown in Figure 7–13. By examining the structure of the chromosomes in the karyotype, geneticists can determine if any are damaged or abnormal and likely to produce genetic defects.

The Human Genome Project

Few of the genes responsible for inherited disorders have been identified or even localized to a specific chromosome. That situation is changing rapidly, however, because of the attention devoted to the **Human Genome Project**. This project, funded by the National Institutes of Health and the Department of Energy, is attempting to transcribe the entire human genome (complement of genes), chromosome by chromosome and gene by gene. The project began in October 1990 and was expected to take 10–15 years. Progress has been more rapid than expected, and it may actually take considerably less time.

The first step in understanding the human genome is to prepare a map of the individual chromosomes. Each chromosome has characteristic banding patterns, and segments can be stained with special dyes (Figure 7–13). The banding patterns are useful as reference points when more detailed genetic maps are prepared. The banding patterns themselves can be useful, as abnormal banding patterns are characteristic of some genetic disorders.

As of 1997, a progress report includes the following:

- Eight chromosomes—chromosomes 3, 11, 12, 16, 19, 21, 22, and the Y chromosome—have been mapped completely, and preliminary maps have been made for all other chromosomes.

- More than 6800 genes have been identified. Although a significant number, this is only a small fraction (about 7 percent) of the estimated 100,000 genes in the human genome.

- The specific genes responsible for more than 60 inherited disorders have been identified, including several of the disorders listed in Table 7–4. Genetic screening can now be done for many of these conditions, as indicated in Figure 7–17.

The Human Genome Project is attempting to determine the normal genetic composition of a "typical" human being. Yet we all are variations on a basic theme. As we improve our abilities to manipulate our own genetic foundations, we will face troubling ethical and legal decisions. For example, few people object to the insertion of a "correct" gene into somatic cells to cure a specific disease. But what if we could insert that modified gene into a gamete and change not only that individual but all of his or her descendants? And what if the gene did not correct or prevent a disorder but "improved" the individual by increasing intelligence, height, or vision or by altering some other phenotypic characteristic? These and other difficult questions will not go away, and in the years to come we will have to find answers we all can live with.

Table 7–4   Fairly Common Inherited Disorders

Autosomal dominants
    Adult polycystic kidney disease
    Marfan's syndrome
    Huntington's disease
Autosomal recessives
    Deafness
    Albinism
    Sickle-cell anemia
    Cystic fibrosis
    Phenylketonuria
    Tay-Sachs disease
X-linked
    Duchenne's muscular dystrophy
    Myotonic muscular dystrophy
    Hemophilia (A and B)
    Testicular feminization syndrome
    Color blindness

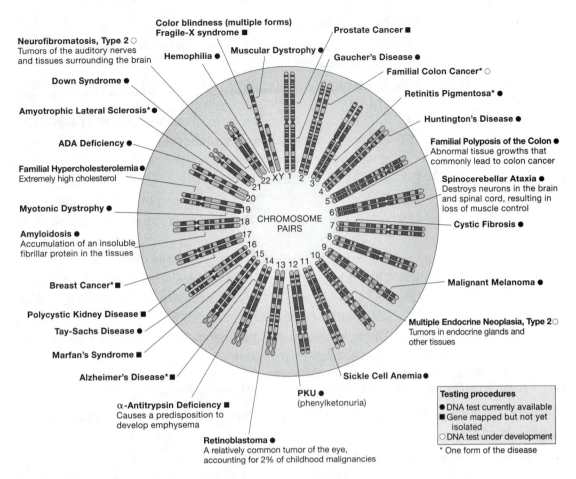

Figure 7–17   A Map of the Human Chromosomes.
The banding patterns of typical chromosomes in a male individual and the locations of the genes responsible for specific inherited disorders. The chromosomes are not drawn to scale.

✏️ Let's Review What You've Just Learned

► **Definitions**

In the space provided, write the term for each of the following definitions.

_____ **136.** The different forms of a gene.

_____ **137.** The term for an individual who possesses a pair of dominant alleles for a trait.

_____ **138.** The chromosome that contains genes responsible for male gender.

_____ **139.** The members of a matched pair of chromosomes.

_____ **140.** A technique used to examine chromosomes.

_____ **141.** An individual's entire genetic composition.

_____ **142.** The term for an individual who has two contrasting alleles for a given trait.

_____ **143.** The term for genes that are located on the X chromosome.

_____ **144.** A random error in the DNA replication process.

_____ **145.** The equal expression of two dominant alleles of a particular gene.

_____ **146.** Nonsex chromosomes.

_____ **147.** The term for an individual who carries a pair of recessive alleles for a given trait.

_____ **148.** The term for chromosomes that are damaged, broken, missing, or represented by extra copies.

_____ **149.** The genetically determined physical characteristics of an individual.

_____ **150.** In simple inheritance, the allele that is expressed in a heterozygous individual.

_____ **151.** The sex chromosome found in ova.

_____ **152.** Inheritance of a trait that is the product of more than one gene.

_____ **153.** A photographic representation of an individual's complement of chromosomes.

_____ **154.** The worldwide attempt to map all of the human chromosomes.

_____ **155.** The chromosomes responsible for determining an individual's sex.

_____ **156.** The term for an individual who possesses a matching pair of alleles for a given trait.

_____ **157.** The masking of one dominant allele by another in the pair that specifies a given trait.

► Word Roots, Prefixes, Suffixes, and Combining Forms

In the space provided, list the boldfaced terms introduced in this section that contain the indicated word part.

Word Part	Meaning	Examples
homo-	same	**158.** _____
hetero-	other	**159.** _____
karyo-	kernel	**160.** _____
som-	body	**161.** _____
auto-	self	**162.** _____
poly-	many	**163.** _____
gen-	to produce	**164.** _____
pheno-	bring to light	**165.** _____

► Completion

Fill in each of the following Punnett squares and answer the questions relating to each one.

166. The ability to curl one's tongue (tongue rolling) is a dominant trait in humans. Use the following Punnett square to determine the possible genotypes of offspring from a father and a mother who are both heterozygous for the trait. (Use R to represent the dominant allele and r to represent the recessive allele.)

_____ **167.** What is the probability that a child from this couple will not be able to roll its tongue?

_____ **168.** What percentage of this couple's offspring can be expected to be heterozygous for the trait?

169. Hemophilia A is an X-linked trait. What percentage of the male offspring of a normal father and a mother heterozygous for hemophilia A can be expected to be hemophiliacs? (Use H to represent a normal allele and h to represent the hemophilia, and complete the following Punnett square to answer this question.)

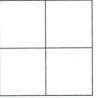

_____ **170.** What percentage of this couple's daughters will be normal but carry the recessive allele for hemophilia?

☑ Self-Check Test

The following test will allow you to determine how well you have mastered the vocabulary and basic concepts of this chapter. It will also help you prepare for the type of questions you are likely to encounter on a test in an anatomy and physiology course. The self-check test will help you assess your understanding of the chapter material and will help you develop good test-taking skills.

The following questions test your ability to use vocabulary and to recall facts.

1. Sperm develop from stem cells called
   a. spermatogonia
   b. primary spermatocytes
   c. secondary spermatocytes
   d. spermatids
   e. spermatozoa

2. During oocyte activation
   a. the metabolic rate of the oocyte increases
   b. the ovum completes meiosis II
   c. the cortical reaction occurs
   d. other sperm are prohibited from fertilizing the egg
   e. all of the above

3. During amphimixis
   a. sperm become capacitated
   b. the ovum finishes meiosis II
   c. the male and female pronuclei fuse
   d. meiosis occurs
   e. gametes are formed

4. Differentiation during the first few days of development is the result of
   a. enzymes produced by the sperm
   b. hormones produced by the egg
   c. an unequal distribution of regulatory molecules in the cytoplasm of the egg
   d. regulator molecules supplied by cells of the uterus
   e. all of the above

5. The penetration of the uterine lining by the blastocyst is referred to as
   a. cleavage
   b. implantation
   c. placentation
   d. embryogenesis
   e. blastulation

6. The solid ball of cells that is formed after several rounds of cell division after fertilization is called a
   a. chorion
   b. blastula
   c. gastrula
   d. morula
   e. blastocyst

7. Separation of the inner cell mass from the trophoblast forms the
   a. blastocoele
   b. lacuna
   c. amniotic cavity
   d. chorion
   e. allantois

8. During gastrulation
   a. the blastodisc is formed
   b. the placenta is formed
   c. the germ layers are formed
   d. cells from the hypoblast move to the epiblast
   e. an embryo becomes a fetus

9. The region known as the primitive streak is the site of
   a. germ cell formation
   b. endoderm formation
   c. ectoderm formation
   d. amnion formation
   e. migration of ectodermal cells into the space between the epiblast and hypoblast

10. The extraembryonic membrane that forms blood is the
    a. yolk sac
    b. amnion
    c. chorion
    d. allantois
    e. decidua

11. Paired chromosomes are called
    a. homologous chromosomes
    b. homozygous chromosomes
    c. heterozygous chromosomes
    d. autosomes
    e. alleles

12. Tetrads form during
    a. metaphase I of meiosis
    b. prophase I of meiosis
    c. anaphase I of meiosis
    d. metaphase II of meiosis
    e. prophase II of meiosis

13. Chromosomes that are not sex chromosomes are called
    a. homologous chromosomes
    b. homozygous chromosomes
    c. heterozygous chromosomes
    d. autosomes
    e. alleles

14. An individual who carries two different alleles for the same trait is
    a. homologous
    b. heterozygous
    c. homozygous
    d. autosomous
    e. polygenic

15. Recessive X-linked traits
    a. are passed from fathers to their sons
    b. are more likely to be expressed in males than in females
    c. always affect some aspect of the reproductive system
    d. are never expressed in females
    e. cannot be passed from mothers to daughters

16. In simple inheritance
    a. phenotypic characters are determined by a single pair of alleles
    b. phenotypic characters are determined by multiple alleles
    c. phenotypic characters are determined by the action of a single gene
    d. phenotypic characters are controlled by regulator genes on several different chromosomes
    e. phenotypic characters are determined by genes on the Y chromosome

17. The period of gestation during which the rudiments of all major organ systems appear is the
    a. first trimester
    b. second trimester
    c. third trimester

The following questions are more challenging and require you to synthesize the information that you have learned in this chapter.

18. A normally pigmented woman whose father was an albino marries a normally pigmented man whose mother was an albino. What is the probability that they will have an albino child?
    a. 1/2
    b. 1/4
    c. 1/8
    d. 1/16
    e. 100%

19. If a sperm cell lacked sufficient quantities of hyaluronidase, it would not be able to
    a. move its flagellum
    b. penetrate the corona radiata of the egg
    c. become capacitated
    d. survive the environment of the female reproductive tract
    e. metabolize sugars

20. Problems involving formation of the chorion would affect
    a. the embryo's ability to produce blood cells
    b. the formation of limbs
    c. the embryo's ability to derive nutrition from its mother
    d. lung formation
    e. formation of the urinary system

☑ Self-Assessment

If your score was

between 18 and 20, you are ready to proceed to the next chapter.

between 15 and 17, you have a good general idea of the chapter content, but you should review sections of the chapter that deal with items that you missed before proceeding to the next chapter.

less than 14, you have not mastered the chapter content well enough to proceed. Reread the chapter and rework the exercises. Then retake the self-check test. Repeat this process until you achieve a score that will allow you to continue.

Answers

1. inheritance
2. spermatogenesis
3. oogonia
4. conception
5. embryology
6. diploid
7. crossing-over
8. secondary oocyte
9. differentiation
10. postnatal development
11. synapsis
12. spermatogonia
13. spermiogenesis
14. embryological development
15. primary oocytes
16. meiosis
17. spermatids
18. atresia
19. spermatozoa
20. genetics
21. reductional division
22. secondary spermatocytes
23. haploid
24. prenatal development

25. seminiferous tubules
26. tetrad
27. gametogenesis
28. senescence
29. equational division
30. fetal development
31. primary spermatocytes
32. oogenesis
33. oocyte, oogenesis, oogonia
34. tetrad
35. oocyte, spermatocyte
36. prenatal, postnatal
37. seminiferous
38. metaphase I
39. chromosomes containing paired chromatids separate randomly
40. nuclear envelope disappears, DNA condenses, chromosomes appear, synapsis occurs
41. anaphase II
42. telophase II
43. chromosomes containing paired chromatids line up on the cell's equatorial plate
44. spermatogonia
45. primary spermatocytes

46. secondary spermatocyte
47. spermatids
48. spermatozoa
49. oogonium
50. primary oocyte
51. secondary oocyte
52. mature ovum
53. amphimixis
54. ooplasm
55. polyspermy
56. zygote
57. uterine tube
58. female pronucleus
59. induction
60. fertilization
61. corona radiata
62. male pronucleus
63. cortical reaction
64. capacitation
65. oocyte activation
66. polyspermy
67. zygote
68. pronucleus
69. corona radiata
70. amphimixis
71. inner cell mass
72. gastrulation
73. amniotic cavity
74. endoderm
75. yolk sac
76. embryogenesis
77. cleavage
78. umbilical arteries
79. gestation
80. morula
81. trophoblast
82. allantois
83. umbilical cord, or umbilical stalk
84. blastodisc
85. placenta
86. trimester
87. epiblast
88. ectoderm
89. amnion
90. body stalk
91. primitive streak
92. implantation
93. blastocoele
94. mesoderm
95. amniotic fluid
96. umbilical vein
97. pediatrics
98. organogenesis
99. blastocyst
100. placentation
101. yolk stalk
102. geriatrics
103. hypoblast
104. lacunae
105. syncytial trophoblast, or syncytiotrophoblast
106. chorionic villi
107. extraembryonic membranes
108. chorion
109. blastocyst, blastocoele, blastodisc, trophoblast, epiblast, hypoblast
110. epiblast
111. gestation
112. neonate
113. trimester
114. trophoblast
115. geriatrics, geriatrician
116. blastocoele
117. hypoblast
118. mesoderm
119. pediatrics
120. extraembryonic membranes
121. ectoderm, mesoderm, endoderm
122. embryogenesis organogenesis
123. syncytial trophoblast
124. ectoderm
125. endoderm
126. rudiments of all major organ systems appear
127. organs and organ systems complete most of their development; body proportions change
128. most of the major organ systems become fully functional; rapid fetal growth
129. secondary oocyte
130. fertilization
131. zygote
132. two-cell stage
133 morula
134. early blastocyst
135. implantation
136. alleles
137. homozygous dominant
138. Y chromosome
139. homologous chromosome
140. karyotyping
141. genotype
142. heterozygous
143. X-linked
144. spontaneous mutation
145. codominance
146. autosomes
147. homozygous recessive
148. chromosomal abnormalities
149. phenotype
150. dominant allele
151. X chromosome
152. polygenic inheritance
153. karyotype
154. Human Genome Project
155. sex chromosomes
156. homozygous
157. suppression
158. homozygous, homologous chromosomes
159. heterozygous
160. karyotyping, karyotype
161. autosome, chromosome
162. autosome

163. polygenic
164. genotype, polygenic, genome
165. phenotype
166.

	R	r
R	RR	Rr
r	Rr	rr

167. 25%
168. 50%

169. 50%

	X^H	X^h
X^H	$X^H X^H$	$X^H X^h$
Y	$X^H Y$	$X^h Y$

170. 50%

Answers to Self-Check Test

1. a 2. e 3. c 4. c 5. b 6. d 7. c 8. c 9. e 10. a 11. a 12. b
13. d 14. b 15. b 16. a 17. a 18. b 19. b 20. c

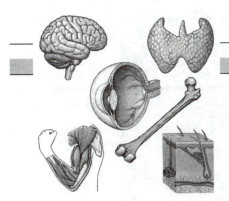

A Survey of Human Body Systems I

In this and the following chapter we will survey the 11 systems of the human body. The systems are presented in the order that they are frequently encountered in a two-semester anatomy and physiology course. Chapter 8 will cover the integumentary system, skeletal system, muscular system, nervous system, and endocrine system. These systems are generally covered in the first semester of a two-semester anatomy and physiology course. Chapter 9 will cover the remaining body systems. The purpose of these two chapters is to give you a general overview of each body system with an emphasis on terminology and general concepts. This background will prepare you for the more detailed study of these systems you will encounter in your future coursework.

THE INTEGUMENTARY SYSTEM

The skin, or **integument** (in-TEG-ū-ment; Latin *integere*, to cover), can be considered as either a large, highly complex organ or a structurally integrated organ system. Most people recognize both possibilities and consider the terms *integument* and *integumentary system* as interchangeable. The components of the integumentary (in-teg-ū-MEN-tuh-rē) system include the epithelium and underlying connective tissue of the skin and the associated hairs, nails, and exocrine glands.

The integumentary system has two major components, the cutaneous membrane and the accessory structures.

1. The **cutaneous membrane** has two components: the **superficial epithelium,** or **epidermis** (ep-i-DER-mis; Greek *epi*, on + *derma*, skin), and the underlying connective tissues of the **dermis** (DER-mis).

2. The accessory structures include hair, nails, and multicellular exocrine glands. These structures are located in the dermis and protrude through the epidermis to the skin surface.

The integument does not function in isolation. An extensive network of blood vessels branches through the dermis, and sensory receptors that monitor touch, pressure, temperature, and pain provide valuable information to the central nervous system about the state of the body. The general structure of the integument is shown in Figure 8–1. Beneath the

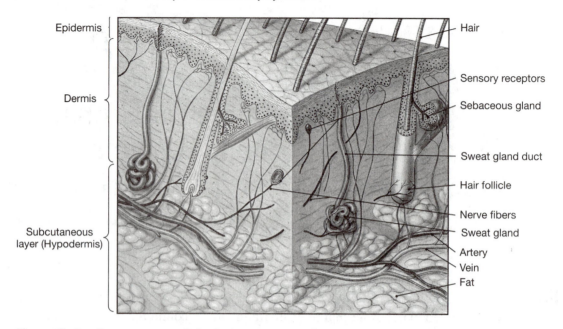

Epidermis

Dermis

Subcutaneous
layer (Hypodermis)

Hair

Sensory receptors

Sebaceous gland

Sweat gland duct

Hair follicle

Nerve fibers

Sweat gland

Artery

Vein

Fat

Figure 8–1   Components of the Integumentary System.
Relationships among the major components of the integumentary system (with the exception of nails).

dermis, the loose connective tissue of the **subcutaneous layer,** also known as the **superficial fascia,** or **hypodermis** (hī-pō-DER-mis; Greek *hypo*, beneath + *derma*, skin), separates the integument from the deep fascia around other organs, such as muscles and bones.

The general functions of the skin include:

1. Protection of underlying tissues and organs.
2. Excretion of salts, water, and organic wastes.
3. Maintenance of normal body temperature.
4. Synthesis of vitamin D_3, that is subsequently converted to a hormone, *calcitriol* (kal-si-TRĪ-ol), which regulates calcium ion absorption and is essential for normal bone maintenance and growth.
5. Storage of nutrients.
6. Detection of touch, pressure, pain, and temperature stimuli and the relay of that information to the nervous system.

The Epidermis

The epidermis consists of a stratified squamous epithelium (see Chapter 6). The most abundant epithelial cells, called **keratinocytes** (ke-RAT-i-nō-sītz; Greek *keras*, horn), form several layers, or **strata** (STRAH-tuh), but the precise boundaries between the layers are often difficult to see in a light micrograph. In thick skin, found on the palms of the hands and the soles of the feet, five layers can be distinguished. Only four layers can be distinguished in the thin skin that covers the rest of the body. The terms *thick* and *thin* refer to the relative thickness of the epidermis, not to the integument as a whole.

Figure 8–2 shows the layers in a section of thick skin. Beginning at the basement membrane and traveling toward the free surface, we find the stratum germinativum, the stratum spinosum, the stratum granulosum, the stratum lucidum, and the stratum corneum.

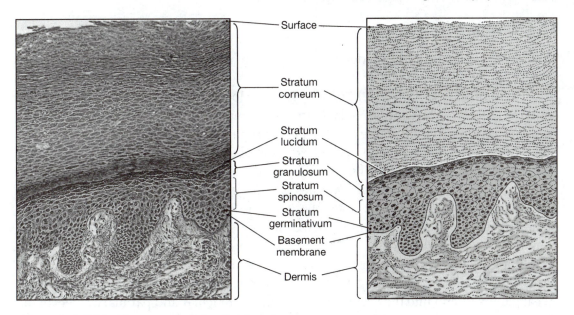

Figure 8–2 The Structure of the Epidermis.
A portion of the epidermis in thick skin, showing the major stratified layers of epidermal cells. (LM × 210)

1. The **stratum germinativum** (STRAH-tum jur-mi-na-TĪ-vum) contains cells that divide periodically to produce new cells that replace those that are lost from the skin surface.

2. The **stratum spinosum** (STRAH-tum spi-NŌ-sum) takes its name from the appearance of cells in a light micrograph. As the cytoplasm shrinks, the desmosomes where the cells are attached to each other appear as spiny projections from the cell surface.

3. The cells of the **stratum granulosum** (STRAH-tum gran-ū-LŌ-sum) manufacture large amounts of a protein called **keratohyalin** (ker-a-tō-HĪ-a-lin) that appear as granules in the cell's cytoplasm.

4. The **stratum lucidum** (STRAH-tum LOO-si-dum) contains cells that are filled with keratohyalin and the fibrous protein keratin, introduced in Chapter 3. Keratin is tough, durable, and water-resistant. In addition to forming the protective barrier in the stratum corneum, keratin is the basic structural component of hair and nails.

5. The **stratum corneum** (STRAH-tum KŌR-nē-um) is the outermost layer of the epidermis, composed of flattened, dead, heavily *keratinized* (KER-a-tin-īzd) cells. These cells are constantly being sloughed off and are the ones replaced by the cells produced in the stratum germinativum.

Skin Color

The color of skin is due to an interaction between (1) pigment composition and concentration and (2) the dermal blood supply.

The epidermis contains variable quantities of two pigments: **carotene** (kar-o-TĒN; Latin *carota*, carrot), an orange-yellow pigment that usually accumulates within epidermal cells, and melanin, a brown to black pigment produced by **melanocytes** (me-LAN-ō-sīts) located in the stratum germinativum.

The Dermis

The dermis lies beneath the epidermis. It has two major components, a superficial papillary layer and a deep reticular layer.

The **papillary** (PAP-i-ler-ē) **layer** consists of loose connective tissue. This region contains the capillaries and sensory neurons that supply the surface of the skin. The papillary layer derives its name from the **dermal papillae** (pa-PIL-ē; Latin *papilla*, nipple) that project between the epidermal ridges as shown in Figure 8–1.

The deeper **reticular** (re-TIK-ū-lar) **layer** consists of an interwoven meshwork of dense irregular connective tissue. Bundles of collagen fibers leave the reticular layer to blend into those of the papillary layer above, so the boundary line between these layers is indistinct. Collagen fibers of the reticular layer also extend into the underlying subcutaneous layer.

In addition to extracellular protein fibers, the dermis contains all the cells of connective tissue proper. Accessory organs of epidermal origin, such as hair follicles and sweat glands extend into the dermis. In addition, the reticular and papillary layers of the dermis contain networks of blood vessels, lymph vessels, and nerve fibers (Figure 8–1).

The Subcutaneous Layer

The connective tissue fibers of the reticular layer are extensively interwoven with those of the subcutaneous layer, or hypodermis, and the boundary between the two is usually indistinct. Although the subcutaneous layer is not a part of the integument, it is important in stabilizing the position of the skin in relation to underlying tissues, such as skeletal muscles or other organs, while permitting independent movement. The subcutaneous layer consists of loose connective tissue with abundant fat cells.

Accessory Structures of the Skin

The **accessory structures** of the integument include hair follicles, sebaceous glands, sweat glands, and nails. During embryological development, these structures originate from the epidermis, and they are also known as **epidermal derivatives.** Although located in the dermis, they project through the epidermis to the integumentary surface.

- **Hair follicles and hair:** Hairs originate in complex organs called **hair follicles** (FOL-i-kulz; Latin *folliculus*, little bag), and hair production is a complex process involving cooperation between the dermis and the epidermis. Hairs on the head protect the scalp from ultraviolet radiation, cushion a blow to the head, and provide insulation. The hairs guarding the entrances to the nostrils and external ear canals help prevent the entry of foreign particles and insects, and eyelashes perform a similar function for the surface of the eye. A group of sensory nerves surrounds the base of each hair follicle. As a result, the movement of even a single hair can be felt at a conscious level. This sensitivity provides an early warning system that may help to prevent injury.

- **Sebaceous glands: Sebaceous** (se-BĀ-shus) **glands,** or oil glands, are holocrine glands that discharge a waxy, oily secretion called **sebum** (SĒ-bum; Latin *sebum*, grease) into hair follicles. Sebum provides lubrication for the skin and inhibits the growth of bacteria.

- **Sweat glands:** The skin contains two groups of sweat glands. (1) **Apocrine sweat glands** are located in the axillae, around the nipples, and in the groin. They are coiled tubular glands that produce a sticky, cloudy, and potentially odorous secretion. (2) **Merocrine sweat glands** are far more numerous and widely distributed than apocrine glands. They are coiled tubular glands that discharge their secretions (mostly water) directly onto the surface of the skin. The clear secretion produced by merocrine sweat glands is called **sweat.** Merocrine sweat glands function in cooling the surface of the skin to reduce body temperature, excreting water and electrolytes, and providing protection from environmental hazards by diluting harmful chemicals and discouraging the growth of microorganisms.

- **Nails:** form on the dorsal surfaces of the tips of fingers and toes. The nails protect the exposed tips of the fingers and toes and help limit their distortion when they are subjected to mechanical stress.

Integration with Other Systems

Although it can function independently, many activities of the integumentary system are integrated with those of other systems. Figure 8–3 diagrams the major functional relationships.

Let's Review What You've Just Learned

▶ Definitions

In the space provided, write the term for each of the following definitions.

_____ **1.** A protein produced by keratinocytes, in addition to keratin.

_____ **2.** The oily secretion from a sebaceous gland.

_____ **3.** The portion of skin that lies beneath the epidermis.

_____ **4.** The outermost layer of the epidermis.

_____ **5.** An orange-yellow pigment that normally accumulates inside epidermal cells.

_____ **6.** The name for the secretion produced by merocrine sweat glands.

_____ **7.** The layer of the epidermis that is found only in thick skin.

_____ **8.** The proper term for skin.

_____ **9.** Another term for layers.

_____ **10.** The layer of the dermis that contains the capillaries and sensory neurons that supply the surface of the skin.

_____ **11.** Another term for the subcutaneous layer.

_____ **12.** Coiled, tubular glands that produce a sticky, cloudy, and potentially odorous secretion.

_____ **13.** A protective structure found on the dorsal surfaces of the tips of fingers and toes.

_____ **14.** The layer of epidermis consisting of three to five layers of keratinocytes containing numerous granules of keratohyalin.

_____ **15.** Cells that produce a brown-black pigment called melanin.

_____ **16.** Complex organs that form hair.

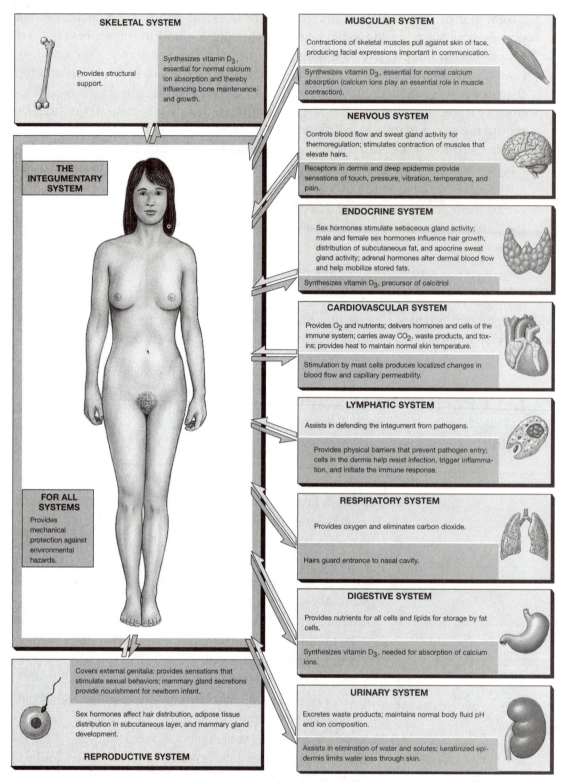

SKELETAL SYSTEM

Provides structural support.

Synthesizes vitamin D_3, essential for normal calcium ion absorption and thereby influencing bone maintenance and growth.

THE INTEGUMENTARY SYSTEM

FOR ALL SYSTEMS

Provides mechanical protection against environmental hazards.

Covers external genitalia; provides sensations that stimulate sexual behaviors; mammary gland secretions provide nourishment for newborn infant.

Sex hormones affect hair distribution, adipose tissue distribution in subcutaneous layer, and mammary gland development.

REPRODUCTIVE SYSTEM

MUSCULAR SYSTEM

Contractions of skeletal muscles pull against skin of face, producing facial expressions important in communication.

Synthesizes vitamin D_3, essential for normal calcium absorption (calcium ions play an essential role in muscle contraction).

NERVOUS SYSTEM

Controls blood flow and sweat gland activity for thermoregulation; stimulates contraction of muscles that elevate hairs.

Receptors in dermis and deep epidermis provide sensations of touch, pressure, vibration, temperature, and pain.

ENDOCRINE SYSTEM

Sex hormones stimulate sebaceous gland activity; male and female sex hormones influence hair growth, distribution of subcutaneous fat, and apocrine sweat gland activity; adrenal hormones alter dermal blood flow and help mobilize stored fats.

Synthesizes vitamin D_3, precursor of calcitriol

CARDIOVASCULAR SYSTEM

Provides O_2 and nutrients; delivers hormones and cells of the immune system; carries away CO_2, waste products, and toxins; provides heat to maintain normal skin temperature.

Stimulation by mast cells produces localized changes in blood flow and capillary permeability.

LYMPHATIC SYSTEM

Assists in defending the integument from pathogens.

Provides physical barriers that prevent pathogen entry; cells in the dermis help resist infection, trigger inflammation, and initiate the immune response.

RESPIRATORY SYSTEM

Provides oxygen and eliminates carbon dioxide.

Hairs guard entrance to nasal cavity.

DIGESTIVE SYSTEM

Provides nutrients for all cells and lipids for storage by fat cells.

Synthesizes vitamin D_3, needed for absorption of calcium ions.

URINARY SYSTEM

Excretes waste products; maintains normal body fluid pH and ion composition.

Assists in elimination of water and solutes; keratinized epidermis limits water loss through skin.

Figure 8–3 Functional Relationships between the Integumentary System and Other Systems.

_____ **17.** The layer of tissues beneath the dermis.

_____ **18.** The layer of the epidermis that produces new skin cells.

_____ **19.** Skin glands that discharge an oily, waxy secretion into hair follicles.

_____ **20.** Nipple-shaped structures that project from the dermis between the epidermal ridges.

_____ **21.** The outermost portion of the skin.

_____ **22.** The most abundant epithelial cells in the epidermis.

_____ **23.** The layer of epidermis composed of layers of epithelial cells that have a spiny appearance when prepared for viewing with a microscope.

_____ **24.** A protein precursor of keratin that is formed in large amounts by the cells of the stratum granulosum.

_____ **25.** The deeper layer of the dermis that is composed of an interwoven meshwork of dense, irregular connective tissue.

_____ **26.** Coiled tubular glands that produce a secretion that is predominantly water.

_____ **27.** Structures such as nails and hair that are derived from the epidermis.

▶ Word Roots, Prefixes, Suffixes, and Combining Forms

In the space provided, list the boldfaced terms introduced in this section that contain the indicated word part.

Word Part	Meaning	Examples
epi-	on	**28.** _____
mero-	part	**29.** _____
-cyte	cell	**30.** _____
apo-	from	**31.** _____
cut-	skin	**32.** _____
derm-	skin	**33.** _____
hypo-	under	**34.** _____
reticul-	net	**35.** _____
sub-	below	**36.** _____
spinos-	spiny	**37.** _____
corn-	horn	**38.** _____

OSSEOUS TISSUE AND THE SKELETAL SYSTEM

The skeletal system includes the bones of the skeleton and the cartilages, ligaments, and other connective tissues that stabilize or connect them. Skeletal elements are more than just racks to hang muscles on: They have a great variety of vital functions. In addition to supporting the weight of the body, bones work together with muscles to maintain body position and to produce controlled, precise movements. Without the skeleton to pull against, contracting muscle fibers would be unable to make us sit, stand, walk, or run. Without something to hold onto, contracting muscles merely get shorter and fatter.

The primary functions of the skeletal system are:

1. Support: The skeletal system provides structural support for the entire body. Individual bones or groups of bones provide a framework for the attachment of soft tissues and organs.

2. **Storage of minerals and lipids:** The calcium salts of bone are a valuable mineral reserve that maintains normal concentrations of calcium and phosphate ions in body fluids. Calcium is the most abundant mineral in the human body. In addition to acting as a mineral reserve, the bones of the skeleton store energy reserves as lipids in areas of yellow bone marrow.

3. **Blood cell production:** Red blood cells, white blood cells, and other blood elements are produced within the red bone marrow that fills the internal cavities of many bones.

4. **Protection:** Many delicate tissues and organs are surrounded by skeletal elements. The ribs protect the heart and lungs, the skull encloses the brain, the vertebrae shield the spinal cord, and the pelvis cradles delicate digestive and reproductive organs.

5. **Leverage:** Many bones of the skeleton function as levers that can change the magnitude and direction of the forces generated by skeletal muscles. The movements produced range from the delicate motion of a fingertip to powerful changes in the position of the entire body.

The bones of the skeleton are actually complex, dynamic organs that contain osseous tissue and other connective tissues, smooth muscle tissue, and neural tissue.

Structure of Bone

Bone tissue, or *osseous tissue*, is one of the supporting connective tissues (see Chapter 6). Like other connective tissues, osseous tissue contains specialized cells and a matrix consisting of extracellular protein fibers and a ground substance. The matrix of bone is solid and sturdy because of the deposition of calcium salts around the protein fibers.

Bone must be very strong, but it also must be able to flex under stress without shattering. These two qualities of bone are provided by its two main components. A hard mineral called **calcium hydroxyapatite** (hī-drok-sē-AP-a-tīt), which contains calcium phosphate $[Ca_3(PO_4)_2]$ and calcium hyroxide $[Ca(OH)_2]$, accounts for almost two-thirds of the weight of bone. Like concrete, the calcium minerals provide strength to the bone. The remaining one-third of a bone's weight is contributed by tough, flexible collagen fibers. Like the iron reinforcing rods in a concrete structure, the collagen fibers allow bone to bend and flex to a slight degree without sacrificing strength.

Four cell types can be found in the matrix of bone (Figure 8–4).

1. **Osteocytes** (OS-tē-ō-sītz; Greek *osteon*, bone + *cyte*, cell) are mature bone cells that account for most of the cell population in a bone.

2. **Osteoblasts** (OS-tē-ō-blasts) are cells that are actively depositing bone matrix.

3. **Osteoprogenitor** (os-tē-ō-prō-GEN-i-tur) **cells** are stem cells whose divisions give rise to osteoblasts.

4. **Osteoclasts** (OS-tē-ō-klasts) are cells that actively remove bone matrix.

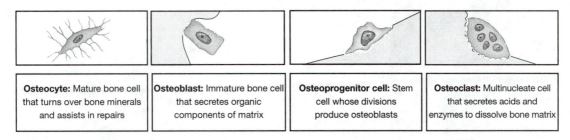

| Osteocyte: Mature bone cell that turns over bone minerals and assists in repairs | Osteoblast: Immature bone cell that secretes organic components of matrix | Osteoprogenitor cell: Stem cell whose divisions produce osteoblasts | Osteoclast: Multinucleate cell that secretes acids and enzymes to dissolve bone matrix |

Figure 8–4   The Cells of Bone.

Compact and Spongy Bone

There are two types of osseous tissue: compact bone, or dense bone, and spongy bone. **Compact bone** is relatively dense and solid, whereas **spongy bone** forms an open network of struts and plates. Both compact and spongy bone are present in a typical bone of the skeleton.

The basic functional unit of mature compact bone is the **osteon** (OS-tē-ōn), or **Haversian** (ha-VUR-zhun) **system** (Figure 8–4). Within an osteon the osteocytes occupy lacunae that are arranged in concentric layers around a **central canal,** or **Haversian canal,** that contains one or more blood vessels that supply the osteon. Osteons in compact bone are all lined up in the same way, making such bones very strong when stressed along that axis. In bones of the upper and lower appendages, osteons are parallel to the long axis of the tubular shaft, or **diaphysis** (dī-AF-i-sis) (Figure 8–5). A layer of compact bone covers the surfaces of bones; the thickness of that layer varies from region to region and from one bone to another. Compact bone is thickest where stresses arrive from a limited range of directions.

There are neither osteons nor blood vessels in spongy bone, or **cancellous** (KAN-sel-us) **bone.** The matrix in spongy bone forms struts or plates called **trabeculae** (tra-BEK-ū-lē; Latin *trabecula*, little beam) (Figure 8–5). The thin trabeculae often branch, creating an open network. Nutrients reach the osteocytes by diffusion along **canaliculi** (kan-uh-LIK-ū-lī; Latin *canaliculus*, small channel) that open onto the surfaces of the trabeculae. Spongy bone is present in the expanded regions of long bones where they connect with other skeletal elements. These expanded regions are the ends, or **epiphyses** (e-PIF-i-sēz), of the bones. Spongy bone is found where bones are not heavily stressed or where stresses arrive from many directions. In addition to being able to withstand stresses applied from many directions, spongy bone is much lighter than compact bone. Spongy bone reduces the weight of the skeleton and makes it easier for muscles to move the bones. Finally, the trabecular framework supports and protects the cells of the bone marrow.

The **marrow cavity,** also known as the **medullary** (MED-ū-ler-ē; Latin *medulla*, marrow) **cavity,** contains **bone marrow,** a loose connective tissue that may be dominated by adipocytes **(yellow marrow)** or by a mixture of mature and immature red and white blood cells and the stem cells that produce them **(red marrow).** In a typical bone, the compact bone on the outside, or **cortex,** encloses the marrow cavity. Compact bone forms the walls, and an internal layer of spongy bone surrounds the marrow cavity and supports the cells of the bone marrow.

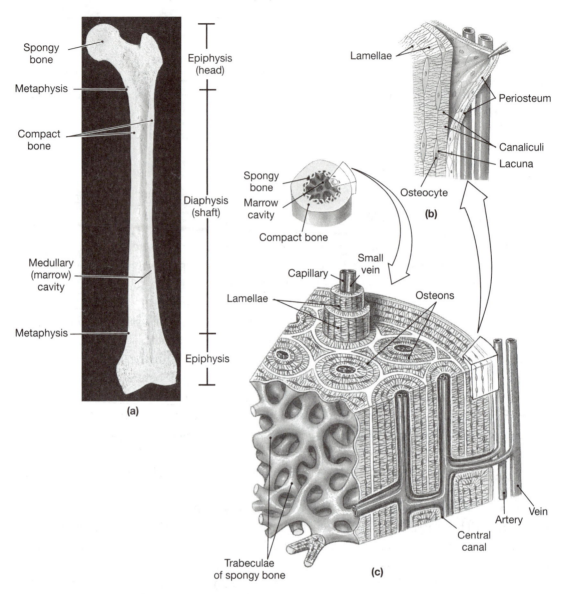

Figure 8–5   Histological Organization of Bone.
(a) Sectional view of a representative limb bone. (b) Diagrammatic view of the structure of the periosteum (c) Diagrammatic view of the structure of a representative bone.

The outer surface of a bone is covered by a membrane called the **periosteum** (per-ē-OS-tē-um) that consists of a fibrous connective tissue outer layer and a cellular inner layer (Figure 8–4). The periosteum (1) isolates the bone from surrounding tissues, (2) provides a route for blood vessels and nerves, and (3) actively participates in bone growth and repair. Inside the bone, a cellular layer called the **endosteum** (en-DOS-tē-um) lines the marrow cavity.

Bone Growth and Development

During development, mesenchyme or cartilage is replaced by bone. This process of replacing other tissues with bone is called **ossification** (os-i-fi-KĀ-shun; Latin *os*, bone + *facere*, to make). Ossification refers specifically to the formation of bone. The process of **calcification** (kal-si-fi-KĀ-shun) refers to the deposition of calcium salts within a tissue.

There are two major forms of ossification. In **intramembranous** (in-tra-MEM-bra-nus) **ossification,** bone develops from mesenchyme or fibrous connective tissue. In **endochondral** (en-dō-KON-drul) **ossification,** bone replaces an existing cartilage model.

Anatomy of Skeletal Elements

The human skeleton contains 206 named bones. We can divide these bones into six broad categories according to their individual shape. Refer to Figure 8–6 as we describe the anatomical classification of bones.

1. **Long bones** are characterized by diaphysis and epiphysis portions and contain a marrow cavity. Long bones are found in the arm and forearm, thigh and leg, palms, soles, fingers, and toes.

2. **Short bones** are boxlike in appearance. Their external surfaces are covered by compact bone, but the interior contains spongy bone. Examples of short bones include bones of the wrists and ankles.

3. **Flat bones** have thin, roughly parallel surfaces of compact bone. In structure, a flat bone resembles a spongy bone sandwich, with a layer of spongy bone between two layers of compact bone. Flat bones are strong but relatively light. Flat bones form the roof of the skull, the sternum, the ribs, and the scapula. They provide protection for underlying soft tissues and offer an extensive surface area for the attachment of skeletal muscles.

4. **Irregular bones** have complex shapes with short, flat, notched, or ridged surfaces. Their internal structure is equally varied. The spinal vertebrae and several bones in the skull are irregular bones.

5. **Sesamoid bones** are usually small, round, and flat. They develop inside tendons and are most often encountered near joints at the knee, the hands, and the feet. Few individuals have sesamoid bones at every possible location, but everyone has sesamoid **patellae** (pa-TEL-ē), or kneecaps.

6. **Sutural bones**, or **Wormian bones**, are small, flat, irregularly shaped bones found between the flat bones of the skull in a suture line (the line where two bones join). There are individual variations in the number, shape, and position of the sutural bones. Their borders are like puzzle pieces, and the bones range in size from a grain of sand to the size of a quarter.

Each bone in the body has not only a distinctive shape but also characteristic external and internal features. Elevations or projections form where tendons and ligaments attach and where adjacent bones connect. Depressions, grooves, and tunnels in bone indicate sites where blood vessels and nerves lie alongside or penetrate the bone. Detailed examination of these bone markings, or surface features, can yield an abundance of anatomical information. For example anthropologists, criminologists, and pathologists often can determine the size, weight, sex, and general appearance of an individual on the basis of incomplete skeletal remains. These markings are useful because they provide fixed landmarks that can help in determining the position of the soft tissue components of other systems. Specific anatomical terms are used to describe the various elevations and depressions. Bone marking terminology is presented in Table 8–1 and illustrated in Figure 8–7.

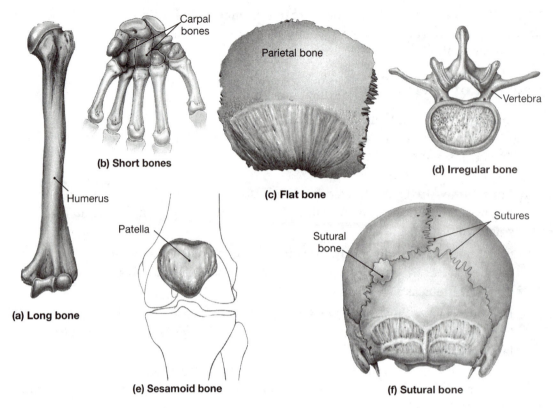

(a) Long bone — Humerus

(b) Short bones — Carpal bones

(c) Flat bone — Parietal bone

(d) Irregular bone — Vertebra

(e) Sesamoid bone — Patella

(f) Sutural bone — Sutures, Sutural bone

Figure 8–6 **Classification of Bones by Shape.**

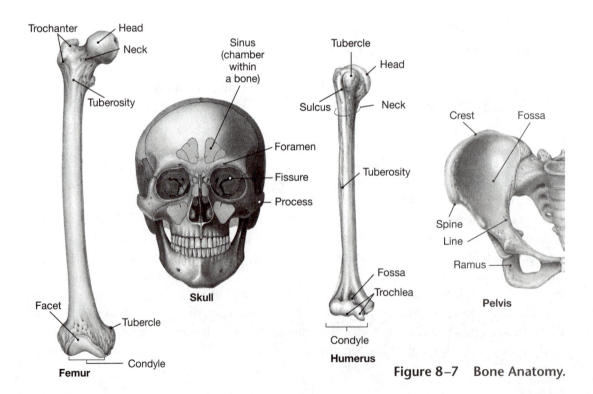

Femur — Trochanter, Head, Neck, Tuberosity, Facet, Tubercle, Condyle

Skull — Sinus (chamber within a bone), Foramen, Fissure, Process

Humerus — Tubercle, Head, Sulcus, Neck, Tuberosity, Fossa, Trochlea, Condyle

Pelvis — Crest, Fossa, Spine, Line, Ramus

Figure 8–7 **Bone Anatomy.**

Table 8–1 An Introduction to Skeletal Terminology

General Description	Anatomical Term	Definition
Elevations and projections (general)	**Process**	Any projection or bump
	Ramus	An extension of a bone making an angle to the rest of the structure
Processes formed where tendons or ligaments attach	**Trochanter**	A large, rough projection
	Tuberosity	A smaller, rough projection
	Tubercle	A small, rounded projection
	Crest	A prominent ridge
	Line	A low ridge
Processes formed for articulation with adjacent bones	**Head**	The expanded articular end of an epiphysis, separated from the shaft by a narrower neck
	Neck	A narrow connection between the epiphysis and diaphysis
	Condyle	A smooth, rounded articular process
	Trochlea	A smooth, grooved articular process shaped like a pulley
	Facet	A small, flat articular surface
	Spine	A pointed process
Depressions	**Fossa**	A shallow depression
	Sulcus	A narrow groove
Openings	**Foramen**	A rounded passageway for blood vessels and/or nerves
	Fissure	An elongate cleft
	Sinus or antrum	A chamber within a bone, normally filled with air

The Skeleton

The skeletal system is divided into axial and appendicular divisions: the components of the axial skeleton are highlighted in Figure 8–8. The **axial** (AK-sē-ul) **skeleton** consists of the bones of the skull, thorax, and vertebral column. These elements form the longitudinal axis of the body. There are 80 bones in the axial skeleton, roughly 40 percent of the bones in the human body.

The function of the axial skeleton is to provide a framework that supports and protects organs in the dorsal and ventral body cavities. In addition, it provides an extensive surface area for the attachment of muscles that (1) adjust the positions of the head, neck, and trunk; (2) perform respiratory movements; and (3) stabilize or position structures of the appendicular skeleton. The joints of the axial skeleton permit limited movement, but they are very strong and heavily reinforced with ligaments.

The **appendicular** (ap-en-DIK-ū-lur) **skeleton** consists of 126 bones. This division includes the bones of the limbs and the supporting elements, or girdles, that connect them to the trunk (Figure 8–9). Each arm articulates with the trunk at the **shoulder**

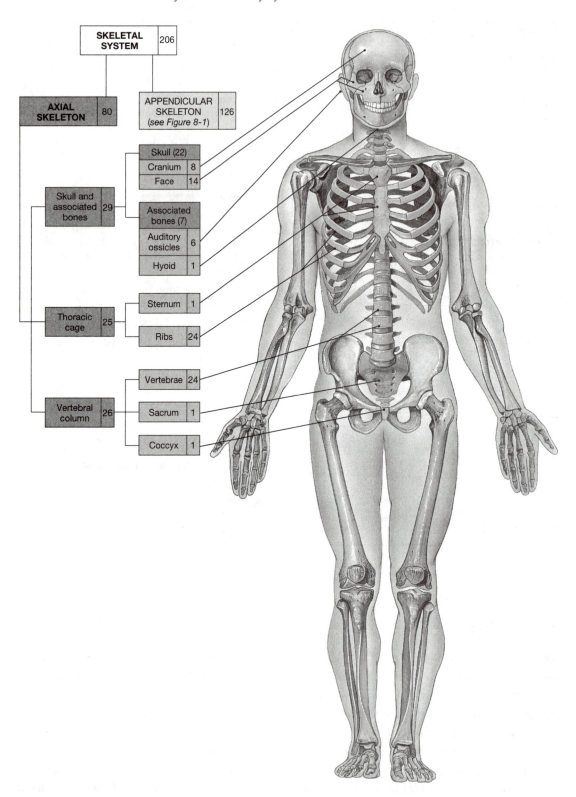

Figure 8–8

Anterior view of the entire skeleton, with the axial components highlighted. The total number of bones of each type or within each category is indicated.

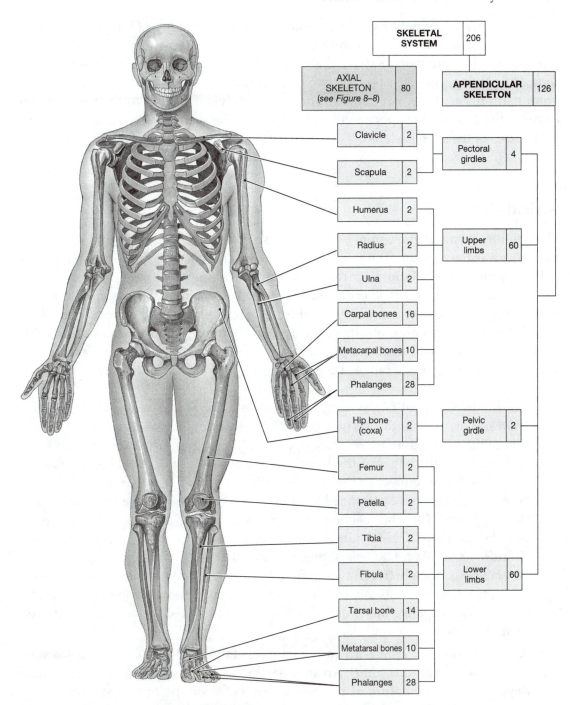

Figure 8–9   The Appendicular Skeleton.
Anterior view of the entire skeleton, with appendicular components highlighted. The total number of bones of each type or within each category is indicated.

girdle or **pectoral** (PEK-tuh-rul) **girdle.** The shoulder girdle consists of the S-shaped **clavicle** (KLAV-i-kul)(collarbone) and a broad flat **scapula** (SKAP-ū-luh)(shoulder blade). The skeleton of the upper limb includes the bones of the arm, forearm, wrist, and hand. Remember that in anatomical descriptions the term *arm* refers only to the proximal portion of the upper limb, not to the entire limb.

The bones of the **pelvic girdle** are more massive than those of the pectoral girdle because of the stresses involved in weight bearing and locomotion. The bones of the lower extremities are more massive than those of the upper extremities for similar reasons. The pelvic girdle consists of the two fused **coxae** (KOK-sē), or **innominate** (i-NOM-i-nāt; Latin *innominatus*, not named) **bones.** The **pelvis** is a composite structure that includes the coxae of the appendicular skeleton and the **sacrum** (SĀ-krum) and **coccyx** (KOK-siks) of the axial skeleton.

Articulations

Most of our daily activities, from breathing or speaking to writing or running, involve movements of the skeleton. The bones of the skeleton are solid and movements can occur only at **joints,** or **articulations** (ar-tik-ū-LĀ-shuns), where two bones interconnect.

The structure of a joint determines the type of movement that can occur. Each joint reflects a workable compromise between the need for strength and the need for mobility.

Three major categories of joints are based on the range of motion permitted (Table 8–2). These functional categories are then subdivided on the basis of the anatomical structure of the joint or the range of motion permitted. The basic categories are:

1. An immovable joint is a **synarthrosis** (sin-ar-THRŌ-sis; Greek, *syn*, together + *arthros*, joint). A synarthrosis may be fibrous or cartilaginous depending on the nature of the connection between the opposing bones. In a **suture** (SOO-chur; Latin *sutura*, seam), the edges of the bones are interlocked and bound together at the suture by dense connective tissue. A **gomphosis** (gom-FŌ-sis; Greek *gomphosis*, a bolting together) is a specialized joint that binds the teeth to the bony sockets in the jaw bones. The fibrous connection between a tooth and its socket is a **periodontal** (pe-rē-ō-DON-tal; Greek *peri*, around + *odontos*, tooth) **ligament.** A **synchondrosis** (sin-kon-DRŌ-sis; Greek *syn*, together + *chondros*, cartilage) is a rigid cartilaginous plate between two articulating bones. A **synostosis** (sin-os-TŌ-sis; Greek *syn*, together + *osteon*, bone) is a totally rigid immovable joint that is created when two separate bones actually fuse together so that the boundary between them disappears.

2. A slightly movable joint is an **amphiarthrosis** (am-fē-ar-THRŌ-sis; Greek *amphi*, on both sides + *arthros*, joint). An amphiarthrosis may be fibrous or cartilaginous depending on the nature of the connection between the opposing bones. At a **syndesmosis** (sin-dez-MŌ-sis; Greek *syn*, together + *desmos*, band or ligament), bones are connected by a ligament. At a **symphysis** (SIM-fi-sis; Greek *sym*, together + *physis*, growth) the articulating bones are separated by a wedge or pad of fibrocartilage.

3. A freely movable joint is a **diarthrosis** (dī-ar-THRŌ-sis; Greek *dia*, through). Diarthroses are also called **synovial** (si-NŌ-vē-ul) **joints.** Their basic structure was introduced in Chapter 6 in the discussion of synovial membranes. Diarthroses are subdivided according to the degree of movement permitted.

Table 8-2 A Functional Classification of Articulations

Functional Category	Structural Category	Description	Example
Synarthrosis (no movement)	**Fibrous**		
	Suture	Fibrous connections plus interdigitation	Between the bones of the skull
	Gomphosis	Fibrous connections plus insertion in alveolar process	Betweeen the teeth and jaws
	Cartilaginous		
	Synchondrosis	Interposition of cartilage plate	Epiphyseal plates
	Bony fusion		
	Synostosis	Conversion of other articular; form a solid mass of bone	Portions of the skull
Amphiarthrosis (little movement)	**Fibrous**		
	Syndesmosis	Ligamentous connection	Between the tibia and fibula
	Cartilaginous		
	Symphysis	Connection by a fibrocartilage pad	Between right and left halves of pelvis; between adjacent vertebral bodies along vertebral column
Diarthrosis (free movement)	**Synovial**	Complex joint bounded by joint capsule and containing synovial fluid	Numerous; subdivided by range of movement
	Monaxial	Permits movement in one plane	Elbow, ankle
	Biaxial	Permits movement in two planes	Ribs, wrist
	Triaxial	Permits movement in all three planes	Shoulder, hip

INTEGRATION WITH OTHER SYSTEMS

Although the bones may seem inert, they are dynamic structures. The entire skeletal system is intimately associated with other systems. The bones of the skeleton are attached to the muscular system, extensively connected to the cardiovascular and lymphatic systems, and largely under the physiological control of the endocrine system. The digestive and excretory systems also play important roles in providing the calcium and phosphate mineral needed for bone growth. In return, the skeleton provides a reserve of calcium, phosphate, and other minerals that can compensate for changes in the dietary supply of those ions. The functional relationships between the skeletal system and other systems are diagrammed in Figure 8-10.

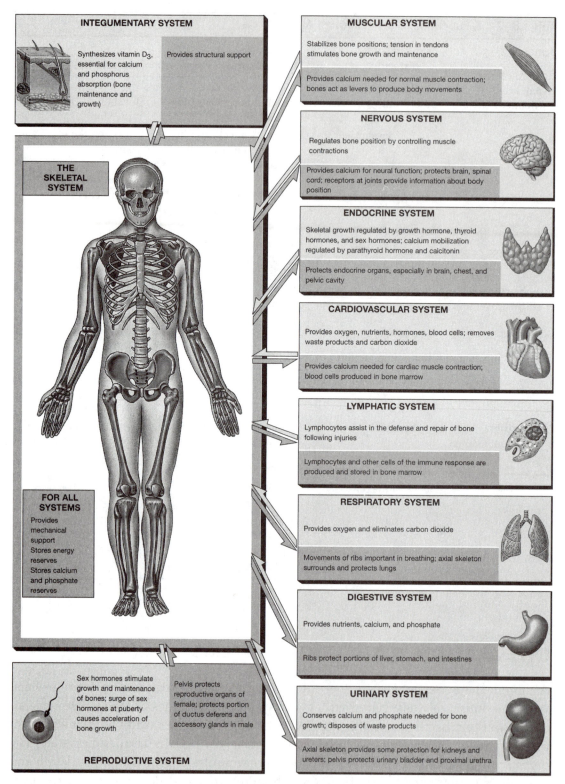

INTEGUMENTARY SYSTEM

Synthesizes vitamin D₃, essential for calcium and phosphorus absorption (bone maintenance and growth)

Provides structural support

THE SKELETAL SYSTEM

FOR ALL SYSTEMS
Provides mechanical support
Stores energy reserves
Stores calcium and phosphate reserves

Sex hormones stimulate growth and maintenance of bones; surge of sex hormones at puberty causes acceleration of bone growth

Pelvis protects reproductive organs of female; protects portion of ductus deferens and accessory glands in male

REPRODUCTIVE SYSTEM

MUSCULAR SYSTEM

Stabilizes bone positions; tension in tendons stimulates bone growth and maintenance

Provides calcium needed for normal muscle contraction; bones act as levers to produce body movements

NERVOUS SYSTEM

Regulates bone position by controlling muscle contractions

Provides calcium for neural function; protects brain, spinal cord; receptors at joints provide information about body position

ENDOCRINE SYSTEM

Skeletal growth regulated by growth hormone, thyroid hormones, and sex hormones; calcium mobilization regulated by parathyroid hormone and calcitonin

Protects endocrine organs, especially in brain, chest, and pelvic cavity

CARDIOVASCULAR SYSTEM

Provides oxygen, nutrients, hormones, blood cells; removes waste products and carbon dioxide

Provides calcium needed for cardiac muscle contraction; blood cells produced in bone marrow

LYMPHATIC SYSTEM

Lymphocytes assist in the defense and repair of bone following injuries

Lymphocytes and other cells of the immune response are produced and stored in bone marrow

RESPIRATORY SYSTEM

Provides oxygen and eliminates carbon dioxide

Movements of ribs important in breathing; axial skeleton surrounds and protects lungs

DIGESTIVE SYSTEM

Provides nutrients, calcium, and phosphate

Ribs protect portions of liver, stomach, and intestines

URINARY SYSTEM

Conserves calcium and phosphate needed for bone growth; disposes of waste products

Axial skeleton provides some protection for kidneys and ureters; pelvis protects urinary bladder and proximal urethra

Figure 8–10 Functional Relationships between the Skeletal System and Other Systems.

✏️ Let's Review What You've Just Learned

▶ Definitions

In the space provided, write the term for each of the following definitions.

_____ **39.** The process of forming bone.

_____ **40.** A cell that deposits bone matrix.

_____ **41.** The proper term for the kneecap.

_____ **42.** The expanded ends of a long bone.

_____ **43.** Bones that are boxlike in appearance.

_____ **44.** The type of joint that permits a wide range of movements.

_____ **45.** The mineral found in the inorganic matrix of bone.

_____ **46.** The term for bone that is relatively dense and solid.

_____ **47.** Bone marrow that is dominated by adipocytes.

_____ **48.** A totally rigid and immovable joint.

_____ **49.** The division of the skeleton that consists of the bones of the skull and vertebral column.

_____ **50.** The term for bones with complex shapes.

_____ **51.** A cell that actively removes bone matrix.

_____ **52.** The deposition of calcium salts within a tissue.

_____ **53.** The functional unit of mature compact bone.

_____ **54.** The lining of the marrow cavity.

_____ **55.** Bones that develop within tendons.

_____ **56.** The proper term for the collarbone.

_____ **57.** The skeletal elements that attach the upper appendages to the axial skeleton.

_____ **58.** A rigid cartilaginous bridge between two articulating bones.

_____ **59.** Bone that forms an open network of struts and plates.

_____ **60.** The membrane that covers the outer surface of a bone.

_____ **61.** The process in which mesenchyme or fibrous connective tissue is replaced by bone.

_____ **62.** Bones that are characterized by diaphysis and epiphysis portions and that contain a marrow cavity.

_____ **63.** The proper term for the shoulderblade.

_____ **64.** The proper term for the hipbone.

_____ **65.** The points in the skeleton where movement can occur.

_____ **66.** The general term for a slightly movable joint.

_____ **67.** A general term for an immovable joint.

_____ **68.** The structure that consists of the coxae, sacrum, and coccyx.

_____ **69.** The struts or plates found in spongy bone.

_____ **70.** The term for the shaft portion of a long bone.

_____ **71.** Mature bone cells.

_____ **72.** The central area of an osteon that contains blood vessels.

_____ **73.** Narrow passageways through the bony matrix.

_____ **74.** The cavity in a bone that contains bone marrow.

_____ **75.** The outer layer of compact bone that encloses the marrow cavity.

_____ **76.** The process by which cartilage is replaced by bone.

_____ **77.** Bones that have thin, roughly parallel surfaces of compact bone with spongy bone sandwiched between.

_____ **78.** The portion of the skeleton composed of the limbs and their supporting elements.

_____ **79.** The skeletal elements that attach the lower limbs to the axial skeleton.

_____ **80.** A synarthrotic joint found between some bones of the skull in which the edges are interlocked and bound by dense connective tissue.

_____ **81.** Stem cells whose divisions give rise to osteoblasts.

_____ **82.** A slightly movable joint in which the bones are attached by ligaments.

_____ **83.** Bone marrow that contains a mixture of mature and immature red and white blood cells and the stem cells that produce them.

_____ **84.** A special synarthrosis that binds teeth to their bony sockets.

_____ **85.** Small, flat, irregularly shaped bones found between the flat bones of the skull.

_____ **86.** An articulation in which the bones are separated by a wedge or pad of fibrocartilage.

_____ **87.** The fibrous connection between a tooth and its socket.

► Word Roots, Prefixes, Suffixes, and Combining Forms

In the space provided, list the boldfaced terms introduced in this section that contain the indicated word part.

Word Part	Meaning	Examples
syn-	together	**88.** _____
-blast	precursor	**89.** _____
peri-	around	**90.** _____
osteo-	bone	**91.** _____
hydro-	water	**92.** _____
endo-	inside	**93.** _____
-clast	broken	**94.** _____
chondro-	cartilage	**95.** _____
arthro-	joint	**96.** _____
sym-	together	**97.** _____
dia-	through	**98.** _____
epi-	on	**99.** _____
pro-	before	**100.** _____
-physis	growth	**101.** _____
amphi-	both	**102.** _____
intra-	within	**103.** _____

MUSCLE TISSUE AND THE MUSCULAR SYSTEM

The muscular system includes all of the skeletal muscles that can be controlled voluntarily. Most of the muscle tissue in the body is part of this system, and approximately 700 skeletal muscles have been identified. Some are attached to bony processes, others to broad sheets of connective tissue, but all are directly or indirectly associated with the skeletal system.

Muscle tissue, one of the four primary tissue types, consists chiefly of muscle cells that are highly specialized for contraction. There are three types of muscle tissue: skeletal muscle, cardiac muscle, and smooth muscle. Without these muscle tissues, introduced in Chapter 6, nothing in the body would move, and no body movement could occur. Skeletal muscles move the body by pulling on bones of the skeleton, making it possible for us to walk, dance, bite into an apple, or play the piano. Cardiac muscle tissue pushes blood through the cardiovascular system. Smooth muscle tissue pushes fluids and solids along the digestive tract, regulates the diameter of small arteries, and performs a variety of other functions.

Skeletal Muscle

Skeletal muscle tissue is found within skeletal muscles, organs that also contain connective tissues, nerves, and blood vessels. As the name implies, skeletal muscles are directly or indirectly attached to the bones of the skeleton. Skeletal muscle tissue gives skeletal muscle the ability to perform the following functions.

1. **Produce skeletal movement:** Skeletal muscle contractions pull on tendons and move the bones of the skeleton. The effects range from simple motions such as extending the arm to the highly coordinated movements of swimming, skiing, and typing.

2. **Maintain posture and body position:** Tension in our skeletal muscles also maintains body posture—for example, holding the head in position when reading a book or balancing the weight of the body above the feet when walking. Without constant muscular activity we could not sit upright without collapsing into a heap or stand without toppling over.

3. **Support soft tissues:** The abdominal wall and the floor of the pelvic cavity consist of layers of skeletal muscle. These muscles support the weight of visceral organs and shield internal tissues from injury.

4. **Guard entrances and exits:** The openings of the digestive and urinary tracts are encircled by skeletal muscles. These muscles provide voluntary control over swallowing, defecation, and urination.

5. **Maintain body temperature:** Muscle contractions require energy, and whenever energy is used in the body, some of it is converted to heat. The heat released by working muscles keeps our body temperature in the range required for normal functioning.

The Structure of Skeletal Muscle

Each skeletal muscle contains three layers of connective tissue: an outer epimysium, a central perimysium, and an inner endomysium. These layers and their relationships are diagrammed in Figure 8–11.

The entire muscle is surrounded by the **epimysium** (ep-i-MĪZ-ē-um; Greek *epi*, on + *mys*, muscle), a dense layer of collagen fibers. The epimysium separates the muscle from surrounding tissues and organs. It is one component of the deep fascia, the dense connective tissue layer described in Chapter 6.

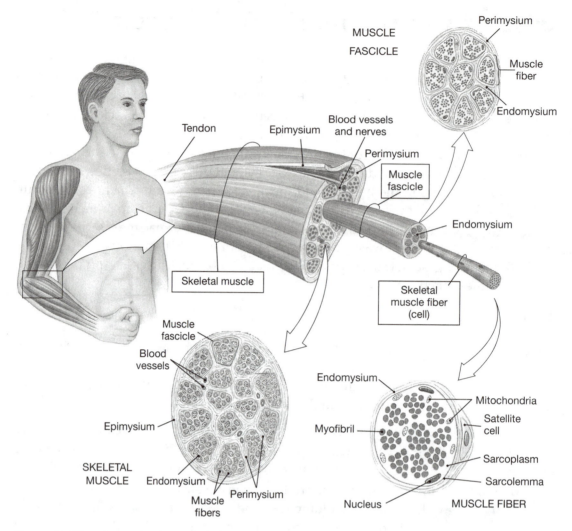

Figure 8–11 Organization of Skeletal Muscles.
A skeletal muscle consists of fascicles (bundles of muscle fibers) enclosed by the epimysium. The bundles are separated by connective tissue fibers of the perimysium, and within each bundle the muscle fibers are surrounded by the endomysium. Each muscle fiber has many superficial nuclei as well as mitochondria.

The connective tissue fibers of the **perimysium** (per-i-MĪZ-ē-um; Greek *peri*, around) divide the skeletal muscle into a series of compartments, each containing a bundle of muscle fibers called a **fascicle** (FA-sik-ul; Latin *fasciculus*, a bundle). Within the fascicle, the delicate connective tissue of the **endomysium** (en-dō-MĪZ-ē-um; Greek *endo*, inside) surrounds the skeletal muscle fibers and ties adjacent muscle fibers together.

The muscle cells, usually called muscle fibers, within a single fascicle are arranged in parallel. The organization of the fascicles in the skeletal muscle can vary, as can the relationship between the fascicles and the associated tendon. There are four patterns of fascicle organization (Figure 8–12).

1. **Parallel muscles:** In a **parallel muscle** the fascicles are parallel to the long axis of the muscle. The functional characteristics of a parallel muscle resemble those of an individual muscle fiber. Most of the skeletal muscles in the body are parallel muscles.

2. **Convergent muscles:** In a **convergent muscle** the muscle fibers are based over a broad area, but all the fibers come together at a common attachment site. Such a

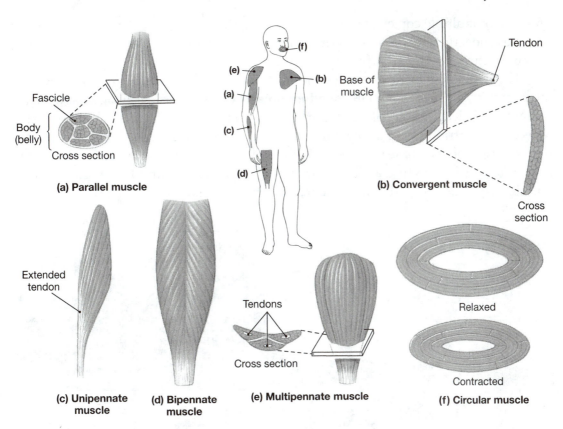

Figure 8–12 **Different Arrangements of Skeletal Muscle Fibers.**

muscle has versatility, for the direction of pull can be changed by stimulating only one group of muscle cells at any one time.

3. **Pennate muscles:** In a **pennate** (PEN-āte; Latin *pennatus*, feathered) **muscle** the fascicles form a common angle with the tendon. Because the muscle cells pull at an angle, contracting pennate muscles do not move their tendons as far as parallel muscles do. But a pennate muscle will contain more muscle fibers than a parallel muscle of the same size. A muscle that has more muscle fibers also has more contractile elements, and as a result contraction of the pennate muscle generates more tension than does a contraction of a parallel muscle of the same size.

4. **Circular muscles:** In a **circular muscle**, or **sphincter** (SFINK-tur; Greek *sphinkter*, to bind tight), the fibers are concentrically arranged around an opening or recess. When the muscle contracts, the diameter of the opening decreases. Circular muscles guard entrances and exits of internal passageways such as those of the digestive and urinary tracts.

Skeletal muscle fibers are quite different from the "typical" cells described in Chapter 4. One obvious difference is size, for skeletal muscle fibers are enormous. A muscle fiber from a thigh muscle could have a diameter of 100 μm and a length equal to that of the entire muscle (30–40 cm, or 10–16 in.). A second obvious difference is that skeletal muscle fibers are multinucleate: Each skeletal muscle fiber contains hundreds of nuclei just beneath the cell membrane. The genes contained in these nuclei direct the production of enzymes and structural proteins required for normal contraction, and the presence of multiple copies of these genes speeds up the process. Rapid production of enzymes and structural proteins is particularly important in skeletal muscle fibers, where metabolic turnover is very rapid.

The distinctive features of size and multiple nuclei are related. During development, groups of embryonic cells called **myoblasts** (MĪ-ō-blasts) fuse together to create individual skeletal muscle fibers (Figure 8–13). Each nucleus in a skeletal muscle fiber reflects the contribution of a single myoblast. Some myoblasts do not fuse with developing muscle fibers. These unfused cells remain in adult skeletal muscle tissue as **satellite cells.** After an injury, satellite cells may enlarge, divide, and fuse with damaged muscle fibers, thereby assisting in the regeneration of tissue.

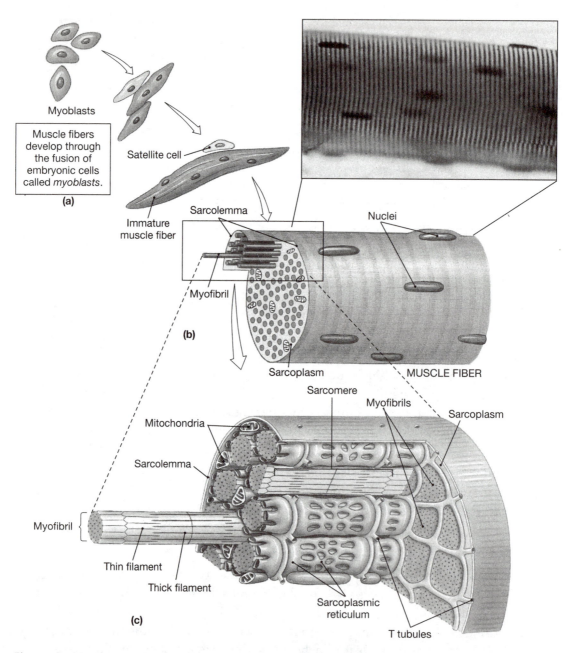

Figure 8–13   Formation and Structure of a Skeletal Muscle Fiber.

(a) The formation of muscle fibers through the fusion of myoblasts. **(b)** Micrograph and diagrammatic view of one muscle fiber. (LM × 612) **(c)** The internal organization of a muscle fiber.

The cell membrane, or **sarcolemma** (sar-kō-LEM-uh; Greek *sarcos*, muscle + *lemma*, husk), of a muscle fiber surrounds the cytoplasm or **sarcoplasm** (SAR-kō-plazm) (Figure 8–13). Like other cell membranes, the sarcolemma has a characteristic transmembrane potential. In a skeletal muscle fiber, a sudden change in the transmembrane potential is the first step that leads to a contraction. Because a skeletal muscle fiber is very large, the signal to contract must be conveyed to the interior of the cell. The signal is conveyed along the **transverse tubules,** or **T tubules.** T tubules are narrow tubes that begin at the sarcolemma and extend into the sarcoplasm at right angles to the membrane surface. They are filled with extracellular fluid, and they form passageways through the muscle fiber.

Inside the muscle fiber, branches of the transverse tubules encircle cylindrical structures called **myofibrils** (mī-ō-FĪ-brilz). A myofibril is a cylindrical structure 1–2 μm in diameter and as long as the entire cell. Each skeletal muscle fiber contains hundreds to thousands of myofibrils. Myofibrils are bundles of **myofilaments** (mī-ō-FIL-a-mentz), protein filaments primarily composed of actin (found in **thin filaments**) and myosin (found in **thick filaments**). Myofilaments are organized in repeating functional units called **sarcomeres** (SAR-kō-mērz; Greek *sarkos*, flesh + *meros*, part) detailed in Figure 8–13.

Myofibrils can actively shorten; they are the organelles responsible for skeletal muscle contraction. Wherever a transverse tubule encircles a myofibril, it makes close contact with the membranes of the **sarcoplasmic reticulum** (sar-kō-PLAZ-mik re-TIK-ū-lum). The sarcoplasmic reticulum (SR) is a membrane complex similar to the smooth endoplasmic reticulum of other cells. In skeletal muscle fibers, the SR forms a tubular network that wraps around each individual myofibril.

Contractions of Skeletal Muscle

Skeletal muscle fibers contract only under the control of the nervous system. Communication between the nervous system and the skeletal muscle fibers occurs at specialized intercellular connections known as **neuromuscular** (noo-rō-MUS-kū-lur) **junctions** (NMJ).

Each skeletal muscle fiber is controlled by a neuron at a single neuromuscular junction midway along its length. A single axon branches within the perimysium to form fine branches. Each of these branches ends at an expanded **synaptic** (si-NAP-tik; Greek *synaptikos*, connective) **knob.** The synaptic knob contains vesicles filled with molecules of **acetylcholine** (as-e-til-KŌ-lēn), usually abbreviated ACh. ACh is an example of a **neurotransmitter,** a chemical released by neurons to change the membrane properties of other cells. The release of ACh from the synaptic knob can result in changes in the sarcolemma's transmembrane potential that trigger the contraction of the muscle fiber.

When a neuron stimulates a muscle fiber, the process occurs in a series of steps (Figure 8–14).

Step 1: *The arrival of an action potential.* The stimulus for ACh release is the arrival of an electrical impulse, or action potential, at the synaptic knob.

Step 2: *The release of ACh.*

Step 3: *ACh binding to receptor molecules on the muscle membrane.*

Step 4: *Formation of an action potential in the sarcolemma.*

Step 5: *Return to the resting state.*

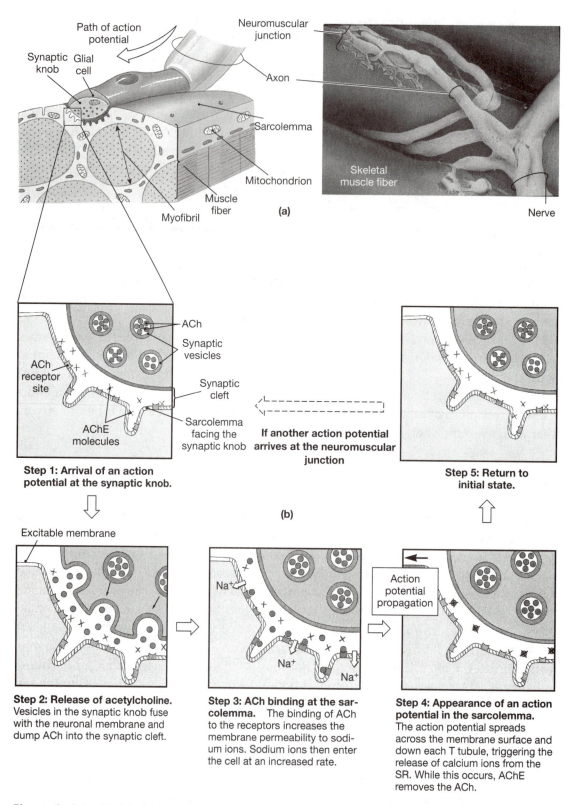

Figure 8–14 Skeletal Muscle Innervation.

(a) Diagrammatic and SEM views of a neuromuscular junction (NMJ). Several neuromuscular junctions are seen on the muscle fibers of the SEM. **(b)** Steps in the transmission of action potentials across the neuromuscular junction.

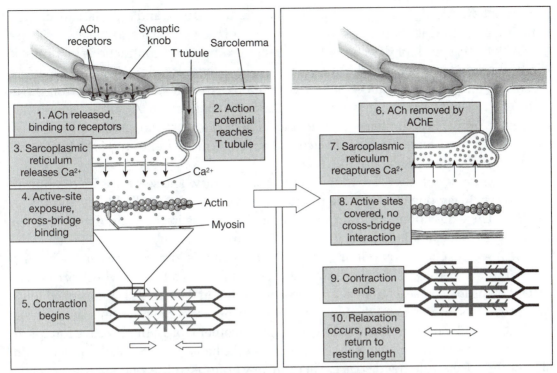

Steps in the initiation of a contraction   **Steps that end the contraction**

Figure 8–15   A Summary of Steps in a Skeletal Muscle Contraction.

The link between the generation of an action potential in the sarcolemma and the start of a muscle contraction is called **excitation-contraction coupling.**

This coupling occurs when an action potential reaches the sarcoplasmic reticulum, triggering a release of calcium ions from the SR (Figure 8–15). The calcium ions diffuse rapidly into the sarcoplasm, where they bind to specialized proteins attached to the actin molecules. This binding results in the exposure of *active sites* on the thin filaments. When the active sites are exposed, they become bound to projections, or myosin *cross-bridges*, that extend outward from the thick filaments. Energy derived from ATP is then used to pull the actin filaments along the length of the thick filaments, toward the center of the sarcomere. This sliding of thin filaments along thick filaments shortens the sarcomere, and ultimately the entire muscle. Relaxation occurs when the calcium ions are actively transported back into the SR. The myosin molecules disengage the actin molecules, and the elastic nature of the muscle tissue and the pull of opposing muscles cause the muscle to return to its precontraction length.

Although most skeletal muscle fibers contract at comparable rates and shorten to the same degree, variations in microscopic and macroscopic organization can dramatically affect the power, range, and speed of movement produced when muscle contracts.

Biomechanics

At the level of the individual skeletal muscle, two factors interact to determine the effects of its contraction: (1) the anatomical arrangement of the muscle fibers and (2) the way the muscle attaches to the bones of the skeletal system. The performance of muscles in the body can be understood in terms of basic mechanical laws. The analysis of biological systems in mechanical terms is the study of **biomechanics.**

Skeletal muscles do not work in isolation. When a muscle is attached to the skeleton, the nature and site of the connection will determine the force, speed, and range of the movement produced. These characteristics are interdependent, and the relationships can explain a great deal about the general organization of the muscular and skeletal systems.

The force, speed, or direction of movement produced by contractions of a muscle can be modified by attaching the muscle to a lever. A **lever** is a rigid structure—such as a board, a crowbar, or a bone—that moves on a fixed point called the **fulcrum** (FUL-krum). In the body, each bone is a lever, and each joint a fulcrum. A child's teeter-totter, or seesaw, provides a familiar example of lever action. Levers can change (1) the direction of an applied force, (2) the distance and speed of movement produced by a force, and (3) the effective strength of the force.

Three classes of levers are found in the human body. The seesaw is an example of a **first-class lever**: one in which the fulcrum lies between the applied force and the resistance. There are not many examples of first-class levers in the body. One, involving the muscles that extend the neck, is shown in Figure 8–16a.

In a **second class lever** (Figure 8–16b) the resistance is located between the applied force and the fulcrum. A familiar example of such a lever is a loaded wheelbarrow. The weight of the load is the resistance, and the upward lift on the handle is the applied force. Because in this arrangement the force is always farther from the fulcrum than the resistance is, a small force can balance a larger weight. In other words, the effective force is increased. Notice, however, that when a force moves the handle, the resistance moves more slowly and covers a shorter distance. There are few examples of second-class levers in the body. When you stand on tiptoe, your calf muscles act via a second-class lever system.

Third class levers are the most common levers in the body. In this lever system, a force is applied between the resistance and the fulcrum (Figure 8–16c). The effect of this arrangement is just the reverse of that produced by a second-class lever: Speed and distance traveled are increased at the expense of effective force. In the example illustrated (the muscle that flexes the forearm), the resistance is six times farther away from the fulcrum than is the applied force. The effective force is reduced accordingly. The muscle must generate 180 kg of tension at its attachment to the forearm to support 30 kg held in the hand. However, the distance traveled and the speed of movement are increased by the same ratio: The resistance will travel 45 cm when the attachment point moves 7.5 cm.

Although not every muscle operates as part of a lever system, the presence of levers provides speed and versatility far in excess of what we would predict on the basis of muscle physiology alone. Skeletal muscle fibers resemble one another closely, and their abilities to contract and generate tension are quite similar. Consider a skeletal muscle that can contract in 500 msec and shorten 1 cm while exerting a 10-kg pull. Without using a lever, this muscle would be performing efficiently only when moving a 10-kg weight a distance of 1 cm. But by using a lever, the same muscle operating at the same efficiency would move 20 kg a distance of 0.5 cm, 5 kg a distance of 2 cm, or 1 kg a distance of 10 cm.

Skeletal Muscle Terminology

Each muscle begins at an **origin,** ends at an **insertion,** and contracts to produce a specific **action.** In general, the origin remains stationary while the insertion moves, or the origin is proximal to the insertion. Such determinations are made during normal movements. When the origins and insertions cannot be determined easily on the basis of movement, other rules are used. If a muscle extends between a broad aponeurosis and a narrow tendon, the aponeurosis is the origin and tendon is the insertion. If there are several tendons at one end and just one at the other, there are multiple origins and a single insertion. These simple rules cannot cover every situation, and knowing which end

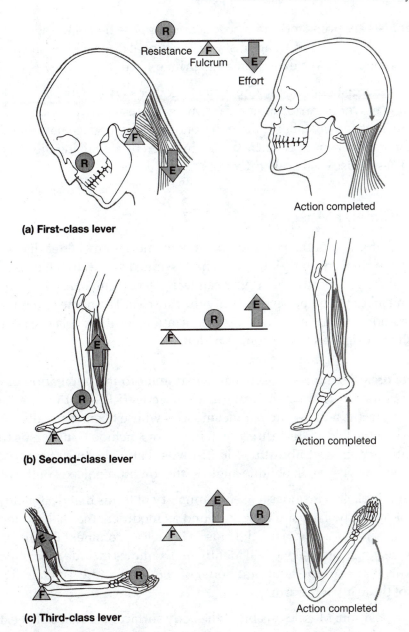

Figure 8–16   The Three Classes of Levers.
(a) In a first-class lever, the effort and the resistance are on opposite sides of the fulcrum. First-class levers can change the amount of force transmitted to the resistance and alter the direction and speed of movement. **(b)** In a second-class lever, the resistance lies between the effort and the fulcrum. This arrangement magnifies force at the expense of distance and speed; the direction of movement remains unchanged. **(c)** In a third-class lever, the effort is applied between the resistance and the fulcrum. This arrangement increases speed and distance moved but requires a larger effort.

is the origin and which is the insertion is ultimately less important than knowing where the two ends attach and what the muscle accomplishes when it contracts.

Almost all skeletal muscles either originate or insert upon the skeleton. When a muscle moves a portion of the skeleton, that movement may involve any number of motions. Muscles may be grouped according to their primary actions.

- **A prime mover,** or **agonist** (AG-o-nist; Greek *agonistes,* competitor), is a muscle whose contraction is chiefly responsible for producing a particular movement.

- **Antagonists** are prime movers whose actions oppose that of the agonist under consideration. Agonists and antagonists are functional opposites; if one produces flexion, the other will have extension as its primary action.

- When a **synergist** (SIN-ur-jist; Greek *syn*, together + *ergon*, work) contracts, it assists the prime mover in performing an action. Synergists may provide additional pull near the insertion or stabilize the point of origin. Synergists may also assist an agonist by preventing movement at a joint and thereby stabilizing the origin of the agonist. These muscles are called **fixators.**

Names of Skeletal Muscles

Fortunately, anatomists of the past did not have memories any better than ours. Rather than writing the answers on their sleeves, they assigned names to the muscles that provided clues to their identification. If you can learn to recognize the clues, you will find it easy to remember the names and identify the muscles. The name of a muscle may include information concerning its fascicle organization, location, relative position, structure, size, shape, origin and insertion, or action.

1. **Fascicle organization:** A muscle name may refer to the orientation of the muscle fibers within a particular skeletal muscle. **Rectus** (REK-tus) means "straight" in Latin, and rectus muscles are parallel muscles whose fibers generally run along the long axis of the body. Other directional indicators include **transversus** (trans-VUR-sus; Latin across) and **obliquus** (ob-LI-kwus; Latin slanting) for muscles whose fibers run across or at an oblique angle to the longitudinal axis of the body.

2. **Location:** Table 8–3 includes a useful summary of terms that designate specific regions of the body. They are usually found as modifiers that help to identify individual muscles. In a few cases, the muscle is such a prominent feature of the region that the regional name alone will identify it. Examples include the temporalis (tem-pō-RĀ-lis; Latin, of the temporal bone) of the head and brachialis (brā-kē-Ā-lis; Latin, of the arm) of the arm.

3. **Relative position:** Muscles visible at the body surface are often called **externus** (ek-STUR-nus; Latin, outward) or **superficialis** (soo-per-fish-ē-AL-is; Latin, of the surface), those lying beneath the surface muscles are termed **internus** (in-TUR-nus; Latin, inward) or **profundus** (prō-FUN-dus; Latin deep). Superficial muscles that position or stabilize an organ are called **extrinsic muscles;** those that operate within the organ are called **intrinsic muscles.**

4. **Structure, size, and shape:** Other muscles were named after specific and unusual structural features. The **biceps** (BĪ-seps; Latin *bi*, two + *caput*, head) **muscle** has two tendons of origin, the **triceps** (TRĪ-seps; Latin tri, three) has three, and the **quadriceps** (KWAH-dri-ceps; Latin *quad*, four) has four. Shape is sometimes an important clue to the name of a muscle. For example **trapezius** (tra-PĒ-zē-us; Latin, little table), **deltoid, rhomboideus** (rom-BOY-dē-us; Latin, rhomboid), and **orbicularis** (or-bik-ū-LAR-is; Latin, circular) refer to prominent muscles that look like a trapezoid, a triangle, a rhomboid, and a circle, respectively. Long muscles are called **longus** (LONG-gus, Latin, long) or **longissimus** (lon-JIS-i-mus; Latin, longest). **Teres** (TER-ēz; Latin, rounded) muscles are both long and round. Short muscles are called **bre-**

Table 8–3 Muscle Terminology

Terms Indicating Direction Relative to Axes of the Body	Terms Indicating Specific Regions of the Body	Terms Indicating Structural Characteristics of the Muscle	Terms Indicating Actions
Anterior (front)	Abdominis (abdomen)	**Origin**	**General**
Externus (superficial)	Anconeus (elbow)	Biceps (two heads)	Abductor
Extrinsic (outside)	Auricularis (auricle of ear)	Triceps (three heads)	Adductor
Inferioris (inferior)	Brachialis (brachium)	Quadriceps (four heads)	Depressor
Internus (deep, internal)	Capitis (head)		Extensor
Intrinsic (inside)	Carpi (wrist)	**Shape**	Flexor
Lateralis (lateral)	Cervicis (neck)	Deltoid (triangle)	Levator
Medialis/medius (medial, middle)	Cleido/clavius (clavicle)	Orbicularis (circle)	Pronator
	Coccygeus (coccyx)	Pectinate (comblike)	Rotator
Obliquus (oblique)	Costalis (ribs)	Piriformis (pear-shaped)	Supinator
Posterior (back)	Cutaneous (skin)	Platys- (flat)	Tensor
Profundus (deep)	Femoris (femur)	Pyramidal (pyramid)	
Rectus (straight, parallel)	Genio- (chin)	Rhomboideus (rhomboid)	**Specific**
Superficialis (superficial)	Glosso/glossal (tongue)	Serratus (serrated)	Buccinator
Superioris (superior)	Halliucis (great toe)	Splenius (bandage)	(trumpeter)
Transversus (transverse)	Ilio- (ilium)	Teres (long and round)	Risorius
	Inguinal (groin)	Trapezius (trapezoid)	(laughter)
	Lumborum (lumbar region)		Sartorius
	Nasalis (nose)	**Other Striking Features**	(like a tailor)
	Nuchal (back of neck)	Alba (white)	
	Oculo-(eye)	Brevis (short)	
	Oris (mouth)	Gracilis (slender)	
	Palpebrae (eyelid)	Lata (wide)	
	Pollicis (thumb)	Latissimus (widest)	
	Popliteus (behind knee)	Longissimus (longest)	
	Psoas (loin)	Longus (long)	
	Radialis (radius)	Magnus (large)	
	Scapularis (scapula)	Major (larger)	
	Temporalis (temples)	Maximus (largest)	
	Thoracis (thoracic region)	Minimus (smallest)	
	Tibialis (tibia)	Minor (smaller)	
	Ulnaris (ulna)	-tendinosus (tendinous)	
	Uro- (urinary)	Vastus (great)	

vis (BREV-is; Latin, short); large ones are called **magnus** (Latin, big), **major** (Latin, bigger), or **maximus** (MAK-si-mus; Latin, biggest); and small ones are called **minor** (Latin, smaller) or **minimus** (Latin, smallest).

5. **Origin and insertion:** Many names tell you the specific origin and insertion of each muscle. In such cases, the first part of the name indicates the origin and the second part the insertion. The **genioglossus** (jē-nē-ō-GLOS-us) for instance originates at the chin (Greek, *geneion*, chin) and inserts in the tongue (Greek, *glossa*, tongue).

6. **Action:** Many muscles are named *flexor, extensor, retractor*, and so on. These are such common actions that the names almost always include other clues concerning the appearance or location of the muscle. A few muscles are named after the specific movements associated with special occupations or habits. The **sartorius** (sar-TŌ-rē-us) muscle is active when crossing the legs. Before sewing machines were invented, a tailor would sit on the floor cross-legged, and the name of the muscle was derived from *sartor,* the latin word for tailor. On the face, the **buccinator** (BŪK-si-nā-tor) muscle compresses the cheeks as when pursing the lips and blowing forcefully. Buccinator translates from Latin as "trumpet player." Finally, another facial muscle, the **risorius** (ri-SŌ-rē-us), was supposedly named after the mood expressed. The Latin term *risor,* however, means laughter; a more appropriate description for the effect would be "grimace."

Cardiac Muscle Tissue

Cardiac muscle tissue was introduced in Chapter 6, and its properties were briefly compared with those of other muscle types. **Cardiac muscle cells** are relatively small, averaging 10–20 μm in diameter and 50–100 μm in length. As the name implies cardiac muscle is found only in the heart.

Smooth Muscle Tissue

Smooth muscle cells range from 5–10 μm in diameter and from 30–200 μm in length. There is a single nucleus, centrally located within each spindle-shaped cell. **Smooth muscle** tissue is found within almost every organ, forming sheets, bundles, or sheaths around other tissues. In the skeletal, muscular, nervous, and endocrine systems, smooth muscle around blood vessels regulates blood flow through vital organs. In the digestive and urinary systems, rings of smooth muscle, called sphincters, regulate movement along internal passageways. Smooth muscles in bundles, layers, or sheets play a variety of other roles.

- **Integumentary system:** Smooth muscles around blood vessels regulate the flow of blood to the superficial dermis; smooth muscles elevate the hairs to form goosebumps.

- **Cardiovascular system:** Smooth muscles encircling vessels of the circulatory system provide control over the peripheral distribution of blood and assist in the regulation of blood pressure.

- **Respiratory system:** Smooth muscle contraction or relaxation alters the diameters of the respiratory passageways and changes the resistance to airflow.

- **Digestive system:** Extensive layers of smooth muscle in the walls of the digestive tract play an essential role in mechanical processing and in moving materials along the tract. Smooth muscle in the walls of the gallbladder contract to eject bile into the digestive tract.

- **Urinary system:** Smooth muscle tissue in the walls of small blood vessels alters the rate of filtration at the kidneys. Layers of smooth muscle in the walls of the ureters transport urine to the urinary bladder; contraction of the smooth muscle in the wall of the urinary bladder forces urine out of the body.

- **Reproductive system:** Layers of smooth muscle are important in the male for the movement of sperm along the reproductive tract and for the ejection of glandular secretions from the accessory glands into the reproductive tract. In the female, layers of smooth muscle are important in the movement of ova (and perhaps sperm) along the reproductive tract, and contraction of the smooth muscle in the walls of the uterus expels the fetus at delivery.

Integration with Other Systems

To operate at maximum efficiency, the muscular system must be supported by many other systems. The changes that occur during exercise provide a good example of such interaction. As noted in earlier sections, active muscles consume oxygen and generate carbon dioxide and heat. Responses of other systems include:

1. **Cardiovascular system:** Dilation of blood vessels in the active muscles and the skin and an increase in the heart rate. These adjustments accelerate oxygen delivery and carbon dioxide removal at the muscle and bring heat to the skin for radiation into the environment.

2. **Respiratory system:** Increased respiratory rate and depth of respiration. Air moves into and out of the lungs more quickly, keeping pace with the increased rate of blood flow through the lungs.

3. **Integumentary system:** Dilation of blood vessels and increased sweat gland secretion. This combination helps promote evaporation at the skin surface and removes the excess heat generated by muscle activity.

4. **Nervous and endocrine systems:** Direct the responses of other systems by controlling heart rate, respiratory rate, and sweat gland activity.

The muscular system has extensive interactions with other systems even at rest. Figure 8–17 summarizes the range of interactions between the muscular system and other vital systems.

Let's Review What You've Just Learned

▶ Definitions

In the space provided, write the term for each of the following definitions.

_____ **104.** The cell membrane of a skeletal muscle fiber.

_____ **105.** A bundle of fibers.

_____ **106.** A muscle whose contraction is chiefly responsible for producing a particular movement.

_____ **107.** A muscle in which the fascicles form a common angle with the tendon.

_____ **108.** A layer of connective tissue that surrounds the skeletal muscle fibers and ties adjacent muscle fibers together.

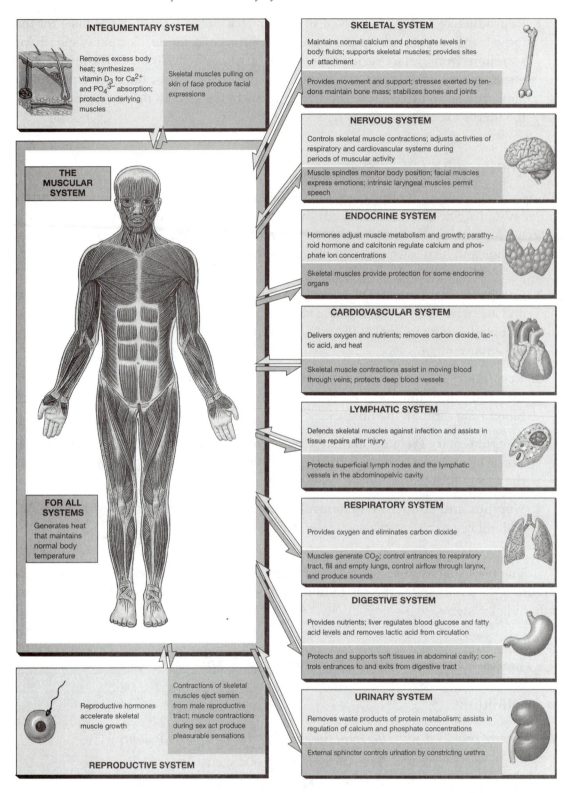

INTEGUMENTARY SYSTEM

Removes excess body heat; synthesizes vitamin D_3 for Ca^{2+} and PO_4^{3-} absorption; protects underlying muscles

Skeletal muscles pulling on skin of face produce facial expressions

THE MUSCULAR SYSTEM

FOR ALL SYSTEMS

Generates heat that maintains normal body temperature

REPRODUCTIVE SYSTEM

Reproductive hormones accelerate skeletal muscle growth

Contractions of skeletal muscles eject semen from male reproductive tract; muscle contractions during sex act produce pleasurable sensations

SKELETAL SYSTEM

Maintains normal calcium and phosphate levels in body fluids; supports skeletal muscles; provides sites of attachment

Provides movement and support; stresses exerted by tendons maintain bone mass; stabilizes bones and joints

NERVOUS SYSTEM

Controls skeletal muscle contractions; adjusts activities of respiratory and cardiovascular systems during periods of muscular activity

Muscle spindles monitor body position; facial muscles express emotions; intrinsic laryngeal muscles permit speech

ENDOCRINE SYSTEM

Hormones adjust muscle metabolism and growth; parathyroid hormone and calcitonin regulate calcium and phosphate ion concentrations

Skeletal muscles provide protection for some endocrine organs

CARDIOVASCULAR SYSTEM

Delivers oxygen and nutrients; removes carbon dioxide, lactic acid, and heat

Skeletal muscle contractions assist in moving blood through veins; protects deep blood vessels

LYMPHATIC SYSTEM

Defends skeletal muscles against infection and assists in tissue repairs after injury

Protects superficial lymph nodes and the lymphatic vessels in the abdominopelvic cavity

RESPIRATORY SYSTEM

Provides oxygen and eliminates carbon dioxide

Muscles generate CO_2; control entrances to respiratory tract, fill and empty lungs, control airflow through larynx, and produce sounds

DIGESTIVE SYSTEM

Provides nutrients; liver regulates blood glucose and fatty acid levels and removes lactic acid from circulation

Protects and supports soft tissues in abdominal cavity; controls entrances to and exits from digestive tract

URINARY SYSTEM

Removes waste products of protein metabolism; assists in regulation of calcium and phosphate concentrations

External sphincter controls urination by constricting urethra

Figure 8–17   Functional Relationships between the Muscular System and Other Systems.

_____ **109.** Embryonic cells that fuse together to form muscle fibers.

_____ **110.** The point of attachment where a skeletal muscle begins.

_____ **111.** Narrow tubes that begin at the sarcolemma and extend into the sarcoplasm at right angles to the membrane surface.

_____ **112.** The expanded end of an axon.

_____ **113.** A protein filament composed primarily of actin and myosin.

_____ **114.** A rigid structure that moves on a fixed point and confers mechanical advantage.

_____ **115.** The dense layer of collagen fibers that surrounds an entire muscle.

_____ **116.** Cells that function in the repair of damaged muscle tissue.

_____ **117.** A prime mover whose action opposes that of a specific agonist.

_____ **118.** The basic functional unit of a myofilament.

_____ **119.** A superficial muscle that positions or stabilizes an organ.

_____ **120.** A muscle in which the fibers are concentrically arranged around an opening or recess.

_____ **121.** Connective tissue that divides a skeletal muscle into compartments each of which contains a bundle of muscle fibers.

_____ **122.** The cytoplasm of a skeletal muscle fiber.

_____ **123.** A chemical released by neurons to change the membrane properties of other cells.

_____ **124.** A muscle in which the fibers are based over a broad area but come together at a common attachment site.

_____ **125.** The specific movement produced when a skeletal muscle contracts.

_____ **126.** A muscle that assists a prime mover in performing a specific action.

_____ **127.** Bundles of myofilaments.

_____ **128.** The link between the generation of an action potential in the sarcolemma and the start of a muscle contraction.

_____ **129.** A muscle that operates within an organ.

_____ **130.** A type of muscle cell found only in the heart.

_____ **131.** A specialized intercellular connection found between a neuron and a muscle cell.

_____ **132.** A muscle in which the fascicles are all parallel to the long axis of the muscle.

_____ **133.** A membrane complex in muscle cells that is similar to the endoplasmic reticulum of other cells.

_____ **134.** The specific chemical released by neurons that stimulates skeletal muscle contraction.

_____ **135.** The analysis of biological systems in mechanical terms.

_____ **136.** The fixed point on which a lever moves.

_____ **137.** The ending attachment point of a skeletal muscle.

_____ **138.** A muscle that stabilizes the origin of an agonist during contraction.

▶ **Word Roots, Prefixes, Suffixes, and Combining Forms**

In the space provided, list the boldfaced terms introduced in this section that contain the indicated word part.

Word Part	Meaning	Examples
myo-	muscle	**139.** _____
syn-	together	**140.** _____
-blast	precursor	**141.** _____
peri-	around	**142.** _____
-lemma	husk	**143.** _____
sarco-	flesh	**144.** _____
endo-	inside	**145.** _____
ant-	against	**146.** _____
-mere	part	**147.** _____
epi-	on	**148.** _____
mys-	muscle	**149.** _____
trans-	across	**150.** _____

▶ **Latin Terms**

Complete the following table by supplying the appropriate Latin term for the word or the meaning of the Latin term.

	Latin Term	Meaning
151.	rectus	
152.		triangle
153.		bundle
154.		long
155.	maximus	
156.	quadriceps	
157.		short
158.	teres	
159.	transversus	
160.		deep
161.		circle
162.	major	
163.		big
164.		trapezoid
165.		two heads
166.	rhomboideus	
167.	minimus	
168.	obliquus	
169.	externus	
170.		small
171.	longissimus	

▶ **Levers**

In the space provided, draw a diagram of the lever system indicated. Use the letters f = *fulcrum,* e = *effort, and* r = *resistance to indicate these three items in your diagram.*

172. A third-class lever system.

173. A first-class lever system.

THE NERVOUS SYSTEM

The nervous system includes all of the neural tissue (introduced in Chapter 6) in the body. Neural tissue with supporting blood vessels and connective tissues forms the organs of the nervous system: the brain, the spinal cord, complex sense organs such as the eye and ear, and the nerves that interconnect those organs and link the nervous system with other systems. The major anatomical subdivisions of the nervous system were introduced in Chapter 1: the central nervous system and the peripheral nervous system.

The **central nervous system (CNS)** consists of the brain and spinal cord. These are complex organs that include not only neural tissue but also blood vessels and the various connective tissues that provide physical protection and support. The CNS is responsible for integrating, processing, and coordinating sensory data and motor commands. Sensory data convey information about conditions inside or outside the body. Motor commands control or adjust the activities of peripheral organs such as skeletal muscles. When you stumble, the CNS processes information concerning balance and limb position and then coordinates your recovery by sending motor commands to appropriate skeletal muscles—all in a split second and without conscious thought. The CNS, specifically the brain, is also the seat of higher functions such as intelligence, memory, learning, and emotion.

The **peripheral nervous system (PNS)** includes all of the neural tissue outside the CNS. The PNS delivers sensory information to the CNS and carries motor commands to peripheral tissues and systems. Bundles of nerve fibers (axons) carry sensory information and motor commands in the PNS. Such bundles, with associated blood vessels and connective tissues, are called **peripheral nerves,** or simply **nerves.** Nerves connected to the brain are called **cranial nerves;** those attached to the spinal cord are called **spinal nerves.**

Figure 8–18 diagrams the functional divisions of the nervous system. The **afferent** (AF-er-ent; Latin *ad,* toward + *ferre,* to carry) **division** of the PNS brings sensory information to the CNS from receptors in peripheral tissues and organs. Receptors are sensory structures, ranging from the processes of single cells to complex organs, that either detect changes in the internal environment or respond to the presence of specific stimuli. Receptors may be neurons or specialized cells of other tissues.

The **efferent** (ĒF-er-ent; Latin *ex,* away + *ferre,* to carry) **division** of the PNS carries motor commands from the CNS to muscles and glands. Because these target organs do something in response to these commands, they are called **effectors.** The efferent division has somatic and visceral components. The **somatic nervous system (SNS)** provides voluntary control over skeletal muscle contractions. The **visceral nervous system,** or **autonomic nervous system (ANS),** provides automatic, involuntary regulation of smooth

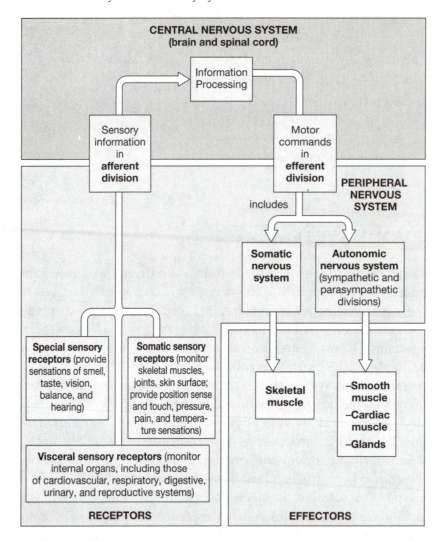

Figure 8–18 Functional Overview of the Nervous System.

muscle, cardiac muscle, and glandular activity or secretions. The ANS includes a sympathetic division and a parasympathetic division. These ANS divisions often have antagonistic effects; for example, activity of the sympathetic division accelerates the heart rate, whereas parasympathetic activity slows the heart rate.

Neuroglia

Neuroglia, or glial cells, were introduced in Chapter 6. These cells function in support of the neurons of the nervous system. There are significant differences between the organization of neural tissue in the CNS and PNS due primarily because of their distinctive glial cell populations.

There are four types of glial cells in the central nervous system (Figure 8–19):

1. **Ependymal** (ep-EN-dī-mul; Greek *ependyma*, an upper garment) **cells** line the fluid-filled central passageways of the spinal cord and brain. The narrow passageway within the spinal cord is termed the **central canal;** the expanded chambers found in portions of the brain are called **ventricles.** The ventricles and central canal are

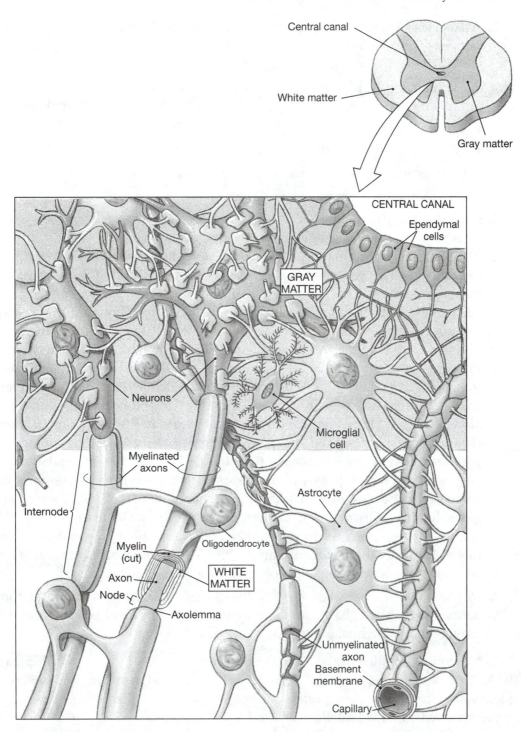

Figure 8–19 Neuroglia in the CNS.
A diagrammatic view of neural tissue in the CNS, showing relationships between neuroglia and neurons.

filled with **cerebrospinal fluid (CSF).** This fluid, which also surrounds the brain and spinal cord, provides a protective cushion and distributes dissolved gases, nutrients, wastes, and other materials. The CSF is formed by specialized ependymal cells in the ventricles of the brain.

2. **Astrocytes** (AS-trō-sītz; Greek *astron*, star + *cyte*, cell) are the largest and most numerous glial cells. They have a variety of functions, many of them poorly understood. These functions can be summarized as:

   - Maintaining the **blood-brain barrier,** a combination of astrocyte processes and capillary endothelium that isolates the CNS from the general circulation.
   - Creating a three-dimensional framework for the CNS.
   - Performing repairs in damaged neural tissue.
   - Guiding neuron development.
   - Controlling the interstitial environment.

3. **Oligodendrocytes** (ō-li-gō-DEN-drō-sītz; Greek *olig*, few + *dendron*, tree + *glia*, glue) possess slender cytoplasmic extensions that usually contact the exposed surfaces of neurons. Many axons in the CNS are completely sheathed in the processes of oligodendrocytes. This covering is so complete that when talking about an axon you have to be quite specific about which "outer membrane" you are referring to. The cell membrane of the axon is the **axolemma** (ak-sō-LEM-uh), but in this case the real outer boundary, or **neurilemma** (noo-ri-LEM-uh) is provided by the glial cell. The composition of the sheath is roughly 80 percent lipid and 20 percent protein, the same as that of any other cell membrane. This multilayered membranous wrapping is called **myelin** (MĪ-e-lin), and the surrounded axon is said to be **myelinated** (MĪ-e-lin-nā-tid). Myelin increases the speed of action potential propagation along an axon. Many oligodendrocytes cooperate in the formation of a myelin sheath around an axon, and small gaps occur between adjacent wrappings. These gaps are called **nodes,** or **nodes of Ranvier** (RAHN-vē-ā), and the relatively large areas wrapped in myelin are called **internodes** (*inter*, between). In dissection, myelinated axons appear a glossy white, primarily because of the lipids present, and regions dominated by myelinated axons constitute the **white matter** of the CNS. In contrast, areas dominated by neuron cell bodies are called **gray matter** because of their dusky gray color. Not all axons in the CNS are myelinated, and unmyelinated axons may not be completely covered by glial cell processes.

4. **Microglia** (mī-KRŌ-glē-uh) are small cells that are capable of migrating through neural tissue. Microglia act as a wandering police force and janitorial service, removing cellular debris, waste products, and pathogens.

Neuron cell bodies in the PNS are clustered together in masses called **ganglia** (GANG-lē-uh, singular *ganglion*). Neuron cell bodies and axons in the PNS are completely insulated from their surroundings by the processes of glial cells. The two glial cell types involved are called satellite cells and Schwann cells.

Satellite cells surround the neuron cell bodies in peripheral ganglia. **Schwann** (shwahn) **cells** form a sheath around every peripheral axon, whether unmyelinated or myelinated. Whereas an oligodendrocyte may myelinate portions of several adjacent axons, a Schwann cell can myelinate only one segment of a single axon. However, a Schwann cell may enclose segments of several unmyelinated axons.

Neurons

Refer to Figure 6–19 for the structure of a representative neuron. Neurons can have a variety of shapes. The neuron pictured in Figure 6–19 is a multipolar neuron, the most common type of neuron in the CNS. The soma, or cell body, contains a relatively large, round nucleus with a prominent nucleolus. The surrounding cytoplasm constitutes the **perikary-on** (per-i-KAR-ē-on; Greek *peri*, around + *karyon*, kernel). The cytoskeleton of the perikary-on contains fibrous elements called **neurofilaments** and **neurotubules.** Bundles of neurofilaments, called **neurofibrils,** extend into the dendrites and axon, providing internal support of these relatively slender processes. The perikaryon also contains organelles that provide energy and synthesize organic materials, especially neurotransmitters.

A variable number of dendrites extend out from the soma. Typical dendrites are highly branched. Dendrites receive information in the form of electrochemical stimuli.

An axon is a long cytoplasmic process capable of propagating an action potential. The **axoplasm** (AK-sō-plazm), or cytoplasm of the axon, contains neurofibrils, neurotubules, small vesicles, lysosomes, mitochondria, and various enzymes. The axolemma is often covered by oligodendrocyte processes in the CNS and invariably is covered by Schwann cells in the PNS. The base, or initial segment, of the axon in a multipolar neuron is attached to the soma at a thickened region known as the **axon hillock.**

An axon may branch along its length, producing branches collectively known as **collaterals.** Collaterals enable a single neuron to communicate with several other cells. The main axon trunk and any collaterals end in a series of fine extensions, or **telodendria** (tē-lō-DEN-drē-uh; Greek *telo*, end + *dendron*, tree). Expanded synaptic knobs at the tips of the telodendria form synaptic connections with other cells. The communication between cells at a synapse most often involves the release of chemicals, called *neurotransmitters*, by the synaptic knob.

The Synapse

A **synapse** (SIN-aps) is a specialized site of intercellular communication. Figure 8–20 shows the structural features of a typical synapse. A synapse may involve two neurons or a neuron and another cell type. When one neuron communicates with another, the synapse may occur on a dendrite, on the soma, or along the length of the axon of the receiving cell. A synapse may also permit communication between a neuron and another cell type. Such a synapse is called a **neuroeffector junction.** There are two major classes of neuroeffector junctions: *neuromuscular junctions* and *neuroglandular junctions.* At a

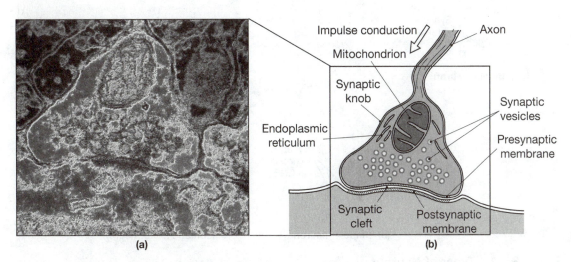

Figure 8–20   Structure of a Chemical Synapse.
(a) Micrograph of a chemical synapse between two neurons. (TEM × 222,000) **(b)** Diagrammatic view of the synapse.

neuromuscular junction, the neuron communicates with a muscle cell. At a **neuroglandular junction,** a neuron controls or regulates the activity of a secretory cell. Neurons also innervate a variety of other cell types, such as fat cells.

Neuron Classification

The billions of neurons in the nervous system are variable in form. Neurons are classified two ways: (1) on the basis of structure and (2) on the basis of function.

The structural classification of neurons is based on the number of processes that project from the cell body (Figure 8–21).

- In a **unipolar neuron** or a **pseudounipolar** (soo-dō-Ū-ni-pō-lar) **neuron,** the dendritic and axonal processes are continuous, and the cell body lies off to one side. Sensory neurons of the peripheral nervous system are usually unipolar.
- **Bipolar neurons** have one dendrite and one axon, with the cell body between them. Bipolar neurons are relatively rare but play an important role in relaying information concerning sight, smell, and hearing.
- **Multipolar neurons** have several dendrites and a single axon that may have one or more branches. Multipolar neurons are the most common type of neuron in the CNS.

Neurons can be categorized into three functional groups: sensory neurons, motor neurons, and interneurons, or association neurons.

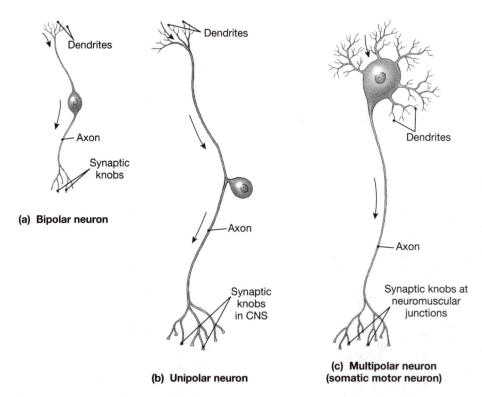

Figure 8–21 Types of Neurons.
The arrows indicate the direction of action potential propagation. The neurons are not drawn to scale; typical bipolar neurons are many times smaller than typical unipolar or multipolar neurons.

1. **Sensory neurons** form the afferent division of the PNS. Their function is to deliver information to the CNS. These are unipolar neurons, and their processes, known as **afferent fibers,** extend between a sensory receptor and the spinal cord or brain. Receptors may be the processes of specialized sensory neurons or cells monitored by sensory neurons. Receptors are broadly categorized as:

   - **Exteroceptors** (ek-stur-ō-SEP-turz; *extero-,* outside) provide information about the external environment in the form of touch, temperature, and pressure sensations and the more complex senses of sight, smell, and hearing.

   - **Proprioceptors** (prō-prē-ō-SEP-turz; *propio,* one's own) monitor the position and movement of skeletal muscles and joints.

   - **Interoceptors** (in-tur-ō-SEP-turz; *intero,* inside) monitor the digestive, respiratory, cardiovascular, urinary, and reproductive systems and provide sensations of taste, deep pressure, and pain.

2. **Motor Neurons:** Motor neurons of the efferent division carry instructions from the CNS to peripheral effectors. A motor neuron stimulates or modifies the activity of a peripheral tissue, organ, or organ system. Axons traveling away from the CNS are called **efferent fibers.**

3. **Interneurons:** Interneurons, or association neurons, may be situated between sensory and motor neurons. Interneurons are located entirely within the brain and spinal cord. There are roughly 20 billion interneurons, outnumbering all other types of neurons combined. Interneurons are responsible for the distribution of sensory information and the coordination of motor activity. The more complex the response to a given stimulus the greater the number of interneurons involved.

Neurophysiology

Chapter 4 introduced the concepts of transmembrane potential and resting potential, two characteristic features of living cells. All of the steps important to neural function involve changes in the transmembrane potentials of individual neurons. Information is conveyed over relatively long distances in the form of action potentials, propagated changes in the transmembrane potential of axons.

Recall from Chapter 4 that intracellular and extracellular fluids differ markedly in ionic composition. The extracellular fluid (ECF) contains relatively high concentrations of sodium and chloride ions, whereas the cytosol (intracellular fluid) contains high concentrations of potassium ions and negatively charged proteins. Because the cell membrane is selectively permeable, the ions are not able to diffuse freely. As a result, there are differences in the distribution of positive and negative charges along the inner and outer surfaces of the cell membrane. The inner surface contains an excess of negative charges with respect to the outer surface.

Action potentials are propagated changes in the transmembrane potential that, once initiated, spread across an entire excitable membrane. In a representative neuron, an action potential usually begins at the initial segment of the axon. It is conducted along the length of the axon until, ultimately, it reaches the synaptic knobs. The stimulus that initiates an action potential is a depolarization large enough to open voltage-regulated sodium channels (see Chapter 4). Sodium ions entering the cytoplasm cause a temporary depolarization of the cell membrane. The electrical changes in one segment of the membrane cause channels in the adjacent segment to open and that segment of membrane depolarizes. While the next section of membrane depolarizes, the initial section repolarizes by allowing positively charged potassium ions to exit to the extracellular fluid. The steps involved in generating an action potential are summarized in Table 8–4.

In the nervous system, messages move from one location to another in the form of action potentials along axons. These electrical events are also known as **nerve impulses.** To be effective, a message must not only be propagated along an axon, it must also be transferred in some way to another cell. At a synapse involving two neurons, the impulse passes from the **presynaptic** (prē-si-NAP-tik) **neuron** (the cell sending the information) to the **postsynaptic** (pōst-si-NAP-tik) **neuron** (the cell receiving the information). A synapse may also involve other types of postsynaptic cells. For example, the neuromuscular junction described earlier in the chapter is an example of a synapse where the postsynaptic cell is a skeletal muscle fiber. At a synapse, a change in the transmembrane potential of the synaptic knob affects the activity of another cell.

The Meninges

The brain and spinal cord are covered by a series of specialized membranes, the **meninges** (me-NIN-jēz; Greek *meninx*, membrane). These membranes provide the necessary physical stability and shock absorption that the nervous system requires. Blood vessels branching within these layers also deliver oxygen and nutrients to the neural tissues. The meninges are composed of three membranes (Figure 8–22).

- **The dura mater:** The tough, fibrous **dura mater** (DOO-ruh MĀ-tur; Latin *dura*, hard + *mater*, mother) forms the outermost covering of the brain and spinal cord.

- **The arachnoid:** The **arachnoid** (a-RAK-noyd; Greek *arachne*, spider) lies beneath the dura mater and is separated from the dura by a narrow **subdural space** that is filled with serous fluid. Beneath the arachnoid epithelium lies the **subarachnoid space,** which contains a delicate network of collagen and elastic fibers. The sub-

---

Table 8–4   Steps in the Generation of an Action Potential

Step 1:

- A stimulus accelerates the movement of sodium ions into the cell, bringing a portion of the membrane to a level known as the **threshold**, typically around –60 mV.

Step 2:

- Voltage-regulated sodium channels open.
- Sodium ions flood into the cell.
- The transmembrane potential goes from –60 mV to +30 mV.

Step 3:

- The voltage-regulated sodium channels close.
- Potassium ions move out of the cell through open voltage-regulated potassium channels.
- Repolarization begins.

Step 4:

- At the end of the action potential, all voltage-regulated channels are closed and the membrane is back to its resting state.

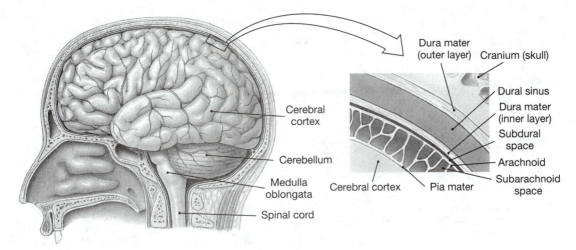

Figure 8–22   Relationship among the Brain, Cranium, and Meninges.
Lateral view of the brain, showing its position in the cranium and the organization of the meninges.

arachnoid space is filled with cerebrospinal fluid that acts as a shock absorber as well as a diffusion medium for dissolved gases, nutrients, chemical messengers, and waste products.

- **The pia mater:** The innermost meningeal layer, the **pia mater** (PĒ-uh MĀ-tur; Latin *pia*, delicate + *mater*, mother), is a meshwork of elastic and collagen fibers that are interwoven with those of the subarachnoid space. The blood vessels servicing the brain and spinal cord are found here, and, unlike more-superficial meninges, the pia mater is firmly bound to the underlying neural tissue.

The Spinal Cord

The central nervous system consists of the spinal cord and brain. The adult human spinal cord extends from the base of the skull to the level of the second lumbar vertebra. The posterior (dorsal) surface of the spinal cord bears a shallow longitudinal groove, the **posterior median sulcus** (Figure 8–23). The **anterior median fissure** is a deeper groove along the anterior (ventral) surface. The anterior median fissure and the posterior median sulcus mark the division between left and right sides of the spinal cord. The peripherally situated white matter contains large numbers of myelinated and unmyelinated axons. The white matter on each side of the spinal cord can be divided into three regions called **columns** or **funiculi** (fū-NIK-ū-lī; Latin *funiculus*, cord). Each column contains tracts, bundles of axons that share functional and structural characteristics. The gray matter dominated by cell bodies of neurons and glial cells surrounds the narrow central canal and forms a rough H or butterfly shape. The projections of gray matter toward the outer surface of the spinal cord are called **horns.**

Nerves originating in the spinal cord are called spinal nerves. Each **spinal nerve** is connected to the spinal cord by a **dorsal root** and a **ventral root**. The **dorsal root ganglion** contains the cell bodies of sensory neurons. A series of connective tissue layers surrounds each spinal nerve and continues along all of its peripheral branches. These layers are comparable to those associated with skeletal muscles. The outermost layer, or **epineurium** (ep-i-NOO-rē-um), consists of a dense network of collagen fibers. The fibers of the **perineurium** (per-i-NOO-rē-um) extend inward from the epineurium, dividing the nerve

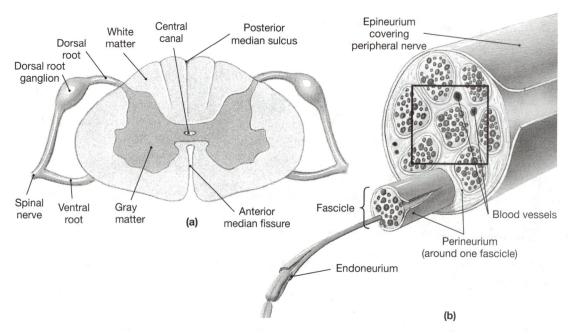

Figure 8–23 **Representative Cross Sectional Views of the Spinal Cord and a Spinal Nerve.**

into a series of compartments that contain bundles of axons or fascicles. Delicate connective tissue fibers of the **endoneurium** (en-dō-NOO-rē-um) extend from the perineurium and surround individual axons.

The Brain

The largest, most obvious part of the human brain is the cerebrum (Figure 8–24). Viewed from the superior surface, the **cerebrum** (SER-e-brum) of the adult brain can be divided into large, paired **cerebral** (SER-ē-brul) **hemispheres.** Conscious thought processes, sensations, intellectual functions, memory storage and retrieval, and complex motor patterns originate in the cerebrum.

Immediately behind the cerebrum are the somewhat smaller hemispheres of the **cerebellum** (ser-e-BEL-um). The cerebellum adjusts voluntary and involuntary motor activities, comparing incoming sensory information with anticipated sensations during the performance of preestablished motor patterns. The surfaces of the cerebral hemispheres and cerebellum are highly folded and covered by **neural cortex**, a superficial layer of gray matter. The term **cerebral cortex** refers to the neural cortex of the cerebral hemispheres as opposed to the **cerebellar cortex** of the cerebellar hemispheres.

The other major regions of the brain—the diencephalon, midbrain, pons, and medulla oblongata—can best be examined after removing the cerebral hemispheres and cerebellum.

The **diencephalon** (dī-en-SEF-a-lon) is a structural and functional link between the cerebral hemispheres and the components of the brain stem. The walls of the diencephalon are composed of the left and right **thalamus** (THAL-a-mus). Each thalamus contains relay and processing centers for sensory information. A narrow stalk, the **infundibulum** (in-fun-DIB-ū-lum; Latin *infundibulum*, funnel) connects the floor of the

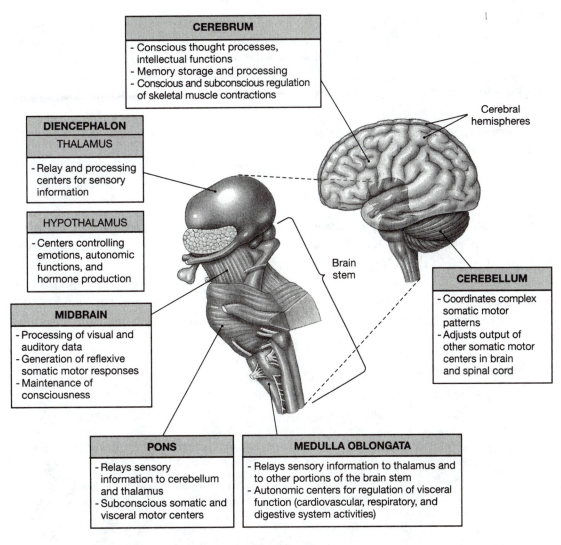

CEREBRUM
- Conscious thought processes, intellectual functions
- Memory storage and processing
- Conscious and subconscious regulation of skeletal muscle contractions

DIENCEPHALON

THALAMUS
- Relay and processing centers for sensory information

HYPOTHALAMUS
- Centers controlling emotions, autonomic functions, and hormone production

MIDBRAIN
- Processing of visual and auditory data
- Generation of reflexive somatic motor responses
- Maintenance of consciousness

Cerebral hemispheres

Brain stem

CEREBELLUM
- Coordinates complex somatic motor patterns
- Adjusts output of other somatic motor centers in brain and spinal cord

PONS
- Relays sensory information to cerebellum and thalamus
- Subconscious somatic and visceral motor centers

MEDULLA OBLONGATA
- Relays sensory information to thalamus and to other portions of the brain stem
- Autonomic centers for regulation of visceral function (cardiovascular, respiratory, and digestive system activities)

Figure 8–24 An Introduction to Brain Functions.

diencephalon, or **hypothalamus** (*hypo*, below), to the pituitary gland, a component of the endocrine system. The hypothalamus contains centers involved with emotions, autonomic function, and hormone production.

The brain stem includes the **midbrain,** the **pons** (ponz), and the **medulla oblongata** (me-DŪL-uh ob-long-AH-tuh). It contains a variety of important processing centers and also provides relay stations for information headed to or from the cerebrum or cerebellum.

Nuclei in the midbrain process visual and auditory information and generate involuntary motor responses involving skeletal muscles. For example, your immediate, reflexive responses to a loud, unexpected noise are directed by nuclei in the mesencephalon. This region also contains centers involved with the maintenance of consciousness.

The term *pons* is Latin for "bridge," and the pons of the brain connects the cerebellum to the brain stem. In addition to tracts and relay centers, the pons also contains nuclei involved with somatic and visceral motor control.

The spinal cord connects to the brain at the medulla oblongata. The caudal portion of the medulla oblongata resembles the spinal cord in having a narrow central canal. The medulla oblongata relays sensory information to the thalamus and to centers in portions of the brain stem. The medulla oblongata also contains major centers concerned with the regulation of autonomic function, such as heart rate, blood pressure, respiration, and digestion.

Nerves that originate in the brain are called cranial nerves. There are 12 pairs of cranial nerves in humans.

The Autonomic Nervous System

Figure 8–25 compares the organization of the SNS (somatic nervous system) and ANS (autonomic nervous system). In the SNS, lower motor neurons exert direct control over skeletal muscles. In the ANS, there is always a synapse between the CNS and the peripheral effector. The visceral motor neurons in the CNS are known as **preganglionic** (prē-gang-lē-ON-ik) **neurons.** The axons of these neurons are called **preganglionic fibers.** The preganglionic fibers leave the CNS and synapse on ganglionic neurons in periph-

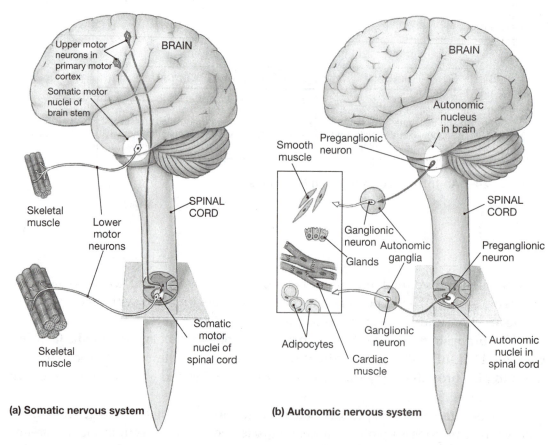

Figure 8–25   Organization of the Somatic and Autonomic Nervous Systems.
(a) In the SNS, an upper motor neuron in the CNS controls a lower motor neuron in the brain stem or spinal cord. The axon of the lower motor neuron has direct control over skeletal muscle fibers. Stimulation of the lower motor neuron always has an excitatory effect on the skeletal muscle fibers. **(b)** In the ANS, the axon of a preganglionic neuron in the CNS controls ganglionic neurons in the periphery. Stimulation of the ganglionic neurons may lead to excitation or inhibition.

eral autonomic ganglia. The axons of ganglionic neurons control peripheral effectors such as cardiac muscle, smooth muscles, glands, and adipose tissue. The axons of ganglionic neurons are called **postganglionic** (post-gang-lē-ON-ik) **fibers** because they conduct impulses away from the ganglion.

The ANS contains two subdivisions, the **sympathetic division** and the **parasympathetic division.** Most often, the two divisions have opposing effects; if the sympathetic division causes excitation, the parasympathetic causes inhibition. Sometimes, however, (1) the two divisions work independently, with some structures innervated only by one division or the other, and sometimes (2) the two divisions work together, each controlling one stage of a complex process.

The sympathetic division prepares the body for heightened levels of somatic activity. An increase in sympathetic activity generally stimulates tissue metabolism, increases alertness, and prepares the body to deal with emergencies. When fully activated, it produces what is known as the "fight or flight" response, which prepares the body for a crisis that may require sudden, intense physical activity. Postganglionic sympathetic neurons communicate with their effectors by way of the neurotransmitter **norepinephrine** (nōr-ep-i-NEF-rin).

The parasympathetic division stimulates visceral activity. It is often called the "rest and repose" system because general parasympathetic activation conserves energy and promotes sedentary activities, such as digestion. Parasympathetic neurons communicate with their effector organs by way of the neurotransmitter acetylcholine.

The two divisions are also anatomically distinct. Preganglionic fibers from the thoracic and upper lumbar spinal segments synapse in ganglia near the spinal cord. These axons and ganglia are part of the sympathetic division, or **thoracolumbar** (thō-ra-kō-LUM-bar) **division,** of the ANS. Preganglionic fibers originating in the brain and the sacral spinal cord segments are part of the parasympathetic division, or **craniosacral** (krā-nē-ō-SĀ-krul) **division,** of the ANS. The preganglionic fibers synapse on neurons of terminal ganglia, or **intramural** (in-truh-MŪ-rul; Latin *intra*, within + *muralis*, wall) **ganglia**, located near or within the tissues of visceral organs.

Sensory Organs

Sensory receptors are specialized cells that provide the central nervous system with information about conditions inside or outside the body. A sensory receptor detects an arriving stimulus and translates it into an action potential that can be conducted to the CNS. This translation process is called **transduction.**

Sensory receptors provide the nervous system with information about the body's internal and external environments. The **general senses** of pain, temperature, touch, pressure, vibration, and proprioception (position sense) are distributed throughout the body. Receptors for the general senses are relatively simple in structure. A simple classification scheme divides them into exteroceptors (receptors that provide the nervous system with information about the external environment) and interoceptors (receptors that provide the nervous system with information about the internal environment). A more detailed classification system divides the general sensory receptors into four types according to the nature of the stimulus that excites them: **nociceptors** (nō-si-SEP-turz; Latin *nocere*, to hurt) (pain), **thermoreceptors** (THUR-mō-rē-sep-turz) (temperature), **mechanoreceptors** (MEK-an-ō-rē-sep-turz) (touch), and **chemoreceptors** (KĒM-ō-rē-sep-turz) (chemical sense). Each class of receptors has distinct structural and functional characteristics.

The **special senses** are **smell (olfaction** [ōl-FACK-shun; Latin *olfacere*, to smell]), **taste (gustation** [gus-TĀ-shun; Latin *gustare*, to taste]), **balance (equilibrium), hearing,** and **sight (vision).** These sensations are provided by receptors that are structurally more complex than those of the general senses. Special sensory receptors are found in sense organs such as the eye and ear, where they are protected by surrounding tissues. The information provided by these receptors is distributed to specific areas of the cerebral cortex and to centers throughout the brain stem.

Reflexes

Reflexes are *rapid, automatic responses to stimuli.* They preserve homeostasis by making rapid adjustments in the function of organs or organ systems. The response shows little variability; activation of a particular reflex usually produces the same motor response. Chapter 1 introduced the basic functional components involved in all types of homeostatic regulation: a receptor, an integration center, and an effector. In neural reflexes, sensory fibers deliver information to the CNS and motor fibers carry motor commands to peripheral effectors. In endocrine reflexes, the commands to peripheral tissues and organs are delivered by hormones in the bloodstream.

The pattern followed by a single reflex is called a **reflex arc** (Figure 8–26). A reflex arc begins at a receptor and ends at a peripheral effector, such as a muscle fiber or gland cell. There are five steps involved in a neural reflex: (1) arrival of a stimulus and activation of a receptor, (2) activation of a sensory neuron, (3) information processing, (4) activation of a motor neuron, and (5) response by an effector (muscle or gland).

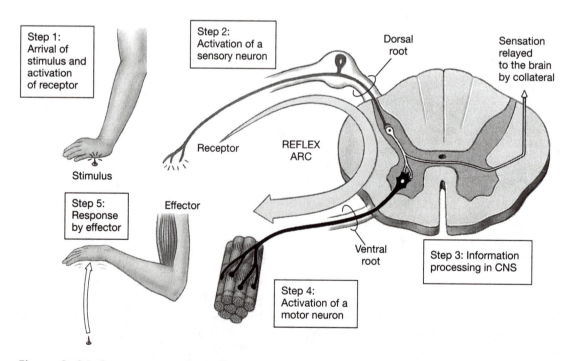

Figure 8–26 Components of a Reflex Arc.

Integration with Other Systems

Figure 8–27 diagrams the relationships between the nervous system and other physio-logical systems.

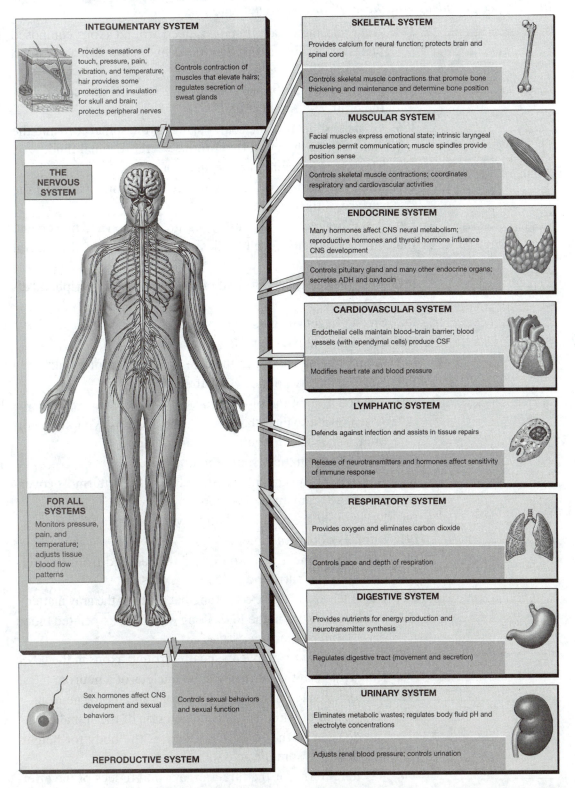

INTEGUMENTARY SYSTEM

Provides sensations of touch, pressure, pain, vibration, and temperature; hair provides some protection and insulation for skull and brain; protects peripheral nerves

Controls contraction of muscles that elevate hairs; regulates secretion of sweat glands

THE NERVOUS SYSTEM

FOR ALL SYSTEMS

Monitors pressure, pain, and temperature; adjusts tissue blood flow patterns

Sex hormones affect CNS development and sexual behaviors

Controls sexual behaviors and sexual function

REPRODUCTIVE SYSTEM

SKELETAL SYSTEM

Provides calcium for neural function; protects brain and spinal cord

Controls skeletal muscle contractions that promote bone thickening and maintenance and determine bone position

MUSCULAR SYSTEM

Facial muscles express emotional state; intrinsic laryngeal muscles permit communication; muscle spindles provide position sense

Controls skeletal muscle contractions; coordinates respiratory and cardiovascular activities

ENDOCRINE SYSTEM

Many hormones affect CNS neural metabolism; reproductive hormones and thyroid hormone influence CNS development

Controls pituitary gland and many other endocrine organs; secretes ADH and oxytocin

CARDIOVASCULAR SYSTEM

Endothelial cells maintain blood–brain barrier; blood vessels (with ependymal cells) produce CSF

Modifies heart rate and blood pressure

LYMPHATIC SYSTEM

Defends against infection and assists in tissue repairs

Release of neurotransmitters and hormones affect sensitivity of immune response

RESPIRATORY SYSTEM

Provides oxygen and eliminates carbon dioxide

Controls pace and depth of respiration

DIGESTIVE SYSTEM

Provides nutrients for energy production and neurotransmitter synthesis

Regulates digestive tract (movement and secretion)

URINARY SYSTEM

Eliminates metabolic wastes; regulates body fluid pH and electrolyte concentrations

Adjusts renal blood pressure; controls urination

Figure 8–27   **Functional Relationships between the Nervous System and Other Systems.**

Let's Review What You've Just Learned

▶ **Definitions**

In the space provided, write the term for each of the following definitions.

_____ **174.** An insulating sheath that is wrapped around axons, composed primarily of lipids and produced by oligodendrocytes and Schwann cells.

_____ **175.** Specialized membranes that provide stability and support for the brain and spinal cord.

_____ **176.** Glial cells that line the central canal of the spinal cord and the ventricles of the brain that produce cerebrospinal fluid.

_____ **177.** The cytoplasm contained in an axon.

_____ **178.** The gray matter of the spinal cord that projects toward the surface of the cord.

_____ **179.** A sensory receptor that monitors limb position and movement.

_____ **180.** Groups of neuron cell bodies that lie outside of the central nervous system.

_____ **181.** Neurons that carry information from the CNS to peripheral effectors.

_____ **182.** Small phagocytic glial cells.

_____ **183.** Neurons that have one dendrite and one axon.

_____ **184.** A propagated change in the transmembrane potential.

_____ **185.** Nerves that are connected to the spinal cord.

_____ **186.** The cell membrane of the axon.

_____ **187.** A synapse in which the presynaptic and postsynaptic membranes are locked together by gap junctions.

_____ **188.** A rapid automatic response to a stimulus.

_____ **189.** A tough, fibrous membrane that forms the outermost covering of the brain and spinal cord.

_____ **190.** Nerves that are connected directly to the brain.

_____ **191.** Bundles of neurofilaments.

_____ **192.** Delicate connective tissue fibers that extend from the perineurium and surround individual axons.

_____ **193.** The outer region of the cerebrum that contains the gray matter.

_____ **194.** Bundles of axons in the PNS along with their associated blood vessels and connective tissues.

_____ **195.** Glial cells that form myelin sheaths around axons in the CNS.

_____ **196.** The cytoplasm that surrounds the nucleus of a neuron.

_____ **197.** Neurons that connect sensory neurons and motor neurons.

_____ **198.** The regions of white matter on each side of the spinal cord.

_____ **199.** The division of the ANS that prepares the body for heightened levels of somatic activity.

_____ **200.** A general term for the target organs and tissues of the efferent division of the nervous system.

_____ **201.** Glial cells that surround neuron cell bodies in peripheral ganglia.

_____ **202.** Neurons that have several dendrites and a single axon.

_____ **203.** A tubular structure containing cerebrospinal fluid that runs along the length of the spinal cord.

_____ **204.** The outer surface of a glial cell that encircles an axon.

_____ **205.** A general term for sensory receptors that provide information about the external environment.

_____ **206.** A synapse in which the cells are not directly connected and communication is by way of a neurotransmitter.

_____ **207.** The path or pattern followed by a single reflex.

_____ **208.** Cavities lined by ependymal cells and filled with cerebrospinal fluid that are located within the brain.

_____ **209.** The thickened region where an axon attaches to the soma of a neuron.

_____ **210.** The innermost layer of the meninges.

_____ **211.** A stalk that connects the floor of the hypothalamus to the pituitary gland.

_____ **212.** The division of the ANS that stimulates visceral activity and is responsible for the state of rest and repose.

_____ **213.** The process of translating a sensory stimulus into an action potential.

_____ **214.** A fluid produced by specialized ependymal cells that surrounds the brain and spinal cord, providing protection and transport of nutrients and wastes.

_____ **215.** A side branch of an axon.

_____ **216.** Neurons that deliver information to the CNS.

_____ **217.** A general term for the electrical events that transmit information in the nervous system.

_____ **218.** The middle layer of the meninges.

_____ **219.** A dense network of collagen fibers that forms the outer layer of a nerve.

_____ **220.** One of the two portions (halves) of the cerebrum.

_____ **221.** The anatomical name for the sympathetic division of the ANS.

_____ **222.** The largest and most numerous glial cells in the CNS.

_____ **223.** Glial cells that form myelin sheaths around axons in the PNS.

_____ **224.** Sensory receptors that monitor the internal organ systems of the body.

_____ **225.** The part of the brain that is surrounded by the cerebrum and plays a vital role in integrating conscious and unconscious sensory information.

_____ **226.** The neurotransmitter released by sympathetic neurons at their effector synapses.

_____ **227.** The combination of capillary endothelium and astrocytes that controls the exchange of chemicals between the blood and the interstitial fluid of the brain.

_____ **228.** Gaps in the myelin sheath.

_____ **229.** A neuron in which the dendritic and axonal processes are continuous and the cell body lies off to one side.

_____ **230.** A membrane that divides a nerve into several compartments, each containing a bundle or fascicle of axons.

_____ **231.** The anatomical name for the parasympathetic division of the ANS.

► Word Roots, Prefixes, Suffixes, and Combining Forms

In the space provided, list the boldfaced terms introduced in this section that contain the indicated word part.

Word Part	Meaning	Examples
dendr-	tree	**232.** _____
neur-	nerve	**233.** _____
ef-	away from	**234.** _____
hypo-	under	**235.** _____
inter-	between	**236.** _____
-lemma	husk	**237.** _____
karyo-	kernel	**238.** _____
astr-	star	**239.** _____
af-	toward	**240.** _____
cephal-	head	**241.** _____
peri-	around	**242.** _____
crani-	head	**243.** _____
oligo-	few	**244.** _____
telo-	end	**245.** _____
pre-	before	**246.** _____
post-	after	**247.** _____

► Completion

For each of the following items fill in the blanks with the appropriate word or phrase.

248. List the five special senses.

a. _____

b. _____

c. _____

d. _____

e. _____

249. For each of the following sensory receptors, identify the type of sensory stimulus to which it responds.

a. nociceptor _____

b. olfactory receptor _____

c. mechanoreceptor _____

d. chemoreceptor _____

e. gustatory receptor _____

f. thermoreceptor _____

► **Concept Mapping**

Using the following terms, fill in the blank spaces next to the circled numbers to complete the concept map. Follow the numbers to comply with the organization of the map.

Brain
Afferent division
Sympathetic nervous system
Motor nervous system

Peripheral nervous system
Smooth muscle
Somatic nervous system

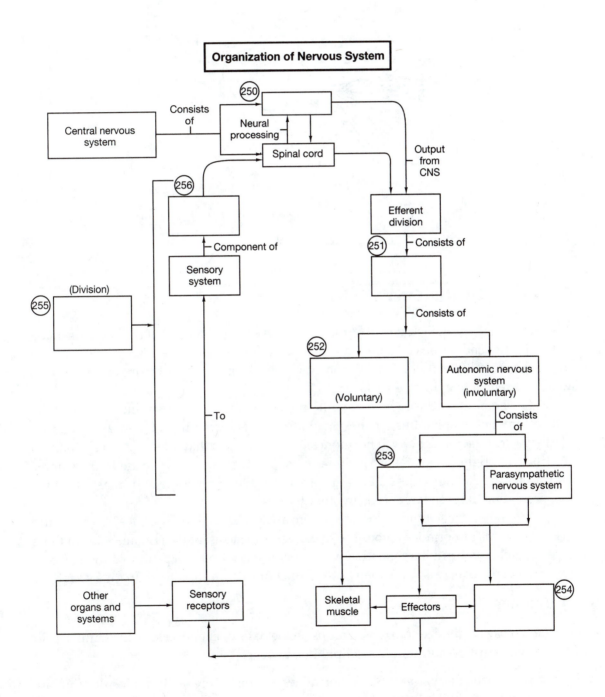

► **Labeling**

Label the regions on this diagram of the brain.

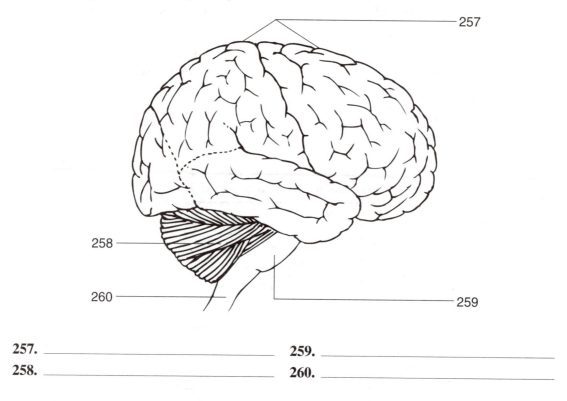

257. _____   259. _____
258. _____   260. _____

THE ENDOCRINE SYSTEM

The endocrine system includes all of the endocrine cells and tissues of the body. As noted in Chapter 6, endocrine cells are glandular secretory cells that release their secretions into the extracellular fluid. This characteristic distinguishes them from exocrine cells, which secrete onto epithelial surfaces.

The chemicals released by endocrine cells may affect only adjacent cells, as in the case of most prostaglandins, or they may affect cells throughout the body. **Paracrine** (PAR-uh-krin) **factors,** or "local hormones," are chemicals that affect other cells only in the tissue of origin. This category includes most prostaglandins and related compounds. **Hormones** are chemical messengers that are released in one tissue and transported via the circulation to reach target cells in other tissues.

The components of the endocrine system are introduced in Figure 8–28. This figure also lists the major hormones produced in each endocrine tissue and organ. Some of these organs, such as the pituitary gland, have endocrine secretion as a primary function; others, such as the pancreas, have many other functions in addition to endocrine secretion.

Hormones

Hormones can be divided into three groups on the basis of chemical structure: amino acid derivatives, peptide hormones, and lipid derivatives.

- **Amino acid derivatives:** Some hormones are relatively small molecules that are structurally similar to amino acids. This group includes epinephrine, norepinephrine, dopamine, thyroid hormones, and the pineal hormone melatonin. Epinephrine,

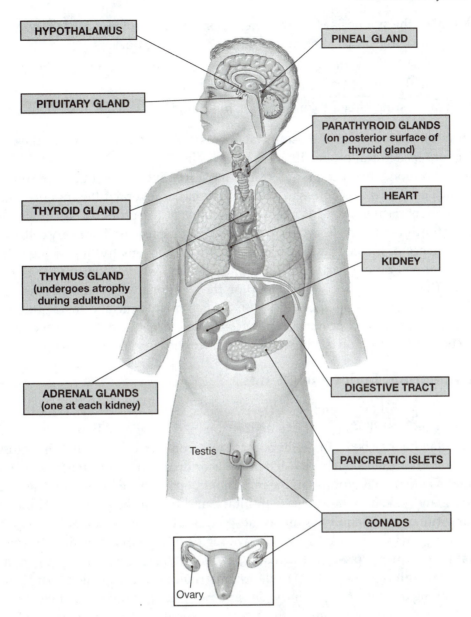

Figure 8–28 **The Endocrine System.**

norepinephrine, and dopamine are structurally similar: these compounds are some-times called **catecholamines** (kat-e-KŌ-la-mēnz).

- **Peptide hormones: Peptide hormones** are chains of amino acids. They range from short amino acid chains, such as ADH and oxytocin (9 amino acids), to polypeptides, such as growth hormone (191 amino acids).

- **Lipid derivatives:** There are two classes of lipid-based hormones: **steroid hormones** derived from cholesterol and **eicosanoids** (ī-KŌ-sa-noyds), derived from *arachidonic acid*, a 20-carbon fatty acid.

All cellular structures and functions depend on proteins. Structural proteins determine the general shape and internal structure of a cell, and enzymes direct its metabolic activities. Hormones alter cellular operations by changing the types, activities, or quantities of important enzymes and structural proteins. In other words, a hormone may:

- Stimulate the synthesis of an enzyme or a structural protein not already present in the cytoplasm by activating appropriate genes in the nucleus.

- Increase or decrease the rate of synthesis of a particular enzyme or other protein by changing the rate of transcription or translation.

- Turn an existing enzyme "on" or "off" by changing its shape or structure.

Through one or more of these mechanisms, a hormone can modify the physical structure or biochemical properties of its target cells.

For a hormone to affect a target cell, it must first interact with an appropriate receptor. Each cell has the receptors needed to respond to several different hormones, but cells in different tissues have different combinations of receptors. This arrangement accounts for the differential effects of hormones on specific tissues. For every cell, the presence or absence of a receptor determines its hormonal sensitivities. If the cell has a receptor that will bind a particular hormone, that cell will respond to the hormone's presence: If the cell lacks the proper receptor, the hormone will have no effect.

Hormone receptors are found both on the cell membrane and inside the cell. The catecholamines, peptide hormones, and eicosanoids target receptors on the cell membrane. The thyroid hormones and steroids interact with intracellular receptors.

Some Important Endocrine Glands

The **pituitary gland,** or **hypophysis** (hī-POF-i-sis; Greek *hypophysis*, outgrowth), is a small oval gland that lies nestled in a depression in the sphenoid bone of the skull. The pituitary gland hangs beneath the hypothalamus, connected by a stalk, the infundibulum. The pituitary gland can be divided into posterior and anterior divisions on anatomical and developmental grounds. Nine important peptide hormones are released by the pituitary gland, seven by the anterior pituitary, and two at the posterior pituitary. The **anterior pituitary,** or **adenohypophysis** (ad-ē-nō-hī-POF-i-sis; Greek *adenos*, gland + *hypophysis*, outgrowth), can be divided into two regions: (1) a large **pars distalis** (dis-TAL-is; distal part), which represents the major portion of the entire pituitary gland, and (2) a slender **pars intermedia** (in-ter-MĒ-dē-uh; intermediate part), which forms a narrow band bordering the posterior pituitary. The anterior pituitary produces seven hormones whose functions and control mechanisms are reasonably well understood. Of the six hormones produced by the pars distalis, four regulate the production of hormones by other endocrine glands. The names of these hormones indicate their activities, but the phrases are often so long that abbreviations are used instead.

- **Thyroid-stimulating hormone (TSH)** targets the thyroid gland and triggers the release of thyroid hormones.

- **Adrenocorticotropic** (a-drē-nō-kōr-ti-kō-TRŌ-pik) **Hormone (ACTH)** stimulates the release of steroid hormones by the adrenal cortex, the outer layer of the adrenal gland.

- **Follicle-stimulating hormone (FSH)** and **luteinizing** (loo-TĒ-i-nī-zing) **hormone (LH)** are called **gonadotropins** (gō-nad-ō-TRŌ-pinz) because they regulate the activities of the male and female sex organs (gonads).

- **Prolactin** (prō-LAK-tin; Latin *pro*, before + *lac*, milk), or **PRL** works with other hormones to stimulate mammary gland development. It also stimulates milk production by the mammary glands.

- **Growth hormone (GH)** or **somatotropin** (sō-ma-tō-TRŌ-pin), stimulates cell growth and replication by accelerating the rate of protein synthesis.

The pars intermedia may secrete two forms of **melanocyte-stimulating hormone (MSH).** As the name indicates, MSH stimulates the melanocytes of the skin, increasing their production of melanin. MSH is not secreted in healthy nonpregnant adults.

The **posterior pituitary** is also called the **neurohypophysis** (noo-rō-hī-POF-i-sis), or **pars nervosa** (nervous part), because it contains the axons of hypothalamic neurons. Neurons in the hypothalamus manufacture **antidiuretic** (an-tē-dī-ū-RET-ik; Greek *anti*, against + *diourein*, to pass urine) **hormone (ADH)** and **oxytocin.** These secretions are transported along axons in the infundibulum to axon terminals located in the posterior pituitary. There, they are stored until released in response to a neural impulse. Antidiuretic hormone (also known as vasopressin) regulates the amount of water lost at the kidneys. Oxytocin stimulates smooth muscle tissue in the wall of the uterus, promoting labor and delivery. After delivery, oxytocin stimulates the movement of milk down ducts from the mammary glands to sinuses beneath the nipple.

The **thyroid gland** is composed of two lobes connected by a slender connection, the **isthmus** (IS-mus). It produces **thyroid hormones** that function in regulating the level of cellular metabolism and **calcitonin** (kal-si-TŌ-nin), a hormone that lowers the concentration of calcium ions in the body fluids. Two pairs of **parathyroid** (par-uh-THĪ-royd) **glands** are found embedded in the posterior surfaces of the thyroid gland. These glands secrete **parathyroid hormone (PTH)**, which raises the level of calcium ions in body fluids.

A yellow, pyramid-shaped **adrenal** (a-DRĒ-nul; Latin *ad*, toward + *ren*, kidney) **gland,** or **suprarenal** (su-pra-RĒ-nal; Latin *supra*, above + *ren*, kidney) **gland,** sits on the superior border of each kidney. The adrenal gland is divided into two parts, a superficial adrenal cortex and an inner adrenal medulla.

The **adrenal cortex** produces more than two dozen steroid hormones, collectively called **adrenocortical** (a-drē-nō-KŌR-ti-kul) **steroids**, or simply **corticosteroids** (kōr-tī-kō-STĒR-oydz). Corticosteroids are vital; if the adrenal glands are destroyed or removed, corticosteroids must be administered or the individual will not survive. Corticosteroids, like other steroid hormones, exert their effects by determining which genes are transcribed in the nuclei of their target cells and at what rates. The resulting changes in the nature and concentration of enzymes in the cytoplasm affect cellular metabolism.

There are three distinct regions, or zones, in the adrenal cortex. Each zone synthesizes different steroid hormones. The outermost zone produces **mineralocorticoids** (min-er-a-lō-KŌR-ti-koydz), steroid hormones that affect the electrolyte composition of body fluids. **Aldosterone** (al-DOS-te-rōn) is the principal mineralocorticoid produced by the human adrenal cortex. The middle zone produces steroid hormones collectively known as **glucocorticoids** (gloo-ko-KŌR-ti-koydz) because of their effects on glucose metabolism. The primary secretion is **cortisol** (KŌR-ti-sol), also called **hydrocortisone** (hī-drō-KŌR-ti-sōn). The innermost zone normally produces small quantities of sex hormones called **androgens** (AN-drō-jinz; Greek *andros*, man).

The secretory activities of the **adrenal medullae** (me-DŪL-ē, plural of *medulla*) are controlled by the sympathetic division of the ANS. The adrenal medullae contain two populations of secretory cells; one produces **epinephrine (adrenaline** [a-DREN-a-lin]) and the other produces **norepinephrine (noradrenaline** [NŌR-a-dren-a-lin]).

The **pancreas** lies within the abdominopelvic cavity. It is a slender, usually pink, organ with a lumpy consistency. The **exocrine pancreas,** roughly 99 percent of the pancreatic volume, produces large quantities of an alkaline, enzyme-rich fluid. This secretion reaches the lumen of the digestive tract by traveling along a network of secretory ducts. The **endocrine pancreas** consists of small groups of cells scattered among the exocrine cells. The endocrine clusters are known as **pancreatic islets**, or the **islets of Langerhans** (LAN-ger-hanz). Pancreatic islets account for the remaining 1 percent of the pancreatic cell population. The endocrine pancreas produces several hormones, most notably insulin, glucagon (GLOO-ka-gon), and pancreatic somatostatin (sō-ma-tō-STĀT-in). **Insulin** acts to lower blood sugar levels, whereas **glucagon** functions to raise blood sugar levels. **Pancreatic somatostatin** suppresses the release of insulin and glucagon and slows the rates of food absorption and enzyme secretion along the digestive tract.

Interactions with Other Systems

The relationships between the endocrine system and other systems are summarized in Figure 8–29.

✎ Let's Review What You've Just Learned

▶ **Definitions**

In the space provided, write the term for each of the following definitions.

_____ **261.** A general term for hormones that stimulate the reproductive organs.

_____ **262.** Another name for the pituitary gland.

_____ **263.** Chemical messengers that are released in one tissue and transported by the circulatory system to target cells in other tissues.

_____ **264.** The secretion of the innermost region of the adrenal cortex.

_____ **265.** Small groups of endocrine cells that are scattered among the exocrine cells of the pancreas.

_____ **266.** Chemicals that act as "local hormones" and affect other cells only in the tissue of origin.

_____ **267.** Another name for the anterior pituitary gland.

_____ **268.** A collective term for all of the steroid hormones produced by the adrenal cortex.

_____ **269.** A collective term for male sex hormones.

_____ **270.** The portion of the pancreas that secretes digestive enzymes.

_____ **271.** A group of similar chemical compounds that includes epinephrine, norepinephrine, and dopamine.

_____ **272.** The part of the anterior pituitary gland that secretes the largest number of hormones.

_____ **273.** Four small glands embedded within the thyroid gland.

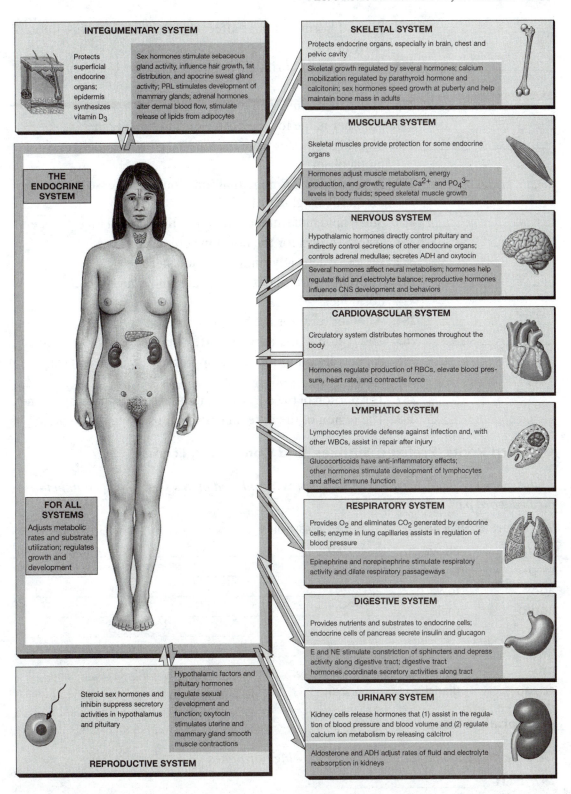

INTEGUMENTARY SYSTEM

Protects superficial endocrine organs; epidermis synthesizes vitamin D₃

Sex hormones stimulate sebaceous gland activity, influence hair growth, fat distribution, and apocrine sweat gland activity; PRL stimulates development of mammary glands; adrenal hormones alter dermal blood flow, stimulate release of lipids from adipocytes

THE ENDOCRINE SYSTEM

FOR ALL SYSTEMS

Adjusts metabolic rates and substrate utilization; regulates growth and development

REPRODUCTIVE SYSTEM

Steroid sex hormones and inhibin suppress secretory activities in hypothalamus and pituitary

Hypothalamic factors and pituitary hormones regulate sexual development and function; oxytocin stimulates uterine and mammary gland smooth muscle contractions

SKELETAL SYSTEM

Protects endocrine organs, especially in brain, chest and pelvic cavity

Skeletal growth regulated by several hormones; calcium mobilization regulated by parathyroid hormone and calcitonin; sex hormones speed growth at puberty and help maintain bone mass in adults

MUSCULAR SYSTEM

Skeletal muscles provide protection for some endocrine organs

Hormones adjust muscle metabolism, energy production, and growth; regulate Ca^{2+} and PO_4^{3-} levels in body fluids; speed skeletal muscle growth

NERVOUS SYSTEM

Hypothalamic hormones directly control pituitary and indirectly control secretions of other endocrine organs; controls adrenal medullae; secretes ADH and oxytocin

Several hormones affect neural metabolism; hormones help regulate fluid and electrolyte balance; reproductive hormones influence CNS development and behaviors

CARDIOVASCULAR SYSTEM

Circulatory system distributes hormones throughout the body

Hormones regulate production of RBCs, elevate blood pressure, heart rate, and contractile force

LYMPHATIC SYSTEM

Lymphocytes provide defense against infection and, with other WBCs, assist in repair after injury

Glucocorticoids have anti-inflammatory effects; other hormones stimulate development of lymphocytes and affect immune function

RESPIRATORY SYSTEM

Provides O_2 and eliminates CO_2 generated by endocrine cells; enzyme in lung capillaries assists in regulation of blood pressure

Epinephrine and norepinephrine stimulate respiratory activity and dilate respiratory passageways

DIGESTIVE SYSTEM

Provides nutrients and substrates to endocrine cells; endocrine cells of pancreas secrete insulin and glucagon

E and NE stimulate constriction of sphincters and depress activity along digestive tract; digestive tract hormones coordinate secretory activities along tract

URINARY SYSTEM

Kidney cells release hormones that (1) assist in the regulation of blood pressure and blood volume and (2) regulate calcium ion metabolism by releasing calcitrol

Aldosterone and ADH adjust rates of fluid and electrolyte reabsorption in kidneys

Figure 8–29   Functional Relationships between the Endocrine System and Other Systems.

_____ **274.** Steroid hormones that affect the electrolyte composition of body fluids.

_____ **275.** A pancreatic hormone that acts to lower blood sugar (glucose) levels.

_____ **276.** Hormones composed of chains of amino acids.

_____ **277.** Another name for the posterior pituitary gland.

_____ **278.** Steroid hormones from the adrenal glands that affect glucose metabolism.

_____ **279.** A pancreatic hormone that functions to increase the levels of blood sugar (glucose).

_____ **280.** Small lipid molecules containing a five-carbon ring at one end.

_____ **281.** Another term for the hormone epinephrine.

_____ **282.** Lipids structurally similar to cholesterol.

_____ **283.** The outer portion of the adrenal gland, which secretes steroid hormones.

_____ **284.** Another term for the hormone norepinephrine.

_____ **285.** The region of the adrenal cortex that secretes aldosterone.

_____ **286.** A pancreatic hormone that suppresses insulin and glucagon release.

_____ **287.** The portion of the adrenal glands that secretes catecholamines.

_____ **288.** The region of the adrenal cortex that secretes cortisol.

▶ Word Roots, Prefixes, Suffixes, and Combining Forms

In the space provided, list the boldfaced terms introduced in this section that contain the indicated word part.

Word Part	Meaning	Examples
supra-	above	**289.** _____
trop-	feed	**290.** _____
ad-	toward	**291.** _____
andro-	male	**292.** _____
para-	beyond	**293.** _____
eicos-	twenty	**294.** _____
pro-	before	**295.** _____
adeno-	gland	**296.** _____

▶ Alphabet Soup

Give the proper name for each of the following hormones.

297. PTH _____

298. FSH _____

299. GH _____

300. LH _____

301. PRL _____

302. ADH _____

303. MSH _____

304. ACTH _____
305. TSH _____

☑ Self-Check Test

The following test will allow you to determine how well you have mastered the vocabulary and basic concepts of this chapter. It will also help you prepare for the type of questions you are likely to encounter on a test in an anatomy and physiology course. The self-check test will help you assess your understanding of the chapter material and help you develop good test-taking skills.

The following questions test your ability to use vocabulary and to recall facts.

1. Accessory structures of the skin include
   a. hair follicles
   b. sweat glands
   c. sebaceous glands
   d. nails
   e. all of these
2. An epidermal layer found only in the skin of the palms of the hands and the soles of the feet is the
   a. stratum corneum
   b. stratun lucidum
   c. stratum germinativum
   d. stratum granulosum
   e. stratum spinosum
3. The layer of skin that contains the blood vessels and nerves that supply the surface of the skin is the
   a. papillary layer
   b. reticular layer
   c. epidermal layer
   d. subcutaneous layer
   e. hypodermal layer
4. Glands that discharge an oily secretion into hair follicles are
   a. ceruminous glands
   b. apocrine sweat glands
   c. merocrine sweat glands
   d. sebaceous glands
   e. mammary glands
5. Mature bone cells are called
   a. osteocytes
   b. osteoblasts
   c. osteoclasts
   d. chondrocytes
   e. osteons

6. The shaft of a long bone is called the
   a. epiphysis
   b. diaphysis
   c. metaphysis
   d. epiphyseal plate
   e. lamella

7. The bone of the arm (humerus) is an example of a
   a. long bone
   b. short bone
   c. flat bone
   d. irregular bone
   e. sesamoid bone

8. A slightly movable joint is a(n)
   a. synarthrosis
   b. diarthrosis
   c. amphiarthrosis
   d. gomphosis
   e. synostosis

9. The dense layer of collagen fibers that surround an entire skeletal muscle is the
   a. tendon
   b. endomysium
   c. perimysium
   d. epimysium
   e. fascicle

10. The cell membrane of skeletal muscle is called the
    a. sarcolemma
    b. sarcomere
    c. sarcosome
    d. sarcoplasm
    e. sarcoplasmic reticulum

11. The _____ contains vesicles filled with acetylcholine.
    a. transverse tubule
    b. synaptic cleft
    c. neuromuscular junction
    d. sarcoplasmic reticulum
    e. synaptic knob

12. Skeletal muscles in which the fascicles are arranged to form a common angle with the tendon are
    a. parallel
    b. circular
    c. pennate
    d. convergent
    e. divergent

13. The myelin sheaths that surround the axons of some of the neurons in the CNS are formed by
    a. astrocytes
    b. satellite cells

   c. Schwann cells

   d. oligodendrocytes

   e. microglia

14. The site of intercellular communication between neurons is the

   a. telodendria

   b. synaptic knob

   c. collateral

   d. axon hillock

   e. synapse

15. Neurons that have several dendrites and a single axon are called

   a. anaxonic

   b. unipolar

   c. bipolar

   d. tripolar

   e. multipolar

16. The projections of gray matter toward the outer surface of the spinal cord are called

   a. columns

   b. fascicles

   c. horns

   d. nerves

   e. ganglia

17. Peptide hormones are

   a. composed of amino acids

   b. produced by cells in the adrenal cortex

   c. lipids

   d. eicosanoids

   e. chemically related to cholesterol

18. The adrenal medulla produces

   a. androgens

   b. mineralocorticoids

   c. glucocorticoids

   d. corticosteroids

   e. catecholamines

19. A gland that has both endocrine and exocrine function is the

   a. pituitary gland

   b. thyroid gland

   c. parathyroid gland

   d. pancreas

   e. adrenal gland

20. The isthmus is part of the

   a. pituitary gland

   b. thyroid gland

   c. parathyroid gland

   d. pancreas

   e. adrenal gland

☑Self-Assessment

If your score was

between 18 and 20, you are ready to proceed to the next chapter.

between 15 and 17, you have a good general idea of the chapter content, but you should review sections of the chapter that deal with items that you missed before proceeding to the next chapter.

less than 14, you have not mastered the chapter content well enough to proceed. Reread the chapter and rework the exercises. Then retake the self-check test. Repeat this process until you achieve a score that will allow you to continue.

Answers

1. keratohyalin
2. sebum
3. dermis
4. stratum corneum
5. carotene
6. sweat
7. stratum lucidum
8. integument
9. strata
10. papillary layer
11. hypodermis
12. apocrine sweat glands
13. nails
14. stratum granulosum
15. melanocytes
16. hair follicles
17. subcutaneous layer
18. stratum germinativum
19. sebaceous glands
20. dermal papillae
21. epidermis
22. keratinocytes
23. stratum spinosum
24. keratohyaline
25. reticular layer
26. merocrine sweat glands
27. epidermal derivative, or accessory structure
28. epidermis
29. merocrine
30. melanocyte, keratinocyte
31. apocrine
32. subcutaneous layer
33. dermis, epidermis, hypodermis
34. hypodermis
35. reticular layer
36. subcutaneous
37. stratum spinosum
38. stratum corneum
39. ossification
40. osteoblast
41. patella
42. epiphyses
43. short bones

44. synovial joint, or diarthrosis
45. hydroxyapatite
46. compact bone
47. yellow bone marrow
48. synostosis
49. axial skeleton
50. irregular bones
51. osteoclast
52. calcification
53. osteon, or Haversian system
54. endosteum
55. sesamoid bones
56. clavicle
57. pectoral girdle
58. synchondrosis
59. spongy bone, or cancellous bone
60. periosteum
61. intramembranous ossification
62. long bones
63. scapula
64. coxa, or innominate bone
65. joints, or articulations
66. amphiarthrosis
67. synarthrosis
68. pelvis
69. trabeculae
70. diaphysis
71. osteocytes
72. central canal, or Haversian canal
73. canaliculi
74. medullary cavity, or marrow cavity
75. cortex
76. endochondral ossification
77. flat bones
78. appendicular skeleton
79. pelvic girdle
80. suture
81. osteoprogenitor cells
82. syndesmosis
83. red bone marrow
84. gomphosis
85. sutural bones, or Wormian bones
86. symphysis

87. periodontal ligament
88. synarthrosis, synostosis, syndesmosis
89. osteoblast
90. periosteum, periodontal
91. osteocyte, osteoblast, osteoclast, osteoprogenitor, osteon
92. hydroxyapatite
93. endosteum, endochondral
94. osteoclast
95. endochondral, synchondrosis
96. amphiarthrosis, synarthrosis, diarthrosis
97. symphysis
98. diaphysis
99. epiphysis
100. progenitor
101. symphysis, diaphysis, epiphysis
102. amphiarthrosis
103. intramembranous
104. sarcolemma
105. fascicle
106. prime mover
107. pennate muscle
108. endomysium
109. myoblasts
110. origin
111. transverse tubules, or T tubules
112. synaptic knob
113. myofilament
114. lever
115. epimysium
116. satellite cells
117. antagonist
118. sarcomere
119. extrinsic muscle
120. circular muscle, or sphincter
121. perimysium
122. sarcoplasm
123. neurotransmitter
124. convergent muscle
125. action
126. synergist
127. myofibrils
128. excitation-contraction coupling
129. intrinsic muscle
130. cardiac muscle
131. neuromuscular junction, or myoneural junction
132. parallel muscle
133. sarcoplasmic reticulum
134. acetylcholine
135. biomechanics
136. fulcrum
137. insertion
138. fixator
139. myofibril, myofilament, myoblast, myoneural
140. synergist, synaptic knob
141. myoblast
142. perimysium
143. sarcolemma
144. sarcomere, sarcoplasm, sarcoplasmic reticulum, sarcolemma
145. endomysium
146. antagonist
147. sarcomere
148. epimysium
149. epimysium, perimysium, endomysium
150. transverse tubule
151. straight
152. deltoid
153. fasciculus
154. longus
155. biggest
156. four heads
157. brevis
158. round
159. transverse
160. profundus
161. orbicularis
162. bigger
163. magnus
164. trapezium
165. biceps
166. rhomboid
167. smallest
168. oblique
169. external
170. minor
171. longest
172. F   E   R → (△ under F)
173. E   R → (△F below)
174. myelin
175. meninges
176. ependymal cells
177. axoplasm
178. horn
179. proprioceptor
180. ganglia
181. motor neurons
182. microglia
183. bipolar neurons
184. action potential
185. spinal nerves
186. axolemma
187. electrical synapse
188. reflex
189. dura mater
190. cranial nerves
191. neurofibrils
192. endoneurium
193. cerebral cortex
194. nerves
195. oligodendrocytes
196. perikaryon
197. interneuron
198. column, or funiculus
199. sympathetic division
200. effector
201. satellite cells
202. multipolar neurons
203. central canal

204. neurilemma
205. exteroceptors
206. chemical synapse
207. reflex arc
208. ventricles
209. axon hillock
210. pia mater
211. infundibulum
212. parasympathetic division
213. transduction
214. cerebrospinal fluid (CSF)
215. collateral
216. sensory neurons
217. nerve impulses
218. arachnoid
219. epineurium
220. cerebral hemisphere
221. thoracolumbar division
222. astrocytes
223. Schwann cells
224. interoceptors
225. diencephalon
226. norepinephrine
227. blood-brain barrier
228. nodes, or nodes of Ranvier
229. unipolar, or pseudounipolar
230. perineurium
231. craniosacral division
232. telodendria, oligodendrocyte
233. neurilemma, neurofibrils, neurofilaments, neurotubules
234. efferent division, efferent fibers
235. hypothalamus
236. interneuron, internode
237. neurilemma, axolemma
238. perikaryon
239. astrocyte
240. afferent division, afferent fibers
241. diencephalon, mesencephalon
242. perineurium, perikaryon
243. cranial nerves
244. oligodendrocytes
245. telodendria
246. presynaptic, preganglionic
247. postsynaptic, postganglionic
248. a. smell
    b. taste
    c. balance
    d. hearing
    e. vision
249. a. pain
    b. odor
    c. movement
    d. chemicals
    e. flavor chemicals
    f. temperature
250. brain
251. motor system

252. somatic nervous system
253. sympathetic nervous system
254. smooth muscle
255. peripheral nervous system
256. afferent division
257. cerebrum
258. cerebellum
259. pons
260. medulla oblongata
261. gonadotropins
262. hypophysis
263. hormones
264. sex hormones
265. pancreatic islets, or islets of Langerhans
266. paracrine factors
267. adenohypophysis
268. adrenocorticosteroids, or corticosteroids
269. androgens
270. exocrine pancreas
271. catecholamines
272. pars distalis
273. parathyroid glands
274. mineralocorticoids
275. insulin
276. peptide hormones
277. neurohypophysis
278. glucocorticoids
279. glucagon
280. eicosanoids
281. adrenaline
282. steroids
283. adrenal cortex
284. noradrenaline
285. zona glomerulosa
286. pancreatic somatostatin
287. adrenal medulla
288. zona fasciculata
289. suprarenal glands
290. gonadotropins
291. adrenal glands
292. androgens
293. parathyroid glands, paracrine factors
294. eicosanoids
295. prolactin
296. adenohypophysis
297. parathyroid hormone
298. follicle-stimulating hormone
299. growth hormone
300. luteinizing hormone
301. prolactin
302. antidiuretic hormone
303. melanocyte-stimulating hormone
304. adrenocorticotrophic hormone
305. thyroid-stimulating hormone

Answers to Self-Check Test

1. e 2. b 3. a 4. d 5. a 6. b 7. a 8. c 9. d 10. a 11. e 12. c
13. d 14. e 15. e 16. c 17. a 18. e 19. d 20. b

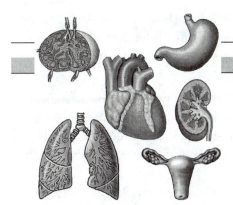

CHAPTER 9

A Survey of Human Body Systems II

In this chapter we will survey the following systems of the human body: cardiovascular system, lymphatic system, respiratory system, digestive system, urinary system, and reproductive system. These are the body systems that are generally covered in the second semester of a two-semester anatomy and physiology course. As in the previous chapter, a general overview of each body system will be presented, with an emphasis on terminology and general concepts.

THE CARDIOVASCULAR SYSTEM

The cardiovascular system consists of the heart, the blood vessels, and the fluid they contain, blood. We will begin our overview of this system by examining the functions and composition of blood.

Blood

Blood is a specialized connective tissue that contains cells suspended in a fluid matrix. The functions of blood include:

1. **The transportation of dissolved gases, nutrients, hormones, and metabolic wastes:** Oxygen is carried from the lungs to the tissues, and carbon dioxide is carried from the tissues to the lungs. Nutrients absorbed at the digestive tract or released from storage in adipose tissue or the liver are distributed throughout the body. Hormones are carried from endocrine glands toward their target tissues, and the wastes produced by the body's cells are absorbed by the blood and carried to the kidneys for excretion.

2. **The regulation of the pH and electrolyte composition of interstitial fluids throughout the body:** The blood absorbs and neutralizes the acids generated by active tissues, such as the lactic acid produced by skeletal muscles. The blood adds and removes ions from the interstitial fluid as necessary.

3. **The restriction of fluid losses through damaged vessels or at other injury sites:** Blood contains enzymes and factors that respond to breaks in the vessel walls by initiating the process of blood clotting. A blood clot acts as a temporary patch and prevents further blood loss.

4. **Defense against toxins and pathogens:** Blood transports white blood cells, specialized cells that migrate into peripheral tissues to fight infections or to remove debris. It also delivers antibodies, special proteins that attack invading organisms or foreign compounds.

5. **Stabilization of body temperature:** Blood absorbs the heat generated by active skeletal muscles and redistributes it to other tissues. When body temperature is already high, that heat will be lost across the surface of the skin. If body temperature is too low, the warm blood is directed to the brain and other temperature-sensitive organs.

Blood has a characteristic and unique composition consisting of plasma and formed elements (Figure 9–1). **Plasma** (PLAZ-mah), the matrix of blood, has a density only slightly greater than that of water. It contains dissolved proteins rather than the network of insoluble fibers found in loose connective tissue or cartilage. **Formed elements** are blood cells and cell fragments that are suspended in the plasma.

Plasma contains significant quantities of dissolved proteins. On average, there are 7.6 g of protein in each 100 ml of plasma. There are three primary classes of plasma proteins, **albumins** (al-BŪ-minz), **globulins** (GLOB-ū-linz), and **fibrinogen** (fī-BRIN-ō-jen).

- Albumins are the most abundant proteins. They are major contributors to the colloid osmotic pressure of the plasma. Albumins are also important in the transport of fatty acids and several other substances useful in metabolism.

- Globulins are important transport proteins. Transport globulins bind small ions, hormones, or compounds that (1) might otherwise be filtered out of the blood at the kidneys or (2) have very low solubility in water. **Immunoglobulins** (i-mū-nō-GLOB-ū-linz), also called **antibodies,** attack foreign proteins and pathogens.

- Fibrinogen functions in blood clotting. Under certain conditions, fibrinogen molecules interact, forming large insoluble strands of **fibrin** (FĪ-brin). These fibers provide the basic framework for a blood clot.

The formed elements of the blood are red blood cells, white blood cells, and platelets.

Red blood cells (RBCs), or **erythrocytes** (e-RITH-rō-sīts; Greek *erythros*, red + *kytos*, container) are the most abundant blood cells and the only cells in the body that lack a nucleus. The primary function of red blood cells is to transport respiratory gases, primarily oxygen. Red blood cells contain the molecule **hemoglobin** (HĒ-mō-glō-bin) **(Hb)** which accounts for 95 percent of the intracellular proteins. Roughly 98.5 percent of the oxygen carried by the blood travels through the circulation bound to hemoglobin molecules inside red blood cells.

The less numerous **white blood cells (WBCs),** or **leukocytes** (LOO-kō-sīts; Greek, *leukos*, white) can easily be distinguished from RBCs because they (1) have nuclei and (2) lack hemoglobin. White blood cells help defend the body gainst invasion by pathogens and remove toxins, wastes, and abnormal or damaged cells. Traditionally, leukocytes have been divided into two groups based on their appearance after staining. On that basis, leukocytes can be divided into **granular leukocytes,** or **granulocytes** (GRAN-yū-lō-sīts) (with abundant stained granules), and **agranular leukocytes,** or **agranulocytes** (A-gran-yoo-lō-sīts) (with few if any stained granules). Granulocytes include neutrophils, eosinophils, and basophils. Monocytes and lymphocytes are agranulocytes.

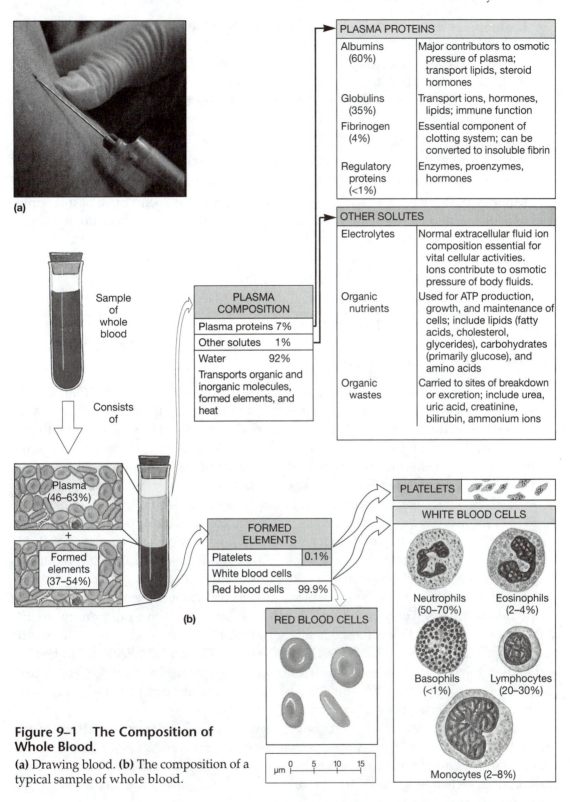

Figure 9–1 The Composition of Whole Blood.
(a) Drawing blood. (b) The composition of a typical sample of whole blood.

- **Neutrophils** (NOO-truh-filz) are highly mobile, and they are usually the first white blood cells to arrive at an injury site. They are very active cells that specialize in attacking and digesting bacteria that have been "marked" with antibodies or complement proteins.

- **Eosinophils** (ē-ō-SIN-uh-filz) were so named because their granules stain darkly with eosin, a red dye. Eosinophils attack objects that have already been coated with antibodies. They are phagocytic cells and will engulf antibody-marked bacteria, protozoa, or cellular debris. Their primary mode of attack, however, involves the release of toxic compounds onto the surface of their targets. Eosinophils are important in defense against large multicellular parasites such as parasitic worms.

- **Basophils** (BĀ-suh-filz) have numerous granules, that stain darkly with basic dyes. Basophils migrate to sites of injury and discharge their granules, which contain histamine and heparin, a chemical that prevents blood clotting, into the interstitial fluid.

- **Monocytes** (MON-ō-sīts) are large white blood cells that spend most of their time outside the bloodstream. Monocytes are aggressive phagocytes, often attempting to engulf items as large or larger than themselves.

- **Lymphocytes** (LIM-fō-sīts) are important in the immune process. They secrete antibodies and recognize and attack foreign cells.

Platelets are small packets of cytoplasm that contain enzymes and factors important to the process of blood clotting.

The Heart and Blood Vessels

The heart is located near the anterior chest wall, directly behind the sternum. It is surrounded by the pericardial cavity. The serous membrane lining the pericardial cavity is called the **pericardium** (per-i-KAR-dē-um). The pericardium can be subdivided into the visceral pericardium and the parietal pericardium. The **visceral pericardium,** or **epicardium** (ep-i-KAR-dē-um), covers the outer surface of the heart; the **parietal pericardium** lines the inner surface of the pericardial sac that surrounds the heart. The pericardial sac, which is reinforced by a dense network of collagen fibers, stabilizes the position of the heart and associated vessels. The space between the opposing parietal and visceral surfaces is the **pericardial cavity.** This cavity normally contains **pericardial fluid** secreted by the pericardial membranes. Pericardial fluid acts as a lubricant, reducing friction between the opposing surfaces as the heart beats.

Blood flows through a network of blood vessels that extend between the heart and the peripheral tissues. Those blood vessels can be subdivided into a **pulmonary circuit** that carries blood to and from the exchange surfaces of the lungs and a **systemic circuit** that transports blood to and from the rest of the body (Figure 9–2). Each circuit begins and ends at the heart, and blood travels through these circuits in sequence. For example, blood returning to the heart from the systemic circuit must complete the pulmonary circuit before reentering the systemic circuit.

Arteries, or **efferent vessels,** carry blood away from the heart; **veins,** or **afferent vessels,** return blood to the heart. **Capillaries** are small, thin-walled vessels between the smallest arteries and veins. Capillaries are called exchange vessels because their thin wall permits exchange of nutrients, dissolved gases, and waste products between the blood and surrounding tissues.

Structure of the Heart

Despite its impressive workload, the heart is a small organ, roughly the size of a clenched fist. The heart contains four muscular chambers, two associated with each circuit (Figure 9–3). The **right atrium** (Ā-trē-um; Latin *atrium,* hall, plural *atria* [Ā-trē-uh]) receives

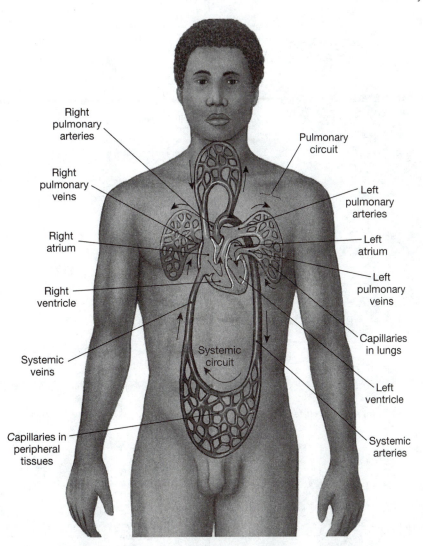

Figure 9–2   An Overview of the Cardiovascular System.
Blood flows through separate pulmonary and systemic circuits, driven by the pumping of the heart. Each circuit begins and ends at the heart and contains arteries, capillaries, and veins.

blood from the systemic circuit and passes it to the **right ventricle** (VEN-tri-kul; Latin *ventriculus*, little belly). The right ventricle discharges blood into the pulmonary circuit. The **left atrium** collects blood from the pulmonary circuit and empties it into the **left ventricle.** Contraction of the left ventricle ejects blood into the systemic circuit. When the heart beats, the two ventricles contract at the same time and eject equal volumes of blood.

The four cardiac chambers can be identified easily in a superficial view of the heart. The two atria have relatively thin muscular walls, and they are highly distensible. When an atrium is not filled with blood, its outer portion deflates and becomes a rather lumpy and wrinkled flap. This expandable extension of an atrium is called an **auricle** (AW-ri-kul; Latin *auricula*, little ear) because it reminded early anatomists of the external ear. A deep groove, the **coronary sulcus,** marks the border between the atria and the ventricles. Shallower depressions, the **anterior interventricular sulcus** and the **posterior interventricular sulcus,** mark the boundary line between the left and right ventricles.

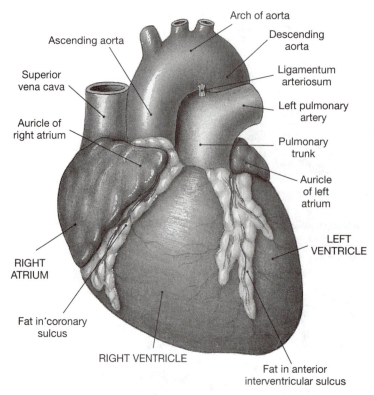

(a) Anterior surface

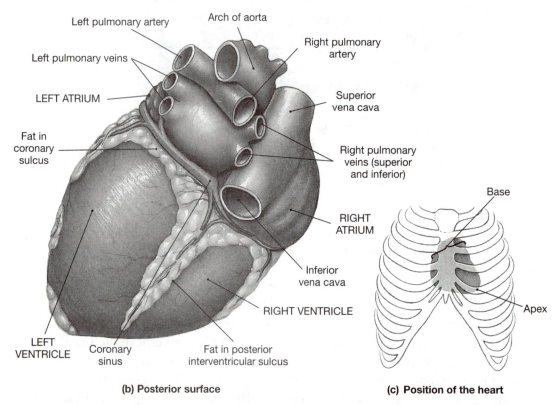

(b) Posterior surface

(c) Position of the heart

Figure 9–3   Superficial Anatomy of the Heart.
(a) Anterior view of the heart, showing major anatomical features. **(b)** The posterior surface of the heart. **(c)** Anterior view of the chest, showing the position of the heart relative to the chest wall.

The right atrium receives blood from the systemic circuit via the two great veins, the **superior vena cava** (VĒ-na CĀ-va) and the **inferior vena cava.** The superior vena cava delivers blood to the right atrium from the head, neck, upper limbs, and chest. The inferior vena cava carries blood to the right atrium from the rest of the trunk, the viscera, and the lower limbs. The **coronary veins** of the heart return blood to the **coronary sinus,** which opens into the right atrium. Blood travels from the right atrium into the right ventricle through a broad opening bounded by three flaps of fibrous tissues. These flaps, or cusps, are part of the **right atrioventricular** (ā-trē-ō-ven-TRIK-ū-lur) **(AV) valve,** also known as the *tricuspid* (trī-KUS-pid; *tri,* three) *valve* (Figure 9–4).

Blood passes from the right ventricle and enters the **pulmonary trunk,** the start of the pulmonary circuit. The opening to the pulmonary trunk is guarded by the **pulmonary semilunar** (sem-ĭ-LOO-nur) **valve.** The pulmonary semilunar valve consists of three semilunar (half-moon–shaped) cusps of thick connective tissue. Once within the pulmonary trunk, blood flows into the **left** and **right pulmonary arteries.** These vessels branch repeatedly within the lungs before supplying the capillaries, where gas exchange occurs.

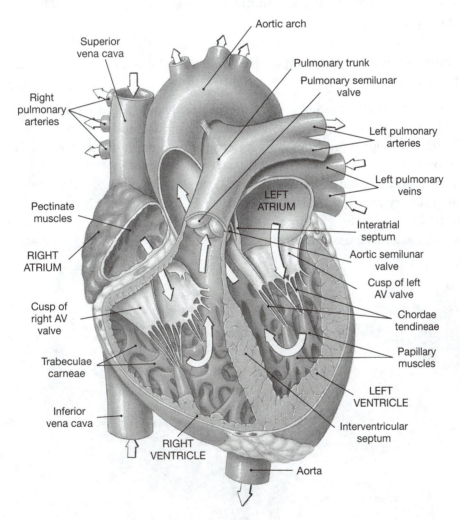

Figure 9–4   Sectional Anatomy of the Heart.
A diagrammatic frontal section through the heart, showing major landmarks and the path of blood flow through the atria, ventricles, and associated vessels.

From the respiratory capillaries, blood collects into small veins that ultimately unite to form the four **pulmonary veins.** The left atrium receives blood from two left and two right pulmonary veins. Like the right atrium, the left atrium has an auricle and a valve, the **left atrioventricular (AV) valve,** or *bicuspid* (bī-KUS-pid; *bi,* two), *valve.* As the name *bicuspid* implies, the left AV valve contains a pair of cusps rather than a trio. Clinicians often use the term *mitral* (MĪ-tral; miter, a bishop's hat) *valve* when referring to this valve. The left atrioventricular valve permits the flow of blood from the left atrium into the left ventricle.

Blood leaves the left ventricle by passing through the **aortic semilunar valve** into the **ascending aorta** (ā-OR-ta). The aortic semilunar valve has the same construction as the pulmonary semilunar valve. From the ascending aorta, blood flows on through the **aortic arch** and into the **descending aorta.**

A section through the wall of the heart reveals three distinct layers: (1) an outer epicardium, (2) a middle myocardium, and (3) an inner endocardium (Figure 9–5).

- The epicardium is the visceral pericardium that covers the outer surface of the heart.
- The **myocardium** (mī-ō-KAR-dē-um), or muscular wall of the heart, forms both atria and ventricles. The myocardium consists of cardiac muscle tissue and associated connective tissue.
- The inner surfaces of the heart, including the valves, are covered by a squamous epithelium, the **endocardium** (en-dō-KAR-dē-um), that is continuous with the lining of the attached blood vessels.

The heart works continuously, and cardiac muscle cells require reliable supplies of oxygen and nutrients. The coronary circulation supplies blood to the muscles of the heart (Figure 9–6). During maximum exertion, the oxygen demand rises considerably, and the blood flow to the heart may increase to nine times that of resting levels. The coronary circulation includes an extensive network of coronary blood vessels. The **left** and **right coronary arteries** originate at the base of the ascending aorta and distribute blood to the heart muscle. The **great** and **middle cardiac veins** carry blood from the coronary capillaries to the coronary sinus, which returns blood to the right atrium.

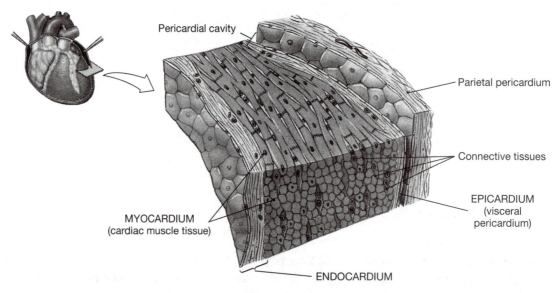

Figure 9–5 The Heart Wall.
A diagrammatic section through the heart wall, showing the relative positions of the epicardium, myocardium, and endocardium.

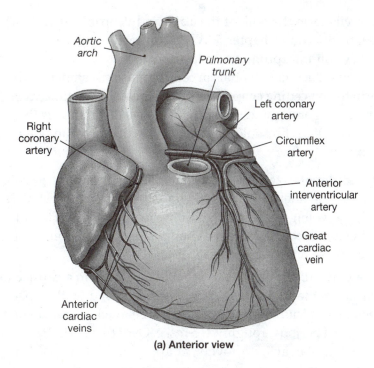

Aortic arch

Pulmonary trunk

Left coronary artery

Right coronary artery

Circumflex artery

Anterior interventricular artery

Great cardiac vein

Anterior cardiac veins

(a) Anterior view

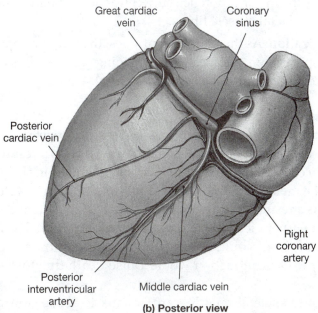

Great cardiac vein

Coronary sinus

Posterior cardiac vein

Posterior interventricular artery

Middle cardiac vein

Right coronary artery

(b) Posterior view

Figure 9–6   Coronary Circulation.
(a) Coronary vessels supplying the anterior surface of the heart. **(b)** Coronary vessels supplying the posterior surface of the heart.

Cardiac Physiology

The myocardium consists of cardiac muscle tissue. Each time the heart beats, the contractions of individual cardiac muscle cells are coordinated and harnessed to ensure that blood flows in the right direction at the proper time. Two types of cardiac muscle cells are involved in a normal heartbeat. **Contractile cells** produce the powerful contractions that propel blood, and specialized muscle cells of the **conducting system** control and coordinate the activities of the contractile cells.

Contractile cells form the bulk of the atrial and ventricular walls. The structure of these cells was introduced in Chapter 5. When contractile cells are stimulated by an action potential, they contract, producing a heartbeat.

The appearance of action potentials in cardiac muscle is similar to that discussed for skeletal muscle in the preceding chapter. An action potential begins when the membrane of the cardiac muscle is brought to threshold. The usual stimulus is the excitation of an adjacent muscle cell. Once threshold has been reached, the action potential proceeds in three basic steps.

Step 1: Rapid depolarization: Rapid depolarization occurs as voltage-regulated sodium channels open. As the transmembrane potential approaches +30 mV, the voltage-regulated sodium channels close. This first step roughly corresponds to the depolarization phase of the action potential in an axon, as discussed in the previous chapter.

Step 2: The plateau: Unlike the situation in a neuron, in a cardiac muscle cell the closing of the sodium ion channels is followed by the opening of voltage-regulated calcium ion channels. These channels remain open for a relatively extended period—roughly 175 msec. Over this period, the transmembrane potential plateaus, or hovers, at approximately 0 mV. The presence of a plateau is the major difference between action potentials in cardiac muscle cells and skeletal muscle fibers.

Step 3: Repolarization: As the plateau continues, the calcium channels begin closing and potassium channels begin opening. The result is a period of repolarization that restores the resting potential.

Until the plateau phase has ended, the cardiac muscle cell cannot respond to further stimulation. By the time the cell membrane has returned to its resting state, the contraction triggered by the action potential has already ended. As a result, cardiac muscle tissue relaxes between contractions. In contrast, action potentials in skeletal muscle fibers are very brief, and the membrane has returned to its resting state well before the contraction has ended. As a result, the arrival of additional action potentials will extend the period of contraction without letting the muscle fiber relax. If cardiac muscle behaved like skeletal muscle, the heart could not function; it must contract and relax to pump blood. A prolonged cardiac contraction would cause death due to cessation of blood flow to the brain.

Also, in contrast to skeletal muscle, cardiac muscle tissue contracts on its own, without neural or hormonal stimulation. This property is called **automaticity.** The cells responsible for initiating and distributing the electrical impulses that stimulate the heart to contract are part of the conducting system of the heart, a network of specialized cardiac muscle cells (Figure 9–7).

The conducting system includes:

1. The **sinoatrial** (sī-nō-Ā-trē-al) **node (SA node)**, which is located in the wall of the right atrium and acts as the heart's natural pacemaker.
2. The **atrioventricular node (AV node)** is located at the junction between the atria and ventricles and is connected to the SA node by **internodal fibers.** The AV node delays the signal from the SA node to the ventricles. This delay allows the atria time to contract before the ventricles begin to contract.

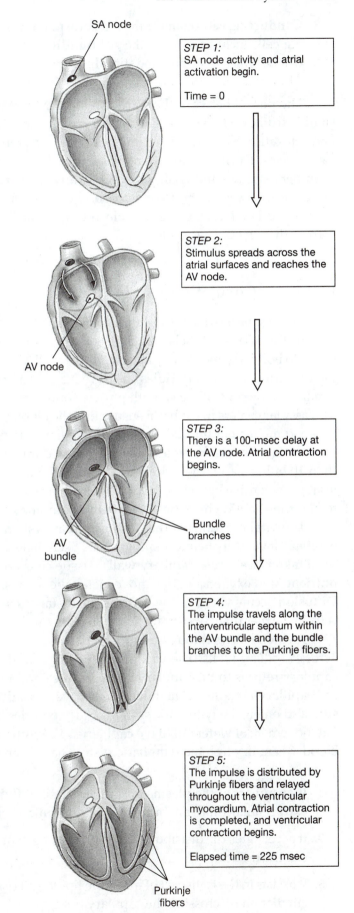

SA node

STEP 1:
SA node activity and atrial activation begin.

Time = 0

STEP 2:
Stimulus spreads across the atrial surfaces and reaches the AV node.

AV node

STEP 3:
There is a 100-msec delay at the AV node. Atrial contraction begins.

Bundle branches

AV bundle

STEP 4:
The impulse travels along the interventricular septum within the AV bundle and the bundle branches to the Purkinje fibers.

STEP 5:
The impulse is distributed by Purkinje fibers and relayed throughout the ventricular myocardium. Atrial contraction is completed, and ventricular contraction begins.

Elapsed time = 225 msec

Purkinje fibers

Figure 9–7   Impulse Conduction through the Heart.

3. **Conducting cells** connect the AV node to the ventricular muscle cells. The conducting cells include those in the **AV bundle**, the **bundle branches**, and the **Purkinje fibers**, which distribute the stimulus to the ventricular myocardium.

The period between the start of one heartbeat and the beginning of the next is a single **cardiac cycle.** The cardiac cycle therefore includes alternate periods of contraction and relaxation. For any one chamber in the heart, the cardiac cycle can be divided into two phases. During contraction, or **systole** (SIS-tō-lē; Greek *systole,* contraction), the chamber contracts and pushes blood into an adjacent chamber or into an arterial trunk. Systole is followed by the second phase, one of relaxation, or **diastole** (dī-AS-tō-lē; Greek *diastole,* a dilatation). During diastole, the chamber fills with blood and prepares for the start of the next cardiac cycle.

Pattern of Circulation

Blood leaves the heart in the pulmonary and aortic trunks, each with a diameter of around 2.5 cm (1 in.). These vessels branch repeatedly, forming the major arteries that distribute blood to body organs. As they approach the capillaries, arteries continue to branch, forming tiny arteries called **arterioles** (ar-TĒ-rē-ōlz). From the arterioles, blood moves into the capillaries. By controlling smooth muscle contractions in the walls of the arterioles, cardiovascular centers in the brain ensure that the blood volume, blood pressure, and speed of blood movement through peripheral capillaries remain within acceptable limits.

Within the various organs, several hundred million arterioles provide blood to more than 10 billion capillaries barely the diameter of a single red blood cell. These capillaries form extensive branching networks; if all the capillaries in the body were placed end to end they would circle the globe, with a combined length of more than 25,000 miles!

The vital functions of the cardiovascular system depend entirely on events at the capillary level. All chemical and gaseous exchanges between the blood and interstitial fluid take place across capillary walls. Tissue cells rely on capillary diffusion to obtain nutrients and oxygen and to remove metabolic wastes, such as carbon dioxide and urea. Diffusion occurs very rapidly because the distances involved are very small; few living cells lie farther than 125 μm (0.005 in.) from a capillary.

As blood flows through peripheral tissues, blood pressure forces water and solutes across capillary walls. The vast majority of the fluid that leaves the arteriole end of a capillary returns to the capillary at the venule end. A small amount of fluid that leaves the capillary remains in the interstitial space. This fluid flows through peripheral tissues and enters the lymphatic system, which empties into the bloodstream. The continual movement of water out of the capillaries, through peripheral tissues, then back to the bloodstream through the lymphatic system has several important functions.

1. It ensures that the plasma and the interstitial fluid, two major components of the extracellular fluid, are in constant communication.

2. It accelerates the distribution of nutrients, hormones, and dissolved gases throughout the tissue.

3. It assists in the transport of insoluble lipids and tissue proteins that cannot enter the circulation by crossing the capillary lining.

4. It has a flushing action that carries bacterial toxins and other chemical stimuli to lymphatic tissues and organs responsible for providing immunity from disease.

As blood leaves the capillaries, it enters tiny veins called **venules** (VEN-yoolz). The venules fuse together to form small veins and, in turn, the small veins fuse to form progressively larger veins that ultimately return the blood to the heart.

Integration with Other Systems

The cardiovascular system is both anatomically and functionally linked to all other systems. Figure 9–8 summarizes the physiological relationships between the cardiovascular system and other organ systems.

The most extensive communication occurs between the cardiovascular and lymphatic systems. Not only are the two systems physically interconnected, but cell populations of the lymphatic system use the cardiovascular system as a highway to move from one part of the body to another. The next section examines the lymphatic system in more detail and considers the role of the lymphatic system in the immune response.

✎ Let's Review What You've Just Learned

▶ Definitions

In the space provided, write the term for each of the following definitions.

_____ **1.** Cell fragments that play an important role in blood clotting.

_____ **2.** The contraction phase of the cardiac cycle.

_____ **3.** The chamber of the heart that receives blood from the pulmonary circuit.

_____ **4.** Plasma proteins that play a role in the transport of fatty acids and other substances and contribute substantially to the colloid osmotic pressure of the blood because they are the most abundant.

_____ **5.** Tiny arteries that connect to capillaries.

_____ **6.** The chamber of the heart that pumps blood to the lungs.

_____ **7.** A protein molecule found in red blood cells that functions in the transport of respiratory gases.

_____ **8.** Blood vessels that carry blood away from the heart, also known as efferent vessels.

_____ **9.** The relaxation phase of the cardiac cycle.

_____ **10.** A type of cardiac muscle cell responsible for generating the force that pumps blood.

_____ **11.** A large vein that returns blood to the heart from the head, neck, and upper appendages.

_____ **12.** The liquid matrix of blood.

_____ **13.** Granulocytic white blood cells that produce histamine and heparin.

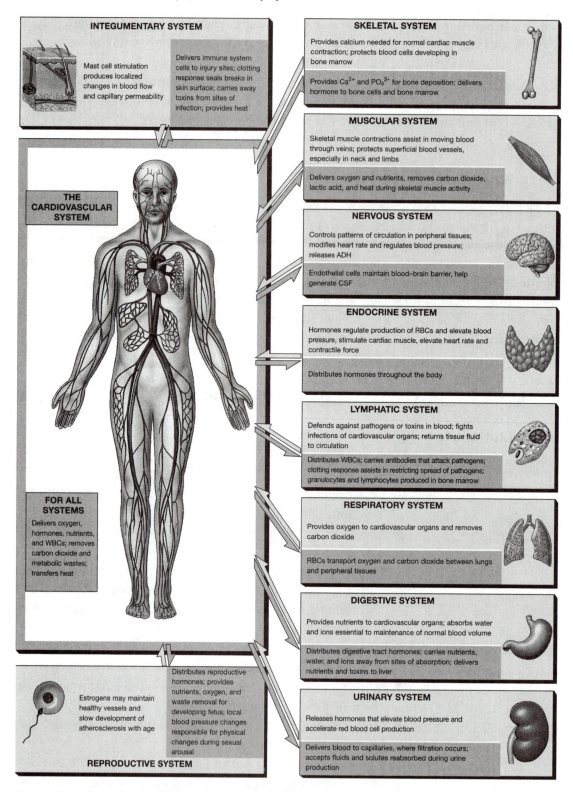

INTEGUMENTARY SYSTEM

Mast cell stimulation produces localized changes in blood flow and capillary permeability

Delivers immune system cells to injury sites; clotting response seals breaks in skin surface; carries away toxins from sites of infection; provides heat

THE CARDIOVASCULAR SYSTEM

FOR ALL SYSTEMS

Delivers oxygen, hormones, nutrients, and WBCs; removes carbon dioxide and metabolic wastes; transfers heat

Estrogens may maintain healthy vessels and slow development of atherosclerosis with age

Distributes reproductive hormones; provides nutrients, oxygen, and waste removal for developing fetus; local blood pressure changes responsible for physical changes during sexual arousal

REPRODUCTIVE SYSTEM

SKELETAL SYSTEM

Provides calcium needed for normal cardiac muscle contraction; protects blood cells developing in bone marrow

Provides Ca^{2+} and PO_4^{3-} for bone deposition; delivers hormone to bone cells and bone marrow

MUSCULAR SYSTEM

Skeletal muscle contractions assist in moving blood through veins; protects superficial blood vessels, especially in neck and limbs

Delivers oxygen and nutrients, removes carbon dioxide, lactic acid, and heat during skeletal muscle activity

NERVOUS SYSTEM

Controls patterns of circulation in peripheral tissues; modifies heart rate and regulates blood pressure; releases ADH

Endothelial cells maintain blood–brain barrier, help generate CSF

ENDOCRINE SYSTEM

Hormones regulate production of RBCs and elevate blood pressure, stimulate cardiac muscle, elevate heart rate and contractile force

Distributes hormones throughout the body

LYMPHATIC SYSTEM

Defends against pathogens or toxins in blood; fights infections of cardiovascular organs; returns tissue fluid to circulation

Distributes WBCs; carries antibodies that attack pathogens; clotting response assists in restricting spread of pathogens; granulocytes and lymphocytes produced in bone marrow

RESPIRATORY SYSTEM

Provides oxygen to cardiovascular organs and removes carbon dioxide

RBCs transport oxygen and carbon dioxide between lungs and peripheral tissues

DIGESTIVE SYSTEM

Provides nutrients to cardiovascular organs; absorbs water and ions essential to maintenance of normal blood volume

Distributes digestive tract hormones; carries nutrients, water, and ions away from sites of absorption; delivers nutrients and toxins to liver

URINARY SYSTEM

Releases hormones that elevate blood pressure and accelerate red blood cell production

Delivers blood to capillaries, where filtration occurs; accepts fluids and solutes reabsorbed during urine production

Figure 9–8   Functional Relationships between the Cardiovascular System and Other Systems.

_____ **14.** The chamber of the heart that receives blood from the systemic circuit.

_____ **15.** A valve composed of three flaps of connective tissue that is located at the opening between the right atrium and right ventricle.

_____ **16.** Tiny veins that connect to capillaries.

_____ **17.** A collective term for the blood cells and cell fragments suspended in blood plasma.

_____ **18.** A phagocytic white blood cell that is the most numerous of the granulocytes.

_____ **19.** The set of blood vessels that carry blood from the heart to the lungs and back again.

_____ **20.** A type of valve that is composed of three half-moon-shaped cusps of thick connective tissue.

_____ **21.** Channels that open and close slowly and produce the plateau phase of the action potential in cardiac muscle cells.

_____ **22.** Globular plasma proteins that function in transport and protection against disease.

_____ **23.** Blood vessels that carry blood toward the heart; also known as afferent vessels.

_____ **24.** A superficial groove that separates the atria of the heart from the ventricles.

_____ **25.** Arteries that carry blood to the lungs.

_____ **26.** The period between the beginning of one heartbeat and the start of the next.

_____ **27.** The muscular layer of the heart wall.

_____ **28.** A plasma protein that when activated forms the basis of a blood clot.

_____ **29.** A serous membrane that lines the pericardial cavity.

_____ **30.** The chamber of the heart that pumps blood into the systemic circuit.

_____ **31.** A group of specialized cardiac muscle cells located in the posterior wall of the right atrium that act as the heart's pacemaker.

_____ **32.** Channels located in the membranes of cardiac muscle cells that open to cause rapid depolarization.

_____ **33.** Specialized globular proteins that attack foreign proteins and pathogens.

_____ **34.** The set of blood vessels that carries blood from the heart to all parts of the body except the lungs and back to the heart.

_____ **35.** A valve composed of two leaflets of connective tissue located in the opening between the left atrium and the left ventricle.

_____ **36.** Cardiac muscle cells that are specialized for conducting impulses through the myocardium of the heart.

_____ **37.** Small blood cells that lack a nucleus and contain the protein hemoglobin.

_____ **38.** A large vein that returns blood to the heart from the lower appendages and abdominal area.

_____ **39.** Large agranular leukocytes.

_____ **40.** A large artery that originates at the left ventricle.

_____ **41.** The outer layer of the heart; also known as the visceral pericardium.

_____ **42.** A general term for white blood cells that contain abundant stained granules in cytoplasm.

_____   **43.** An expanded extension of the atrium visible from an anterior view of the heart.

_____   **44.** Blood cells that have a nucleus and do not contain hemoglobin.

_____   **45.** Small, thin-walled vessels that are located between the smallest arteries and smallest veins.

_____   **46.** White blood cells that contain granules that stain well with the dye *eosin*.

_____   **47.** The membrane that lines the inner surface of the heart and covers the heart valves.

_____   **48.** The artery that originates from the right ventricle.

_____   **49.** White blood cells that produce antibodies and function in the immune response.

_____   **50.** The ability of cardiac muscle tissue to contract on its own without neural or hormonal stimulation.

_____   **51.** White blood cells that do not contain stainable granules in their cytoplasm.

▶ Word Roots, Prefixes, Suffixes, and Combining Forms

In the space provided, list the boldfaced terms introduced in this section that contain the indicated word part.

Word Part	Meaning	Examples
erythro-	red	**52.** _____
a-	without	**53.** _____
cardi-	heart	**54.** _____
hem-	blood	**55.** _____
leuko-	white	**56.** _____
peri-	around	**57.** _____
-phil	love	**58.** _____
mono-	one	**59.** _____
pulmo-	lung	**60.** _____
myo-	muscle	**61.** _____
endo-	inside	**62.** _____

THE LYMPHATIC SYSTEM

Lymphocytes, the primary cells of the lymphatic system were introduced in the preceding section. These cells are vital to our ability to resist or overcome infection and disease. Lymphocytes respond to the presence of (1) invading pathogens, such as bacteria and viruses, (2) abnormal body cells, such as virus-infected cells and cancer cells, and (3) foreign proteins, such as the toxins released by some bacteria. They attempt to eliminate these threats or render them harmless by a combination of physical and chemical attack.

Lymphocytes respond to specific threats. If bacteria invade peripheral tissues, the lymphocytes organize a defense against that particular type of bacterium. For this reason, lymphocytes are said to provide a specific defense, known as the **immune response. Immunity** is the ability to resist infection and disease through the activation of specific defenses. All of the cells and tissues involved with the production of immunity are sometimes considered to be part of an **immune system,** a physiological system that includes not only the lymphatic system but also components of the integumentary, cardiovascular, respiratory, digestive, and other systems. This section begins by examining the organization of the lymphatic system. We will then consider how the lymphatic system interacts with cells and tissues of other systems to defend the body against infection and disease.

ORGANIZATION OF THE LYMPHATIC SYSTEM

The lymphatic system includes:

1. A network of lymphatic vessels that begin in peripheral tissues and end at connections to the venous system (Figure 9–9).
2. A fluid, called **lymph** (limf), resembling plasma but containing a much lower concentration of suspended proteins.
3. Lymphoid tissues and organs connected to the lymphatic vessels and containing large numbers of lymphocytes. Lymphoid tissues, such as the **tonsils**, consist of connective tisues dominated by lymphocytes. Lymphoid organs are separated from surrounding tissues by a fibrous connective tissue capsule. Important lymphoid organs include the lymph nodes, the thymus, and the spleen.

- **Lymph glands**, also known as **lymph nodes**, are small, oval lymphoid organs ranging in diameter from 1 to 25 mm. A lymph node functions like a kitchen water filter: It filters and purifies lymph before it reaches the venous system.

- The **thymus gland** lies behind the sternum, in the anterior portion of the mediastinum. The thymus secretes hormones that control the development of lymphocytes.

- The **spleen** is a somewhat oval, dark-colored organ that lies along the curving lateral border of the stomach. The functions of the spleen can be summarized as (1) the removal of abnormal blood cells and other blood components through phagocytosis, (2) the storage of iron from recycled red blood cells, and (3) the initiation of immune responses by B cells and T cells in response to antigens in the circulating blood.

The primary functions of the lymphatic system are:

- **The production, maintenance, and distribution of lymphocytes:** Lymphocytes, the primary cells involved in the immune response, are produced and stored within (1) lymphoid tissues and organs, such as the spleen and thymus, and (2) areas of red bone marrow.

- **The return of fluid and solutes from peripheral tissues to the blood:** Capillaries normally deliver more fluid to the tissues than they carry away. The return of tissue fluids though lymphatic vessels maintains normal blood volume and eliminates local variation in the composition of the interstitial fluid.

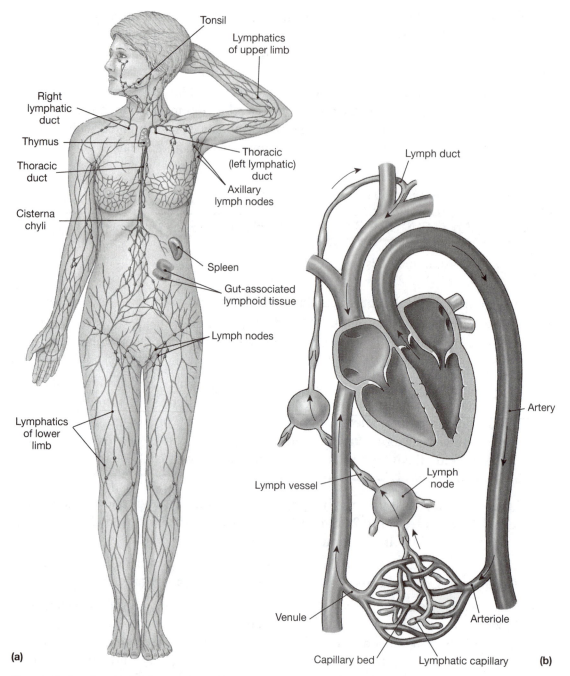

Figure 9–9 **Components and Organization of the Lymphatic System.**
(a) Anatomy of the lymphatic system. **(b)** Relationship between the blood vessels in peripheral tissues.

- The distribution of hormones, nutrients, and waste products from their tissues of origin to the general circulation: Substances that originate in the tissues but are for some reason unable to enter the bloodstream directly may do so via the lymphatic vessels. For example, lipids absorbed by the digestive tract often fail to enter the circulation at the capillary level. However, they still reach the bloodstream through passage along the lymphatic vessels.

Types of Lymphocytes

There are three classes of lymphocytes in the blood: **T cells** (thymus-dependent), **B cells** (bone marrow-derived), and **NK cells** (natural killer). Each type has distinctive biochemical and functional characteristics.

There are several types of T cells. They include:

- **Cytotoxic T cells** attack foreign cells or body cells infected by viruses. Their attack often involves direct contact. These lymphocytes are the primary cells involved in **cell-mediated immunity,** or **cellular immunity.**
- **Helper T cells** stimulate the activation and function of both T cells and B cells.
- **Suppressor T cells** inhibit the activation and function of both T cells and B cells.

B cells, when stimulated, can differentiate into **plasma cells.** Plasma cells, introduced in Chapter 6, are responsible for the production and secretion of antibodies, soluble proteins that are also known as immunoglobulins. These proteins react with specific chemical targets, called **antigens.** Antigens are usually pathogens, parts or products of pathogens, or other foreign compounds. Most antigens are proteins, but some lipids, polysaccharides, and nucleic acids can also stimulate antibody production. Binding of an antibody to its target antigen starts a chain of events leading to the destruction of the target compound or organism. B cells are responsible for **antibody-mediated immunity,** which is also known as **humoral** ("liquid") **immunity,** because antibodies are found in body fluids.

NK cells are also known as **large granular lymphocytes.** These lymphocytes will attack foreign cells, normal cells infected with viruses, and cancer cells that appear in normal tissues. Their continuous policing of peripheral tissues has been called **immunological surveillance.**

The Lymphatic System and Body Defenses

The human body has multiple defense mechanisms, but these can be sorted into two general categories.

1. **Nonspecific defenses** do not discriminate between one threat and another. These defenses, which are present at birth, include physical barriers, phagocytic cells, immunological surveillance, interferon, complement, inflammation, and fever. They provide the body with a defensive capability known as **nonspecific resistance.**
2. **Specific defenses** provide protection against threats on an individual basis. For example, a specific defense may protect against infection by one type of bacteria but ignore other bacteria and viruses. Many specific defenses develop after birth, as a result of accidental or deliberate exposure to environmental hazards. Specific defenses are dependent upon the activities of lymphocytes. The body's specific defenses produce a state of protection known as **immunity,** or **specific resistance**.

Nonspecific and specific resistance are complementary, and both must function normally to provide adequate resistance to infection and disease.

Nonspecific Defenses

Nonspecific defenses prevent the approach of, deny entrance to, or limit the spread of microorganisms or other environmental hazards. The major categories of nonspecific defenses are summarized in Figure 9–10.

- **Physical barriers** keep hazardous organisms and materials outside the body. For example, a mosquito that lands on a full head of hair may be unable to reach the surface of the scalp.

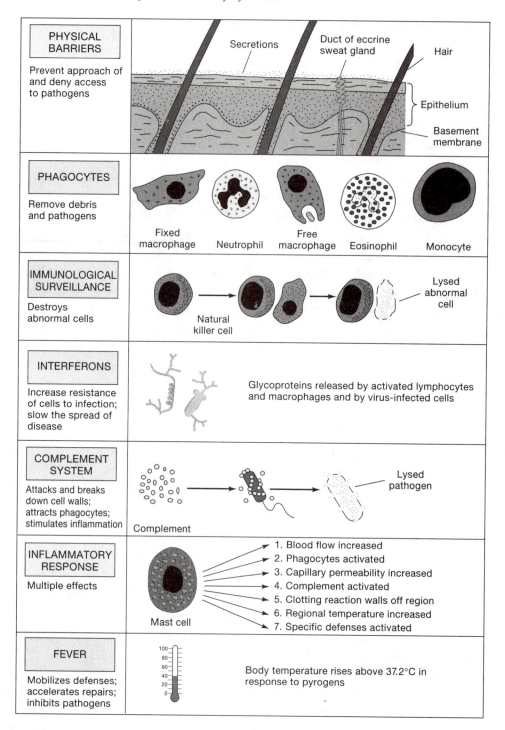

Figure 9–10 Nonspecific Defenses.

- **Phagocytes** are cells that engulf pathogens and cell debris. Examples of phagocytes are the macrophages of peripheral tissues and the neutrophils and eosinophils of the blood.

- **Immunological surveillance** is the destruction of abnormal cells by NK cells in peripheral tissues.

- **Interferons** are chemical messengers that coordinate the defenses against viral infection.

- **Complement** is a system of circulating proteins that assist antibodies in the destruction of pathogens.

- **Inflammation** is a local response to injury or infection that is directed at the tissue level. Inflammation tends to restrict the spread of an injury and to combat infection.
- **Fever** is an elevation in body temperature that accelerates tissue metabolism and defenses.

Specific Resistance: The Immune Response

Specific resistance, or immunity, is provided by the coordinated activities of T cells and B cells that respond to the presence of specific antigens. The basic functional relationship can be summarized as follows:

1. T cells are responsible for cell-mediated immunity, our defense against abnormal cells and pathogens inside living cells.
2. B cells provide antibody-mediated immunity, our defense against antigens and pathogenic organisms in body fluids.

Both mechanisms are important because activated T cells do not respond to antigenic material in solution, and the antibodies produced by activated B cells cannot cross cell membranes. Moreover, helper T cells play a crucial role in antibody-mediated immunity by stimulating the activity of B cells.

Immunity may be either innate or acquired.

- **Innate immunity** is genetically determined; it is present at birth and has no relationship to previous exposure to the antigen involved. For example, people are not subject to the same diseases as goldfish.

Innate immunity breaks down only in the case of AIDS or other conditions that depress all aspects of specific resistance.

- **Active immunity** appears after exposure to an antigen, as a consequence of the immune response. The immune system has the capability of defending against a large number of antigens. However, the appropriate defenses are mobilized only after an individual encounters a particular antigen. Active immunity may develop as a result of natural exposure to an antigen in the environment or from deliberate exposure to an antigen. Active immunity normally begins to develop after birth, and it is continually enhanced as the individual encounters "new" pathogens or other antigens. You might compare this process to vocabulary development; a child begins with a few basic common words and learns new ones on an as-needed basis. The purpose of deliberate exposure to an antigen is to stimulate antibody production under controlled conditions. As a result, antibody production occurs, and the individual will be able to overcome natural exposure to the pathogen at some time in the future. This is the basic principle behind immunization to prevent disease.
- **Passive immunity** is produced by the transfer of antibodies from another individual. Throughout a pregnancy, antibodies produced by the mother provide protection against infections during development (across the placenta) and in early infancy, maternal antibodies are provided in breast milk. Antibodies from humans or animals can be administered to fight infection, neutralize toxins, or prevent disease.

Finally, immunity can be characterized by four general properties:

1. **Specificity:** A specific defense is activated by an antigen, and the response targets that particular antigen and not others. Specificity results from the activation of appropriate lymphocytes and the production of antibodies with targeted effects.

2. **Versatility:** In the course of a normal lifetime, an individual encounters tens of thousands of antigens. The immune system can differentiate among them, producing appropriate and specific responses to each. Versatility results in part from the large diversity of lymphocytes present in the body and in part from variability in the structure of synthesized antibodies.

3. **Memory:** The immune system "remembers" antigens that it encounters. As a result, the immune response that occurs after a second exposure to an antigen is stronger and lasts longer than the response to the first exposure.

4. **Tolerance:** Tolerance is said to exist when the immune system does not respond to a particular antigen. For example, all cells and tissues in the body contain antigens that normally fail to stimulate an immune response.

Integration with Other Systems

Figure 9–11 summarizes the interactions between the lymphatic system and other physiological systems. The relationships among the cells of the immune response and the nervous and endocrine systems are now the focus of intense research. It is now apparent that there is substantial interaction between these systems.

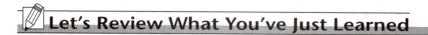

Let's Review What You've Just Learned

► **Definitions**

In the space provided, write the term for each of the following definitions.

_____ **63.** T cells that stimulate the activation and function of both B cells and other T cells.

_____ **64.** An elevation in body temperature that accelerates tissue metabolism and defenses.

_____ **65.** A fluid found in lymph vessels that resembles plasma but has a lower concentration of proteins.

_____ **66.** Immunity that results from antibodies produced by the mother being passed across the placenta or by breast milk to her offspring.

_____ **67.** Defenses that prevent the approach of, deny entrance to, or limit the spread of microorganisms or other environmental hazards.

_____ **68.** A system of circulating proteins that assist antibodies in the destruction of pathogens.

_____ **69.** Small, oval lymphoid organs that filter circulating lymph.

_____ **70.** A type of B cell that is responsible for the production of circulating antibodies.

_____ **71.** The ability to resist infection and disease through the activation of specific defenses.

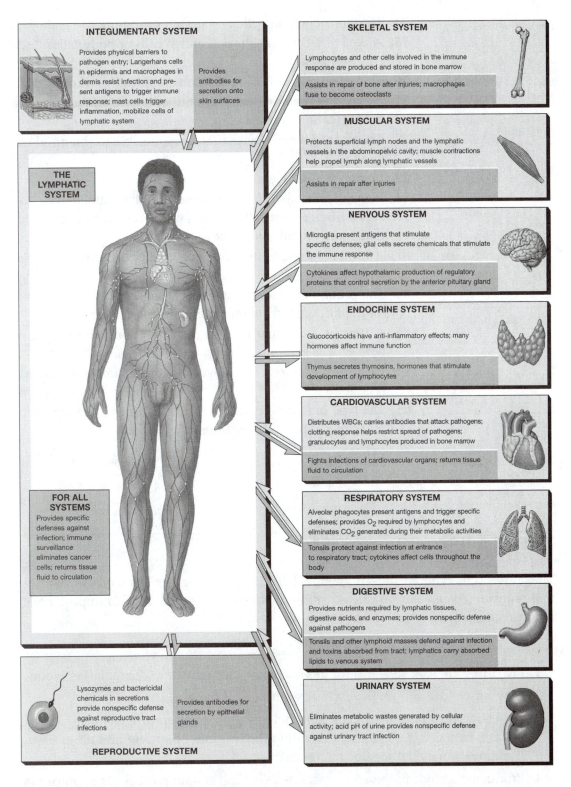

Figure 9–11   Functional Relationships between the Lymphatic System and Other Systems.

_____ **72.** The class of lymphocytes responsible for cell-mediated immunity.

_____ **73.** Chemical messengers that coordinate the defenses against viral infections.

_____ **74.** The type of immunity that occurs after exposure to a pathogen.

_____ **75.** A type of T cell that attacks foreign cells or body cells infected by viruses.

_____ **76.** The constant monitoring of normal tissues by NK cells.

_____ **77.** A type of immunity in which antibodies are administered to fight infection or disease.

_____ **78.** The class of lymphocytes that is responsible for humoral immunity.

_____ **79.** Immunity that is genetically determined.

_____ **80.** Lymphocytes, also known as large granular lymphocytes, that attack foreign cells, cells infected with viruses, and cancer cells that appear in normal tissue.

_____ **81.** A local response to injury or infection that is directed at the tissue level.

_____ **82.** The general term for immunity that is produced by the transfer of antibodies from one individual to another.

_____ **83.** A type of T cell that inhibits the activation and function of both B cells and other T cells.

_____ **84.** Pathogens or parts of pathogens that can stimulate antibody production.

_____ **85.** The type of immunity that is produced when an individual is purposely exposed to an antigen.

THE RESPIRATORY SYSTEM

The body's cells generate most of their ATP by aerobic respiration, a metabolic pathway that requires oxygen and produces carbon dioxide (see Chapter 5). This important cellular process is supported by the respiratory system.

The functions of the respiratory system include:

1. Providing an extensive area for gas exchange between air and circulating blood.
2. Moving air to and from the exchange surfaces of the lungs.
3. Protecting respiratory surfaces from dehydration, temperature changes, or other environmental variations and defending the respiratory system and other tissues from invasion by pathogenic microorganisms.
4. Producing sounds involved in speaking, singing, and nonverbal communication.
5. Providing olfactory sensations to the CNS from the olfactory epithelium in the superior portions of the nasal cavity.
6. Assisting in the regulation of body fluid pH.

The respiratory system (Figure 9–12) can be divided into an upper respiratory system and a lower respiratory system.

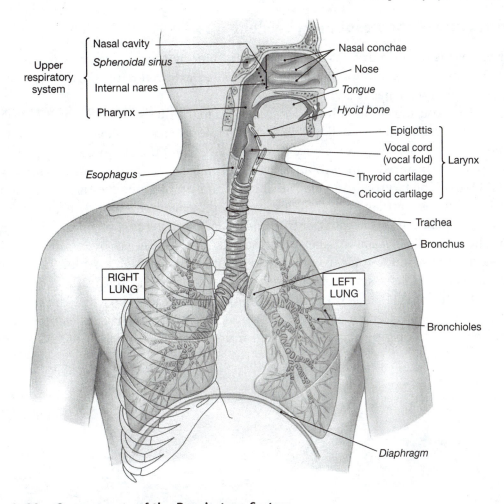

Figure 9–12 Components of the Respiratory System.
The conducting portion of the respiratory system is shown here. At this scale, the alveoli are not visible.

- The **upper respiratory system** consists of the nose, nasal cavity, paranasal sinuses, and pharynx. These passageways filter, warm, and humidify the air, protecting the more delicate surfaces of the lower respiratory system.
- The **lower respiratory system** includes the larynx (voicebox), trachea (windpipe), bronchi, bronchioles, and alveoli of the lungs.

The **respiratory tract** consists of the airways that carry air to and from the exchange surfaces of the lungs. The respiratory tract can be divided into a conduction portion and a respiratory portion. The conduction portion begins at the entrance to the nasal cavity and extends through the pharynx and larynx and along the trachea, bronchi, and bronchioles to the terminal bronchioles. The respiratory portion of the tract includes the delicate respiratory bronchioles and the alveoli, which are the site of gas exchange.

Filtering, warming, and humidifying of the inspired air begin at the entrance to the upper respiratory system and continue throughout the rest of the conducting system. By the time air reaches the alveoli, most foreign particles and pathogens have been removed, and the humidity and temperature are within acceptable limits. The success of this "conditioning process" is due primarily to the properties of the **respiratory mucosa** (mū-KŌ-sa) that lines the respiratory system (see mucous membranes in Chapter 6).

Structure of the Respiratory System

The nose is the primary passageway for air entering the respiratory system. Air normally enters the respiratory system via the paired **external nares** (NĀR-ēz), or nostrils, that open into the **nasal cavity** (Figure 9–13).

The nose, mouth, and throat are connected to the **pharynx** (FAR-inks). The pharynx is a chamber shared by the digestive and respiratory systems. It extends between the internal openings of the nasal cavity (**internal nares**) and the entrances to the larynx and esophagus. Inspired (inhaled) air leaves the pharynx by passing through the **glottis** (GLOT-is). The **larynx** (LAR-inks) surrounds and protects the glottis. It is essentially a cylinder whose cartilaginous walls are stabilized by ligaments and skeletal muscles. The larynx contains the **vocal folds,** or **true vocal cords,** which function in sound production, or **phonation** (fō-NĀ-shun; Greek *phone,* sound or voice). Phonation is one component of speech production, but clear speech also requires **articulation** (ar-tik-ū-LĀ-shun), the modification of those sounds by other structures, such as the lips, teeth, and nose.

The **trachea** (TRĀ-kē-a), or windpipe, is a tough flexible tube with a diameter around 2.5 cm (1 in.) and a length of approximately 11 cm (4.25 in.). The trachea branches within the mediastinum, giving rise to the right and left **primary bronchi** (BRONG-kī; singular

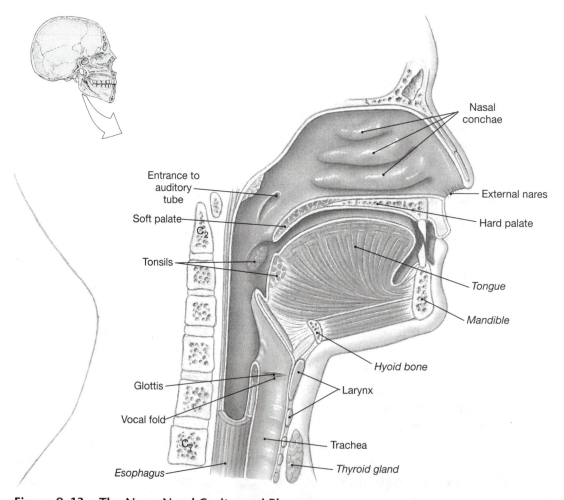

Figure 9–13   The Nose, Nasal Cavity, and Pharynx.
The nasal cavity and pharynx as seen in sagittal section, with the nasal septum removed.

Figure 9–14   The Bronchi and Lobules of the Lung.
(a) Branching pattern of bronchi in the left lung, simplified. (b) The structure of a single lobule.

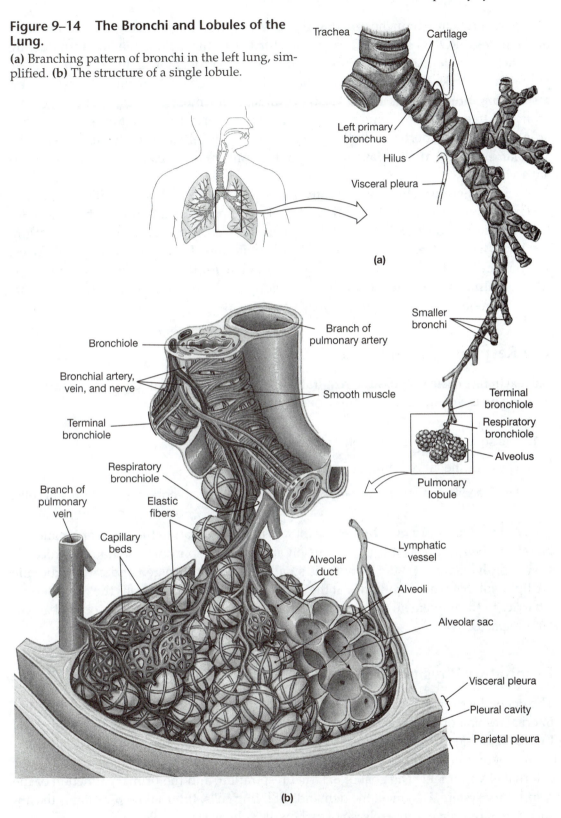

(a)

(b)

bronchus) (Figure 9–14). Each primary bronchus travels to a groove along the medial surface of its lung before branching further. This groove, the **hilus** (HĪ-lus), also provides access for entry to pulmonary vessels and nerves.

Each bronchus branches several times within the lungs, giving rise to multiple **bronchioles** (BRONG-kē-ōlz). These branch further, until reaching the finest conducting branches, called **terminal bronchioles.** Each terminal bronchiole delivers air to a single pulmonary lobule. Within the lobule, the terminal bronchiole branches to form several **respiratory bronchioles**. These are the thinnest and most delicate branches of the bronchial tree, and they deliver air to the exchange surfaces of the lungs. Respiratory bronchioles are connected to individual **alveoli** (al-VĒ-ō-lī) and to **alveolar ducts.** The alveolar ducts end at **alveolar sacs,** common chambers connected to multiple individual alveoli.

The left and right lungs are situated in the left and right pleural cavities (see Chapter 1). Each lung is a blunt cone, with the tip, or **apex,** pointing superiorly. The broad concave inferior portion, or **base,** of each lung rests on the superior surface of the diaphragm. The lungs have distinct **lobes** separated by deep fissures. The right lung has three lobes, and the left lung has only two lobes to accommodate for the heart. The lobes are divided into **pulmonary lobules** (LOB-ūlz), each supplied by branches of the pulmonary arteries, pulmonary veins, and respiratory passageways.

The Respiratory Membrane

Gas exchange occurs across the respiratory membrane of the alveoli. The **respiratory membrane** is a composite structure consisting of

1. The squamous epithelial cell lining of the alveolus.

2. The endothelial cell lining of an adjacent capillary.

3. The fused basement membranes that lie between the alveolar and endothelial cells.

At the respiratory membrane, the total distance separating the alveolar air and the blood can be as little as 0.1 μm. Diffusion across the respiratory membrane proceeds very rapidly because (1) the distance is small and (2) both oxygen and carbon dioxide are lipid-soluble. The membranes of the epithelial and endothelial cells thus do not pose a barrier to the movement of oxygen and carbon dioxide between the blood and alveolar air spaces.

Respiratory Physiology

The general term *respiration* refers to two integrated processes, external respiration and internal respiration. The precise definitions of these terms vary from reference to reference. In this discussion, **external respiration** includes all of the processes involved in the exchange of oxygen and carbon dioxide between the interstitial fluids of the body and the external environment. The goal of external respiration, and the primary function of the respiratory system, is to meet the demands of living cells. **Internal respiration** is the absorption of oxygen and the release of carbon dioxide by those cells.

Respiratory physiology involves four integrated steps that are involved in external respiration.

1. **Pulmonary ventilation,** or **breathing,** which involves the physical movement of air into and out of the lungs.

2. Gas diffusion across the respiratory membrane, between the alveolar air spaces and the alveolar capillaries.

3. The storage and transport of oxygen and carbon dioxide between the alveolar capillaries and capillary beds in other tissues.

4. The exchange of dissolved gases between the blood and interstitial fluids.

Abnormalities affecting any one of these steps will ultimately affect the gas concentrations of the interstitial fluids, and thereby affect cellular activities. If the oxygen content declines (**hypoxia**; [hī-POK-sē-uh]; *hypo*, below + *ox*, oxygen), the affected tissues will become oxygen-starved. Hypoxia places severe limits on the metabolic activities of the tissue involved. If the supply of oxygen is cut off completely, the condition of **anoxia** (a-NOKS-ē-uh; *a*, without + *ox*, oxygen) results. Anoxia kills cells very quickly. Much of the damage caused by strokes and heart attacks is the result of localized anoxia.

Gas Laws Affecting Respiratory Function

To understand the mechanical and physical processes of respiration, we need to know some basics concerning the behavior of gases. The physical behavior of gases under a variety of conditions is described by various gas laws. Three important gas laws that will help you better understand the process of respiration are Boyle's law, Dalton's law, and Henry's law.

Boyle's Law: Gas Pressure and Volume

The primary differences between liquids and gases such as air reflect the interactions between individual molecules. Although the molecules in a liquid are in constant motion, they are held closely together by weak interactions such as hydrogen bonding between the atoms of one molecule and those of another. As a result, liquids are relatively dense and viscous. But because the electrons of adjacent atoms tend to repel one another, liquids tend to resist compression. If you squeeze a balloon filled with water, it will distort into a different shape, but the volume of the new shape will be the same as that of the original.

In a gas, the molecules are bouncing around as independent entities. At normal atmospheric pressures, the molecules are fairly far apart, and the density (mass of substance in a given volume, usually measured in grams per cubic centimeter [cc]) of air is rather low. At such distances, the forces acting between the molecules are minimal, so an applied pressure can push them closer together. For example, suppose we have a sealed container of air at atmospheric pressure, such as the one depicted in Figure 9–15. The pressure exerted by the enclosed gas results from the collision of gas molecules with the walls of the container. The greater the number of collisions, the higher the pressure.

The gas pressure within a container can be changed by altering the volume of the container, thereby giving the gas molecules more or less room in which to bounce around. Decreasing the volume of the container will result in more frequent collisions, and thus elevate the pressure of the gas (Figure 9–15a). If the volume is increased, there will be fewer collisions per unit time, because it will take longer for a gas molecule to travel from one wall to another. As a result, the gas pressure inside the container will decline (Figure 9–15b).

An inverse relationship thus exists between pressure and volume: If you decrease the volume of a gas its pressure rises; if you increase the volume of a gas its pressure falls. The relationship between pressure and volume is reciprocal: If you double the external pressure on a flexible container, its volume will decrease by one-half. If you reduce the

Figure 9–15 Pressure and Volume Relationships.

Gas molecules within a container bounce off the walls and off one another, traveling the distance indicated in a given period of time. **(a)** If the volume decreases, each molecule will travel the same distance in that same time period but will strike the walls more frequently. The pressure exerted by the gas increases. **(b)** Alternatively, if the volume of the container increases, the gas molecules will strike the walls less often, lowering the pressure in the container.

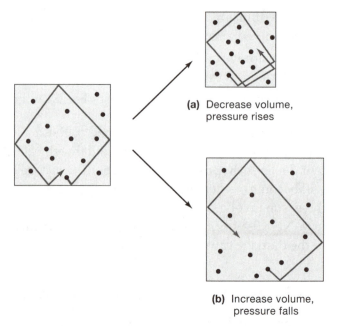

(a) Decrease volume, pressure rises

(b) Increase volume, pressure falls

external pressure by one-half, the volume of the container will double. Because temperature also affects gas pressure (P) and volume (V), the relationship is true only if the gas is at constant temperature (as it is in the human body). This relationship, $P \propto 1/V$, first recognized by Robert Boyle in the 1600s, is called **Boyle's law.**

Dalton's Law and Partial Pressures

The air we breathe is not a single gas but a mixture of gases. Nitrogen molecules (N_2) are the most abundant, accounting for about 78.6 percent of the atmospheric gas molecules. Oxygen molecules (O_2), the second most abundant, account for roughly 20.8 percent of the atmospheric gas molecules. Most of the remaining 0.6 percent consists of water molecules, with carbon dioxide (CO_2) contributing a mere 0.04 percent to the atmospheric total.

Gas pressures are frequently measured in millimeters of mercury (mm Hg). A device called a barometer is used to measure air pressure. As the air presses down on a reservoir of mercury in the device, it forces some of the mercury up a tube. The higher the pressure, the higher the mercury rises in the tube. The height of the mercury column is measured in millimeters and is an indication of the gas pressure.

Atmospheric pressure at sea level, 760 mm Hg, represents the combined effects of collisions involving each type of molecule. At any given moment, 78.6 percent of those collisions will involve nitrogen molecules, 20.8 percent oxygen molecules, and so on. Thus, each of the gases contributes to the total pressure in proportion to its relative abundance. This relationship is known as **Dalton's law.**

The **partial pressure** of a gas is the pressure contributed by a single gas within a mixture of gases. The partial pressure is abbreviated by the prefix P or p. All of the partial pressures added together equal the total pressure exerted by the gas mixture. In the case of the atmosphere, this relationship can be summarized as:

$$P_{N_2} + P_{O_2} + P_{H_2O} + P_{CO_2} = 760 \text{ mm Hg}$$

Because we know the individual percentages, the partial pressure for each gas can be calculated easily. For example, the partial pressure of oxygen, P_{O_2}, is 20.8 percent of 760 mm Hg, or roughly 159 mm Hg. The partial pressures for other atmospheric gases are included in Table 9–1.

Table 9–1   Partial Pressures (mm Hg) and Normal Gas Concentrations (%) in Air

Source of Sample	Nitrogen (N₂)	Oxygen (O₂)	Carbon Dioxide (CO₂)	Water Vapor (H₂O)
Inspired air (dry)	597 (78.6%)	159 (20.9%)	0.3 (0.04%)	3.7 (0.5%)
Alveolar air (saturated)	573 (75.4%)	100 (13.2%)	40 (5.2%)	47 (6.2%)
Expired air (saturated)	569 (74.8%)	116 (15.3%)	28 (3.7%)	47 (6.2%)

Henry's Law: Diffusion between Liquids and Gases

Differences in pressure move gas molecules from one place to another. Pressure differences also affect the movement of gas molecules into and out of solution. At a given temperature, the amount of a particular gas in solution is directly proportional to the partial pressure of that gas. This principle is known as **Henry's law.**

When a gas under pressure contacts a liquid, the pressure tends to force gas molecules into solution. At a given pressure, the number of dissolved gas molecules rises until an equilibrium becomes established. At equilibrium, gas molecules are diffusing out of the liquid as quickly as they are arriving, and the total number of gas molecules in solution remains constant. If the partial pressure goes up, more gas molecules go into solution. If the partial pressure goes down, gas molecules will come out of solution. These relationships are diagrammed in Figure 9–16.

You see Henry's law in action whenever you grab a can of soda. The soda was put into the can under pressure, and the gas (carbon dioxide) is in solution. When you open the can, the pressure falls and the gas molecules begin coming out of solution. The process will theoretically continue until an equilibrium develops between the air and the gas in solution. In fact, the volume of the can is so small and the volume of the atmosphere is so great that over the course of a half-hour or so virtually all of the carbon dioxide comes out of solution. You are then left with a "flat" soda.

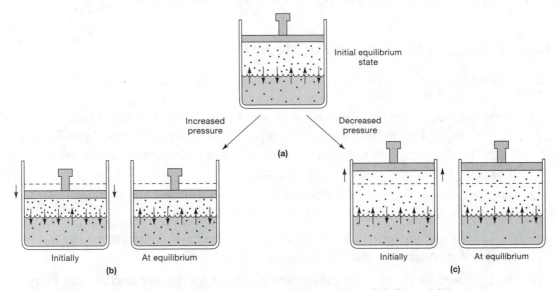

Figure 9–16   Henry's Law and the Relationship between Solubility and Pressure.
(a) A solution containing dissolved gas molecules at equilibrium with air under a given pressure. **(b)** Increasing the pressure drives additional gas molecules into solution until a new equilibrium becomes established. **(c)** When the pressure decreases, some of the dissolved gas molecules leave the solution until equilibrium is restored.

The actual amount of gas in solution at a given partial pressure and temperature depends on the solubility of the gas in the particular liquid. Carbon dioxide is very soluble, oxygen is somewhat less soluble, and nitrogen has very limited solubility in body fluids. The dissolved gas content is usually reported in terms of milliliters of gas per 100 ml of solution. For example, blood in a pulmonary vein, which has a P_{N_2} of 573 mm Hg, usually contains around 1.25 ml of nitrogen per 100 ml of blood.

Pulmonary Ventilation

The primary function of pulmonary ventilation is to maintain adequate **alveolar ventilation,** air movement into and out of the alveoli. Alveolar ventilation prevents the buildup of carbon dioxide in the alveoli and ensures a continual supply of oxygen that keeps pace with absorption by the bloodstream. Air will flow from an area of higher pressure to an area of relatively lower pressure. This tendency for directed airflow plus the pressure-volume relationships of Boyle's law provide the basis for pulmonary ventilation.

A single **respiratory cycle** consists of an inhalation, or *inspiration*, and an exhalation, or *expiration*. Inhalation and exhalation involve changes in the volume of the lungs, and these changes create pressure gradients that move air into or out of the respiratory tract.

At the start of a breath, pressures inside and outside the thoracic cavity are identical, and there is no movement of air into or out of the lungs. During inspiration, the contraction of muscles in the thorax causes the thoracic cavity to enlarge, and the pleural cavities and lungs expand to fill the additional space. This expansion lowers the pressure inside the lungs (Boyle's law). Air now enters the respiratory passageways because the pressure inside the lungs is lower than atmospheric pressure (pressure outside). Air continues to enter until the volume stops increasing and the internal pressure is the same as the outside pressure. When the thoracic cavity decreases in volume, pressures rise inside the lungs (Boyle's law again), forcing air out of the respiratory tract. The alternating changes in pressure that occur as the result of the respiratory cycle continuously move oxygen toward the lungs and carbon dioxide out of the body.

Gas Exchange at the Respiratory Membrane

Gas exchange at the respiratory membrane is efficient because:

1. The differences in partial pressure across the respiratory membrane are substantial. This fact is important because the greater the difference in partial pressure, the faster the rate of gas diffusion. Conversely, if the P_{O_2} in the alveoli decreases, the rate of oxygen diffusion into the blood will decline.

2. The distances involved are small. The fusion of capillary and alveolar basement membranes reduces the distance to an average of 0.5 μm.

3. The gases are lipid-soluble. Both oxygen and carbon dioxide diffuse readily through the alveolar and endothelial cell membranes.

4. The total surface area is large. The combined alveolar surface area at peak inspiration is approximately 140 m^2.

5. Blood flow and airflow are coordinated. This arrangement improves the efficiency of both pulmonary ventilation and pulmonary circulation. For example, blood flow

is greatest around alveoli with the highest P_{O_2}, where oxygen uptake can proceed with maximum efficiency.

Gas Pickup and Delivery

Oxygen and carbon dioxide have limited solubilities in blood plasma. For example, of the total amount of oxygen that needs to be transported in the blood only a very small amount, about 1.5 percent, will actually dissolve in blood plasma. (The remaining 98.5 percent is carried by the hemoglobin in red blood cells.) The limited solubilities of these gases are a problem because peripheral tissues need more oxygen and generate more carbon dioxide than the plasma can absorb and transport.

The problem is solved by the red blood cells, which remove dissolved oxygen and carbon dioxide molecules and either tie them up (in the case of oxygen) or use them to manufacture soluble compounds (in the case of carbon dioxide). Because the reactions remove dissolved gas from the plasma, gas will continue to diffuse into the blood but will never reach equilibrium.

The important thing about these reactions is that they are (1) temporary and (2) completely reversible. When plasma oxygen (in the lungs) or carbon dioxide (in the tissues) concentrations are high, the excess molecules are removed from the plasma by the red blood cells; when the plasma concentrations are falling (carbon dioxide in the lungs and oxygen in the tissues), the red blood cells release their stored reserves.

Control of Respiration

Peripheral cells are continuously absorbing oxygen from the interstitial fluids and generating carbon dioxide. Under normal conditions, the cellular rates of absorption and generation are matched by the capillary rates of delivery and removal. These rates are identical to those of oxygen absorption and carbon dioxide excretion at the lungs. If these rates become unbalanced, homeostatic mechanisms intervene to restore equilibrium. Those mechanisms involve (1) changes in blood flow and oxygen delivery that are regulated at the local level and (2) variations in the depth and rate of respiration under the control of the respiratory centers of the brain.

Integration with Other Systems

The respiratory system has extensive anatomical connections to the cardiovascular system, and the functional ties are just as extensive.

The goal of respiratory activity is the maintenance of homeostatic oxygen and carbon dioxide levels in peripheral tissues. Changes in respiratory activity alone are seldom sufficient to accomplish this. For example, during exercise, when tissue oxygen demands are high, alveolar ventilation increases through stimulation of the respiratory muscles. This response, which actually increases the demand for oxygen, serves no purpose unless the amount of blood being pumped by the heart increases simultaneously, so that oxygen delivery to active tissues can be improved.

Of course, the respiratory system is functionally linked to all other systems, and Figure 9–17 details some of those interrelationships.

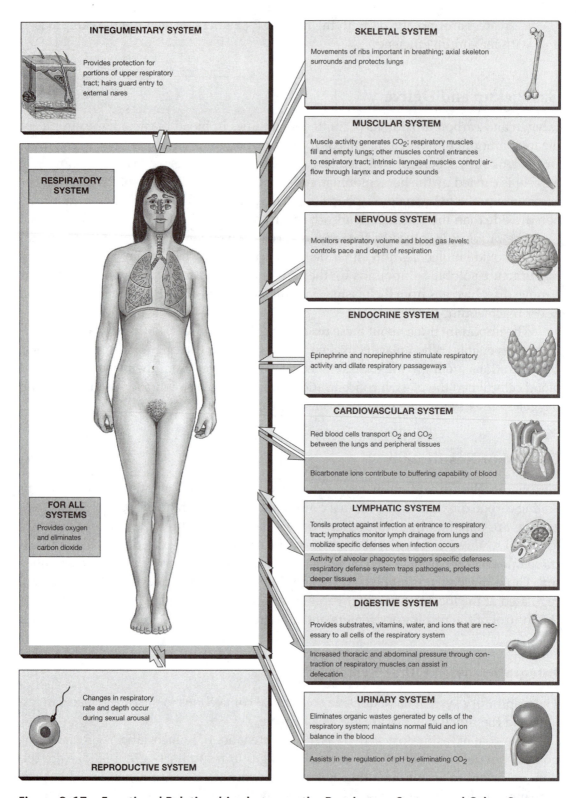

INTEGUMENTARY SYSTEM

Provides protection for portions of upper respiratory tract; hairs guard entry to external nares

RESPIRATORY SYSTEM

FOR ALL SYSTEMS

Provides oxygen and eliminates carbon dioxide

Changes in respiratory rate and depth occur during sexual arousal

REPRODUCTIVE SYSTEM

SKELETAL SYSTEM

Movements of ribs important in breathing; axial skeleton surrounds and protects lungs

MUSCULAR SYSTEM

Muscle activity generates CO_2; respiratory muscles fill and empty lungs; other muscles control entrances to respiratory tract; intrinsic laryngeal muscles control airflow through larynx and produce sounds

NERVOUS SYSTEM

Monitors respiratory volume and blood gas levels; controls pace and depth of respiration

ENDOCRINE SYSTEM

Epinephrine and norepinephrine stimulate respiratory activity and dilate respiratory passageways

CARDIOVASCULAR SYSTEM

Red blood cells transport O_2 and CO_2 between the lungs and peripheral tissues

Bicarbonate ions contribute to buffering capability of blood

LYMPHATIC SYSTEM

Tonsils protect against infection at entrance to respiratory tract; lymphatics monitor lymph drainage from lungs and mobilize specific defenses when infection occurs

Activity of alveolar phagocytes triggers specific defenses; respiratory defense system traps pathogens, protects deeper tissues

DIGESTIVE SYSTEM

Provides substrates, vitamins, water, and ions that are necessary to all cells of the respiratory system

Increased thoracic and abdominal pressure through contraction of respiratory muscles can assist in defecation

URINARY SYSTEM

Eliminates organic wastes generated by cells of the respiratory system; maintains normal fluid and ion balance in the blood

Assists in the regulation of pH by eliminating CO_2

Figure 9–17 **Functional Relationships between the Respiratory System and Other Systems.**

✎ Let's Review What You've Just Learned

► **Definitions**

In the space provided, write the term for each of the following definitions.

_____ **86.** Blind pockets at the end of the respiratory tree that are the site of gas exchange with the blood.

_____ **87.** The gas law that states that gas volume and gas pressure are inversely proportional at constant temperature.

_____ **88.** A structure that serves as a common passageway for air and food.

_____ **89.** The lining of the respiratory system.

_____ **90.** The process of physically moving air into and out of the lungs.

_____ **91.** The external openings into the nasal cavity.

_____ **92.** The modification of sounds by various structures to produce speech.

_____ **93.** A tough, flexible tube that connects the larynx with the two primary bronchi.

_____ **94.** The gas law that states that the total pressure exerted by a mixture of gases is equal to the sum of the individual partial pressures of the gases in the mixture.

_____ **95.** Tiny airways that branch directly from a bronchus.

_____ **96.** The opening into the larynx.

_____ **97.** Distinct units of a lung that are separated by deep fissures.

_____ **98.** A single cycle of inhalation and exhalation.

_____ **99.** The general term for the airways that carry air to and from the exchange surfaces of the lungs.

_____ **100.** Connections between respiratory bronchioles and individual or multiple alveoli.

_____ **101.** The gas law that states that at a given temperature, the amount of a particular gas in solution is directly proportional to the partial pressure of the gas.

_____ **102.** The openings of the nasal cavity into the pharynx.

_____ **103.** A condition in which there is no oxygen available for tissues.

_____ **104.** One of the two structures that connects the trachea to the lungs.

_____ **105.** All of the processes involved in the exchange of oxygen and carbon dioxide between the interstitial fluids of the body and the external environment.

_____ **106.** The process of sound production.

_____ **107.** The branches of terminal bronchioles that occur within lobules of the lungs.

_____ **108.** The condition of lower than normal amounts of oxygen for the body's tissues.

_____ **109.** The pressure contributed by a single gas in a mixture of gases.

_____ **110.** A cartilaginous structure that surrounds and protects the glottis and contains the vocal folds.

_____ **111.** Common chambers that are connected to multiple individual alveoli.

_____ **112.** Divisions of the lobes of a lung.

_____ **113.** The absorption of oxygen and the release of carbon dioxide by the cells of the body.

_____ **114.** The amount of air reaching the alveoli each minute.

_____ **115.** The membrane composed of the epithelial lining of an alveolus, the endothelial cells of adjacent capillaries, and the fused basement membranes that lie in between.

▶ **Word Roots, Prefixes, Suffixes, and Combining Forms**

In the space provided, list the boldfaced terms introduced in this section that contain the indicated word part.

Word Part	Meaning	Examples
pulmo-	lung	**116.** _____
hypo-	under	**117.** _____
bronch-	windpipe	**118.** _____
a-	without	**119.** _____
oxi-	oxygen	**120.** _____

THE DIGESTIVE SYSTEM

The digestive system consists of a muscular tube, the **digestive tract,** and various accessory organs. Accessory digestive organs include the teeth, tongue, and various glands, such as the salivary glands, liver, and pancreas, that secrete into ducts emptying into the digestive tract. Food enters the digestive tract and passes along its length. On the way, the secretions of the glandular organs are discharged into the digestive tract. These secretions, which contain water, enzymes, buffers, and other components, assist in preparing organic and inorganic nutrients for absorption across the epithelium of the digestive tract.

Digestive functions can be considered as a series of integrated steps.

1. **Ingestion** occurs when materials enter the digestive tract through the mouth. Ingestion is an active process involving conscious choice and decision making.

2. **Mechanical processing** is physical manipulation and distortion that make materials easier to swallow and increase the surface area for enzymatic attack. Mechanical processing may or may not be required; liquids can be swallowed immediately, but solids must usually be processed first. Squashing with the tongue and tearing and crushing with the teeth are examples of mechanical processing that occurs before ingestion. Swirling, mixing, and churning motions of the digestive tract provide mechanical processing after ingestion.

3. **Digestion** refers to the chemical breakdown of food into small organic fragments suitable for absorption by the digestive epithelium. Simple molecules in food, such as glucose, can be absorbed intact, but epithelial cells have no way to deal with molecules the size and complexity of proteins, polysaccharides, and triglycerides.

Those molecules must be disassembled by digestive enzymes before absorption. For example, the starches in a potato are of no value until enzymes have broken them down to simple sugars that can be absorbed and distributed to our cells.

4. **Secretion** is the release of water, acids, enzymes, buffers, and salts by the epithelium of the digestive tract and by glandular organs.

5. **Absorption** is the movement of organic substrates, electrolytes, vitamins, and water across the digestive epithelium and into the interstitial fluid of the digestive tract.

6. **Excretion** is the elimination of waste products from the body. The digestive tract and glandular organs secrete waste products in secretions discharged into the lumen of the tract. Most of these waste products will leave the body through the process of **defecation** (def-e-KĀ-shun), which also eliminates the indigestible residue of the digestive process.

The lining of the digestive tract plays a protective role by safeguarding surrounding tissues against (1) the corrosive effects of digestive acids and enzymes, (2) mechanical stresses, such as abrasion, and (3) bacteria that are either swallowed with food or reside inside the digestive tract. The digestive epithelium and its secretions provide a nonspecific defense against these bacteria.

An Overview of the Digestive Tract

The major components of the digestive system are shown in Figure 9–18. The digestive tract begins at the oral cavity and continues through the pharynx, esophagus, stomach, small intestine, and large intestine before ending at the rectum and anus. Although these structures have overlapping functions, each has certain areas of specialization and shows distinctive histological characteristics.

The major layers of the digestive tract include (1) the mucosa, (2) the submucosa, (3) the muscularis externa, and (4) the serosa. Sectional and diagrammatic views of these layers are presented in Figure 9–19. There are regional variations in the structure of the layers; Figure 9–19 is a composite view that most closely resembles the appearance of the small intestine, the longest segment of the digestive tract.

1. **The mucosa:** The inner lining, or **mucosa,** of the digestive tract is an example of a mucous membrane. Mucous membranes were described in Chapter 6.

2. **The submucosa:** The **submucosa** is a layer of dense connective tissue. Large blood vessels and lymphatics are found in this layer, and in some regions the submucosa also contains exocrine glands that secrete buffers and enzymes into the lumen of the digestive tract. Along its outer margin, the submucosa contains a network of nerve fibers and scattered neurons.

3. **The muscularis externa.** The **muscularis externa** is a region dominated by smooth muscle fibers. The smooth muscle fibers are arranged in an inner, circular layer and an outer, longitudinal layer. These layers play an essential role in mechanical processing and in the movement of materials along the digestive tract.

4. **The serosa:** Along most portions of the digestive tract inside the peritoneal cavity, the muscularis externa is covered by a serous membrane known as the **serosa.** There is no serosa covering the muscularis externa of the oral cavity, pharynx, esophagus, and rectum, where a dense network of collagen fibers firmly attaches the digestive tract to adjacent structures. This fibrous sheath is called an **adventitia.**

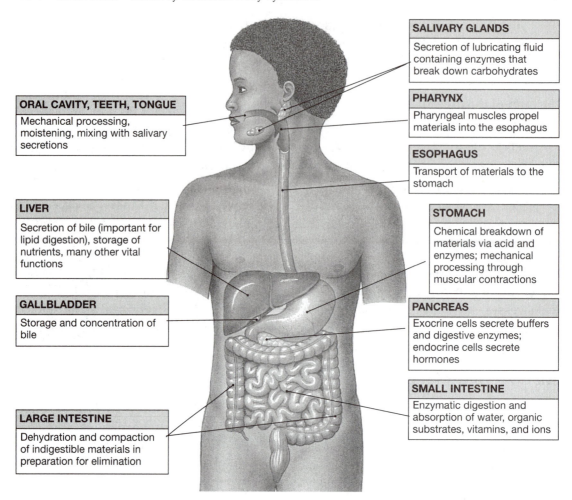

SALIVARY GLANDS
Secretion of lubricating fluid containing enzymes that break down carbohydrates

PHARYNX
Pharyngeal muscles propel materials into the esophagus

ESOPHAGUS
Transport of materials to the stomach

STOMACH
Chemical breakdown of materials via acid and enzymes; mechanical processing through muscular contractions

PANCREAS
Exocrine cells secrete buffers and digestive enzymes; endocrine cells secrete hormones

SMALL INTESTINE
Enzymatic digestion and absorption of water, organic substrates, vitamins, and ions

ORAL CAVITY, TEETH, TONGUE
Mechanical processing, moistening, mixing with salivary secretions

LIVER
Secretion of bile (important for lipid digestion), storage of nutrients, many other vital functions

GALLBLADDER
Storage and concentration of bile

LARGE INTESTINE
Dehydration and compaction of indigestible materials in preparation for elimination

Figure 9–18   Components of the Digestive System.
The major regions and accessory organs of the digestive tract, together with their primary functions.

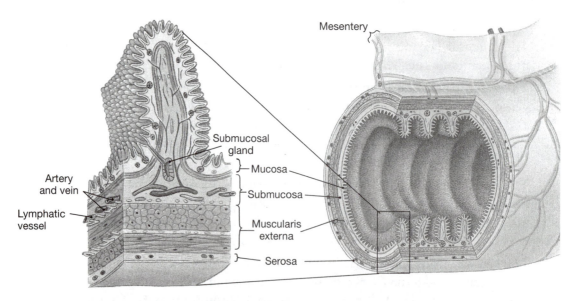

Mesentery

Submucosal gland

Mucosa

Submucosa

Muscularis externa

Serosa

Artery and vein

Lymphatic vessel

Figure 9–19   Structure of the Digestive Tract.
Diagrammatic view of a representative portion of the digestive tract. The features illustrated are those of the small intestine.

The Movement of Digestive Materials

The digestive tract contains layers of smooth muscle tissue (smooth muscle was introduced in Chapter 6) that shows rhythmic cycles of activity due to the presence of pacesetter cells. **Pacesetter cells** are smooth muscle cells that undergo spontaneous depolarization. Their contraction triggers a wave of contraction that spreads through the entire muscular sheet. The coordinated contractions of smooth muscle cells play a vital role in the movement of materials along the digestive tract, through peristalsis, and in mechanical processing, through segmentation.

- The muscularis externa propels materials from one portion of the digestive tract to another through the contractions of **peristalsis** (per-i-STAL-sis) (Figure 9–20). Peristalsis consists of waves of muscular contractions that move along the length of the digestive tract.

- Most areas of the small intestine and some portions of the large intestine undergo **segmentation.** These movements churn and fragment the digestive materials, mixing the contents with intestinal secretions. Because they do not follow a set pattern, segmentation movements do not produce directional movement of materials along the tract.

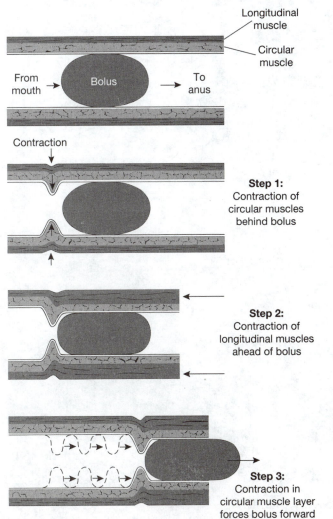

Longitudinal muscle

Circular muscle

From mouth → Bolus → To anus

Contraction

Step 1:
Contraction of circular muscles behind bolus

Step 2:
Contraction of longitudinal muscles ahead of bolus

Step 3:
Contraction in circular muscle layer forces bolus forward

Figure 9–20 Peristalsis.
Peristalsis propels materials along the length of the digestive tract.

The activities of the digestive system are regulated in three basic ways: (1) by neural mechanisms, (2) by hormonal mechanisms, and (3) by local mechanisms.

Structure and Function of the Digestive Tract

Our exploration of the digestive tract will follow the path of food from the mouth to the anus. The mouth opens into the **oral cavity,** or **buccal** (BŪK-al), **cavity** (Figure 9–21a). The oral cavity is bounded laterally by the cheeks, superiorly by the hard and soft palate, and inferiorly by the floor of the mouth. The functions of the oral cavity may be summarized as follows: (1) analysis of material before swallowing; (2) mechanical processing through the actions of the teeth, tongue, and surfaces of the palate; (3) lubrication by mixing with mucus and salivary secretions; and (4) limited digestion of carbohydrates and lipids.

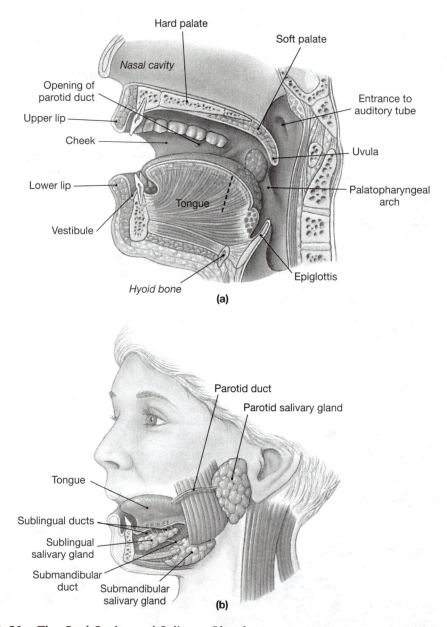

Figure 9–21   The Oral Cavity and Salivary Glands.

(a) The oral cavity as seen in sagittal section. **(b)** A laterial view showing the relative positions of the salivary glands on the left side of the head.

The tongue manipulates materials inside the mouth and may occasionally be used to bring foods into the oral cavity. The primary functions of the tongue are: (1) mechanical processing by compression, abrasion, and distortion; (2) manipulation to assist in chewing and to prepare the materials for swallowing; (3) sensory analysis by touch, temperature, and taste receptors; and (4) secretion of mucus and an enzyme, lingual lipase.

Three pairs of salivary glands secrete into the oral cavity (Figure 9–21b):

1. The large **parotid** (pa-ROT-id) **salivary glands** are located inferior to the ear and secrete a thick, serous secretion containing large amounts of **salivary amylase** (AM-i-lāce), an enzyme that breaks down complex carbohydrates.

2. The **sublingual** (sub-LING-gwal) **salivary glands** are located in the floor of the mouth and produce a watery, mucous secretion that acts as a buffer and lubricant.

3. The **submandibular** (sub-man-DIB-ū-lur) **salivary glands** are found in the floor of the mouth along the inner surface of the lower jaw. They secrete a mixture of buffers, mucus, and salivary amylase.

The collective secretions of the salivary glands are called **saliva.** The saliva produced at mealtimes has a variety of functions, including:

- Lubricating the mouth.
- Moistening and lubricating materials in the mouth.
- Dissolving chemicals that can stimulate the taste buds and provide sensory information about the material.
- Initiating the digestion of complex carbohydrates before the material is swallowed.

Movements of the tongue are important in passing food across the opposing surfaces of the teeth. The opposing, or **occlusal** (uh-KLOO-zul; Latin *occlusus*, shut), **surfaces** of the teeth perform chewing, or **mastication** (mas-ti-KĀ-shun), of food. Mastication breaks down tough connective tissues in meat and the plant fibers in vegetable matter, and it helps saturate the materials with salivary secretions and enzymes. During mastication, food is forced back and forth across the occlusal surfaces. Once the material has been shredded or torn to a satisfactory consistency and moistened with salivary secretions, the tongue begins compacting the debris into a small oval mass, or **bolus.** A compact, moist, cohesive bolus can be swallowed relatively easily.

The pharynx (see Figure 9–21a) serves as a common passageway for solid food, liquids, and air. Food passes through the pharynx on the way to the esophagus. Several muscles associated with the pharynx cooperate with muscles of the oral cavity and esophagus to initiate the process of swallowing, or **deglutition** (dē-gloo-TISH-un; Latin *deglutire*, swallow down), which delivers the bolus along the esophagus and into the stomach.

The **esophagus** is a hollow muscular tube (see Figure 9–18). The primary function of the esophagus is to carry solid food and liquids to the stomach. Waves of peristaltic contractions force food down the length of the esophagus and into the stomach.

The **stomach** is a J-shaped, muscular organ (see Figure 9–18). It performs four major functions: (1) the bulk storage of ingested food, (2) the mechanical breakdown of ingested food, (3) the disruption of chemical bonds through the action of acids and enzymes, and (4) the production of intrinsic factor, a glycoprotein whose presence in the digestive tract is required for the absorption of vitamin B_{12}. The mixing of ingested substances with the gastric juices secreted by the glands of the stomach produces a viscous, highly acid, soupy mixture of partially digested food. This material is called **chyme** (kīm).

Two types of secretory cells dominate in the mucosa of the stomach: parietal cells and chief cells. **Parietal cells** secrete intrinsic factor and hydrochloric acid (HCl). The secretory activities of the parietal cells can keep the stomach contents at a pH of 1.5 to 2.0. This highly acid environment does not by itself digest the chyme, but it has several important functions.

- The extreme acidity of gastric juice kills most of the microorganisms ingested with food.
- The acidity denatures proteins and inactivates most of the enzymes in food.
- The acid helps break down plant cell walls and the connective tissues in meat.
- An acid environment is essential for the activation and function of pepsin, a **protease** (PRŌ-tē-ās) (protein-digesting enzyme) secreted by chief cells.

Chief cells secrete an inactive proenzyme, **pepsinogen** (pep-SIN-ō-jen), that is converted by the acid in the stomach to an active enzyme, **pepsin.** The stomach performs preliminary digestion of proteins by pepsin and, for a variable period, permits the digestion of carbohydrates and lipids by salivary amylase and lingual lipase. As the stomach contents become more fluid and the pH approaches 2.0, pepsin activity increases and protein disassembly begins. Protein digestion is not completed in the stomach, because (1) time is limited, and (2) pepsin attacks only specific types of peptide bonds, not all peptide bonds. No nutrient absorption occurs in the stomach.

From the stomach, food passes to the small intestine (see Figure 9–18). The **small intestine** plays the primary role in the digestion and absorption of nutrients. It occupies all abdominal regions except the right and left hypochondriac and epigastric regions (see Chapter 1). Ninety percent of nutrient absorption occurs in the small intestine, and most of the rest occurs in the large intestine.

The small intestine has three subdivisions: the duodenum, the jejunum, and the ileum.

- The **duodenum** (doo-ō-DĒ-num or doo-AH-de-num; Latin *duodecim*, twelve) is the section closest to the stomach. This portion of the small intestine is a "mixing bowl" that receives chyme from the stomach and digestive secretions from the pancreas and liver. From the connection with the stomach, the duodenum curves in a C that encloses the pancreas.
- A rather abrupt bend marks the boundary between the duodenum and the **jejunum** (je-JOO-num; Latin *jejunus*, fasting or empty). The bulk of chemical digestion and nutrient absorption occurs in the jejunum.
- The **ileum** (IL-ē-um; Greek *eileos*, twisted) is the third and last segment of the small intestine. The ileum ends at a sphincter, the **ileocecal** (il-ē-ō-SĒ-kal) **valve,** which controls the flow of chyme from the ileum into the cecum of the large intestine.

The small intestine secretes a watery intestinal juice. Intestinal juice moistens the chyme, assists in buffering acids, and dissolves both the digestive enzymes provided by the pancreas and the products of digestion.

The **pancreas** lies behind the stomach, extending laterally from the duodenum toward the spleen (Figure 9–22). It is primarily an exocrine organ, producing digestive enzymes and buffers. The large pancreatic duct delivers these secretions to the duodenum.

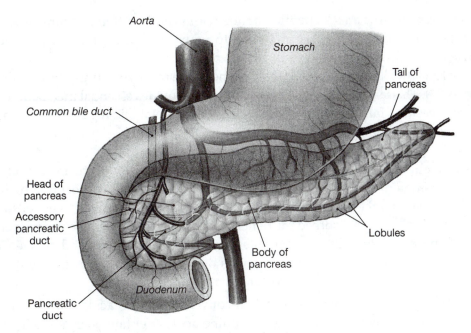

Aorta

Stomach

Tail of pancreas

Common bile duct

Head of pancreas

Accessory pancreatic duct

Lobules

Body of pancreas

Duodenum

Pancreatic duct

Figure 9–22   The Pancreas.
Gross anatomy of the pancreas. The head of the pancreas is tucked into a curve of the duodenum.

The secretory activities of the pancreas are controlled primarily by hormones from the duodenum. When acid chyme arrives in the duodenum, **secretin** (se-KRĒ-tin) is released. This hormone triggers the pancreatic secretion of a watery buffer solution with a pH of 7.5 to 8.8. Among its other components, this secretion contains sodium bicarbonate, a buffer that helps elevate the pH of the chyme. A different duodenal hormone, **cholecystokinin** (kōl-ē-sis-tō-KĪ-nin) **(CCK)**, stimulates the production and secretion of pancreatic enzymes. The specific pancreatic enzymes involved include:

- **Pancreatic amylase: Pancreatic amylase** is a carbohydrase (kar-bō-HĪ-drās), an enzyme that breaks down starches. Pancreatic amylase is almost identical to salivary amylase.

- **Pancreatic lipase: Pancreatic lipase** breaks down complex lipids, releasing fatty acids and other products that can be easily absorbed.

- **Nucleases: Nucleases** break down nucleic acids.

- **Proteolytic enzymes: Proteolytic enzymes** break proteins apart. The proteolytic enzymes of the pancreas include proteases and peptidases; **proteases** break apart large protein complexes, whereas **peptidases** (PEP-ti-dā-sēz) break small peptide chains into individual amino acids.

As in the stomach, release of a proenzyme rather than an active enzyme protects the secretory cells from the destructive effects of their own products. Among the proenzymes secreted by the pancreas are **trypsinogen** (trip-SIN-ō-jen), **chymotrypsinogen** (kī-mō-trip-SIN-ō-jen), **procarboxypeptidase** (prō-kar-bok-sē-PEP-ti-dās), and **proelastase** (prō-ē-LAS-tās).

Once inside the duodenum, **enterokinase** (en-ter-ō-KĪ-nās) produced by the small intestine triggers the conversion of trypsinogen to **trypsin,** an active protease. Trypsin then activates the other proenzymes, producing **chymotrypsin, carboxypeptidase,** and

elastase. Each enzyme attacks peptide bonds with slightly different characteristics. Together, they break down complex proteins into a mixture of dipeptides, tripeptides, and amino acids.

The **liver,** the largest visceral organ, is one of the most versatile organs in the body (Figure 9–23). This large, firm, reddish brown organ provides essential metabolic and synthetic services that fall into three general categories: metabolic regulation, hematological regulation, and bile production.

1. **Metabolic regulation.** The liver is the primary organ involved in regulating the composition of the circulating blood. All blood leaving the absorptive surfaces of the digestive tract flows into the liver. This arrangement gives liver cells the opportunity to extract absorbed nutrients or toxins from the blood before it reaches the systemic circulation. Excess nutrients are removed and stored, and deficiencies are corrected, by mobilizing stored reserves or performing appropriate synthetic activities. Other important metabolic regulation includes:

   - **Removal of waste products:** When converting amino acids to lipids or carbohydrates, or when breaking down amino acids to obtain energy, the liver strips off the amino groups, a process called **deamination.** This process produces ammonia, a toxic waste product that the liver neutralizes through conversion to **urea,** a relatively harmless compound that is excreted at the kidneys. Other waste products, circulating toxins, and drugs are also removed from the blood for subsequent inactivation, storage, or excretion.

   - **Vitamin storage.** Fat-soluble vitamins (A, D, E, and K) and vitamin B_{12} are absorbed from the blood and stored in the liver. These reserves are called upon when the diet contains inadequate amounts of these vitamins.

   - **Mineral storage:** The liver contains important reserves of iron.

   - **Drug inactivation:** The liver removes and breaks down circulating drugs, thereby limiting the duration of their effects.

2. **Hematological regulation:** The liver, the largest blood reservoir in the body, receives about 25 percent of the blood pumped into the systemic circuit. As blood passes through, the liver performs the following functions.

   - Phagocytosis and antigen presentation.

   - Plasma protein synthesis.

   - Removal of circulating hormones.

   - Removal of antibodies.

   - Removal or storage of toxins.

3. **Bile production: Bile** is synthesized in the liver and excreted into the lumen of the duodenum. Bile consists mostly of water, with minor amounts of ions, **bilirubin** (bil-i-ROO-bin) (a pigment derived from hemoglobin), cholesterol, and an assortment of lipids collectively known as bile salts. Bile salts are synthesized from cholesterol in the liver. The water and ions assist in the dilution and buffering of acids in chyme as it enters the small intestine.

Most dietary lipids are not water-soluble. Mechanical processing in the stomach creates large drops containing a variety of lipids. Pancreatic lipase is not lipid-soluble, so the enzymes can interact with lipids only at the surface of a lipid drop. The larger the drop, the more lipids are found inside, isolated and protected from these enzymes. **Bile salts**

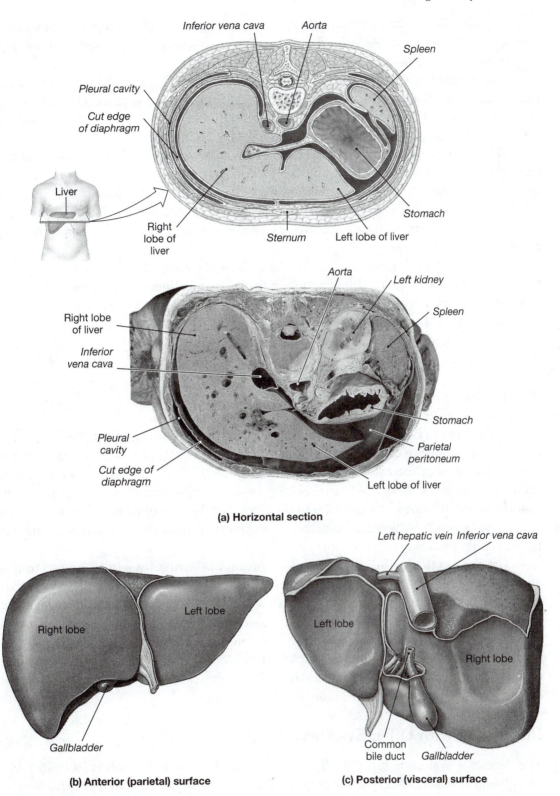

Figure 9–23   Anatomy of the Liver.
(a) Horizontal sectional views (diagrammatic and actual) through the upper abdomen. (b) The anterior surface of the liver. (c) The posterior surface of the liver.

break the drops apart, a process called **emulsification** (ē-mul-si-fi-KĀ-shun). Emulsification creates tiny emulsion droplets with a superficial coating of bile salts. The formation of tiny droplets increases the surface area available for enyzmatic attack. In addition, the layer of bile salts facilitates interaction between the lipids and lipid-digesting enzymes provided by the pancreas. After lipid digestion has been completed, bile salts promote absorption of lipids by the intestinal epithelium.

Bile is stored in a saclike organ called the **gall bladder** (Figure 9–23) until it is needed for digestion. Bile is released from the gallbladder in response to the hormone CCK secreted by the small intestine. Contractions of the muscular walls of the gall bladder force the bile along the common bile duct and into the duodenum.

The horseshoe-shaped **large intestine** begins at the end of the ileum and ends at the anus (Figure 9–24). The large intestine lies inferior to the stomach and liver and almost completely frames the small intestine. The major functions of the large intestine include: (1) the reabsorption of water and compaction of chyme into **feces** (FĒ-sēz), (2) the absorption of important vitamins liberated by bacterial action, and (3) the storing of fecal material before defecation.

The large intestine, often called the **large bowel**, can be divided into three parts: (1) the pouchlike cecum, the first portion of the large intestine; (2) the colon, the largest portion of the large intestine; and (3) the rectum, the last 15 cm (6 in.) of the large intestine and the end of the digestive tract.

Material arriving from the ileum first enters an expanded pouch called the **cecum** (SĒ-kum; Latin *caecus*, blind). The ileum attaches to the medial surface of the cecum and opens into the cecum at the ileocecal valve. The cecum collects and stores chyme and begins the process of compaction. The slender, hollow **vermiform appendix** (Latin *vermis*, a worm) is attached to the posteromedial surface of the cecum.

The **colon** can be subdivided into four regions: the **ascending colon,** the **transverse colon,** the **descending colon,** and the **sigmoid colon.** The reabsorption of water is an important function of the colon. Although roughly 1500 ml of material enters the colon each day, only about 200 ml of feces is ejected. In addition to reabsorbing water, the colon absorbs other substances that remain in the chyme or that were secreted into the chyme as it passed along the digestive tract; these substances include vitamin K, biotin, vitamin B_5, bile salts, and toxins.

The **rectum** (REK-tum) forms the last portion of the digestive tract. The rectum is an expandable organ for the temporary storage of fecal material. Movement of fecal materials into the rectum triggers the urge to defecate. The last portion of the rectum is the **anorectal** (ā-nō-REK-tal) **canal.** The circular muscle layer of the muscularis externa in this region forms the **internal anal sphincter.** The smooth muscle fibers of the internal anal sphincter are not under voluntary control. The **external anal sphincter** guards the exit of the anorectal canal, termed **anal orifice.** This sphincter, which consists of a ring of skeletal muscle fibers, is under voluntary control.

Integration with Other Systems

The digestive system is functionally linked to all other systems, and it has extensive anatomical connections to the nervous, cardiovascular, endocrine, and lymphatic systems. Figure 9–25 summarizes the physiological relationships between the digestive system and other organ systems.

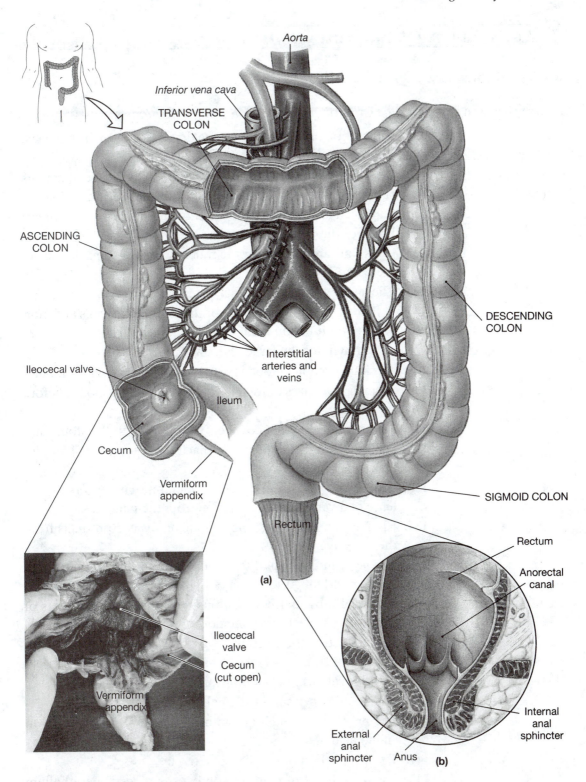

Aorta

Inferior vena cava

TRANSVERSE COLON

ASCENDING COLON

Ileocecal valve

Ileum

Cecum

Vermiform appendix

Interstitial arteries and veins

DESCENDING COLON

SIGMOID COLON

Rectum

(a)

Ileocecal valve

Cecum (cut open)

Vermiform appendix

Rectum

Anorectal canal

External anal sphincter

Anus **(b)**

Internal anal sphincter

Figure 9–24   The Large Intestine.
(a) Gross anatomy and regions of the large intestine. **(b)** Detailed anatomy of the rectum and anus.

Let's Review What You've Just Learned

▶ **Definitions**

In the space provided, write the term for each of the following definitions.

_____ **121.** The section of the small intestine that is closest to the stomach.

_____ **122.** Another term for the oral cavity.

_____ **123.** The chemical breakdown of food into small organic fragments suitable for absorption by the digestive epithelium.

_____ **124.** Salivary glands that are located beneath the mucous membrane of the floor of the mouth.

_____ **125.** Cells that are located in the mucosa of the stomach and secrete pepsinogen.

_____ **126.** The last segment of the small intestine.

_____ **127.** A fluid synthesized by the liver that contains wastes and molecules that function in fat emulsification.

_____ **128.** A synonym for the large intestine.

_____ **129.** The introduction of food into the digestive tract via the mouth.

_____ **130.** A small oval mass of food that is formed in the mouth before swallowing.

_____ **131.** A muscular tube that connects the pharynx to the stomach.

_____ **132.** Cells in the mucosa of the stomach that secrete HCl and intrinsic factor.

_____ **133.** A hormone produced by the duodenum that triggers the release of a watery buffer solution from the pancreas.

_____ **134.** Elimination of indigestible residue and waste products from the digestive tract.

_____ **135.** The layer in the wall of the digestive tract that contains both circular and longitudinal smooth muscle.

_____ **136.** Waves of muscular contractions that propel the contents of the digestive tract from one portion to another.

_____ **137.** The collective fluid produced by the three pairs of salivary glands.

_____ **138.** A technical term for swallowing.

_____ **139.** The middle portion of the small intestine.

_____ **140.** The process by which an amino group is removed from an amino acid.

_____ **141.** The last portion of the digestive tract.

_____ **142.** The movement of materials across the digestive epithelium and into the interstitial fluid of the digestive tract.

_____ **143.** Another term for chewing.

_____ **144.** A viscous, highly acid, soupy mixture of partially digested food.

_____ **145.** A hollow, pear-shaped, muscular organ that stores bile.

_____ **146.** An expanded pouch that receives material from the ileum.

_____ **147.** The circular layer of the muscularis externa in the anorectal canal.

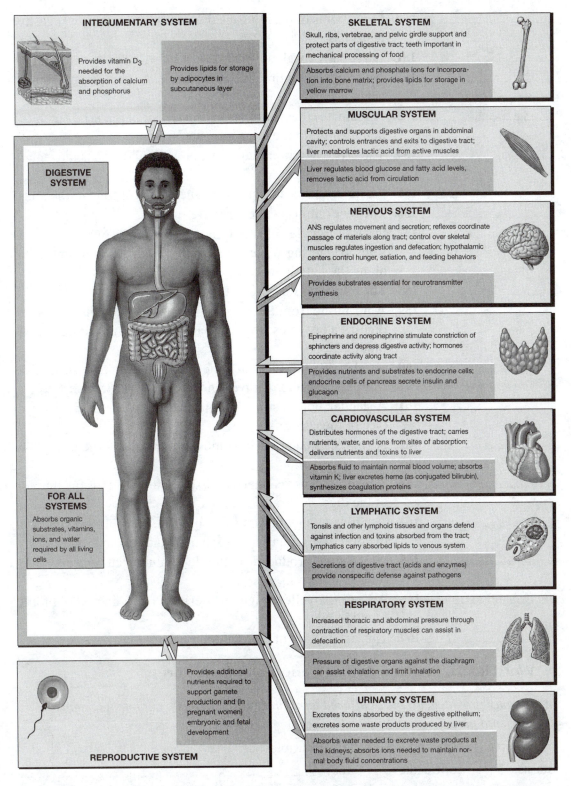

INTEGUMENTARY SYSTEM

Provides vitamin D₃ needed for the absorption of calcium and phosphorus

Provides lipids for storage by adipocytes in subcutaneous layer

SKELETAL SYSTEM

Skull, ribs, vertebrae, and pelvic girdle support and protect parts of digestive tract; teeth important in mechanical processing of food

Absorbs calcium and phosphate ions for incorporation into bone matrix; provides lipids for storage in yellow marrow

MUSCULAR SYSTEM

Protects and supports digestive organs in abdominal cavity; controls entrances and exits to digestive tract; liver metabolizes lactic acid from active muscles

Liver regulates blood glucose and fatty acid levels, removes lactic acid from circulation

NERVOUS SYSTEM

ANS regulates movement and secretion; reflexes coordinate passage of materials along tract; control over skeletal muscles regulates ingestion and defecation; hypothalamic centers control hunger, satiation, and feeding behaviors

Provides substrates essential for neurotransmitter synthesis

ENDOCRINE SYSTEM

Epinephrine and norepinephrine stimulate constriction of sphincters and depress digestive activity; hormones coordinate activity along tract

Provides nutrients and substrates to endocrine cells; endocrine cells of pancreas secrete insulin and glucagon

CARDIOVASCULAR SYSTEM

Distributes hormones of the digestive tract; carries nutrients, water, and ions from sites of absorption; delivers nutrients and toxins to liver

Absorbs fluid to maintain normal blood volume; absorbs vitamin K; liver excretes heme (as conjugated bilirubin), synthesizes coagulation proteins

LYMPHATIC SYSTEM

Tonsils and other lymphoid tissues and organs defend against infection and toxins absorbed from the tract; lymphatics carry absorbed lipids to venous system

Secretions of digestive tract (acids and enzymes) provide nonspecific defense against pathogens

RESPIRATORY SYSTEM

Increased thoracic and abdominal pressure through contraction of respiratory muscles can assist in defecation

Pressure of digestive organs against the diaphragm can assist exhalation and limit inhalation

URINARY SYSTEM

Excretes toxins absorbed by the digestive epithelium; excretes some waste products produced by liver

Absorbs water needed to excrete waste products at the kidneys; absorbs ions needed to maintain normal body fluid concentrations

DIGESTIVE SYSTEM

FOR ALL SYSTEMS

Absorbs organic substrates, vitamins, ions, and water required by all living cells

REPRODUCTIVE SYSTEM

Provides additional nutrients required to support gamete production and (in pregnant women) embryonic and fetal development

Figure 9–25   Functional Relationships between the Digestive System and Other Systems.

_____ **148.** The elimination of waste products from the body.

_____ **149.** The covering of the muscularis externa in the digestive tract with the exception of the oral cavity, pharynx, esophagus, and rectum.

_____ **150.** Movements of the intestine that churn and fragment digestive materials.

_____ **151.** Large salivary glands that lie just inferior to the ear.

_____ **152.** An enzyme that breaks down proteins to peptides and amino acids.

_____ **153.** A sphincter that controls the movement of material out of the ileum and into the large intestine.

_____ **154.** The process of breaking down large lipid droplets into smaller ones.

_____ **155.** Waste products eliminated by the digestive tract at the anus.

_____ **156.** The inner lining of the digestive tract.

_____ **157.** Smooth muscle cells that undergo spontaneous depolarizations, triggering waves of muscular contractions that move along the length of the digestive tract.

_____ **158.** The opposing surfaces of the teeth.

_____ **159.** A hormone from the duodenum that triggers the release of digestive enzymes from the pancreas and bile from the gallbladder.

_____ **160.** A relatively harmless organic compound that is synthesized from ammonia in the liver and excreted by the kidneys.

_____ **161.** A slender, hollow structure attached to the posteromedial surface of the cecum.

_____ **162.** A ring of circular skeletal muscle that guards the exit of the anorectal canal.

_____ **163.** A layer of dense connective tissue that surrounds the mucosa of the digestive tract.

_____ **164.** The fibrous sheath that surrounds the muscularis externa of the oral cavity, pharynx, esophagus, and rectum.

_____ **165.** An enzyme produced by the duodenum that converts trypsinogen to trypsin.

_____ **166.** An orange-yellow pigment derived from hemoglobin and found in bile.

_____ **167.** The last portion of the rectum.

▶ Word Roots, Prefixes, Suffixes, and Combining Forms

In the space provided, list the boldfaced terms introduced in this section that contain the indicated word part.

Word Part	Meaning	Examples
-stalsis	contractile	**168.** _____
trans-	across	**169.** _____
ile-	ileum	**170.** _____
sub-	under	**171.** _____
chole-	bile	**172.** _____
vermi-	worm	**173.** _____

► **Completion**

Complete the following table by indicating the substrate for each of the digestive enzymes listed.

	Enzyme	Substrate
174.	pepsin	
175.	amylase	
176.	nuclease	
177.	trypsin	
178.	elastase	
179.	lipase	
180.	carboxypeptidase	
181.	chymotrypsin	

THE URINARY SYSTEM

The urinary system performs vital excretory functions and eliminates waste products generated by cells throughout the body. But it also has other essential functions that are often overlooked. A more complete list of urinary system functions includes the following:

1. Regulating blood volume and blood pressure by (1) adjusting the volume of water lost in the urine and (2) releasing hormones that control blood pressure and red blood cell formation.

2. Regulating plasma concentrations of sodium, potassium, chloride, and other ions by controlling the quantities lost in the urine and controlling calcium ion levels by the synthesis of calcitriol.

3. Contributing to the stabilization of blood pH by controlling the loss of hydrogen ions and bicarbonate ions in the urine.

4. Conserving valuable nutrients by preventing their excretion in the urine, while eliminating organic waste products, especially nitrogenous wastes such as urea and uric acid.

5. Assisting the liver in detoxifying poisons and deaminating amino acids so that they can be broken down by other tissues.

These activities are carefully regulated to keep the composition of the blood within acceptable limits. A disruption of any one of these functions will have immediate and potentially fatal consequences.

Organization of the Urinary System

The urinary system includes the kidneys, ureters, urinary bladder, and urethra (Figure 9–26). The excretory functions of the urinary system are performed by the two kidneys. These organs produce urine, a fluid containing water, ions, and small soluble compounds. Urine leaving the kidneys travels along the paired **ureters** (ū-RĒ-terz) to the urinary

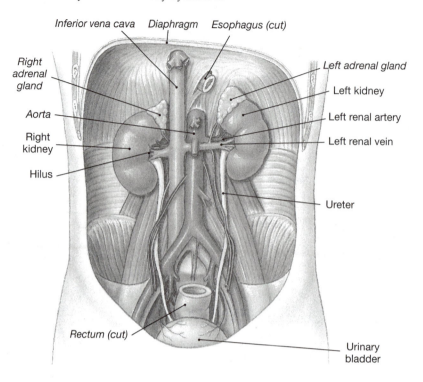

Inferior vena cava   Diaphragm   Esophagus (cut)

Right adrenal gland

Aorta

Right kidney

Hilus

Left adrenal gland

Left kidney

Left renal artery

Left renal vein

Ureter

Rectum (cut)

Urinary bladder

Figure 9–26   The Urinary System.
Diagrammatic view of the abdominopelvic cavity, showing the kidneys, ureters, urinary bladder, and the blood supply to the urinary structures.

bladder for temporary storage. When **urination,** or **micturition** (mik-tū-RI-shun; Latin *micturire,* to urinate), occurs, contraction of the muscular urinary bladder forces urine through the urethra and out of the body.

The **kidneys** are located on either side of the vertebral column between the last thoracic and third lumbar vertebrae. Each brownish red kidney has the shape of a kidney bean. A prominent medial indentation, the **hilus** (HĪ-lus; Latin *hilum,* a little thing), is the point of entry for the renal artery and of exit for the renal vein and ureter (Figure 9–27). A fibrous **renal capsule** covers the kidney and folds inward at the hilus to line an internal cavity, the **renal sinus.** The **renal cortex** is the outer layer of the kidney in contact with the capsule. The **renal medulla** consists of 6 to 18 distinct conical or triangular structures called **renal pyramids.** The base of each pyramid faces the cortex, and the tip, or **renal papilla,** projects into the renal sinus.

Each renal papilla discharges urine into a cup-shaped drain, called a **minor calyx** (KĀ-liks; Greek *kalyx,* cup). Four or five minor **calyces** (KĀL-i-sēz) merge to form a **major calyx,** and two of the major calyces combine to form a large, funnel-shaped chamber, the renal pelvis. The **renal pelvis,** which fills most of the renal sinus, is connected to the ureter at the hilus of the kidney.

Urine production begins in the cortex of each renal lobe, at microscopic structures called **nephrons** (NEF-ronz) (Figure 9–28). There are roughly 1.25 million nephrons in each kidney, with a combined length of around 145 km (85 miles). Each nephron consists of a **renal tubule.** The tubule has two convoluted (coiled or twisted) segments separated by a simple U-shaped tube. The convoluted segments are in the cortex, and the tube extends partially or completely into the medulla.

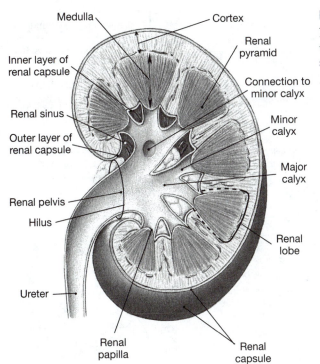

Figure 9–27   Structure of the Kidney.
Diagrammatic view of a frontal section through the left kidney, showing major structures

The renal tubule begins at an expanded chamber called a **renal corpuscle** (KŌR-pus-ul). The renal corpuscle includes (1) a capillary knot, or **glomerulus** (glō-MER-ū-lus; Latin *glomerulus*, little ball), and (2) the expanded initial segment of the renal tubule, a region known as **Bowman's capsule.** Blood arrives at the glomerulus via the **afferent arteriole** and departs the glomerulus through the **efferent arteriole.**

Filtration occurs in the renal corpuscle as blood pressure forces fluid and dissolved solutes out of the glomerular capillaries and into the capsular space. Filtration produces an essentially protein-free solution known as a **filtrate** that is otherwise very similar to blood plasma. Filtration is a passive process that permits or prevents movement across a barrier solely on the basis of solute size. A filter with pores large enough to permit the passage of organic waste products is unable to prevent the passage of water, ions, and other organic molecules, such as glucose, fatty acids, and amino acids. These useful substances must be reclaimed and the waste products excreted. The segments of the nephron distal to the renal corpuscle are responsible for:

- Reabsorbing all of the useful organic substances from the filtrate.
- Reabsorbing over 90 percent of the water in the filtrate.
- Secreting into the tubular fluid any waste products that were missed by the filtration process.

From the renal corpuscle, the filtrate enters a long tubular passageway that is subdivided into regions with varied structural and functional characteristics. Major subdivisions include the proximal convoluted tubule, the loop of Henle (HEN-lē), and the distal convoluted tubule. As it travels along the tubule, the filtrate, now called **tubular fluid**, gradually changes its composition. The changes that occur and the characteristics of the urine that result depend on the specialized activities under way in each segment of the nephron.

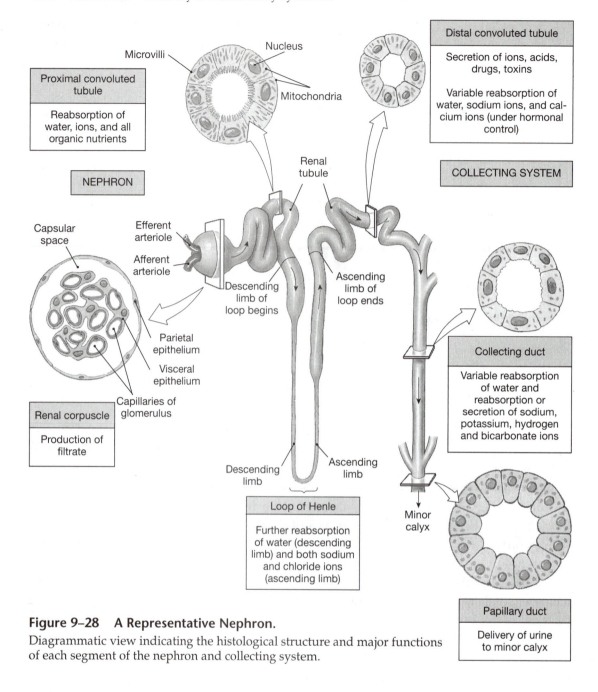

Figure 9–28 A Representative Nephron.
Diagrammatic view indicating the histological structure and major functions of each segment of the nephron and collecting system.

The **proximal convoluted tubule (PCT)** is a twisted portion of the renal tubule that is lined by a simple cuboidal epithelium with a microvillous surface. The cuboidal tubular cells actively absorb organic nutrients, ions, and plasma proteins (if any) from the tubular fluid and release them into the **peritubular fluid,** the interstitial fluid surrounding the renal tubule. As these solutes are absorbed and transported, osmotic forces pull water across the wall of the PCT and into the peritubular fluid. Although reabsorption represents the primary function of the PCT, the epithelial cells can also secrete substances into the lumen.

The proximal convoluted tubule ends at a bend that turns the renal tubule toward the medulla. This bend marks the start of the **loop of Henle.** The loop of Henle can be divided into a descending limb and an ascending limb. The **descending limb** travels in the medulla toward the renal pelvis, and the **ascending limb** returns toward the cortex. The ascending limb, which begins deep in the medulla, contains active transport mechanisms that pump sodium and chloride ions out of the tubular fluid. As a result of these transport activities, the interstitial fluid of the medulla contains an unusually high concentration of solutes. The ascending limb of the loop of Henle ends where it forms a sharp angle that places the tubular wall in close contact with the glomerulus and its accompanying vessels.

The **distal convoluted tubule (DCT)** begins at the end of the loop of Henle. The distal convoluted tubule is an important site for:

- The active secretion of ions, acids, and other materials.
- The selective reabsorption of sodium ions from the tubular fluid.

In the distal portions of the DCT an osmotic flow of water may assist in concentrating the tubular fluid.

Each nephron empties into the collecting system. A **collecting tubule** connected to the distal convoluted tubule carries the tubular fluid toward a nearby collecting duct. The **collecting duct,** which receives tubular fluid from many different nephrons, leaves the cortex and enters the medulla carrying fluid toward a **papillary duct** that drains into a minor calyx.

Additional water and salts will be removed in the collecting system before the urine is released into the renal sinus. You will find an overview of important information concerning the regions of the nephron and collecting system in Figure 9–28 and Table 9–2.

Basic Principles of Urine Formation

The goal in urine production is the maintenance of homeostasis by regulating the volume and composition of the blood. This process involves the excretion and elimination of solutes, specifically metabolic waste products. The most noteworthy organic waste products are:

- **Urea:** Urea is the most abundant organic waste, and roughly 1800 mg of urea is generated each day. Most of it is produced during the breakdown of amino acids.
- **Creatinine: Creatinine** (krē-AT-i-nēn) is generated in skeletal muscle tissue through the breakdown of creatine phosphate, a high-energy compound that plays an important role in muscle contraction.
- **Uric acid:** Approximately 40 mg of **uric** (ū-rik) **acid** is produced each day during the recycling of nitrogenous bases from RNA molecules.

These waste products must be excreted in solution, so their elimination is accompanied by an unavoidable water loss. The normal kidneys are capable of producing a concentrated urine with an osmotic concentration more than four times that of plasma. If the kidneys were not able to concentrate the filtrate produced by glomerular filtration, fluid losses would lead to a fatal dehydration in hours. At the same time, the kidneys ensure that the fluid that is lost does not contain potentially useful organic substances, such as sugars or amino acids, that are found in blood plasma. These valuable materials must be reabsorbed and retained for use by other tissues.

Table 9–2 The Organization of the Nephron and Collecting System in the Kidney

Region	Primary Function	Histological Characteristics
NEPHRON		
Renal corpuscle	Filtration of plasma	Glomerulus (capillary knot), enclosed by capsular space within Bowman's capsule
Renal tubule		
Proximal convoluted tubule (PCT)	Reabsorption of ions, organic molecules, vitamins, water; secretion of drugs, toxins, acids	Cuboidal cells with microvilli
Loop of Henle	Descending limb: reabsorption of water from tubular fluid Ascending limb: reabsorption of ions; assists in creation of a concentration gradient in the medulla	Low cuboidal or squamous cells
Distal convoluted tubule (DCT)	Reabsorption of sodium ions and calcium ions; secretion of acids, ammonia, drugs, toxins	Cuboidal cells with few microvilli
COLLECTING SYSTEM		
Connecting tubule	Reabsorption of water, sodium ions; secretion or reabsorption of hydrogen ions or bicarbonate ions	Cuboidal cells without microvilli
Collecting duct	Reabsorption of water, sodium ions; secretion or reabsorption of bicarbonate ions or hydrogen ions	Cuboidal to columnar cells
Papillary duct	Conduction of tubular fluid to minor calyx; contributes to concentration gradient of the medulla	Columnar cells

To accomplish these goals, the kidneys rely on three distinct processes.

1. In **filtration,** blood pressure forces water across a filtration membrane. At the kidneys, the filtration membrane includes the glomerular endothelium and the lining of Bowman's capsule. Solute molecules small enough to pass through this filtration complex are carried along by the surrounding water molecules.

2. **Reabsorption** is the removal of water and solute molecules from the filtrate after it enters the renal tubules. Materials reabsorbed from the filtrate are usually nutrients that can be used by the body. Whereas filtration occurs solely on the basis of size, reabsorption is a selective process. Solute reabsorption may involve simple diffusion or the activity of carrier proteins in the tubular epithelium. The reabsorbed substances pass into the peritubular fluid and eventually reenter the blood. Water reabsorption occurs passively through osmosis.

3. **Secretion** is the transport of solutes from the peritubular fluid, across the tubular epithelium, and into the tubular fluid. Secretion is necessary because filtration does not force all of the dissolved materials out of the plasma. Tubular secretion pro-

vides a backup for the filtration process and can further lower the plasma concentrations of undesirable materials. Secretion can represent the primary method of excretion of some compounds, including many drugs.

All segments of the nephron and collecting system participate in the process of urine formation. Most regions of the nephron perform a combination of reabsorption and secretion, but the balance between the two shifts from one region to another.

1. Filtration occurs exclusively in the renal corpuscle, across the glomerular walls.
2. Nutrient reabsorption occurs primarily at the proximal convoluted tubule.
3. Active secretion occurs primarily at the distal convoluted tubule.
4. The loop of Henle and the collecting system interact to regulate the amount of water and the number of sodium and potassium ions lost in the urine.

The final composition and concentration of the tubular fluid will be determined by the events under way in the DCT and the collecting system. Although the DCT, collecting tubule, and collecting duct are generally impermeable to solute molecules, the osmolarity of the tubular fluid can be adjusted through active transport.

The osmotic concentration of the urine is controlled by variations in water permeabilities of the distal portions of the DCT, the collecting tubules, and the collecting ducts. These segments are impermeable to water unless exposed to **antidiuretic hormone (ADH)** from the posterior pituitary. At normal concentrations of ADH, the distal portions of the DCT and the collecting tubules and ducts are somewhat permeable to water, and there is an osmotic flow of water out of the tubular fluid as it passes along the collecting ducts. If the ADH levels rise, the water permeability increases, and additional water leaves the fluid in the DCT and collecting system. The urine thus becomes more concentrated. If ADH levels decline, the amount of water reclaimed by these regions decreases, and the urine becomes more dilute.

Normal kidney function can continue only as long as the processes of filtration, reabsorption, and secretion function within relatively narrow limits. A disruption in kidney function has immediate effects on the composition of the circulating blood. If both kidneys are affected, death will occur within a few days unless medical assistance is provided.

Urine Transport, Storage, and Elimination

The ureters are a pair of muscular tubes that carry the urine formed in the kidneys to the urinary bladder (Figure 9–29). The **urinary bladder** is a hollow muscular organ that functions as a temporary "storage reservoir" for urine. The dimensions of the urinary bladder vary depending on the state of distension, but the full urinary bladder can contain about a liter of urine. The opening to the urethra lies at the most inferior point of the bladder. The region surrounding the urethral opening, known as the **neck** of the urinary bladder, contains a muscular **internal urethral sphincter.** The smooth muscle fibers of the internal urethral sphincter provide involuntary control over the discharge of urine from the bladder.

The **urethra** (ū-RĒ-thra) extends from the neck of the urinary bladder to the exterior. In the female, the urethra is very short. The **external urethral opening,** or **external urethral meatus,** is situated near the anterior wall of the vagina. In the male, the urethra extends from the neck of the urinary bladder to the tip of the penis. The external urethral

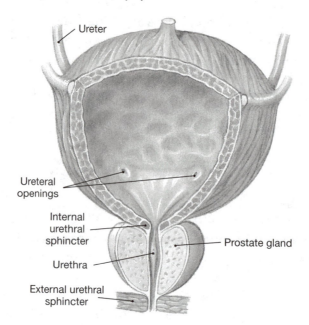

Figure 9–29   The Organs for the Conduction and Storage of Urine.
The urinary bladder of a male.

meatus is located at the tip of the penis. In both sexes, as the urethra passes through the floor of the pelvis, a circular band of skeletal muscle forms the **external urethral sphincter.** The contractions of both the external and internal urethral sphincters are controlled by the nervous system. Only the external urethral sphincter is under voluntary control.

Urine reaches the urinary bladder by the peristaltic contractions of the ureters. The process of urination is coordinated by the **micturition reflex.** Stretch receptors in the wall of the urinary bladder are stimulated as it fills with urine. Afferent fibers in the pelvic nerves carry the impulses generated to the sacral spinal cord. As a result, we become consciously aware of the fluid pressure in the urinary bladder. The micturition reflex begins to function when the stretch receptors have provided adequate stimulation to parasympathetic motor neurons. Activity in these motor neurons generates efferent impulses that produce a sustained contraction of the urinary bladder. This contraction elevates fluid pressure in the urinary bladder, but urine ejection does not occur unless both the internal and external sphincters are relaxed. Relaxation of the external sphincter occurs under voluntary control. When the external sphincter relaxes so does the internal sphincter. If the external sphincter does not relax the internal sphincter remains closed. Once the volume of the urinary bladder exceeds 500 ml, the micturition reflex may generate enough pressure to force open the internal sphincter. This opening leads to a reflexive relaxation in the external sphincter, and urination occurs despite voluntary opposition or the potential inconvenience.

Integration with Other Systems

The urinary system is not the only organ system concerned with excretion. The urinary, integumentary, respiratory, and digestive systems are sometimes considered to form an anatomically diverse excretory system. The components of this system perform all of the excretory functions of the body that affect the composition of body fluids. Examples of excretory activities discussed earlier include:

1. **Integumentary system:** Water and electrolyte losses in perspiration can affect plasma volume and composition. The effects are most apparent when losses are extreme, as in maximal sweat production. Small amounts of metabolic wastes, including urea, are also excreted in perspiration.

2. **Respiratory system:** The lungs excrete the carbon dioxide generated by living cells. Small amounts of other compounds, such as acetone and water, evaporate into the alveoli and are eliminated during exhalation.

3. **Digestive system:** Small amounts of metabolic waste products are excreted by the liver in bile, and a variable amount of water is lost in feces.

These excretory activities have an impact on the composition of body fluids. The respiratory system, for example, is the primary site of carbon dioxide excretion. But the excretory functions of these systems are not regulated as closely as are those of the kidneys, and under normal circumstances the effects of integumentary and digestive excretory activities are minor compared with those of the urinary system. Figure 9–30 summarizes the functional relationships between the urinary system and other systems.

Let's Review What You've Just Learned

▶ **Definitions**

In the space provided, write the term for each of the following definitions.

_____ **182.** The basic functional unit of a kidney.

_____ **183.** An indentation on the medial surface of the kidney.

_____ **184.** A pair of muscular tubes that carry urine from the kidneys to the urinary bladder.

_____ **185.** A layer of collagen fibers that covers the outer surface of the kidney.

_____ **186.** The expanded initial segment of the renal tubule.

_____ **187.** The structure that connects a nephron to a collecting duct.

_____ **188.** The tube that carries urine from the urinary bladder to the exterior.

_____ **189.** Triangular structures that make up the renal medulla.

_____ **190.** The interstitial fluid that surrounds the renal tubule.

_____ **191.** A hollow muscular organ that serves as a temporary storage reservoir for urine.

_____ **192.** The structure formed by the fusion of the major calyces.

_____ **193.** The blood vessel that carries blood into the glomerulus.

_____ **194.** The external opening of the urethra.

_____ **195.** The tip of a renal pyramid that projects into the renal sinus.

_____ **196.** A duct of the collecting system that drains directly into a minor calyx.

_____ **197.** A ring of smooth muscle located in the neck of the urinary bladder.

_____ **198.** The outer layer of the kidney.

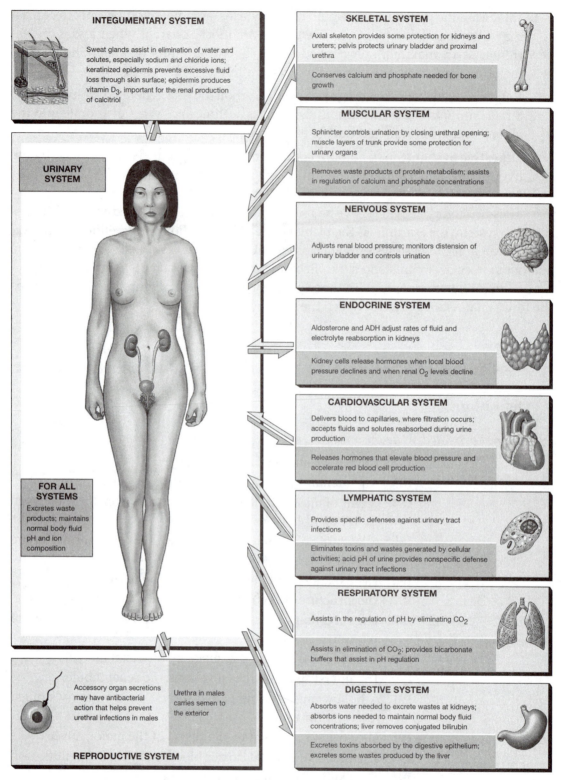

INTEGUMENTARY SYSTEM

Sweat glands assist in elimination of water and solutes, especially sodium and chloride ions; keratinized epidermis prevents excessive fluid loss through skin surface; epidermis produces vitamin D₃, important for the renal production of calcitriol

URINARY SYSTEM

FOR ALL SYSTEMS
Excretes waste products; maintains normal body fluid pH and ion composition

SKELETAL SYSTEM

Axial skeleton provides some protection for kidneys and ureters; pelvis protects urinary bladder and proximal urethra

Conserves calcium and phosphate needed for bone growth

MUSCULAR SYSTEM

Sphincter controls urination by closing urethral opening; muscle layers of trunk provide some protection for urinary organs

Removes waste products of protein metabolism; assists in regulation of calcium and phosphate concentrations

NERVOUS SYSTEM

Adjusts renal blood pressure; monitors distension of urinary bladder and controls urination

ENDOCRINE SYSTEM

Aldosterone and ADH adjust rates of fluid and electrolyte reabsorption in kidneys

Kidney cells release hormones when local blood pressure declines and when renal O_2 levels decline

CARDIOVASCULAR SYSTEM

Delivers blood to capillaries, where filtration occurs; accepts fluids and solutes reabsorbed during urine production

Releases hormones that elevate blood pressure and accelerate red blood cell production

LYMPHATIC SYSTEM

Provides specific defenses against urinary tract infections

Eliminates toxins and wastes generated by cellular activities; acid pH of urine provides nonspecific defense against urinary tract infections

RESPIRATORY SYSTEM

Assists in the regulation of pH by eliminating CO_2

Assists in elimination of CO_2; provides bicarbonate buffers that assist in pH regulation

Accessory organ secretions may have antibacterial action that helps prevent urethral infections in males

Urethra in males carries semen to the exterior

DIGESTIVE SYSTEM

Absorbs water needed to excrete wastes at kidneys; absorbs ions needed to maintain normal body fluid concentrations; liver removes conjugated bilirubin

Excretes toxins absorbed by the digestive epithelium; excretes some wastes produced by the liver

REPRODUCTIVE SYSTEM

Figure 9–30   Functional Relationships between the Urinary System and Other Systems.

_____ **199.** A cup-shaped drain that receives urine from the renal papilla.

_____ **200.** A capillary knot located in the renal corpuscle.

_____ **201.** The twisted portion of the nephron that drains filtrate from Bowman's capsule.

_____ **202.** A hormone from the posterior pituitary gland that regulates the permeability of the DCT and the collecting system to water.

_____ **203.** The portion of the kidney that is made up of renal pyramids.

_____ **204.** A waste product produced in skeletal muscle tissue when creatine phosphate is broken down.

_____ **205.** Another term for urination.

_____ **206.** A structure that receives tubular fluid from several different nephrons and carries it to a papillary duct.

_____ **207.** The region of a kidney where you find the renal artery, renal vein, and ureter.

_____ **208.** A blood vessel that carries blood away from the glomerulus.

_____ **209.** A U-shaped segment of a nephron that descends from the cortex to the medulla then ascends back into the cortex.

_____ **210.** A circular band of skeletal muscle that surrounds the urethra where it passes through the floor of the pelvis.

_____ **211.** An internal cavity formed by inward folding of the renal capsule at the hilus.

_____ **212.** A structure formed by the fusion of four or five minor calyces.

_____ **213.** The expanded origin of a renal tubule.

_____ **214.** An essentially protein-free solution that collects in Bowman's capsule.

_____ **215.** The twisted portion of the nephron that lies between the loop of Henle and the collecting tubule.

_____ **216.** A waste product produced from the recycling of nitrogenous bases from RNA.

_____ **217.** A large, funnel-shaped chamber formed from the fusion of major calyces.

_____ **218.** The term applied to the filtrate as it passes along the renal tubule.

▶ Word Roots, Prefixes, Suffixes, and Combining Forms

In the space provided, list the boldfaced terms introduced in this section that contain the indicated word part.

Word Part	Meaning	Examples
nephr-	kidney	**219.** _____
affer-	carry toward	**220.** _____
peri-	around	**221.** _____
effer-	carry away	**222.** _____

THE REPRODUCTIVE SYSTEM

The reproductive system includes:

- Reproductive organs, or **gonads** (GŌ-nadz; Greek _gonos_, seed), that produce gametes and hormones.

- Ducts that receive and transport the gametes.

- Accessory glands and organs that secrete fluids into these or other excretory ducts.

- Perineal structures associated with the reproductive system. These perineal structures are collectively known as the **external genitalia** (jen-i-TĀ-lē-uh).

The male and female reproductive systems are functionally quite different. In the adult male, the gonads, or **testes** (TES-tēz; singular *testis*), secrete androgens, principally testosterone, and produce one-half billion sperm each day. After storage, mature sperm travel along a lengthy duct system, where they are mixed with the secretions of accessory glands. The mixture created is known as **semen** (SĒ-men). During *ejaculation* the semen is expelled from the body.

The female gonads, or **ovaries,** typically release only one immature ovum a month. This gamete travels along short uterine tubes (oviducts) that end in the muscular **uterus** (Ū-ter-us). A short passageway, the **vagina** (va-JĪ-na; Latin *vagina*, sheath), connects the uterus with the exterior. During the sexual act, male ejaculation introduces semen into the vagina, and the sperm cells ascend the female reproductive tract. If fertilization occurs, the uterus will enclose and support a developing embryo as it grows into a fetus and prepares for eventual delivery.

The Reproductive System of the Male

The principal structures of the male reproductive system are shown in Figure 9–31. Proceeding from the testes, the sperm cells, or spermatozoa, travel along the **epididymis** (ep-i-DID-i-mus), the **ductus deferens** (DUK-tus DEF-e-renz), the **ejaculatory** (ē-JAK-ū-la-tō-rē) **duct,** and the urethra before leaving the body. Accessory organs, notably the **seminal** (SEM-i-nal) **vesicles,** the **prostate** (PROS-tāt) **gland,** and the **bulbourethral** (bul-

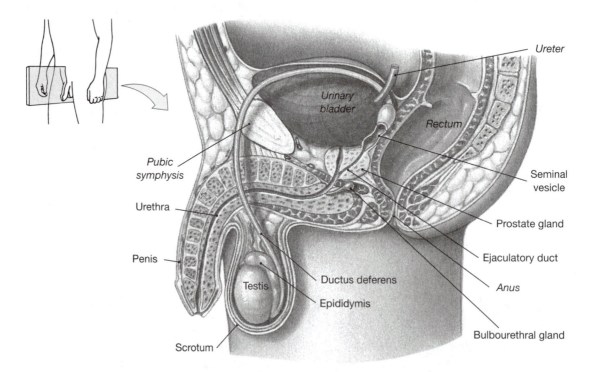

Figure 9–31 The Male Reproductive System.
The male reproductive organs, diagrammatic sagittal section.

bō-ū-RĒ-thral) **glands,** secrete into the ejaculatory ducts and urethra. The external genitalia include the **scrotum** (SKRŌ-tum), which encloses the testes, and the **penis** (PĒ-nis), an erectile organ that surrounds the distal portion of the urethra.

Each testis has the shape of a flattened oval and hangs within the scrotum. Beneath the serous membrane covering the testis lies the **tunica albuginea** (TOO-ni-ka al-bū-JIN-ē-uh), a dense layer of connective tissue. The collagen fibers of the tunica albuginea extend into the substance of the testis, forming fibrous partitions, or **septa** (SEP-ta). The septa subdivide the testis into a series of **lobules.** Roughly 800 slender, tightly coiled **seminiferous** (se-mi-NIF-er-us) **tubules** are distributed among the lobules. Sperm production occurs within these tubules (see Chapter 7). Each seminiferous tubule contains spermatogonia, spermatocytes at various stages of meiosis, spermatids, spermatozoa, and large **sustentacular** (sus-ten-TAK-ū-lar) **cells.** Within the spaces between seminiferous tubules are found large **interstitial cells.** Interstitial cells are responsible for the production of sex hormones called **androgens.** Testosterone is the most important androgen.

The testes produce physically mature spermatozoa that are, as yet, incapable of fertilizing an ovum. The other portions of the male reproductive system are concerned with the functional maturation, nourishment, storage, and transport of spermatozoa. Although sperm in the seminiferous tubules have most of the physical characteristics of mature sperm cells, they are still functionally immature and incapable of coordinated locomotion or fertilization. Fluid currents transport the spermatozoa into the epididymis, which lies along the posterior border of the testis. The epididymis has the following functions.

1. It monitors and adjusts the composition of the fluid that surrounds the spermatozoa.

2. It acts as a recycling center for damaged spermatozoa.

3. It stores spermatozoa and facilitates their functional maturation.

Transport along the epididymis involves some combination of fluid movement and peristaltic contractions of smooth muscle. After passing along the epididymis, the spermatozoa enter the ductus deferens.

The ductus deferens begins at the epididymis and ascends through the **inguinal canal,** a passage through the abdominal wall, in the spermatic cord. The **spermatic cords** consist of layers of fascia, tough connective tissue, and muscle enclosing the ductus deferens, and the blood vessels, nerves, and lymphatics supplying the testes. Inside the abdominal cavity, the ductus deferens passes along the posterior of the urinary bladder toward the prostate gland. Just before it reaches the prostate and seminal vesicles, the ductus deferens becomes enlarged, and the expanded portion is known as the **ampulla** (am-PŪ-luh; Latin *ampulla*, small flask). Peristaltic contractions propel spermatozoa and fluid along the ductus deferens. In addition to transporting sperm, the ductus deferens can store spermatozoa for several months. During this time the spermatozoa remain in a state of suspended animation, with low metabolic rates.

The junction of the ampulla with the base of the seminal vesicle marks the start of the ejaculatory duct. This relatively short passageway penetrates the muscular wall of the prostate gland and empties into the urethra near the ejaculatory duct from the opposite side. The urethra in the male is a passageway used by both the urinary and reproductive systems.

The fluids contributed by the seminiferous tubules and the epididymis account for only about 5 percent of the final volume of semen. The **seminal fluid** is a mixture of the secretions of many different glands; each secretion has distinctive biochemical characteristics. Important glands include the seminal vesicles, the prostate gland, and the bulbourethral glands. Major functions of these glandular organs include: (1) activating the spermatozoa; (2) providing the nutrients spermatozoa need for motility; (3) propelling spermatozoa and fluids along the reproductive tract, primarily through peristaltic contractions; and (4) producing buffers that counteract the acidity of the urethral and vaginal contents.

The penis is a tubular organ that surrounds the urethra. It conducts urine to the exterior and introduces semen into the female vagina during sexual intercourse. The penis is divided into three regions.

- The **root of the penis** is the fixed portion that attaches the penis to the body wall.
- The **body (shaft) of the penis** is the tubular movable portion. Masses of erectile tissue are found within the body.
- The **glans** (glanz; Latin *glans*, acorn) of the penis is the expanded distal end that surrounds the external urethral meatus.

The major hormones that regulate male reproduction are follicle-stimulating hormone (FSH), luteinizing hormone (LH), and androgens. In the male, **FSH** targets primarily the sustentacular cells of the seminiferous tubules. Under FSH stimulation and in the presence of the male hormone testosterone from the interstitial cells, sustentacular cells (1) promote spermatogenesis and spermiogenesis and (2) secrete a protein called *androgen-binding protein* that binds testosterone and concentrates high levels of the hormone in the seminiferous tubules for the support of sperm production and (3) secrete **inhibin**, a hormone that suppresses secretion of FSH. (Inhibin secretion thus regulates FSH production through negative feedback.) **LH** causes the secretion of testosterone and other androgens by the interstitial cells of the testes. **Testosterone,** the most important androgen, has numerous functions that include:

1. Stimulating spermatogenesis and promoting the functional maturation of spermatozoa.
2. Maintaining the accessory organs of the male reproductive tract.
3. Determining the secondary sexual characteristics, such as the distribution of facial hair, increased muscle mass and body size, and the quantity and location of characteristic adipose tissue deposits.
4. Stimulating metabolism throughout the body, especially pathways concerned with protein synthesis and muscle growth.
5. Affecting **libido** (li-BĒ-dō) (sexual drive) and related behaviors.

The Reproductive System of the Female

A woman's reproductive system must produce sex hormones and functional gametes and also protect and support a developing embryo. The principal organs of the female reproductive system (Figure 9–32) include the ovaries, the uterine tubes (Fallopian tubes, or oviducts), the uterus, the vagina, and the components of the external genitalia. As in the male, a variety of accessory glands secrete into the reproductive tract.

The **ovaries** are small, almond-shaped organs located near the lateral walls of the pelvic cavity. The ovaries are responsible for (1) the production of female gametes, or ova; (2) the secretion of female sex hormones, including estrogens and progestins; and (3) the secretion of **inhibin** (in-HIB-in), involved in the feedback control of pituitary FSH production.

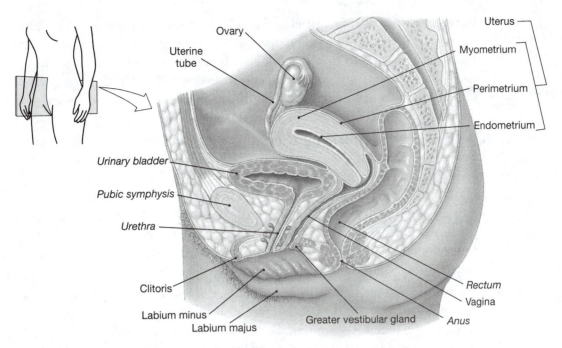

Figure 9–32   The Female Reproductive System.
The female reproductive organs, diagrammatic sagittal section.

Ovarian follicles are specialized structures where oocyte growth and meiosis I occur. The ovarian follicles are located in the outer layer (cortex) of the ovary. Each primary oocyte (see Chapter 7) is surrounded by a simple squamous layer of **follicular cells**, and the combination is known as a **primordial** (prī-MOR-dē-al) **follicle.** After sexual maturation has occurred, a different group of primordial follicles is activated approximately every 28 days. This process is known as the **ovarian cycle** (Figure 9–33). Important steps in the ovarian cycle are summarized on following page.

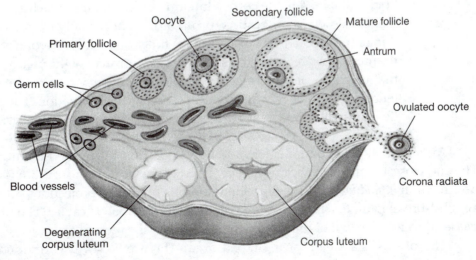

Figure 9–33   The Ovarian Cycle.
Primordial follicles are present in the ovaries of a female from the time of birth. During each ovarian cycle, as many as two dozen of these follicles will begin to develop and grow. Usually only one of the follicles eventually develops into a mature follicle. After ovulation, the remaining cells of the follicle from a corpus luteum that is responsible for secreting the hormone progesterone and maintaining the uterus if pregnancy occurs.

Step 1: **Formation of primary follicles:** Follicle formation is stimulated by **FSH** from the anterior pituitary. The ovarian cycle begins as activated primordial follicles develop into primary follicles. In a **primary follicle** the follicular cells enlarge and undergo repeated cell divisions. This division creates several layers of follicular cells around the oocyte. These follicle cells are now called **granulosa** (gran-ū-LŌ-suh) **cells.**

Step 2: **Formation of secondary follicles:** Although many primordial follicles develop into primary follicles, only a few will proceed to the next step. The transformation begins as the wall of the follicle thickens and the deeper follicular cells begin secreting small amounts of fluid. This **follicular fluid** accumulates in small pockets that gradually expand. At this stage, the complex is known as a **secondary follicle.** Although the primary oocyte continues to grow at a steady pace, the follicle as a whole now enlarges rapidly because of the accumulation of follicular fluid.

Step 3: **Formation of a tertiary follicle:** Eight to ten days after the start of the ovarian cycle, the ovaries usually contain only a single secondary follicle destined for further development. By the tenth to fourteenth day of the cycle it has formed a **tertiary follicle.** Until this time, the primary oocyte has been suspended in prophase of the first meiotic division. As the tertiary follicle completes its development, **LH** levels begin rising, and the primary oocyte now completes meiosis, producing a secondary oocyte and a small, nonfunctional polar body.

Step 4: **Ovulation:** At ovulation the tertiary follicle releases the secondary oocyte.

Step 5: **Formation and degeneration of the corpus luteum:** The empty tertiary follicle initially collapses, and ruptured vessels bleed into it. The remaining granulosa cells then invade the area, proliferating to create an endocrine structure known as the **corpus luteum** (LOO-tē-um; Latin *luteus,* yellow), named for its yellow color. This process occurs under LH stimulation. The lipids contained in the corpus luteum are used to manufacture steroid hormones known as **progestins** (prō-JES-tinz), principally the steroid **progesterone** (prō-JES-ter-ōn). The primary function of progesterone is to prepare the uterus for pregnancy by stimulating the growth of the uterine lining and the secretions of uterine glands. Unless pregnancy occurs, the corpus luteum begins to degenerate roughly 12 days after ovulation. The disintegration, or **involution,** of the corpus luteum marks the end of the ovarian cycle.

After ovulation, an ovum enters a hollow, muscular tube called the **uterine tube.** The end closest to the ovary forms an expanded funnel, or **infundibulum** (in-fun-DIB-ū-lum; Latin *infundibulum,* funnel), with numerous fingerlike projections called **fimbriae** (FIM-brē-ē; Latin *fimbria,* fringe) that extend into the pelvic cavity. The uterine tube passes through the wall of the uterus and opens into the uterine cavity.

The **uterus** is a small, pear-shaped organ (Figure 9–34). It is divided into two anatomical regions: the body and the cervix. The **uterine body,** or **corpus** (KOR-pus; Latin *corpus,* body), is the largest division of the uterus. The **cervix** (SER-viks; Latin *cervix,* neck) is the tubular, inferior portion of the uterus that projects into the vagina. The uterus provides mechanical protection, nutritional support, and waste removal for the developing embryo and fetus. In addition, contractions in the muscular wall of the uterus are important in ejecting the fetus at the time of birth.

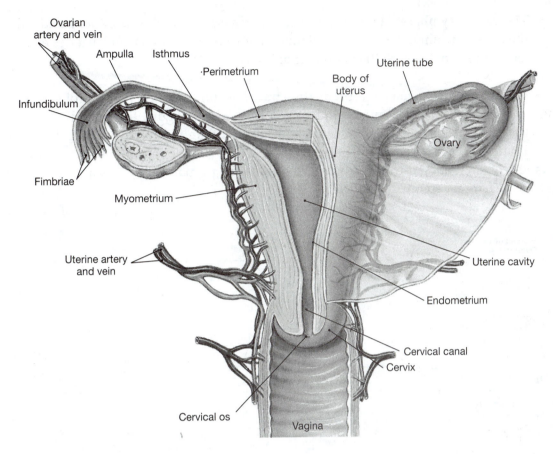

Figure 9–34   The Uterus.
A posterior view of the uterus with the left uterus, uterine tube, and ovary shown in section.

The uterine wall has an outer, muscular **myometrium** (mī-ō-MĒ-trē-um; Greek *myos*, muscle + *metra*, womb) and an inner glandular **endometrium** (en-dō-MĒ-trē-um). The superior and posterior surfaces of the uterine body are covered by a serous membrane continuous with the peritoneal lining. This incomplete serosal layer is called the **perimetrium** (per-i-MĒ-trē-um). The glandular and vascular tissues of the endometrium support the physiological demands of the growing fetus. The smooth muscle of the myometrium provides much of the force needed to move a large fetus out of the uterus and into the vagina.

The **uterine cycle,** or **menstrual** (MEN-stroo-al; Latin *menstrualis*, monthly) **cycle,** is a repeating series of changes in the structure of the endometrium. It is intimately related to the ovarian cycle and occurs in synchrony with the events of the ovarian cycle. Like the ovarian cycle, the uterine cycle averages 28 days in length, but it can range from 21 to 35 days in normal individuals. The cycle can be divided into three phases.

1. **Menses:** The uterine cycle begins with the onset of **menses** (MEN-sēz; Latin *menses*, months), a period marked by the degeneration of the outer layer of the endometrium. Blood cells and degenerating tissues break away and enter the uterine lumen. The sloughing of tissue is gradual and is called **menstruation** (men-stroo-Ā-shun).

2. **The proliferative phase:** In the days following the completion of menses, the epithelial cells of the remaining layer of endometrium multiply and spread across the endometrial surface, restoring it. Further growth and vascularization will result in the complete restoration of the endometrial lining. As this reorganization proceeds, the endometrium is said to be in the **proliferative phase.**

3. **The secretory phase:** During the secretory phase of the uterine cycle, glands in the endometrium enlarge and accelerate their rates of secretion, and arteries elongate and spiral through the endometrial lining.

The activity of the female reproductive tract falls under hormonal control involving an interplay between pituitary and gonadal secretions (Figure 9–35). But the regulatory pattern of females is much more complicated than in males, because it must coordinate the ovarian and uterine cycles to ensure proper reproductive function. Changes in circulating estrogen concentrations are the primary mechanism for coordinating the female reproductive cycle.

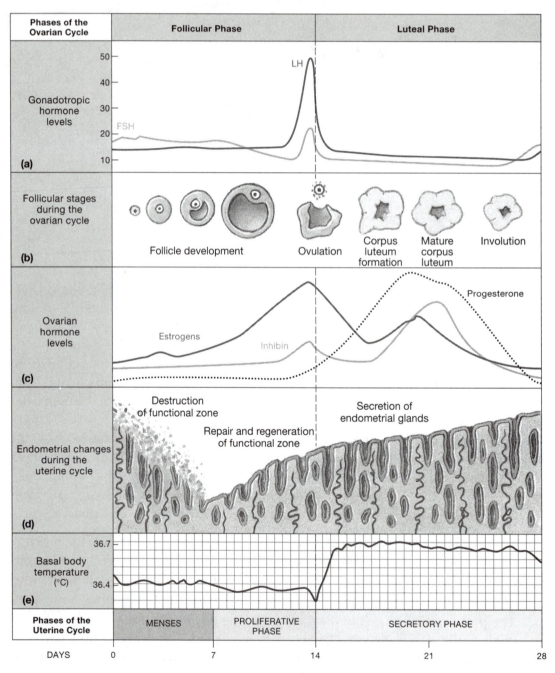

Figure 9–35   Hormonal Regulation of the Female Reproductive Cycle.

As noted previously, follicular development begins under FSH stimulation. As the follicles enlarge they start secreting estrogens. The hormone **estradiol** (es-tra-DĪ-ol) is the most important estrogen, and it is the dominant hormone before ovulation. Estrogens have multiple functions, affecting the activities of many different tissues and organs throughout the body. Important general functions include (1) stimulating bone and muscle growth, (2) maintaining female secondary sex characteristics such as body hair distribution and the location of adipose tissue deposits, (3) affecting CNS activity, (4) maintaining functional accessory reproductive glands and organs, and (5) initiating repair and growth to the endometrium.

After ovulation, LH stimulates the formation of the corpus luteum and its secretion of progestins. Although moderate amounts of estrogens are also secreted by the corpus luteum, progesterone is the principal hormone of the period following ovulation. Its primary function is to prepare the uterus for pregnancy by stimulating the growth and development of the blood supply and secretory glands of the endometrium.

The hormonal changes involved with the ovarian cycle in turn affect the activities of other reproductive tissues and organs. For instance, at the uterus, the hormonal changes are responsible for maintenance of the uterine cycle.

The vagina is an elastic, muscular tube extending between the cervix of the uterus and the vaginal opening into the vestibule (see Figure 9–34). The vagina has three major functions.

1. It serves as a passageway for the elimination of menstrual fluids.

2. It receives the penis during sexual intercourse and holds spermatozoa before they pass into the uterus.

3. It forms the lower portion of the birth canal through which the fetus passes during delivery.

The region enclosing the female genitalia is usually called the **vulva** (VUL-va; Latin *vulva*, womb), or **pudendum** (pū-DEN-dum; Latin *pudere*, to be ashamed). The vagina opens into the **vestibule,** a central space bounded by the **labia minora** (LĀ-bē-a mi-NŌR-a; Latin, small lips; singular *labium minus*). The urethra opens into the vestibule just anterior to the vaginal entrance. Anterior to the urethral opening, the **clitoris** (KLI-tō-ris) projects into the vestibule. The clitoris is the female equivalent of the penis, derived from the same embryonic structures.

A variable number of small **lesser vestibular glands** discharge their secretions onto the exposed surface of the vestibule, keeping it moistened. During arousal, a pair of ducts discharges the secretions of the **greater vestibular glands** into the vestibule near the posterolateral margins of the vaginal entrance.

The outer limits of the vulva are established by the mons pubis and the labia majora. The prominent bulge of the **mons pubis** is created by adipose tissue beneath the skin anterior to the pubic symphysis. Adipose tissue also accumulates within the fleshy **labia majora** (LĀ-bē-uh ma-JŌR-a; Latin, large lips; singular *labium majus*) which encircle and partially conceal the labia minora and vestibular structures.

Integration with Other Systems

Figure 9–36 summarizes the relationships between the reproductive system and other physiological systems. Normal human reproduction is a complex process that requires the participation of multiple systems. Hormones play a major role in coordinating these

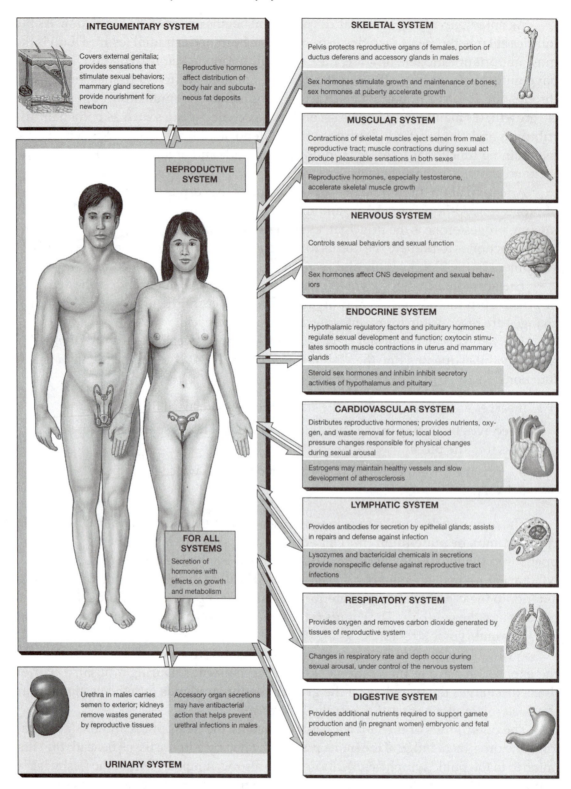

INTEGUMENTARY SYSTEM

Covers external genitalia; provides sensations that stimulate sexual behaviors; mammary gland secretions provide nourishment for newborn

Reproductive hormones affect distribution of body hair and subcutaneous fat deposits

SKELETAL SYSTEM

Pelvis protects reproductive organs of females, portion of ductus deferens and accessory glands in males

Sex hormones stimulate growth and maintenance of bones; sex hormones at puberty accelerate growth

MUSCULAR SYSTEM

Contractions of skeletal muscles eject semen from male reproductive tract; muscle contractions during sexual act produce pleasurable sensations in both sexes

Reproductive hormones, especially testosterone, accelerate skeletal muscle growth

NERVOUS SYSTEM

Controls sexual behaviors and sexual function

Sex hormones affect CNS development and sexual behaviors

ENDOCRINE SYSTEM

Hypothalamic regulatory factors and pituitary hormones regulate sexual development and function; oxytocin stimulates smooth muscle contractions in uterus and mammary glands

Steroid sex hormones and inhibin inhibit secretory activities of hypothalamus and pituitary

CARDIOVASCULAR SYSTEM

Distributes reproductive hormones; provides nutrients, oxygen, and waste removal for fetus; local blood pressure changes responsible for physical changes during sexual arousal

Estrogens may maintain healthy vessels and slow development of atherosclerosis

LYMPHATIC SYSTEM

Provides antibodies for secretion by epithelial glands; assists in repairs and defense against infection

Lysozymes and bactericidal chemicals in secretions provide nonspecific defense against reproductive tract infections

RESPIRATORY SYSTEM

Provides oxygen and removes carbon dioxide generated by tissues of reproductive system

Changes in respiratory rate and depth occur during sexual arousal, under control of the nervous system

DIGESTIVE SYSTEM

Provides additional nutrients required to support gamete production and (in pregnant women) embryonic and fetal development

REPRODUCTIVE SYSTEM

FOR ALL SYSTEMS

Secretion of hormones with effects on growth and metabolism

URINARY SYSTEM

Urethra in males carries semen to exterior; kidneys remove wastes generated by reproductive tissues

Accessory organ secretions may have antibacterial action that helps prevent urethral infections in males

Figure 9–36 Functional Relationships between the Reproductive System and Other Systems.

events. The reproductive process depends on a variety of physical, physiological, and psychological factors, many of which require intersystem cooperation. For example, the male's sperm count must be adequate, the semen must have the correct pH and nutrients, and erection and ejaculation must occur in the proper sequence. For these steps to occur the reproductive, digestive, endocrine, nervous, cardiovascular, and urinary systems must all be functioning normally.

Let's Review What You've Just Learned

▶ **Definitions**

In the space provided, write the term for each of the following definitions.

_____ **223.** The expanded distal end of the penis.

_____ **224.** A general term for reproductive organs.

_____ **225.** The structure composed of a primary oocyte and a simple squamous layer of follicle cells.

_____ **226.** A collective term for the external female genitals.

_____ **227.** The fingerlike projections that surround the infundibulum of the uterine tube.

_____ **228.** The sac that encloses the testes.

_____ **229.** The male gonads.

_____ **230.** Tightly coiled tubules in which spermatozoa are formed.

_____ **231.** An endocrine structure that is formed from the empty tertiary follicle.

_____ **232.** An elastic muscular tube that extends between the cervix and the vestibule.

_____ **233.** The female equivalent of the penis.

_____ **234.** Cells of the testes that are located outside of the seminiferous tubules and secrete androgens.

_____ **235.** The hormone that promotes spermatogenesis and spermiogenesis in males and follicle development in females.

_____ **236.** A central space bounded by the labia minora.

_____ **237.** A general term for the dominant sex hormones in males.

_____ **238.** The fluid found within a secondary or tertiary follicle.

_____ **239.** A collective term for the perineal structures associated with the reproductive system.

_____ **240.** A mature follicle that is ready for ovulation.

_____ **241.** The process of endometrial sloughing.

_____ **242.** The muscular layer in the wall of the uterus.

_____ **243.** A mound of fatty tissue anterior to the pubic symphysis of a female.

_____ **244.** An erectile organ found in males that surrounds the distal portion of the urethra and functions to deposit sperm in the vagina.

_____ **245.** The female gonads.

_____ **246.** The pituitary hormone that stimulates ovulation and the formation of a corpus luteum in females and secretion of androgens by the interstitial cells in males.

_____ **247.** Folds of tissue that form the border of the vestibule.

_____ **248.** The combination of spermatozoa and secretions produced by the male accessory glands of reproduction.

_____ **249.** The period of endometrial degeneration that marks the beginning of the uterine cycle.

_____ **250.** A hollow muscular tube that carries ova to the body of the uterus.

_____ **251.** A repeating series of changes in the endometrium of the uterus.

_____ **252.** A serous membrane that covers the testis.

_____ **253.** A passage through the abdominal wall through which the spermatic cord passes.

_____ **254.** Fleshy, fat-filled folds that surround the labia minora.

_____ **255.** The fluid component of semen.

_____ **256.** The funnel-shaped end of the uterine tube.

_____ **257.** An incomplete serosal layer that covers the superior and posterior portion of the body of the uterus.

_____ **258.** Large cells located within the seminiferous tubules that support spermatogenesis and spermiogenesis.

_____ **259.** A long twisted tubule that lies along the posterior border of the testis and functions in the storage and maturation of spermatozoa.

_____ **260.** Sexual drive.

_____ **261.** A hormone from the gonads that functions in feedback inhibition of FSH.

_____ **262.** The phase of the uterine cycle during which the endometrium is restored.

_____ **263.** The expanded end of the ductus deferens.

_____ **264.** Specialized structures where oocyte growth and meiosis I occur.

_____ **265.** The name given to follicle cells that are produced in the primary follicle.

_____ **266.** A muscular organ that provides mechanical protection, nutritional support, and waste removal for the developing embryo and fetus.

_____ **267.** The phase in the uterine cycle during which the endometrial glands enlarge and increase their rate of secretion and arteries elongate and spiral through the tissue of the endometrium.

_____ **268.** A pair of glands that release a mucous secretion into the vestibule during sexual arousal.

_____ **269.** A tubular structure that carries sperm from the epididymis to the ejaculatory duct.

_____ **270.** A structure consisting of layers of fascia, tough connective tissue, and muscle that encloses the blood vessels, nerves, lymphatics, and ductus deferens that serves a testis.

_____ **271.** The principal male hormone.

_____ **272.** A repeating series of changes involving the activation and development of groups of ovarian follicles.

_____ **273.** The largest division of the uterus.

_____ **274.** Small glands that discharge secretions onto the surface of the vestibule and keep it moistened.

_____ **275.** The most important estrogen.

_____ **276.** A structure formed by the fusion of the duct of a seminal vesicle and the ampulla of a ductus deferens.

_____ **277.** The most important progestin.

_____ **278.** The mucosal lining of the uterus.

_____ **279.** The tubular, inferior portion of the uterus.

_____ **280.** A term for the disintegration of the corpus luteum.

_____ **281.** The cells that form a layer around an oocyte in a primordial follicle.

► Word Roots, Prefixes, Suffixes, and Combining Forms

In the space provided, list the boldfaced terms introduced in this section that contain the indicated word part.

Word Part	Meaning	Examples
gest-	to bear	**282.** _____
myo-	muscle	**283.** _____
corp-	body	**284.** _____
men-	month	**285.** _____
peri-	around	**286.** _____
andro-	male	**287.** _____
-metria	uterus	**288.** _____
cerv-	neck	**289.** _____
lute-	yellow	**290.** _____

☑ Self-Check Test

The following test will allow you to determine how well you have mastered the vocabulary and basic concepts of this chapter. It will also help you prepare for the type of questions you are likely to encounter on a test in an anatomy and physiology course. The self-check test will help you assess your understanding of the chapter material and will help you develop good test-taking skills.

The following questions test your ability to use vocabulary and to recall facts.

1. Plasma proteins that are important in body defense are the
   a. albumins
   b. fibrinogens
   c. immunoglobulins
   d. metalloproteins
   e. lipoproteins

2. Red blood cells are also known as
   a. leukocytes
   b. erythrocytes
   c. granulocytes
   d. agranulocytes
   e. thrombocytes

3. Cell fragments that function in clotting are
   a. leukocytes
   b. lymphocytes

   c. phagocytes

   d. platelets

   e. neutrophils

4. The chamber collecting venous blood from the heart itself is the

   a. ventricle

   b. coronary sinus

   c. interatrial septum

   d. auricle

   e. mitral valve

5. The left ventricle pumps blood to

   a. the lungs

   b. the right ventricle

   c. the right atrium

   d. the systemic circuit

   e. the pulmonary trunk

6. The myocardium is primarily composed of

   a. elastic tissue

   b. fibrous connective tissue

   c. epithelial tissue

   d. cardiac muscle tissue

   e. smooth muscle tissue

7. Blood vessels that carry blood away from the heart are called

   a. capillaries

   b. veins

   c. arteries

   d. venules

   e. vena cavae

8. The lymphatic system is composed of

   a. lymphatic vessels

   b. lymph

   c. the spleen

   d. lymph nodes

   e. all of the above

9. The cells known as lymphocytes

   a. are actively phagocytic

   b. destroy red blood cells

   c. produce proteins called antibodies

   d. are primarily found in red bone marrow

   e. decrease in number during most infections

10. The openings to the nostrils are the

   a. external nares

   b. internal nares

   c. vestibules

   d. glottises

   e. palates

11. The structure that carries air from the trachea to a lung is the

   a. pharynx

   b. larynx

  c. bronchiole

  d. alveolar duct

  e. primary bronchus

12. Boyle's law states that gas volume is

  a. directly proportional to pressure at constant temperature

  b. directly proportional to temperature at constant pressure

  c. inversely proportional to pressure at constant temperature

  d. inversely proportional to its solubility in water at constant temperature

  e. directly proportional to the sum of the partial pressures of the gas in a mixture

13. Which of the following is not a digestive function?

  a. mechanical processing

  b. absorption

  c. compaction

  d. ingestion

  e. filtration

14. Which of the following is an accessory organ of digestion?

  a. stomach

  b. pancreas

  c. esophagus

  d. jejunum

  e. colon

15. Which of the following processes takes place in the oral cavity?

  a. defecation

  b. mastication

  c. micturition

  d. deglutition

  e. flatulation

16. The basic functional unit of the kidney is the

  a. nephron

  b. renal corpuscle

  c. glomerulus

  d. loop of Henle

  e. renal pyramid

17. The process of filtration in the kidneys occurs at

  a. the loop of Henle

  b. the collecting duct

  c. the minor calyces

  d. Bowman's capsule

  e. the ureter

18. A waste product produced in the liver from amino groups removed from amino acids is

  a. uric acid

  b. urea

  c. creatinine

  d. bile

  e. bilirubin

19. The reproductive system includes

  a. gonads

    b. ducts that receive and transport gametes

    c. accessory glands and organs that secrete fluids

    d. external genitalia

    e. all of the above

20. Which of the following is not part of the female reproductive system?

    a. clitoris

    b. epididymis

    c. vulva

    d. cervix

    e. vagina

☑ Self-Assessment

If your score was

between 18 and 20, you are ready to proceed to the next chapter.

between 15 and 17, you have a good general idea of the chapter content, but you should review sections of the chapter that deal with items that you missed before proceeding to the next chapter.

less than 14, you have not mastered the chapter content well enough to proceed. Reread the chapter and rework the exercises. Then retake the self-check test. Repeat this process until you achieve a score that will allow you to continue.

Answers

1. platelets
2. systole
3. right atrium
4. albumin
5. arterioles
6. right ventricle
7. hemoglobin
8. arteries
9. diastole
10. contractile cell
11. superior vena cava
12. plasma
13. basophils
14. left atrium
15. right atrioventricular (AV) valve, or tricuspid valve
16. venules
17. formed elements
18. neutrophil
19. pulmonary circuit
20. semilunar valve
21. calcium channels
22. globulins
23. veins
24. coronary sulcus
25. pulmonary arteries
26. cardiac cycle
27. myocardium
28. fibrinogen

29. pericardium
30. left ventricle
31. sinoatrial (SA) node
32. sodium ion channels
33. immunoglobulins, or antibodies
34. systemic circuit
35. left atrioventricular (AV) valve, or mitral valve, or bicuspid valve
36. conducting cells
37. red blood cells, or erythrocytes
38. inferior vena cava
39. monocytes
40. aorta
41. epicardium
42. granulocytes, or granular leukocytes
43. auricle
44. white blood cells, or leukocytes
45. capillaries
46. eosinophils
47. endocardium
48. pulmonary trunk
49. lymphocytes
50. automaticity
51. agranulocytes, or agranular leukocytes
52. erythrocytes
53. agranular
54. pericardium, epicardium, endocardium, myocardium, cardiac cycle
55. hemoglobin

56. leukocytes
57. pericardium, pericardial fluid, pericardial cavity
58. neutrophil, basophil, eosinophil
59. monocyte
60. pulmonary circuit, pulmonary trunk, pulmonary arteries, pulmonary veins
61. myocardium
62. endocardium
63. helper T cells
64. fever
65. lymph
66. passive immunity
67. nonspecific defenses
68. complement
69. lymph glands, or lymph nodes
70. plasma cells
71. immunity
72. T cells
73. interferons
74. active immunity
75. cytotoxic T cells
76. immunological surveillance
77. induced passive immunity
78. B cells
79. innate immunity
80. NK cells
81. inflammation
82. passive immunity
83. suppressor T cell
84. antigens
85. active immunity
86. alveoli
87. Boyle's law
88. pharynx
89. respiratory mucosa
90. pulmonary ventilation, or breathing
91. external nares
92. articulation
93. trachea
94. Dalton's law of partial pressure
95. bronchioles
96. glottis
97. lobes
98. respiratory cycle
99. respiratory tract
100. alveolar ducts
101. Henry's law
102. internal nares
103. anoxia
104. primary bronchus
105. external respiration
106. phonation
107. respiratory bronchioles
108. hypoxia
109. partial pressure
110. larynx
111. alveolar sacs
112. lobules
113. internal respiration
114. alveolar ventilation
115. respiratory membrane
116. pulmonary lobule, pulmonary ventilation
117. hypoxia
118. bronchi, bronchioles
119. anoxia
120. hypoxia, anoxia
121. duodenum
122. buccal cavity
123. digestion
124. sublingual salivary glands
125. chief cells
126. ileum
127. bile
128. colon
129. ingestion
130. bolus
131. esophagus
132. parietal cells
133. secretin
134. defecation
135. muscularis externa
136. peristalsis
137. saliva
138. deglutition
139. jejunum
140. deamination
141. rectum
142. absorption
143. mastication
144. chyme
145. gallbladder
146. cecum
147. internal anal sphincter
148. excretion
149. serosa
150. segmentation
151. parotid salivary glands
152. protease
153. ileocecal valve
154. emulsification
155. feces
156. mucosa
157. pacesetter cells
158. occlusal surfaces
159. cholecystokinin (CCK)
160. urea
161. vermiform appendix
162. external anal sphincter
163. submucosa
164. adventitia
165. enterokinase
166. bilirubin
167. anorectal canal
168. peristalsis
169. transverse colon
170. ileocecal valve
171. submucosa, submandibular salivary glands
172. cholecystokinin
173. vermiform appendix
174. protein
175. starch

176. nucleic acids
177. proteins
178. elastic proteins
179. lipids
180. peptides
181. proteins
182. nephron
183. hilus
184. ureters
185. renal capsule
186. Bowman's capsule
187. collecting tubule
188. urethra
189. pyramids
190. peritubular fluid
191. urinary bladder
192. renal pelvis
193. afferent arteriole
194. external urethral opening, or external urethral meatus
195. renal papilla
196. papillary duct
197. internal urethral sphincter
198. renal cortex
199. minor calyx
200. glomerulus
201. proximal convoluted tubule (PCT)
202. antidiuretic hormone (ADH)
203. renal medulla
204. creatinine
205. micturition
206. collecting duct
207. renal hilus
208. efferent arterioles
209. loop of Henle
210. external urethral sphincter
211. renal sinus
212. major calyx
213. renal corpuscle
214. filtrate
215. distal convoluted tubule (DCT)
216. uric acid
217. renal pelvis
218. tubular fluid
219. nephron
220. afferent arteriole
221. peritubular fluid
222. efferent arteriole
223. glans
224. gonads
225. primordial follicles
226. vulva, or pudendum
227. fimbriae
228. scrotum
229. testes
230. seminiferous tubules
231. corpus luteum
232. vagina
233. clitoris
234. interstitial cells

235. follicle-stimulating hormone (FSH)
236. vestibule
237. androgens
238. follicular fluid
239. external genitals
240. tertiary follicle
241. menstruation
242. myometrium
243. mons pubis
244. penis
245. ovaries
246. luteinizing hormone (LH)
247. labia minora
248. semen
249. menses
250. uterine tube (oviduct, Fallopian tube)
251. uterine cycle (menstrual cycle)
252. tunica albuginea
253. inguinal canal
254. labia majora
255. seminal fluid
256. infundibulum
257. perimetrium
258. sustentacular cells
259. epididymis
260. libido
261. inhibin
262. proliferative phase
263. ampulla
264. ovarian follicle
265. granulosa cells
266. uterus
267. secretory phase
268. greater vestibular glands
269. ductus deferens
270. spermatic cord
271. testosterone
272. ovarian cycle
273. body, or corpus
274. lesser vestibular glands
275. estradiol
276. ejaculatory duct
277. progesterone
278. endometrium
279. cervix
280. involution
281. follicle cells
282. progestins, progesterone
283. myometrium
284. corpus luteum, corpus of the uterus
285. menses, menstruation, menstrual cycle
286. perimetrium
287. androgens
288. myometrium, endometrium, perimetrium
289. cervix
290. corpus luteum

Answers to Self-Check Test

1. c 2. b 3. d 4. b 5. d 6. d 7. c 8. e 9. c 10. a 11. e 12. c
13. e 14. b 15. b 16. a 17. d 18. b 19. e 20. b

abdominal cavity: The cavity that extends from the inferior surface of the diaphragm to an imaginary plane extending from the inferior surface of the lowest spinal vertebra to the anterior and superior margin of the pelvic girdle, 41

abdominopelvic cavity: The portion of the ventral body cavity that contains abdominal and pelvic subdivisions; also contains the *peritoneal cavity*, 41

abdominopelvic quadrants, 29

abduction: Movement away from the midline of the body, as viewed in the anatomical position, 359

absorption: The active or passive uptake of gases, fluids, or solutes, 433

accessory structures, 332

acetylcholine (ACh) (as-ē-til-KŌ-lēn)**:** A chemical neurotransmitter in the brain and peripheral nervous system; dominant neurotransmitter in the peripheral nervous system, released at neuromuscular junctions and synapses of the parasympathetic division, 353

acetyl-CoA: An acetyl group bound to coenzyme A, a participant in the anabolic and catabolic pathways for carbohydrates, lipids, and many amino acids, 188

acetyl group: —CH_3C=O, 189

acid: A compound whose dissociation in solution releases a hydrogen ion and an anion; an acid solution has a pH below 7.0 and contains an excess of hydrogen ions, 87

acidic, 86

acidosis (a-sid-Ō-sis)**:** An abnormal physiological state characterized by a plasma pH below 7.35, 86

acinus/acini (AS-i-nī)**:** A histological term referring to a blind pocket, pouch, or sac.

actin: The protein component of microfilaments that forms thin filaments in skeletal muscles and produces contractions of all muscles through interaction with thick (myosin) filaments; *see also* **sliding filament theory,** 145

action potential: A conducted change in the transmembrane potential of excitable cells, initiated by a change in the membrane permeability to sodium ions; *see also* **nerve impulse,** 371

action, 356

activation energy: The energy required to initiate a specific chemical reaction, 78

active immunity: Immunity that appears following an exposure to antigen, 417

active processes, 159

active site: The region of an enzyme that binds the substrate, 115

active transport: The ATP-dependent absorption or excretion of solutes across a cell membrane, 167

adduction: Movement toward the axis or midline of the body, as viewed in the anatomical position, 359

adenine: A purine; one of the nitrogenous bases in the nucleic acids RNA and DNA, 122

adenohypophysis (ad-e-nō-hī-POF-i-sis)**:** The anterior portion of the pituitary gland, also called the **anterior pituitary,** 386

adenosine diphosphate (ADP): A compound consisting of adenosine with two phosphate groups attached, 124

adenosine monophosphate (AMP): A nucleotide consisting of adenine plus a phosphate group (PO_4^{3-}); also known as adenosine phosphate, 124

adenosine triphosphate (ATP): A high-energy compound consisting of adenosine with three phosphate groups attached; the third is attached by a high-energy bond, 124

adipocyte (AD-i-pō-sīt)**:** A fat cell, 251

adipose tissue: Loose connective tissue dominated by adipocytes, 253

adolescence: The period of life from puberty to physical maturity, 309

adrenal cortex: The superficial portion of the adrenal gland that produces steroid hormone, 387

adrenal gland: A small endocrine gland that secretes steroids and catecholamines and is located superior to each kidney; also called the *suprarenal gland*, 387

adrenal medulla: The core of the adrenal gland; a modified sympathetic ganglion that secretes catecholamines into the blood after sympathetic activation, 387

adrenocortical hormone (a-drē-nō-KOR-ti-kul)**:** Any of the steroids produced by the adrenal cortex, 387

adrenocortical steroids: *See* **corticosteroids,** 387

adrenocorticotropic hormone (ACTH): The hormone that stimulates the production and secretion of glucocorticoids by the zona fasciculata of the adrenal cortex; released by the anterior pituitary in response to CRH, 386

adventitia (ad-ven-TISH-a)**:** The superficial layer of connective tissue surrounding an internal organ; fibers are continuous with those of surrounding tissues, providing support and stabilization, 433

aerobic: Requiring the presence of oxygen.

aerobic metabolism: The complete breakdown of organic substrates into carbon dioxide and water, via pyruvic acid; a process that yields large amounts of ATP but requires mitochondria and oxygen, 184

afferent: Toward.

afferent arteriole: An arteriole that brings blood to a glomerulus of the kidney, 449

afferent division of PNS: The division of the peripheral nervous system that carries sensory information to the central nervous system, 367

afferent fibers, 371

agonist: A muscle responsible for a specific movement, 357

agranular: Without granules; *agranular leukocytes* are monocytes and lymphocytes; the *agranular reticulum* is an intracellular organelle that synthesizes and stores carbohydrates and lipids.

agranulocytes (A-gran-yoo-lō-sītz)**:** White blood cells that lack visibly staining granules in their cytoplasm. Also known as agranular leuckocytes, 398

albumin (al-BU-min)**:** A class of plasma proteins, 398

aldosterone: A mineralocorticoid produced by the zona glomerulosa of the adrenal cortex; stimulates sodium and water conservation at the kidneys; secreted in response to the presence of angiotensin II, 387

alkaline: The condition of being basic; the opposite of acidic, 86

alkalosis (al-ka-LŌ-sis)**:** The condition characterized by a plasma pH of greater than 7.45; associated with relative deficiency of hydrogen ions or an excess of bicarbonate ions, 86

allantois (a-LAN-tō-is)**:** One of the four extraembryonic membranes; provides vascularity to the chorion and is therefore essential to placenta formation; the proximal portion becomes the urinary bladder, 303

alleles (a-LĒLZ)**:** Alternate forms of a particular gene, 314

alpha particle: A particle consisting of a helium nucleus: 2 protons and 2 neutrons, 60

alpha-helix, 113

alveolar ducts, (al-VE-ō-lar) 424

alveolar gland, 244

alveolar sac: An air-filled chamber that supplies air to several alveoli, 424

alveolar ventilation: The movement of air into and out of the alveoli, 428

alveolus/alveoli (al-VĒ-o-lī): Blind pockets at the end of the respiratory tree, lined by a simple squamous epithelium and surrounded by a capillary network; sites of gas exchange with the blood; bony socket that holds the root of a tooth, 424

amino acids: Organic compounds whose chemical structure can be summarized as R—$CHNH_2$—COOH, 112

amino group: —NH_2, 112

amnesia: Temporary or permanent memory loss.

amniocentesis: Sampling of amniotic fluid for analytical purposes; used to detect certain genetic abnormalities, 112

amnion (AM-nē-on): One of the four extraembryonic membranes; surrounds the developing embryo/fetus, 300, 302

amniotic cavity: A fluid-filled chamber formed by the separation of the inner cell mass from the trophoblast, 300

amniotic fluid (am-nē-OT-ik): Fluid that fills the amniotic cavity; cushions and supports the embryo/fetus, 303

amphiarthrosis (am-fē-ar-THRŌ-sis): An articulation that permits a small degree of independent movement; *see* **interosseous membrane** and **pubic symphysis**, 344

amphicytes (AM-fi-sīts): Supporting cells that surround neurons in the peripheral nervous system; also called *satellite cells*.

amphimixis (am-fi-MIK-sis): The fusion of male and female pronuclei after fertilization, 295

ampulla/ampullae (am-PŪL-la): A localized dilation in the lumen of a canal or passageway, 459

amylase: An enzyme that breaks down polysaccharides; produced by the salivary glands and pancreas, 440

anabolism (a-NAB-ō-lizm): The synthesis of complex organic compounds from simpler precursors, 76, 183

anaerobic: Without oxygen.

anal orifice: *See* **anus**, 442

anaphase (AN-a-fāz): The mitotic stage in which the paired chromatids separate and move toward opposite ends of the spindle apparatus, 217

anaplasia (a-nuh-PLA-zē-uh): The breakdown of tissue organization, 275

anatomical position: An anatomical reference position; the body viewed from the anterior surface with the palms facing forward; supine, 29

anatomy (a-NAT-o-mē): The study of the structure of the body, 1

androgen (AN-drō-jen): A steroid sex hormone primarily produced by the interstitial cells of the testis and manufactured in small quantities by the adrenal cortex in either gender, 387, 459

anion (AN-ī-on): An ion bearing a negative charge, 64

anorectal canal (ā-nō-REC-tal): The distal portion of the rectum that contains the rectal columns and ends at the anus, 444

anoxia (a-NOKS-ē-uh): Tissue oxygen deprivation, 425

antagonist: A muscle that opposes the movement of an agonist, 358

antebrachium: The forearm, 32

anteflexion (an-tē-FLEK-shun): The normal position of the uterus, with the superior surface bent forward.

anterior: On or near the front, or ventral surface, of the body, 29

anterior interventricular sulcus, 401

anterior median fissure: A deep longitudinal groove lying along the anterior surface of the spinal cord, 373

anterior pituitary: *See* **pituitary gland**, 386

antiangiogenesis factor (an-tē-an-jē-ō-JEN-eh-sis): A chemical produced by chondrocytes that inhibits the formation of blood vessels, 261

antibody (AN-ti-bod-ē): A globular protein produced by plasma cells that will bind to specific antigens and promote their destruction or removal from the body, 349, 398

antibody-mediated immunity: Immunity resulting from the presence of circulating antibodies produced by plasma cells; also called *humoral immunity*, 415

anticodon: Three nitrogenous bases on a tRNA molecule that interact with an appropriate codon on a strand of mRNA, 208

antidiuretic hormone (ADH) (an-tī-dī-ū-RET-ik): A hormone synthesized in the hypothalamus and secreted at the posterior pituitary; causes water retention at the kidneys and an elevation of blood pressure, 387, 453

antigen: A substance capable of inducing the production of antibodies, 415

anus: The external opening of the anorectal canal, 444

aorta: The large, elastic artery that carries blood away from the left ventricle and into the systemic circuit, 404

aortic arch, 404

aortic semilunar valve, 404

apex: The tip of a conical-shaped organ, 424

apocrine secretion: A mode of secretion in which the glandular cell sheds portions of its cytoplasm, 242

apocrine sweat glands, 333

aponeurosis/aponeuroses (ap-ō-nū-RŌ-sis): A broad tendinous sheet that may serve as the origin or insertion of a skeletal muscle, 255

apoptosis (ap-op-TO-sis): The genetically controlled death of cells, 214

appendicular (ap-en-DIK-ū-lur): Pertaining to the upper or lower limbs.

appendicular skeleton: The division of the skeleton consisting of the bones of the limbs and the supporting elements or girdles, 341

appendix: A blind tube connected to the cecum of the large intestine, 442

aqueous solution: A solution in which water is the solvent, 82

arachnoid (a-RAK-noyd): The middle meninges that encloses cerebrospinal fluid and protects the central nervous system, 372

areolar: Containing minute spaces, as in areolar connective tissue.

arteriole (ar-TĒ-rē-ōl): A small arterial branch that delivers blood to a capillary network, 408

artery: A blood vessel that carries blood away from the heart and toward a peripheral capillary, 261, 400

articulation (ar-tik-ū-LĀ-shun): A joint; the formation of words, 344, 422

ascending aorta, 404

ascending colon, 442

ascending limb, 451

astral rays: Small microtubules that radiate from centrioles into the cytoplasm during mitosis, 216

astrocyte (AS-trō-sīt): One of the glial cells in the central nervous system; responsible for maintaining the blood–brain barrier by stimulation of endothelial cells, 368

atom: The smallest stable unit of matter, 12, 55, 59

atomic mass unit (amu): The unit used to measure the atomic weight of atoms. Also known as a dalton, 60

atomic number: The number of protons in the nucleus of an atom, 59

atomic weight: Roughly, the average total number of protons and neutrons in the atoms of a particular element, 60

atresia (a-TRĒ-zē-uh): The closing of a cavity, or its incomplete development; used to refer to the degeneration of developing ovarian follicles, 290

atria: Thin-walled chambers of the heart that receive venous blood from the pulmonary or systemic circuit, 400

atrioventricular (AV) node (ā-trē-ō-ven-TRIK-ū-lar): Specialized cardiocytes that relay the contractile stimulus to the bundle of His, the bundle branches, the Purkinje fibers, and the ventricular myocardium; located at the boundary between the atria and ventricles, 406

atrioventricular (AV) valve: One of the valves that prevent backflow into the atria during ventricular systole, 403

auricle (AW-ri-kul): the expandable extension of an atrium of the heart, 401

autolysis: The destruction of a cell due to the rupture of lysosomal membranes in its cytoplasm, 153

automaticity: Spontaneous depolarization to threshold, a characteristic of cardiac pacemaker cells, 406

autonomic nervous system (ANS): Centers, nuclei, tracts, ganglia, and nerves involved in the unconscious regulation of visceral functions; includes components of the central nervous system and the peripheral nervous system, 365

autoregulation, 22

autosomal (aw-to-SŌ-mal): Chromosomes other than the X or Y chromosome.

AV bundle, 408

avascular (ā-VAS-kū-lar)**:** Without blood vessels, 230

axial skeleton (AK-sē-ul)**:** The division of the skeleton consisting of the bones of the skull, thorax, and vertebral column, 341

axolemma: The cell membrane of an axon, continuous with the cell membrane of the soma and dendrites and distinct from any glial cell coverings, 368

axon: The elongate extension of a neuron that conducts an action potential, 274

axon hillock: In a multipolar neuron, the portion of the neural soma adjacent to the initial segment, 369

axoplasm (AK-sō-plazm)**:** The cytoplasm within an axon, 369

B cells: Lymphocytes capable of differentiating into the plasma cells that produce antibodies, 414

basal body: A structure similar to a centriole that anchors a cilium to a cell membrane, 148

basal lamina: The layer of the basement membrane closest to the epithelium, 235

base: A compound whose dissociation releases a hydroxide ion (OH⁻) or removes a hydrogen ion (H⁺) from the solution, 87

base: The broad portion of a conical-shaped organ.

basement membrane: A layer of filaments and fibers that attach an epithelium to the underlying connective tissue, 235

basophils (BĀ-sō-filz)**:** Circulating granulocytes (white blood cells) similar in size and function to tissue mast cells, 251, 400

benign tumor: A tumor in which the cells remain contained within a connective tissuecapsule, 219

beta oxidation: Fatty acid catabolism that produces molecules of acetyl-CoA, 197

beta particle: An electron that is emitted from the nucleus of a radioisotope.

bicarbonate ions: HCO₃⁻; anion components of the carbonic acid–bicarbonate buffer system, 87

biceps muscle, 358

bicuspid valve: The left atrioventricular valve, also known as the *mitral valve*, 404

bile: The exocrine secretion of the liver that is stored in the gallbladder and ejected into the duodenum, 440

bile salts: Steroid derivatives in the bile; responsible for the emulsification of ingested lipids, 106, 440

bilirubin (bil-ē-ROO-bin)**:** A pigment, the byproduct of hemoglobin catabolism, 440

biomechanics: The analysis of biological systems in mechanical terms, 355

biopsy: The removal of a small sample of tissue for pathological analysis, 274

bipennate: A muscle whose fibers are arranged on either side of a common tendon, 351

bipolar neuron: A neuron that has only one dendrite and one axon, 370

bladder: A muscular sac that distends as fluid is stored and whose contraction ejects the fluid at an appropriate time; used alone, the term usually refers to the urinary bladder, 453

blastocoele (BLAS-tō-sēl)**:** A fluid-filled cavity within a blastocyst, 297

blastocyst (BLAS-tō-sist)**:** An early stage in the developing embryo, consisting of an outer trophoblast and an inner cell mass, 297

blastodisc (BLAS-tō-disk)**:** A late stage in the development of the inner cell mass; includes the cells that will form the embryo, 300

blood: A fluid connective tissue composed of formed elements and plasma, 260, 397

blood–brain barrier: The isolation of the central nervous system from the general circulation; primarily the result of astrocyte regulation of capillary permeabilities, 368

body cavities, 39

body (shaft) of the penis: The tubular movable portion of the penis, 460

body stalk: The connection between the embryo and the chorion, 303

bolus: A compact mass; usually refers to compacted ingested material on its way to the stomach, 437

bowel: The intestinal tract, 442

Bowman's capsule: The cup-shaped initial portion of the renal tubule; it surrounds the glomerulus and receives the glomerular filtrate, 449

Boyle's law: The principle that, in a gas, pressure and volume are inversely related, 426

brachium: The arm, 29

branched gland, 244

brevis: Short, 358

bronchioles (BRONG-kē-ōlz)**:** Tiny airways that branch from the bronchi, 424

bronchus/bronchi: One of the branches of the bronchial tree between the trachea and bronchioles, 422

buccal cavity (BUK-al)**:** *See* **oral cavity**, 436

buccinator, 360

buffer: A compound that stabilizes the pH of a solution by removing or releasing hydrogen ions, 87

buffer system: Interacting compounds that prevent increases or decreases in the pH of body fluids; includes the carbonic acid–bicarbonate buffer system, the phosphate buffer system, and the protein buffer system, 87

bulbourethral glands (bul-bō-ū-RĒ-thral)**:** Mucous glands at the base of the penis that secrete into the penile urethra; the equivalent of the greater vestibular glands of the female; also called *Cowper's glands*, 458

bulk flow: The movement of large numbers of water molecules through a membrane at at one time, 163

bulk transport, 169

bundle branches, 408

calcification, 339

calcified: Containing calcium salts, 249

calcitonin (kal-si-TŌ-nin)**:** The hormone secreted by C cells of the thyroid when calcium ion concentrations are abnormally high; restores homeostasis by increasing the rate of bone deposition and the renal rate of calcium loss, 387

calcitriol (kal-si-TRI-ol)**:** A hormone important in regulating calcium levels in the body. Also known as vitamin D, 106

calcium hydroxyapatite, 336

Calorie (C): The amount of heat that is required to raise the temperature of one kilogram of water 1°C; also called the *kilocalorie*, 78

calorie (c) (KAL-o-rē)**:** The amount of heat that is required to raise the temperature of one gram of water 1°C, 78

calyx/calyces (KĀL-i-sēz)**:** Cup-shaped divisions of the renal pelvis, 448

canaliculi (kan-a-LIK-ū-lī)**:** Microscopic passageways between cells; bile canaliculi carry bile to bile ducts in the liver; in bone, canaliculi permit the diffusion of nutrients and wastes to and from osteocytes, 264, 337

cancellous bone (KAN-sel-us)**:** Spongy bone, composed of a network of bony struts, 337

cancer: A malignant tumor that tends to undergo metastasis, 220

capacitation (ka-pas-i-TĀ-shun)**:** The activation process that must occur before a spermatozoon can successfully fertilize an oocyte; occurs in the vagina after ejaculation, 293

capillary: A small blood vessel, interposed between an arteriole and a venule, whose thin wall permits the diffusion of gases, nutrients, and wastes between the plasma and interstitial fluids, 261, 400

capsule: The thick fibrous layer that surrounds internal organs, 257

carbohydrate (kar-bō-HĪ-drāt)**:** An organic compound containing carbon, hydrogen, and oxygen in a ratio that approximates 1:2:1, 95

carbon dioxide: CO₂; a compound produced by the decarboxylation reactions of aerobic metabolism.

carboxyl group: —COOH, 102

carboxypeptidase (kar-bok-sē-PEP-ti-dās)**:** A protease that breaks down proteins and releases amino acids, 439

cardiac: Pertaining to the heart.

cardiac cycle: One complete heartbeat, including atrial and ventricular systole and diastole, 408

cardiac muscle cells, 360

cardiac muscle tissue: A specialized muscle tissue found only in the heart, 271

cardiac myocyte: A heart muscle cell, 271

cardiocyte (KAR-dē-ō-sīt)**:** A cardiac muscle cell, 271

carotene (KAR-ō-tēn)**:** A yellow-orange pigment found in carrots and in green and orange leafy vegetables; a compound that the body can convert to vitamin A, 331

carrier-mediated transport: A transport process that requires the presence of specializedintegral proteins; it may be active or passive, 165

cartilage: A connective tissue with a gelatinous matrix that contains an abundance of fibers, 261

catabolism (ka-TAB-ō-lizm)**:** The breakdown of complex organic molecules into simpler components, accompanied by the release of energy, 76, 183

catalyst (KAT-uh-list)**:** A substance that accelerates a specific chemical reaction but that is not altered by the reaction, 78

catecholamine (kat-e-KŌL-am-ēn)**:** Epinephrine, norepinephrine, dopamine, and related compounds, 385

cation (KAT-ī-on)**:** An ion that bears a positive charge, 64

caudal/caudally: Closest to or toward the tail (coccyx), 33

cecum (SĒ-kum)**:** An expanded pouch at the start of the large intestine, 442

cell: The smallest living unit in the human body, 125, 133

cell adhesion molecule (CAM): A transmembrane protein specialized for attaching cells to each other, 232

cell division: The process of cellular reproduction in which a single cell duplicates itself, 213

cell junction: A specialized attachment site between cells, 232

cell-mediated immunity: Resistance to disease through the activities of sensitized T cells that destroy antigen-bearing cells by direct contact or through the release of lymphotoxins; also called *cellular immunity*, 415

cell membrane: A phospholipid bilayer that separates the cell contents from the environment. Also known as a plasma membrane, 136

cell physiology, 9

cell theory: The concept that cells are the fundamental units of all plant and animal tissues, 133

cellulose: A polysaccharide that is a structural component of plants, 98

central canal: Longitudinal canal in the center of an osteon that contains blood vessels and nerves, also called the *Haversian canal*; a passageway along the longitudinal axis of the spinal cord that contains cerebrospinal fluid, 337, 366

central nervous system (CNS): The brain and spinal cord, 365

centriole: A cylindrical intracellular organelle composed of nine groups of microtubules, three in each group; functions in mitosis or meiosis by organizing the microtubules of the spindle apparatus, 148

centromere (SEN-trō-mēr)**:** The localized region where two chromatids remain connected after chromosome replication; site of spindle fiber attachment, 216

centrosome: A region of cytoplasm that contains a pair of centrioles oriented at right angles to one another, 148

cephalic: Pertaining to the head.

cerebellar cortex: The neural cortex of the cerebellar hemispheres, 374

cerebellum (ser-e-BEL-um)**:** The posterior portion of the metencephalon, containing the cerebellar hemispheres; includes the arbor vitae, cerebellar nuclei, and cerebellar cortex, 374

cerebral cortex: An extensive area of neural cortex covering the surfaces of the cerebral hemispheres, 374

cerebral hemispheres: Expanded portions of the cerebrum covered in neural cortex, 374

cerebrospinal fluid (CSF): Fluid bathing the internal and external surfaces of the central nervous system; secreted by the choroid plexus, 367

cerebrum (SER-ē-brum)**:** The largest portion of the brain, composed of the cerebral hemispheres; includes the cerebral cortex, the cerebral nuclei, and the internal capsule, 374

cervix: The lower part of the uterus, 462

chalones (KA-lōnz)**:** Peptides that inhibit cell division, 219

chemical bond: A force that holds atoms together, 64

chemical elements, 57

chemical energy: Energy that is stored in a chemical bond, 76

chemical notation: The use of symbols, subscripts, superscripts, and numerical coefficients to describe chemical compounds and chemical reactions, 69

chemistry: The branch of science that deals with atoms and their interactions, 55

chemoreception: The detection of alterations in the concentrations of dissolved compounds or gases, 377

chemoreceptors, 377

chief cells: Cells in the gastric mucosa that secrete pepsinogen, 438

childhood: The period of life from two years until puberty, 306

cholecystokinin (CCK) (kō-lē-sis-tō-KĪ-nin)**:** A duodenal hormone that stimulates the contraction of the gallbladder and the secretion of enzymes by the exocrine pancreas; also called *pancreozymin*, 439

cholesterol: A steroid component of cell membranes and a substrate for the synthesis of steroid hormones and bile salts, 106

chondrocyte (KON-drō-sīt)**:** A cartilage cell, 261

chondroitin sulfate (kon-DROI-tin)**:** The predominant proteoglycan in cartilage, responsible for the gelatinous consistency of the matrix, 261

chorion/chorionic (KOR-ē-on) (ko-rē-ON-ik)**:** An extraembryonic membrane, consisting of the trophoblast and underlying mesoderm, that forms the placenta, 303

chorionic villus: A fingerlike extension formed from the trophoblast, 303

chromatid (KRŌ-ma-tid)**:** One complete copy of a DNA strand and its associated nucleoproteins, 216

chromatin (KRŌ-ma-tin)**:** A histological term referring to the grainy material visible in cell nuclei during interphase; the appearance of the DNA content of the nucleus when the chromosomes are uncoiled, 204

chromosomal abnormalities, 319

chromosomal microtubules: Spindle fibers that attach to chromatids during mitosis, 216

chromosomes: Dense structures, composed of tightly coiled DNA strands and associated histones, that become visible in the nucleus when a cell prepares to undergo mitosis or meiosis; normal human somatic cells contain 46 chromosomes apiece, 155, 204

chyme (kīm)**:** A semifluid, acidic mixture of ingested food and digestive secretions that is found in the stomach in the early phases of digestion, 437

chymotrypsin (kī-mō-TRIP-sin)**:** A protease found in the small intestine, 439

chymotrypsinogen: The inactive proenzyme secreted by the pancreas that is subsequently converted to chymotrypsin, 439

ciliated epithelium, 232

cilium/cilia: A slender organelle that extends above the free surface of an epithelial cell and generally undergoes cycles of movement; composed of a basal body and microtubules in a 9×2 array, 148

circular muscle: *See* sphincter, 351

circulatory system: The network of blood vessels that are components of the cardiovascular system.

circumduction (sir-kum-DUK-shun)**:** A movement at a synovial joint in which the distal end of the bone describes a circle but the shaft does not rotate.

citric acid: A six-carbon acid that forms at the beginning of the citric acid cycle, 188

citric acid cycle: The aerobic reaction sequence that occurs in the mitochondrial matrix; in the process organic molecules are broken down, carbon dioxide molecules are released, and hydrogen atoms are transferred to coenzymes that deliver them to the electron transport system, 188

clavicle, 343

cleavage (KLĒ-vij)**:** Mitotic divisions that follow fertilization of the ovum and lead to the formation of a blastocyst, 297

clitoris (KLI-to-ris)**:** A small erectile organ of the female that is the developmental equivalent of the male penis, 465

coated vesicle: A vesicle containing ligands and receptors clustered together, 170

coccyx (KOK-siks)**:** The terminal portion of the spinal column, consisting of relatively tiny, fused vertebrae, 344

coding strand, 206

codominance: A genetic system in which both alleles in a pair are fully expressed, 318

codon (KŌ-don)**:** A sequence of three nitrogenous bases along an mRNA strand that will specify the location of a single amino acid in a peptide chain, 207

coelom (SĒ-lōm)**:** The ventral body cavity, lined by a serous membrane and subdivided during fetal development into the pleural, pericardial, and abdominopelvic (peritoneal) cavities, 39

coenzyme A: A coenzyme involved in carrying acetyl groups in cellular metabolism, 187

coenzyme Q, 190

coenzymes (kō-EN-zīmz)**:** Complex organic cofactors; most are structurally related to vitamins, 115

cofactor: Ions or molecules that must be attached to the active site before an enzyme can function; examples include mineral ions and several vitamins, 115

collagen: A strong, insoluble protein fiber common in connective tissues, 114

collagen fibers, 252

collagenous tissue: Another term for dense connective tissue, 255

collateral axon: A branch of an axon.

collaterals, 369

collecting duct: A duct that collects tubular fluid from many different nephrons and carries it to a papillary duct, 451

collecting tubule: A tubule that connects the distal convoluted tubule to a collecting duct, 451

colloid/colloidal suspension: A solution containing large organic molecules in suspension, 84

colon: The large intestine, 442

columnar epithelial cell: An epithelial cell that is taller and more slender than a cuboidal epithelial cell, 237

compact bone: Dense bone that contains parallel osteons, 337

Competitive inhibition: The process in which molecules resembling normal substrate bind to a receptor site on an active molecule preventing the binding of normal substrate, 117

complement: A system of 11 plasma proteins that interact in a chain-reaction after exposure to activated antibodies or the surfaces of certain pathogens; complement proteins promote cell lysis, phagocytosis, and other defense mechanisms, 416

complementary base pairs: The pairing of a purine and a pyrimidine base in the DNA molecule, 122

compound: A molecule containing two or more elements in combination, 64

compound gland, 244

concentration gradient: The difference between the high and low concentrations of a substance in a given area, 159

conception: Fertilization, 285

conducting cells: Heart muscle cells that are adapted for conducting action potentials, 408

conducting system: A system of specialized cardiac muscle cells that control and coordinate the activities of contractile cells, 405

contractile cells: Cardiac muscle cells that produce the force of a cardiac contraction, 405

control center, 23

convergent muscle: A muscle in which the fibers are based over a large area, but they all come together at a common attachment site, 350

corona radiata (ko-RŌ-na rā-dē-A-ta): A layer of follicle cells surrounding a secondary oocyte at ovulation, 293

coronary arteries: Blood vessels that supply blood to the heart muscle, 405

coronary sinus: A structure that collects venous blood from the heart muscle before returning to the right atrium, 403

coronary sulcus: A shallow depression marking the border between the atrium and the ventricle, 401

coronary vein: A vein that drains blood from the heart muscle, 403

corpus/corpora: Body.

corpus luteum (LOO-tē-um): The progestin-secreting mass of follicle cells that develops in the ovary after ovulation, 462

cortex: The outer layer or portion of an organ, 337

cortical reaction: A chemical process that occurs when a sperm cell enters an oocyte that prevents other sperm from penetrating, 295

corticosteroid: A steroid hormone produced by the adrenal cortex, 106, 387

cortisol (KOR-ti-sol): One of the corticosteroids secreted by the zona fasciculata of the adrenal cortex; a glucocorticoid, 387

cotransport: The membrane transport of a nutrient, such as glucose, in company with the movement of an ion, normally sodium; transport requires a carrier protein but does not involve direct ATP expenditure and can occur regardless of the concentration gradient for the nutrient, 168

countertransport: Secondary active transport that moves two substances each in an opposite direction. Also known as antiport, 168

covalent bond (kō-VĀ-lent): A chemical bond between atoms that involves the sharing of electrons, 66

coxa/coxae: A bone of the hip, 344

cranial: Pertaining to the head.

cranial cavity: The space that encloses the brain, 39

cranial nerves: Peripheral nerves originating at the brain, 365

craniosacral division (krā-nē-ō-SAK-ral): *See* **parasympathetic division,** 377

cranium, 39

creatinine: A breakdown product of creatine metabolism, 452

crenation: Cellular shrinkage due to an osmotic movement of water out of the cytoplasm, 165

cristae, 150

crossing over: The exchange of genetic material between adjacent chromatids during prophase I of meiosis, 287

CT, 43

cuboidal epithelium: Epithelium composed of cells that appear to be square in typical sectional views, 237

cutaneous membrane: The epidermis and papillary layer of the dermis, 269, 329

cytochrome (SĪ-tō-krōm): A pigment component of the electron transport system; a structural relative of heme, 191

cytokinesis (sī-tō-ki-NĒ-sis): The cytoplasmic movement that separates two daughter cells at the completion of mitosis, 216

cytology (sī-TOL-o-jē): The study of the structure and function of cells, 7, 134

cytoplasm: The material between the cell membrane and the nuclear membrane; cell contents, 136

cytosine: A pyrimidine; one of the nitrogenous base in the nucleic acids RNA and DNA, 122

cytoskeleton: A network of microtubules and microfilaments in the cytoplasm, 141, 145

cytosol: The fluid portion of the cytoplasm, 144

cytotoxic T cells: Lymphocytes of the cellular immune response that kill target cells by direct contact or through the secretion of lymphotoxins; also called *killer T cells* and T_C *cells*, 415

Dalton's law: The relationship that the total gas pressure exerted by a mixture of gases is equal to the sum of the individual partial pressures of the gases, 426

daughter cells: Genetically identical cells produced by somatic cell division, 213

daughter chromosomes: Structures that result from the separation of paired chromatids during anaphase of mitosis, 217

deamination (dē-am-i-NĀ-shun): The removal of an amino group from an amino acid, 201, 440

decarboxylation (dē-kar-boks-i-LĀ-shun): The removal of a molecule of CO_2, 187

decidua basalis: The disc-shaped area of the placenta that functions in nutrient exchange.

decidua capsularis: The thin portion of the placenta that does not participate in nutrient exchange.

decidua parietalis: The portion of the uterine lining that has no connection with the chorion.

decomposition reaction: A chemical reaction that breaks a molecule into smaller fragments, 71

deep fascia, 270

defecation (def-e-KĀ-shun): The elimination of fecal wastes, 433

deglutition: Swallowing, 437

degree Celsius, 56

dehydration synthesis: The joining of two molecules associated with the removal of a water molecule, 97

deltoid, 358

denaturation: Irreversible alteration in the three-dimensional structure of a protein, 117

dendrite (DEN-drīt): A sensory process of a neuron, 274

dense irregular connective tissue, 256

dense regular connective tissue, 255

deoxyribonucleic acid (DNA) (dē-ok-sē-rī-bō-noo-KLĀ-ik): A nucleic acid consisting of a chain of nucleotides that contain the sugar deoxyribose and the nitrogenous bases adenine, guanine, cytosine, and thymine, 121

deoxyribose: A five-carbon sugar resembling ribose but lacking an oxygen atom, 121

depolarization: A change in the transmembrane potential from a negative value toward 0 mV, 406

dermal papillae, 332

dermis: The connective tissue layer beneath the epidermis of the skin, 329

descending aorta, 404

descending colon, 442

descending limb, 450

desomosome (DEZ-mō-sōm): A very thin proteoglycan layer between two opposing cell membranes reinforced by a network of intermediate filaments that lock the cells together, 233

development: The growth and the acquisition of increasing structural and functional complexity; includes the period from conception to maturity, 285

developmental anatomy, 7

diaphragm (DĪ-a-fram): Any muscular partition; often used to refer to the respiratory muscle that separates the thoracic cavity from the abdominopelvic cavity, 39

diaphysis (dī-A-fi-sis): The shaft of a long bone, 337

diarthrosis (dī-ar-THRŌ-sis): A synovial joint, 344

diastole (dī-AS-tō-lē): The period of cardiac relaxation, 408

diencephalon (dī-en-SEF-a-lon): A division of the brain that includes the epithalamus, thalamus, and hypothalamus, 374

differentiation: The gradual appearance of characteristic cellular specializations during development as the result of gene activation or repression, 220, 229

diffusion: Passive molecular movement from an area of relatively high concentration to an area of relatively low concentration, 159

digestion: The chemical breakdown of ingested materials into simple molecules that can be absorbed by the cells of the digestive tract, 432

digestive system: The digestive tract and associated glands, 19

digestive tract: *See* **gastrointestinal tract**, 432

diglyceride: A molecule composed of glycerol and two fatty acids, 104

dipeptide, 112

diploid (DIP-loyd): Having a complete somatic complement of chromosomes (23 pairs in human cells), 286

disaccharide (di-SAK-a-rīd): A compound formed by the joining of two simple sugars by dehydration synthesis, 97

disease: The failure to maintain homeostatic conditions in the body, 27

dissociation (di-sō-sē-Ā-shun): *See* **ionization**, 82

distal: Movement away from the point of attachment or origin; for a limb, away from its attachment to the trunk, 33

distal convoluted tubule (DCT): The portion of the nephron closest to the connecting tubules and collecting duct; an important site of active secretion, 451

DNA fingerprint: The pattern of DNA in segments composed of repeating DNA sequences, 205

DNA molecule: Two DNA strands wound in a double helix and held together by weak bonds between complementary nitrogenous base pairs, 121

DNA polymerase: The enzyme that forms new molecules of DNA, 215

DNA replication: The process of producing two identical copies of a DNA molecule, 215

dominant: A gene whose presence will determine the phenotype, regardless of the nature of its allelic companion, 314

dorsal: Toward the back, posterior, 33

dorsal body cavity: The body cavity that surrounds the brain and spinal cord, 39

dorsal root, 373

dorsal root ganglion, 373

dorsiflexion: The elevation of the superior surface of the foot through movement at the ankle.

double covalent bond, 67

duct: A passageway that delivers exocrine secretions to an epithelial surface, 241

ductus deferens (DUK-tus DEF-e-renz): A passageway that carries sperm from the epididymis to the ejaculatory duct, 458

duodenum (doo-AH-de-num): The proximal 25 cm of the small intestine that contains short villi and submucosal glands, 438

dura mater (DŪ-ra MĀ-ter): The outermost component of the meninges that surround the brain and spinal cord, 372

dysplasia (dis-PLA-zē-uh): A change in the normal shape, size, and organization of tissue cells, 274

echogram, 43f

ectoderm: One of the three primary germ layers; covers the surface of the embryo and gives rise to the nervous system, the epidermis and associated glands, and a variety of other structures, 301

effector: A peripheral gland or muscle cell innervated by a motor neuron, 23, 365

efferent (EF-er-ent): Away from.

efferent arteriole: An arteriole carrying blood away from a glomerulus of the kidney, 449

efferent division of PNS: The division of the peripheral nervous system that carries motor commands from the central nervous system to muscles and glands, 365

efferent fibers, 371

eicosanoid (ī-KO-sa-noyd): A molecule derived from the polyunsaturated acid arachidonic acid that consists of 20 carbon atoms folded in the shape of a hairpin, 105, 385

ejaculatory ducts (ē-JAK-ū-la-to-rē): Short ducts that pass within the walls of the prostate gland and connect the ductus deferens with the prostatic urethra, 458

elastase (ē-LAS-tās): A pancreatic enzyme that breaks down elastin fibers, 440

elastic cartilage: A type of cartilage that has a matrix containing numerous elastin fibers, 264

elastic fibers: Fibers that contain the protein elastin, 252

elastic tissue: Tissue that contains large numbers of elastic fibers, 255

elastin: Connective tissue fibers that stretch and recoil, providing elasticity to connective tissues, 252

electric current: A flow of charged particles, 75

electrical energy: Energy that results from the interactions between charged particles and involves the movement of ions or electrons, 75

electrochemical gradient: The net result of the chemical and electrical forces acting on a particular ion, 161

electrolytes (ē-LEK-trō-līts): Soluble inorganic compounds whose ions will conduct an electrical current in solution, 83

electromagnetic energy: A form of energy that travels through space as a wave, 74

electromagnetic spectrum: A continuum formed by energy waves of different wavelengths, 75

electron: One of the three fundamental particles; a subatomic particle that bears a negative charge and normally orbits the protons of the nucleus, 59

electron microscopy, 135

electron transport system (ETS): The cytochrome system responsible for most of the energy production in living cells; a complex bound to the inner mitochondrial membrane, 191

element: All the atoms with the same atomic number, 57

embryo (EM-brē-ō): The developmental stage beginning at fertilization and ending at the start of the third developmental month, 302

embryogenesis (em-brē-ō-JEN-e-sis): The formation of a viable embyro, 297

embryological development, 285

embryology (em-brē-OL-o-jē): The study of embryonic development, focusing on the first 2 months after fertilization, 7, 265

emulsification (ē-mul-si-fi-KĀ-shun): The physical breakup of fats in the digestive tract, forming smaller droplets accessible to digestive enzymes; normally the result of mixing with bile salts, 441

endergonic reaction: A reaction that absorbs energy, 77

endocardium (en-dō-KAR-dē-um): The simple squamous epithelium that lines the heart and is continuous with the endothelium of the great vessels, 404

endochondral ossification, 339

endocrine gland: A gland that secretes hormones into the blood, 241

endocrine pancreas: the portion of the pancreas composed of the islets of Langerhans, 388

endocytosis (EN-dō-sī-tō-sis): The movement of relatively large volumes of extracellular material into the cytoplasm via the formation of a membranous vesicle at the cell surface; includes pinocytosis and phagocytosis, 169

endoderm: One of the three primary germ layers; the layer on the undersurface of the embryonic disc; gives rise to the epithelia and glands of the digestive system, the respiratory system, and portions of the urinary system, 301

endometrium (en-dō-MĒ-trē-um): The mucous membrane lining the uterus, 463

endomysium (en-dō-MĪS-ē-um): A delicate network of connective tissue fibers that surrounds individual muscle cells, 350

endoneurium: A delicate network of connective tissue fibers that surrounds individual nerve fibers, 374

endoplasmic reticulum (en-dō-PLAZ-mik re-TIK-ū-lum): A network of membranous channels in the cytoplasm of a cell that function in intracellular transport, synthesis, storage, packaging, and secretion, 150

endosteum: An incomplete cellular lining on the inner (medullary) surfaces of bones, 338

endothelium (en-dō-THĒ-lē-um): The simple squamous epithelium that lines blood and lymphatic vessels, 237

energy: The capacity to perform work, 73

energy level: The specific amount of energy associated with an electron orbital, 61

enterokinase: An enzyme in the lumen of the small intestine that activates the proenzymes secreted by the pancreas, 439

enzyme: A protein that catalyzes a specific biochemical reaction, 78

eosinophil (ē-ō-SIN-ō-fil): A microphage (white blood cell) with a lobed nucleus and red-staining granules; participates in the immune response and is especially important during allergic reactions, 261, 400

ependyma (ep-EN-di-mah): The layer of cells lining the ventricles and central canal of the central nervous system.

ependymal cells (ependyma), 366

epiblast: The epithelial layer of the blastodisc that faces the amniotic cavity, 300

epicardium: A serous membrane covering the outer surface of the heart; also called the *visceral pericardium,* 400

epidermal derivatives, 332

epidermis: The epithelium covering the surface of the skin, 329

epididymis (ep-i-DID-i-mus): A coiled duct that connects the rete testis to the ductus deferens; site of functional maturation of spermatozoa, 458

epimysium (ep-i-MIS-ē-um): A dense layer of collagen fibers that surrounds a skeletal muscle and is continuous with the tendons/aponeuroses of the muscle and with the perimysium, 349

epinephrine: A catecholamine secreted from the adrenal medullae, 387

epineurium: A dense layer of collagen fibers that surrounds a peripheral nerve, 373

epiphysis (e-PIF-i-sis): The head of a long bone, 337

epithelial tissue, 230

epithelium (e-pi-THĒ-lē-um): One of the four primary tissue types; a layer of cells that forms a superficial covering or an internal lining of a body cavity or vessel, 230

eponyms, 3

equational division: The second meiotic division, 287, 378

equilibrium (ē-kwi-LIB-rē-um): A dynamic state in which two opposing forces or processes are in balance, 72

erythrocyte (e-RITH-rō-sīt): A red blood cell; a blood cell that has no nucleus and contains large quantities of hemoglobin, 260, 398

esophagus: A muscular tube that connects the pharynx to the stomach, 437

essential amino acids: Amino acids that cannot be synthesized in the body in adequate amounts and must be obtained from the diet.

essential fatty acids: Fatty acids that cannot be synthesized in the body and must be obtained from the diet, 199

estradiol (es-tra-DI-ol): The most important of the estrogens in humans, 465

estrogens (ES-trō-jenz): A class of steroid sex hormones that includes estradiol, 106

exchange pump: An ion pump that moves two different ions in opposite directions across a cell membrane, 167

exchange reaction: A chemical reaction in which parts of the reacting substances are exchanged with each other, 72

excitation-contraction coupling: The link between the generation of an action potential in the sarcolemma and the start of a muscle contraction, 355

excretion: Elimination from the body, 433

exergonic reaction: A reaction that releases energy, 77

exfoliative cytology: The study of cells shed or collected from an epithelial surface, 240

exocrine gland: A gland that secretes onto the body surface or into a passageway connected to the exterior, 241

exocrine pancreas: The largest part of the pancreas (roughly 99%) that secretes digestive enzymes and alkaline fluid, 388

exocytosis (EK-sō-sī-tō-sis): The ejection of cytoplasmic materials by the fusion of a membranous vesicle with the cell membrane, 172

exon: The region of a gene that codes for a polypeptide, 207

expiration: Exhalation; breathing out, 428

extension: An increase in the angle between two articulating bones; the opposite of flexion, 359

external anal sphincter, 442

external genitalia, 458

external nares: The nostrils; the external openings into the nasal cavity, 422

external respiration: The diffusion of gases between the alveolar air and the alveolar capillaries and between the systemic capillaries and peripheral tissues, 424

external urethral meatus: *See* **external urethral opening,** 453

external urethral opening: The opening of the urethra to the outside of the body, 453

external urethral sphincter, 454

externus, 358

exteroceptors: General sensory receptors in the skin, mucous membranes, and special sense organs that provide information about the external environment and about our position within it, 371

extracellular fluid: All body fluids other than that contained within cells; includes plasma and interstitial fluid, 136, 261

extraembryonic membranes: The yolk sac, amnion, chorion, and allantois, 301

extrinsic muscles, 358

extrinsic regulation, 22

facilitated diffusion: The passive movement of a substance across a cell membrane by means of a protein carrier, 166

fasciae (FASH-ē-ē): Connective tissue fibers, primarily collagenous, that form sheets or bands beneath the skin to attach, stabilize, enclose, and separate muscles and other internal organs, 269

fascicle: *See* fasciculus, 350

fasciculus (fa-SIK-ū-lus): A small bundle; usually referring to a collection of nerve axons or muscle fibers, 350

fast channels: Ion channels in heart muscle cells that depolarize quickly, 406

fatty acids: Hydrocarbon chains that end in a carboxylic acid group, 102

feces: Waste products eliminated by the digestive tract at the anus; contains indigestible residue, bacteria, mucus, and epithelial cells, 442

female pronucleus, 295

fertilization: The fusion of oocyte and sperm to form a zygote, 292

fetal development, 285

fetus: The developmental stage lasting from the start of the third developmental month to delivery, 306

fever: An elevation in body temperature, 417

fibrin (FĪ-brin): Insoluble protein fibers that form the basic framework of a blood clot, 398

fibrinogen (fī-BRIN-ō-jen): A plasma protein that is the soluble precursor of the fibrous protein fibrin, 398

fibroblasts (FĪ-brō-blasts): Cells of connective tissue proper that are responsible for the production of extracellular fibers and the secretion of the organic compounds of the extracellular matrix, 251

fibrocartilage: A type of cartilage that contains little ground substance and many tightly packed collagen fibers, 264

fibrous proteins, 114

filtrate: The fluid produced by filtration at a glomerulus in the kidney, 449

filtration: The movement of a fluid across a membrane whose pores restrict the passage of solutes on the basis of size, 165, 452

fimbriae (FIM-brē-ē): Fringes; the fingerlike processes that surround the entrance to the uterine tube, 462

first-class lever: A lever in which the fulcrum lies between the applied force and the resistance, 356

first trimester, 297

fixator: A muscle that prevents movement at a joint.

fixed macrophages, 251

fixed ribosomes, 149

flagellum/flagella (fla-JEL-uh): An organelle structurally similar to a cilium but used to propel a cell through a fluid.

flat bones, 339

flavin adenine dinucleotide: A coenzyme important in oxidative phosphorylation; it cycles between the oxidized ($FADH_2$) and reduced (FAD) states.

flavin adenine mononucleotide: A coenzyme important in oxidative phosphorylation; cycles between the oxidized ($FMNH_2$) and reduced (FMN) states.

flexion (FLEK-shun): A movement that reduces the angle between two articulating bones; the opposite of extension, 359

fluid shift: The osmotic movement of water into or out of cells, 165

FMN (flavin mononucleotide), 190

follicle (FOL-i-kul): A small secretory sac or gland.

follicle-stimulating hormone (FSH): A hormone secreted by the anterior pituitary; stimulates oogenesis (female) and spermatogenesis (male), 386, 460

follicular cells: The squamous cells that surround the oocyte in a primordial follicle, 461

follicular fluid: The fluid secreted by granulosa cells that fills the antrum of a secondary follicle, 462

formed elements: The blood cells and fragments of cells found in blood, 260, 398

free macrophages, 251

free radical: A molecule that contains unpaired electrons in its outer shell, 67

free ribosomes, 149

freely permeable, 159

frequency: The number of wave cycles (peak to peak) that occur per second, 74

frontal plane: A sectional plane that divides the body into an anterior portion and a posterior portion; also called the *coronal plane*, 37

fructose: A hexose (six-carbon simple sugar) found in foods and in semen, 97

fulcrum: The fixed point on which a lever moves, 356

funiculus (fū-NIK-ū-lus): One of the divisions of the white matter on each side of the spinal cord. Also known as a *column*, 373

G0 phase: The period of interphase during which a cell performs normal functions, 215

G1 phase: The period of interphase during which a cell manufactures cellular components in preparation for cell division, 215

G2 phase: The period of interphase that precedes mitosis, 215

gallbladder: The pear-shaped reservoir for the bile secreted by the liver, 442

gametes (GAM-ēts): Reproductive cells (sperm or oocytes) that contain half the normal chromosome complement.

gametogenesis (ga-me-tō-JEN-e-sis): The formation of gametes, 286

gamma rays: Electromagnetic waves with very high energy, 60

ganglion/ganglia: A collection of neuron cell bodies outside the central nervous system, 368

gap junctions: Connections between cells that permit electrical coupling, 232

gastric: Pertaining to the stomach.

gastrointestinal (GI) tract: An internal passageway that begins at the mouth, ends at the anus, and is lined by a mucous membrane; also known as the *digestive tract*.

gastrulation (gas-troo-LĀ-shun): The movement of cells of the inner cell mass that creates the three primary germ layers of the embryo, 300

gated channel: A pore in a cell membrane that can open or close to regulate ion passage, 140

gene: A portion of a DNA strand that functions as a hereditary unit and is found at a particular site on a specific chromosome, 205

general senses: The senses of pain, temperature, touch, pressure, vibration, and proprioception, 377

genetic code: The method of information storage within the DNA strands in the nucleus, 205

genetic recombination: The formation of new combinations of alleles on a chromosome, 318

genetics: The study of mechanisms of heredity, 286

genioglossus, 359

genitalia (jen-i-TĀ-lē-uh): The reproductive organs, 458

genotype (JĒN-ō-tīp): An individual's genetic complement, which determines the individual's phenotype, 312

geriatricians, 309

geriatrics: A medical specialty concerned with the mechanics of the aging process, 309

germinative cells: Stem cells that through continual division maintain an epithelium, 235

gestation (jes-TĀ-shun): The period of intrauterine development, 296

gland: Cells that produce exocrine or endocrine secretions, 243

gland cell: An epithelial cell that produces secretions, 231

glans: The expanded tip of the penis that surrounds the external urethral meatus; continuous with the corpus spongiosum, 460

globular proteins, 113

globulins (GLOB-ū-linz): A class of plasma proteins that includes antibodies, 398

glomerulus (glo-MER-ū-lus): A ball or knot; in the kidneys, a knot of capillaries that projects into the enlarged, proximal end of a nephron; the site of filtration, the first step in the production of urine, 449

glottis (GLOT-is): Passageway from the pharynx to the larynx, 422

glucagon (GLOO-ka-gon): A hormone secreted by the alpha cells of the pancreatic islets; elevates blood glucose concentrations, 388

glucocorticoids: Hormones secreted by the zona fasciculata of the adrenal cortex to modify glucose metabolism; cortisol, cortisone, and corticosterone are important examples, 387

gluconeogenesis (gloo-kō-nē-ō-JEN-e-sis): The synthesis of glucose from protein or lipid precursors, 195

glucose (GLOO-kōs): A six-carbon sugar, $C_6H_{12}O_6$; the preferred energy source for most cells and the only energy source for neurons under normal conditions, 95

glucose-6-phosphate, 186

glycerides: Lipids composed of glycerol bound to fatty acids, 104

glycerol (GLI-se-rōl): A three-carbon alcohol found in simple fats, 104

glycocalyx (glī-kō-KAL-iks): A layer on the outer surface of a cell membrane formed by the carbohydrate portions of glycolipids and glycoproteins, 142

glycogen (GLĪ-kō-jen): A polysaccharide that represents an important energy reserve; a polymer consisting of a long chain of glucose molecules, 98

glycogenesis: The synthesis of glycogen from glucose molecules, 197

glycolipids (glī-cō-LIP-idz): Compounds created by the combination of carbohydrate and lipid components, 107

glycolysis (glī-KOL-i-sis): The anaerobic cytoplasmic breakdown of glucose into lactic acid by way of pyruvic acid, with a net gain of two ATP, 186

glycoprotein (glī-kō-PRŌ-tēn): A compound containing a relatively small carbohydrate group attached to a large protein, 119

goblet cell: A goblet-shaped, mucus-producing, unicellular gland in certain epithelia of the digestive and respiratory tracts, 243

Golgi apparatus (gol-jē): A cellular organelle consisting of a series of membranous plates that give rise to lysosomes and secretory vesicles, 152

gomphosis (gom-FŌ-sis): A fibrous synarthrosis that binds a tooth to the bone of the jaw; see **periodontal ligament**, 344

gonadotropins: Gonadotropic hormones, 386

gonads (GŌ-nads): Reproductive organs that produce gametes and hormones, 457

gout: A condition resulting from elevated uric acid concentrations in the blood and peripheral tissues, 202

Graafian follicle: See **mature follicle**.

gram, 56

granulocytes (GRAN-ū-lō-sīts): White blood cells containing granules visible with the light microscope; includes eosinophils, basophils, and neutrophils; also called *granular leukocytes*, 398

granulosa cells (GRAN-ū-lō-suh): secreting cells that surround the primary oocyte in a growing follicles, 462

gray matter: Areas in the central nervous system dominated by neuron bodies, glial cells, and unmyelinated axons, 368

great cardiac veins, 404

greater vestibular glands, 465

gross anatomy: The study of the structural features of the human body without the aid of a microscope, 4

ground substance: The fluid component of connective tissue, 249

growth hormone (GH): An anterior pituitary hormone that stimulates tissue growth and anabolism when nutrients are abundant and restricts tissue glucose dependence when nutrients are in short supply, 387

GTP, 125

guanine: A purine; one of the nitrogenous bases in the nucleic acids RNA and DNA, 122

gustation (gus-Tā-shun): Taste, 378

hair: A keratinous strand produced by epithelial cells of the hair follicle, 332

hair follicle: An accessory structure of the integument; a tube lined by a stratified squamous epithelium that begins at the surface of the skin and ends at the hair papilla, 332

half-life: The time required for a 50% reduction in the amount of radiation emitted by a a radioisotope or the time required for the 50% reduction in the amount a substance in the body, 60

haploid (HAP-loyd): Possessing half the normal number of chromosomes; a characteristic of gametes, 286

Haversian system: *See* osteon, 337

head fold, 304

hearing, 378

heat capacity: The ability of a substance to absorb and retain heat, 81

heat energy: Energy that results from the random motion of atoms and molecules, 77

helper T cells: Lymphocytes (T_H cells) whose secretions and other activities coordinate the cell-mediated and antibody-mediated immune responses, 415

hemoglobin (hē-mō-GLŌ-bin): A protein composed of four globular subunits, each bound to a heme molecule; gives red blood cells the ability to transport oxygen in the blood, 398

hemolysis: The breakdown (lysis) of red blood cells, 164

Henrys law: The relationship that the amount of a gas in a solution is directly proportional to the partial pressure of the gas, 427

heparin (HEP-a-rin): An anticoagulant released by activated basophils and mast cells, 251

heptose, 95

hertz (Hz): The unit used to measure frequency. It is equal to one cycle per second, 75

heterozygous (het-er-ō-ZĪ-gus): Possessing two different alleles at corresponding sites on a chromosome pair; the individual's phenotype may be determined by one or both of the alleles, 314

hexose: A six-carbon simple sugar, 95

high-energy bond: A covalent bond that when broken release a useful amount of energy, 122

high-energy compound: An organic molecule containing a phosphate group attached by a high-energy bond, 124

hilum/hilus (HĪ-lum): A localized region where blood vessels, lymphatics, nerves, and/or other anatomical structures are attached to an organ, 448

histamine (HIS-tuh-mēn): Chemical released by stimulated mast cells or basophils to initiate or enhance an inflammatory response, 251

histology (his-TOL-o-jē): The study of tissues, 7, 230

histones: Proteins associated with the DNA of the nucleus; the DNA strands are wound around them, 204

holocrine (HO-lō-krin): A form of exocrine secretion in which the secretory cell becomes swollen with vesicles and then ruptures, 242

homeostasis (hō-mē-ō-STĀ-sis): The maintenance of a relatively constant internal environment, 22

homeostatic regulation, 22

homologous chromosomes (hō-MOL-o-gus): The members of a chromosome pair, 313

homozygous (hō-mō-ZĪ-gus): Having the same allele for a given phenotypic character on two homologous chromosomes, 314

homozygous dominant, 314

homozygous recessive, 314

hormone: A compound secreted by one cell that travels through the circulatory system to affect the activities of cells in another portion of the body, 22, 384

horn: A projection of gray matter in the central spinal cord, 373

Human Genome Project, 319

humoral immunity: *See* **antibody-mediated immunity,** 415

hyaline cartilage (HI-a-lin): The most common type of cartilage composed of a matrix of tightly packed collagen fibers, 262

hyaluronidase (hī-uh-loo-RON-ik), 252

hyaluronic acid: A polysaccharide substance thatt is the major component of intercellular cement, 233

hydration sphere: A zone of water molecules that surrounds an ion in solution, 82

hydrogen bond: A weak interaction between the hydrogen atom on one molecule and a negatively charged portion of another molecule, 68

hydrolysis (hī-DROL-i-sis): The breakage of a chemical bond through the addition of a water molecule; the reverse of dehydration synthesis, 72

hydrophilic (hī-drō-PHIL-ik): Freely associating with water; readily entering into solution, 83

hydrophobic: Incapable of freely associating with water molecules; insoluble, 83

hydrostatic pressure: Fluid pressure, 163

hydroxide ion (hī-DROK-sīd): OH—, 85

hydroxyapatite: A hard mineral found in bone, 336

hydroxyl group (hī-DROK-sil): OH, 102

hypertension: Abnormally high blood pressure.

hypertonic: In comparing two solutions, the solution with the higher osmolarity, 165

hyperuricemia (hī-per-ū-ri-SE-mē-ah): A condition characterized by an abnormally high level of uric acid in the blood, 202

hypoblast (HI-pō-blast): The epithelial layer of the blastodisc that lies beneath the epiblast, 300

hypodermis: *See* **subcutaneous layer,** 269, 330

hypophysis (hī-POF-i-sis): The anterior pituitary gland, which is subdivided into the pars distalis and the pars intermedia, 386

hypothalamus: The floor of the diencephalon; the region of the brain containing centers involved with the unconscious regulation of visceral functions, emotions, drives, and the coordination of neural and endocrine functions, 375

hypotonic: In comparing two solutions, the one with the lower osmolarity, 164

hypoxia (hī-POKS-ē-uh): Low tissue oxygen concentrations, 425

ileocecal valve (il-ē-ō-SĒ-kal): A fold of mucous membrane that guards the connection between the ileum and the cecum, 438

ileum (IL-ē-um): The last 2.5 m of the small intestine, 438

immune response: A specific body defense provided by lymphocytes, 413

immune system, 413

immunity: Resistance to injuries and diseases caused by foreign compounds, toxins, and pathogens, 413, 415

immunoglobulin (i-mū-nō-GLOB-ū-lin): A circulating antibody, 398

immunological surveillance: The policing of peripheral tissues by white blood cells, 415, 416

impermeable, 159

implantation (im-plan-TĀ-shun): The erosion of a blastocyst into the uterine wall, 297

inclusion: A mass of insoluble material that is located in the cytosol of a cell, 145

incomplete dominance: A genetic system in which a dominant allele and a recessive allele interact to produce a phenotype different from that resulting from either allele by itself, 318

induced active immunity, 417

induced passive immunity, 417

induction: The chemical interplay between developing cells whereby chemical signals from one cell influence the development of another cell, 295

infancy: The period of life from one month until two years, 306

infection: The invasion and colonization of body tissues by pathogenic organisms, 274

inferior: Below, in reference to a particular structure, with the body in the anatomical position, 33

inferior vena cava: The vein that carries blood from the parts of the body below the heart to the right atrium, 403

inflammation: A nonspecific defense mechanism that operates at the tissue level, characterized by swelling, redness, warmth, pain, and some loss of function, 274, 417

infrared (IR) radiation: Electromagnetic energy in the range adjacent to red light with longer wavelengths and lower frequencies than red light, 75

infundibulum (in-fun-DIB-ū-lum): A tapering, funnel-shaped structure; in the nervous system, the connection between the pituitary gland and the hypothalamus; in the uterine tube, the entrance bounded by fimbriae that receives the oocytes at ovulation, 374, 462

ingestion: The introduction of materials into the digestive tract by way to the mouth, 432

inguinal canal: A passage through the abdominal wall that marks the path of testicular descent and that contains the testicular arteries, veins, and ductus deferens, 459

inheritance: The transfer of genetically determined characters from one generation to the next generation, 286

lipid: An organic compound containing carbons, hydrogens, and oxygens in a ratio that does not approximate 1:2:1; includes fats, oils, and waxes, 102

lipogenesis (li-pō-JEN-e-sis): The synthesis of lipids from nonlipid precursors, 198

lipolysis: The catabolism of lipids as a source of energy, 197

liposuction (LI-pō-suk-shen): The surgical removal of unwanted fat, 255

liquor folliculi: *See* **follicular fluid,** 462

liter, 56

liver: An organ of the digestive system with varied and vital functions, including the production of plasma proteins, the excretion of bile, the storage of energy reserves, the detoxification of poisons, and the interconversion of nutrients, 440

lobe: A subdivision of an organ, 424

lobule (LOB-ūl): The basic organizational unit of the liver at the histological level, 424, 459

logissimus, 358

long bones, 339

loop of Henle: The portion of the nephron responsible for the creation of the concentration gradient in the renal medulla, 450

loose connective tissue, 253

lower respiratory system, 421

luteinizing hormone (LH) (LOO-tē-in-ī-zing): An anterior pituitary hormone that, in the female, assists FSH in follicle stimulation, triggers ovulation, and promotes the maintenance and secretion of the endometrial glands; in the male, stimulates spermatogenesis; formerly known as *interstitial cell–stimulating hormone* in males, 386, 460, 462

lymph: The fluid contents of lymphatic vessels, similar in composition to interstitial fluid, 260, 413

lymph gland: *See* lymph node, 413

lymph nodes: Lymphatic organs that monitor the composition of lymph, 413

lymphatics: The vessels of the lymphatic system, 261

lymphocyte (LIM-fō-sīt): A cell of the lymphatic system that participates in the immune response, 251, 400

lysis (LĪ-sis): The destruction of a cell through the rupture of its cell membrane.

lysosomal storage disease: A disorder characterized by problems with lysosomal enzyme production resulting in the accumulation of wastes and/or debris in the affected cells, 154

lysosome (LĪ-sō-sōm): An intracellular vesicle containing digestive enzymes, 153

M phase: The period of the cell cycle during which mitosis occurs, 215

macrophage: A phagocytic cell of the monocyte–macrophage system, 251

macroscopic anatomy, 4

magnus, 359

major, 359

major calyx, 448

male pronucleus, 295

malignant tumor: A tumor composed of cells that no longer respond to normal control mechanisms, 219

manus: The hand, 32

marrow: A tissue that fills the internal cavities in a bone; may be dominated by hemopoietic cells (red marrow) or adipose tissue (yellow marrow), 337

mass: A measure of the amount of matter in an object, 57

mass number: The total number of protons and neutrons in the nucleus of an atom, 60

mast cell: A connective tissue cell that when stimulated releases histamine, serotonin, and heparin, initiating the inflammatory response, 251

mastication (mas-ti-KĀ-shun): Chewing, 437

matrix: The ground substance of a connective tissue, 249

matter: Anything that has mass and occupies space, 57

maximus, 359

mechanoreception: The detection of mechanical stimuli, such as touch, pressure, or vibration, 377

mechanoreceptors (mechanoreception), 377

medial: Toward the midline of the body, 33

mediastinum (mē-dē-as-TĪ-um or mē-dē-AS-ti-num): The central tissue mass that divides the thoracic cavity into two pleural cavities; includes the aorta and other great vessels, the esophagus, trachea, thymus, the pericardial cavity and heart, and a host of nerves, small vessels, and lymphatics; area of connective tissue attaching

a testis to the epididymis, proximal portion of ductus deferens, and associated vessels, 41

medical anatomy, 7

medulla: The inner layer or core of an organ.

medulla oblongata: The most caudal of the five brain regions, also known as the *myelencephalon,* 375

medullary cavity: The space within a bone that contains the marrow, 337

meiosis (mī-Ō-sis): Cell division that produces gametes with half the normal somatic chromosome complement.

meiosis I, 214, 286

melanin (ME-la-nin): The yellow-brown pigment produced by the melanocytes of the skin, 251

melanocyte (me-LAN-ō-sīt): A specialized cell in the deeper layers of the stratified squamous epithelium of the skin; responsible for the production of melanin, 251, 331

melanocyte-stimulating hormone (MSH): A hormone of the pars intermedia of the anterior pituitary that stimulates melanin production, 387

membrane flow: The movement of sections of membrane surface to and from the cell surface and components of the endoplasmic reticulum, the Golgi apparatus, and vesicles, 155

membranous organelles, 145

meninges (men-IN-jēz): Three membranes that surround the surfaces of the central nervous system; the dura mater, the pia mater, and the arachnoid, 372

menses (MEN-sēz): The first portion of the uterine cycle, the portion in which the endometrial lining sloughs away, 463

menstrual cycle (MEN-stroo-al): *See* **uterine cycle,** 463

menstruation: The cyclic sloughing of the uterine lining, 463

merocrine (MER-ō-krin): A method of secretion in which the cell ejects materials through exocytosis, 241

merocrine sweat glands, 241, 333

mesencephalon (mez-en-SEF-a-lon): The midbrain; the region between the diencephalon and pons, 375

mesenchyme: Embryonic/fetal connective tissue, 252

mesoderm: The middle germ layer that lies between the ectoderm and endoderm of the embryo, 301

mesothelium (mez-ō-THĒ-lē-um): A simple squamous epithelium lining one of the divisions of the ventral body cavity, 237

messenger RNA (mRNA): RNA formed at transcription to direct protein synthesis in the cytoplasm, 206

metabolic turnover: The continuous breakdown and replacement of organic materials within living cells, 125

metabolism (me-TAB-ō-lizm): The sum of all biochemical processes under way within the human body at a given moment; includes anabolism and catabolism, 9, 71

metabolites (me-TAB-ō-līts): Compounds produced in the body as the result of metabolic reactions, 80

metalloproteins (met-al-ō-PRŌ-tēnz): Plasma proteins that transport metal ions, 191

metaphase (MET-a-fāz): The stage of mitosis in which the chromosomes line up along the equatorial plane of the cell, 216

metaphase plate: The region of the cell where chromosomes line up during metaphase of mitosis, 217

metaplasia (me-tuh-PLA-zē-uh): A structural change that dramatically alters the character of a tissue, 274

metastasis (me-TAS-ta-sis): The spread of cancer cells from one organ to another, leading to the establishment secondary tumors, 219

meter, 56

micelle (mī-SEL): A droplet with hydrophilic portions on the outside; spherical aggregation of bile salts, monoglycerides, and fatty acids in the lumen of the intestinal tract, 108

microfilaments: Fine protein filaments visible with the electron microscope; components of the cytoskeleton, 145

microglia (mī-KROG-lē-uh): Phagocytic glial cells in the central nervous system, 368

micrometer, 135

microphages: Neutrophils and eosinophils, 251

microscopic anatomy, 4

microtubules: Microscopic tubules that are part of the cytoskeleton and are found in cilia, flagella, the centrioles, and spindle fibers, 146

microvilli: Small, fingerlike extensions of the exposed cell membrane of an epithelial cell, 147

micturition (mik-tū-RI-shun): Urination, 448

micturition reflex, 454

midbrain: The mesencephalon, 375

middle cardiac veins, 404

midsagittal plane, 37

milliliters, 56

millivolt, 76

mineralocorticoid: Corticosteroids produced by the zona glomerulosa of the adrenal cortex; steroids such as aldosterone that affect mineral metabolism, 387

minimus, 359

minor, 359

minor calyx, 448

mitochondrion (mī-tō-KON-drē-on)**:** An intracellular organelle responsible for generating most of the ATP required for cellular operations, 150

mitosis (mī-TŌ-sis)**:** The division of a single cell nucleus that produces two identical daughter cell nuclei; an essential step in cell division, 214, 216

mitotic rate: The rate of cell division, 217

mitral valve (MĪ-tral)**:** *See* **bicuspid valve,** 404

mixed gland: A gland that contains exocrine and endocrine cells, or an exocrine gland that produces serous and mucous secretions.

mole: A quantity of an element or compound having a mass in grams equal to the element's atomic weight or to the compound's molecular weight.

molecular weight: The sum of the atomic weights of the atoms in a molecule, 70

molecule: A chemical structure containing two or more atoms that are held together by chemical bonds, 12, 66

monocytes (MON-ō-sīts)**:** Phagocytic agranulocytes (white blood cells) in the circulating blood, 261, 400

monoglyceride (mo-nō-GLI-se-rīd)**:** A lipid consisting of a single fatty acid bound to a molecule of glycerol, 104

monosaccharide (mon-ō-SAK-uh-rīd)**:** A simple sugar, such as glucose or ribose, 95

mons pubis: A prominent bulge of fatty tissue beneath the skin and anterior to the pubic symphysis in females, 465

morula (MOR-ū-la)**:** A mulberry-shaped collection of cells produced through the mitotic divisions of a zygote, 297

motor neuron: A neuron that carries instructions from the central nervous system to effectors, 371

MRI, 43f

mucosa (mū-KŌ-sa)**:** A mucous membrane; the epithelium plus the lamina propria, 433

mucous: The presence or production of mucus.

mucuous connective tissue: Loose connective tissue found in many portions of the embryo, 252

mucous membranes: *See* **mucosa.**

mucus: A lubricating fluid composed of water and mucins produced by unicellular and multicellular glands along the digestive, respiratory, urinary, and reproductive tracts, 241

multicellular exocrine gland, 243

multicellular glands, 243

multipolar neuron: A neuron with many dendrites and a single axon; the typical form of a motor neuron, 370

muscle: A contractile organ composed of muscle tissue, blood vessels, nerves, connective tissues, and lymphatics, 349

muscle tissue: A tissue characterized by the presence of cells capable of contraction; includes skeletal, cardiac, and smooth muscle tissues, 270

muscularis externa (mus-kū-LAR-is)**:** Concentric layers of smooth muscle responsible for peristalsis, 433

mutation: A change in the nucleotide sequence of the DNA in a cell, 210

myelin (MĪ-e-lin)**:** An insulating sheath around an axon; consists of multiple layers of glial cell membrane; significantly increases conduction rate along the axon, 368

myelinated (myelination), 368

myelination: The formation of myelin, 368

myoblast (MI-ō-blast)**:** Embryonic cells that fuse together to form muscle fibers, 352

myocardium: The cardiac muscle tissue of the heart, 404

myofibril: Organized collections of myofilaments in skeletal and cardiac muscle cells, 353

myofilaments: Fine protein filaments composed primarily of the proteins actin (thin filaments) and myosin (thick filaments), 353

myometrium (mī-ō-MĒ-trē-um)**:** The thick layer of smooth muscle in the wall of the uterus, 463

myoneural junction: *See* **neuromuscular junction.**

Na⁺—K⁺ ATPase: The protein involved in the Na+-K+ exchange pump, 168

Na⁺—K⁺ exchange pump: An active transport process that moves 3 Na+ out of a cell while while moving 2 K+ back into the cell, 168

NADH, 186

nail: A keratinous structure produced by epithelial cells of the nail root, 333

nanometer, 61

nares, external (NA-rēz)**:** The entrance from the exterior to the nasal cavity, 422

nares, internal: The entrance from the nasal cavity to the nasopharynx, 422

nasal cavity: A chamber in the skull bounded by the internal and external nares, 422

natural killer (NK) cells: Lymphocytes that are specialized for killing pathogens and other cells. Also known as large granular lymphocytes, 414

natural passive immunity, 417

naturally acquired immunity, 417

neck of bladder, 453

negative feedback: A corrective mechanism that opposes or negates a variation from normal limits, 24

neonatal period, 306

neonate: A newborn infant, or baby, 307

neoplasm: A tumor, or mass of abnormal tissue, 219

nephron (NEF-ron)**:** The basic functional unit of the kidney, 448

nerve: A bundle of axons located in the peripheral nervous system. Also known as a *peripheral nerve,* 365

nerve fibers, 274

nerve impulse: An action potential in a neuron cell membrane, 372

net diffusion, 159

neural cortex: An area where gray matter is found at the surface of the central nervous system, 374

neural tissue: Tissue that is specialized for the conduction of electrical impulses, 273

neurilemma (noo-ri-LEM-muh)**:** The outer surface of a glial cell that encircles an axon, 368

neuroeffector junction: A synapse between a motor neuron and a peripheral effector, such as a muscle, gland cell, or fat cell, 369

neuroepithelium: An epithelium that contains sensory cells, 231

neurofibrils: Microfibrils in the cytoplasm of a neuron, 369

neurofilaments: Microfilaments in the cytoplasm of a neuron, 146, 369

neuroglandular junction: A specific type of neuroeffector junction, 370

neuroglia (noo-RŌ-glē-ah)**:** Cells of the central nervous system and peripheral nervous system that support and protect the neurons, 273

neurohypophysis (NOO-rō-hī-pof-i-sis)**:** The posterior pituitary, or pars nervosa, 387

neuromuscular junction: A type of neuroeffector junction, 353

neuron (NOO-ron)**:** A cell in neural tissue specialized for intercellular communication via (1) changes in membrane potential and (2) synaptic connections, 273

neurotransmitter: A chemical compound released by one neuron to affect the transmembrane potential of another, 353

neurotubules: Microtubules in the cytoplasm of a neuron, 369

neutral fat: *See* **triglyceride,** 104

neutron: A fundamental particle that does not carry a positive or a negative charge, 59

neutrophil (NOO-trō-fil)**:** A microphage that is very numerous and normally the first of the mobile phagocytic cells to arrive at an area of injury or infection, 261, 399

nicotinamide adenine dinucleotide (NAD): A coenzyme that removes hydrogen atoms from certain molecules during an enzyme-catalyzed reaction, 186

nitrogenous wastes: Organic waste products of metabolism that contain nitrogen, such as urea, uric acid, and creatinine, 202

nociception (nō-sē-SEP-shun)**:** Pain perception, 377

node of Ranvier: The area between adjacent glial cells where the myelin covering of an axon is incomplete, 368

nonmembranous organelles, 145

nonspecific resistance, 415

ly responsible for activities that conserve energy and lower the metabolic rate, 377

parathyroid glands: Four small glands embedded in the posterior surface of the thyroid; responsible for parathyroid hormone secretion, 387

parathyroid hormone (PTH): A hormone secreted by the parathyroid gland when plasma calcium levels fall below the normal range; causes increased osteoclast activity, increased intestinal calcium uptake, and decreased calcium ion loss at the kidneys, 387

parietal: Referring to the body wall or outer layer.

parietal cells: Cells of the gastric glands that secrete HCl and intrinsic factor, 438

parietal pericardium: The membrane that lines the inner surface of the pericardial sac, 400

parotid salivary glands (pa-ROT-id)**:** Large salivary glands that secrete a saliva containing high concentrations of salivary (alpha) amylase, 437

pars distalis (dis-TAL-is)**:** The large, anterior portion of the anterior pituitary gland, 386

pars intermedia (in-ter-ME-dē-uh)**:** The portion of the anterior pituitary immediately adjacent to the posterior pituitary and the infundibulum, 386

pars nervosa: The posterior pituitary gland, 387

partial pressure: The pressure exerted by a single gas within a mixture of gases, 426

passive immunity: Immunity produced by the transfer of antibodies from one individual to another, 417

passive processes, 159

patella (pa-TEL-uh)**:** The sesamoid bone of the kneecap, 339

pathogen: An organism that causes disease, 27, 251

pathologist (pa-THO-lo-jist)**:** An M.D. specializing in the identification of diseases on the basis of characteristic structural and functional changes in tissues and organs, 274

pathology: The study of disease, 27

pathophysiology, 9

pathway, 79

pediatrics: A medical specialty focusing on postnatal development from infancy through adolesence, 307

pelvic cavity: The inferior subdivision of the abdominopelvic (peritoneal) cavity; encloses the urinary bladder, the sigmoid colon and rectum, and male or female reproductive organs, 41

pelvic girdle, 344

pelvis: A bony complex created by the articulations among the coxae, the sacrum, and the coccyx, 344

penis (PĒ-nis)**:** A component of the male external genitalia; a copulatory organ that surrounds the urethra and serves to introduce semen into the female vagina; the developmental equivalent of the female clitoris, 459

pennate muscle (PEN-āte)**:** A muscle in which the fascicles form a common angle with the tendon, 351

pentapeptide, 112

pentose, 95

pepsin: A proteolytic enzyme secreted by the chief cells of the gastric glands in the stomach, 438

pepsinogen (pep-SIN-ō-jen)**:** The inactive form of the enzyme pepsin, 438

peptidases: Enzymes that split peptide bonds and release amino acids, 439

peptide: A chain of amino acids linked by peptide bonds, 112

peptide bond: A covalent bond between the amino group of one amino acid and the carboxyl group of another, 112

peptide hormone: A hormone composed of a chain of amino acids, 385

pericardial cavity (per-i-KAR-dē-al)**:** The space between the parietal pericardium and the epicardium (visceral pericardium) that covers the outer surface of the heart, 41, 400

pericardial fluid: The fluid found in the pericardial cavity, 400

pericardium (per-i-KAR-dē-um)**:** The fibrous sac that surrounds the heart and whose inner, serous lining is continuous with the epicardium, 41, 400

perichondrium (per-i-KON-drē-um)**:** The layer that surrounds a cartilage, consisting of an outer fibrous and an inner cellular region, 261

perikaryon (per-i-KAR-ē-on)**:** The cytoplasm that surrounds the nucleus in the soma of a nerve cell, 369

perimetrium (per-i-ME-trē-um)**:** The incomplete serosal layer of the uterus, 463

perimysium (pe-ri-MĪS-ē-um)**:** A connective tissue partition that separates adjacent fasciculi in a skeletal muscle, 350

perineurium: A connective tissue partition that separates adjacent bundles of nerve fibers in a peripheral nerve, 373

perinuclear space: The space between the two membranes of the nuclear envelope, 155

periodontal ligament (per-ē-ō-DON-tal)**:** Collagen fibers that bind the cementum of a tooth to the periosteum of the surrounding alveolus, 344

periosteum (per-ē-OS-tē-um)**:** The layer that surrounds a bone, consisting of an outer fibrous and inner cellular region, 264, 338

peripheral nervous system (PNS): All neural tissue outside the central nervous system, 365

peripheral protein: A protein bound to the inner or outer surface of a cell membrane, 140

peristalsis (per-i-STAL-sis)**:** A wave of smooth muscle contractions that propels materials along the axis of a tube such as the digestive tract, the ureters, or the ductus deferens, 435

peritoneal cavity: See **abdominopelvic cavity,** 39

peritoneum (per-i-tō-NĒ-um)**:** The serous membrane that lines the peritoneal (abdominopelvic) cavity, 41

peritubular fluid: The interstitial fluid that surrounds a renal tubule, 450

permeability: The ease with which dissolved materials can cross a membrane; if the membrane is freely permeable, any molecule can cross it; if impermeable, nothing can cross; most biological membranes are selectively permeable, 159

peroxisome: A membranous vesicle containing enzymes that break down hydrogen peroxide (H_2O_2), 154

pH: The negative exponent of the hydrogen ion concentration, expressed in moles per liter, 85

phagocyte: A cell that performs phagocytosis, 416

phagocytosis (fa-gō-sī-TŌ-sis)**:** The engulfing of extracellular materials or pathogens; movement of extracellular materials into the cytoplasm by enclosure in a membranous vesicle, 172

pharynx: The throat; a muscular passageway shared by the digestive and respiratory tracts, 422

phenotype (FĒN-ō-tīp)**:** Physical characteristics that are genetically determined, 313

phenylketonuria: A genetic disease in which a person is unable to convert the amino acid phenylalanine to tyrosine resulting in the accumulation of toxic byproducts called phenylketones, 201

phonation (fō-NĀ-shun)**:** Sound production at the larynx, 422

phosphate group: PO_4^{3-}, 121

phospholipid (fos-fō-LIP-id)**:** An important membrane lipid whose structure includes both hydrophilic and hydrophobic regions, 107

phosphorylation (fos-for-i-LĀ-shun)**:** The addition of a high-energy phosphate group to a molecule, 124, 186

photoreceptors: Specialized nerve cells that can respond to the stimulus of visible light, 75

physiology (fiz-ē-OL-o-jē)**:** Literally, the study of function; deals with the ways organisms perform vital activities, 1

pia mater: The tough, outer meningeal layer that surrounds the central nervous system, 373

pinocytosis (pi-nō-sī-TŌ-sis)**:** The introduction of fluids into the cytoplasm by enclosing them in membranous vesicles at the cell surface, 171

pituitary gland: An endocrine organ situated in the sella turcica of the sphenoid bone and connected to the hypothalamus by the infundibulum; includes the posterior pituitary (pars nervosa) and the anterior pituitary (pars intermedia and pars distalis), 386

placenta (pla-SENT-uh)**:** A temporary structure in the uterine wall that permits diffusion between the fetal and maternal circulatory systems; see **afterbirth,** 297

placentation (plas-en-TA-shun)**:** The process of forming a placenta, 297

plasma (PLAZ-muh)**:** The fluid ground substance of whole blood; what remains after the cells have been removed from a sample of whole blood, 261, 398

plasma cell: Activated B cells that secrete antibodies, 251, 415

plasmalemma (plaz-ma-LEM-a)**:** A cell membrane, 136

platelets (PLĀT-lets)**:** Small packets of cytoplasm that contain enzymes important in the clotting response; manufactured in the bone marrow by megakaryocytes, 261, 400

pleated sheet, 113

substrate: A participant (product or reactant) in an enzyme-catalyzed reaction, 115

sucrose: A disaccharide composed of glucose and fructose. Table sugar, 97

sulcus (SUL-kus): A groove or furrow.

superficial fascia: *See* **subcutaneous layer**.

superficialis, 358

superior: Above, in reference to a portion of the body in the anatomical position, 33

superior vena cava (SVC): The vein that carries blood from the parts of the body above the heart to the right atrium, 403

supination (soo-pi-NĀ-shun): Rotation of the forearm so that the palm faces anteriorly, 359

supine (SOO-pīn): Lying face up, with palms facing anteriorly, 29

suppression: A genetic system in which one allele suppresses the expression of another, 317

suppressor T cells: Lymphocytes that inhibit B cell activation and plasma cell secretion of antibodies, 415

suprarenal gland (soo-pra-RĒ-nal): *See* **adrenal gland**, 387

surface anatomy, 4

surface tension, 68

surgical anatomy, 7

suspension, 84

sustentacular cells (sus-ten-TAK-ū-lar): Supporting cells of the seminiferous tubules of the testis; responsible for the differentiation of spermatids, the maintenance of the blood–testis barrier, and the secretion of inhibin, androgen-binding protein, and Müllerian-inhibiting factor, 459

sutural bones: Irregular bones that form in fibrous tissue between the flat bones of the developing cranium; also called *Wormian bones*, 339

suture: A fibrous joint between flat bones of the skull, 344

sweat, 333

sympathetic division: The division of the autonomic nervous system responsible for "fight or flight" reactions; primarily concerned with the elevation of metabolic rate and increased alertness, 377

symphysis: A fibrous amphiarthrosis, such as that between adjacent vertebrae or between the pubic bones of the coxae, 344

synapse: The site of communication between a nerve cell and some other cell; if the other cell is not a neuron, the term *neuroeffector junction* is often used, 369

synapsis (SIN-ap-sis): The coming together of paired maternal and paternal chromosomes during prophase I of meiosis, 286

synaptic knob (si-NAP-tik): The expanded terminal end of an axon fiber, 353

synarthrosis (sin-ar-THRŌ-sis): A joint that does not permit relative movement between the articulating elements; *see* **lambdoidal suture**, 344

synchondrosis (sin-kon-DRŌ-sis): A cartilaginous synarthrosis, such as the articulation between the epiphysis and diaphysis of a growing bone, 344

syncytial trophoblast: The multinucleate cytoplasmic layer that covers the blastocyst; responsible for uterine erosion and implantation, 298

syndesmosis (sin-dez-MŌ-sis): A fibrous amphiarthrosis, 344

synergist (SIN-er-jist): A muscle that assists a prime mover in performing its primary action, 358

synostosis (sin-os-TŌ-sis): A synarthrosis formed through the fusion of the articulating elements, 344

synovial joint: A freely movable joint where the opposing bone surfaces are separated by synovial fluid; a diarthrosis, 344

synovial membrane: An incomplete layer of fibroblasts confronting the synovial cavity, plus the underlying loose connective tissue, 269

synthesis reaction: A chemical reaction that assembles larger compounds from smaller components. The opposite of a decomposition reaction, 72

system: An interacting group of organs that performs one or more specific functions.

systemic anatomy, 4

systemic circuit: The vessels between the aortic semilunar valve and the entrance to the right atrium; the circulatory system other than vessels of the pulmonary circuit, 400

systemic physiology, 9

systole (SIS-tō-lē): The period of cardiac contraction, 408

T cells: Lymphocytes responsible for cell-mediated immunity and for the coordination and regulation of the immune response; includes regulatory T cells (helpers and suppressors) and cytotoxic (killer) T cells, 414

T tubules: The transverse, tubular extensions of the sarcolemma that extend deep into the sarcoplasm to contact cisternae of the sarcoplasmic reticulum; also called *transverse tubules*, 353

tail fold, 304

telodendria (te-lō-DEN-drē-uh): Terminal axonal branches that end in synaptic knobs, 369

telophase (TĒL-ō-fāz): The final stage of mitosis, characterized by the disappearance of the spindle apparatus, the reappearance of the nuclear membrane, the disappearance of the chromosomes, and the completion of cytokinesis, 217

temperature: An indicator of the direction of heat flow, 77

template strand, 206

tendon: A collagenous band that connects a skeletal muscle to an element of the skeleton, 255

teres: Long and round, 358

terminal: Toward the end.

terminal bronchioles, 424

tertiary follicle: A mature ovarian follicle, containing a large, fluid-filled chamber, 462

testes (TES-tēz): The male gonads, sites of gamete production and hormone secretion, 458

testosterone (tes-TOS-te-rōn): The principal androgen produced by the interstitial cells of the testes, 106, 460

tetrad (TET-rad): Paired, duplicated chromosomes visible at the start of meiosis I, 287

tetrapeptide, 112

tetrose, 95

thalamus: The walls of the diencephalon, 374

thermal energy, 77

thermal inertia: The property of a substance that determines how rapidly it will change temperature, 82

thermoreception: Sensitivity to temperature changes, 377

thermoreceptors (thermoreception), 377

thermoregulation: Homeostatic maintenance of body temperature, 24

thick filament: A cytoskeletal filament in a skeletal or cardiac muscle cell; composed of myosin, with a core of titin, 146, 353

thin filaments, 353

third-class lever: A lever in which the applied force lies between the fulcrum and the resistance, 356

third trimester, 297

thoracic cavity: The portion of the ventral body cavity enclosed by the chest wall, 41

thoracolumbar division (tho-ra-kō-LUM-bar): The sympathetic division of the autonomic nervous system, 377

thromboxanes (throm-BOX-ānz): Eicosanoids released by platelets when blood clotting occurs, 106

thymine: A pyrimidine; one of the nitrogenous bases in the nucleic acid DNA, 122

thymus: A lymphoid organ, the site of T cell formation, 413

thyroid gland: An endocrine gland whose lobes sit lateral to the thyroid cartilage of the larynx, 387

thyroid hormones: Thyroxine (T_4) and triiodothyronine (T_3), hormones of the thyroid gland; hormones that stimulate tissue metabolism, energy utilization, and growth, 387

thyroid-stimulating hormone (TSH): The anterior pituitary hormone that triggers the secretion of thyroid hormones by the thyroid gland, 386

tight junction: A connection between cells formed by the partial fusion of the lipid portions of the two cell membranes, 232

tissue: A collection of specialized cells and cell products that perform a specific function, 7, 229

tonicity (tō-NIS-eh-tē): The effect of an osmotic solution on a living cell, 164

trabecula (tra-BEK-ū-la): A connective tissue partition that subdivides an organ, 337

trachea (TRĀ-kē-a): The windpipe, an airway extending from the larynx to the primary bronchi, 422

trans-fatty acid: A fatty acid produced in the manufacture of margarine or vegetable shortening from polyunsaturated fatty acids, 104